ESSENTIAL NOTES IN PSYCHIATRY

Edited by **Victor Olisah**

Essential Notes in Psychiatry
Edited by Victor Olisah

Published by InTech
Janeza Trdine 9, 51000 Rijeka, Croatia

Publishing Process Manager Petra Nenadic

Technical Editor Teodora Smiljanic

Cover Designer InTech Design Team

Additional hard copies can be obtained from orders@intechopen.com

Essential Notes in Psychiatry, Edited by Victor Olisah
p. cm.
ISBN 978-953-51-0574-9

For EU product safety concerns:
IN TECH d.o.o., Prolaz Marije Krucifikse Kozulić 3, 51000 Rijeka, Croatia,
info@intechopen.com or visit our website at intechopen.com.

Meet the editor

Dr Victor Olisah is a Lecturer and Consultant Psychiatrist at the Ahmadu Bello University Teaching Hospital, Zaria, Nigeria. He obtained his Bachelor of Medicine and Surgery (MB,BS) degree in 1993 from Ahmadu Bello University, Zaria, Nigeria and Fellowship of the West African College of Physicians FWACP(Psych.) in 2007. Dr Olisah is a researcher of repute with several publications in local and international journals. His research interest is in the mental health of people living with HIV/AIDS. He is also interested in Drug Addiction and Social Psychiatry.

Contents

Preface

This book is essentially a review of the current state of psychiatric knowledge in selected areas of mental health. It is comprised of numerous chapters, each written by contributors considered to be authorities in their fields who provide comprehensive and up-to-date information on relevant mental health topics. The purpose is to translate the numerous advances and new discoveries in psychiatry into a form useful to clinicians, residents, and others interested in this field.

Coverage in this book is quite thorough and is divided into five sections. In section 1 comprises of chapters 1 to 4 and contributors discuss the psychosocial consequences of stressful work environment on employees in a few selected organizations. Chapter 1 highlights the causes and psychosocial consequences of mobbing in the workplace and also describes the special qualities of victims and the aggressors. Chapter 2 is quite interesting and examines the effects of social support, psychological safety and Organizational civility in moderating the effects of stress in the workplace. Chapter 3 examines workplace stress in a rural community and addresses issues specified by the community mental health team by empowering them to become active agents of change through action research. Chapter 4 discusses the psychosocial determinants of work stress, effort-reward imbalance and their effects on productivity and perceptions of quality of life among Nurses at a general hospital in Japan.

Section 2 covers chapters 5 to 11 and contributors discuss various aspects of post traumatic stress disorder and an overview of anxiety disorder. The definition, measures, and risk factors for depression in women experiencing intimate partner violence is examined and factors encouraging Resident to Resident aggression in long term care facility is presented. A review of literatures examining the links between cigarette smoking and anxiety/depression among adolescents in the Americas is also discussed.

Section 3 is very interesting and covers chapters 12 to 18. Contributors discuss the effectiveness of selected mental health therapies and interventions. A review of evidence for different pharmacological treatment options of psychotic symptoms in Alzheimer's disease is presented and the effectiveness of inter-professional and inter-cultural competence training in promoting collaboration and efficiency in encountering new refugees is discussed. The section also discusses the effectiveness of a computer-aided exposure technique in treating spider phobia by comparing the results of treatment using this method with the conventional treatment methods of "live exposure" and "live exposure and modeling. Other interventions or therapies discussed in this section include the effectiveness of participative community singing on promoting resilience and mental health, home visit to mothers with children between 0-4 years as an effective mental health intervention strategy and a review of relevant literature on the development of preventive intervention programmes aimed at reducing suicide rates in the world and Slovania as a case study. This section also discusses reasons why substance abusers don't seek treatment; factors associated with treatment entry and proposes effective models for treatment entry.

Section 4 covers chapters 19 to 22. Contributors to this section discuss psychosocial factors in the development of mental disorders in children. Chapter 19 examines the effects of maternal depression on child development and chapter 20 is a review of the literature examining the links between parental mental health (especially that of the mother) and child development. Chapter 21 is a balanced detail of the multicultural issues that may promote or protect against mental health problems in children from different cultures while chapter 22 examines the different types of lifestyles (morning versus evening-type) and the connection between evening-type lifestyle and mental disorders in children. The chapter also discusses the environmental factors that promote evening-type lifestyle and intervention programs that promote morning-type lifestyle.

Section 5 is made up of chapters 23 to 25 and deals with the inter-relationship between personality, mental health and mental disorders. Contributors highlights some very important correlates of mental health such as resilience, emotional intelligence, stress, coping/defense style, religion and spirituality. Factors associated with positive mental health such as sociodemographic, lifestyle and psychosocial issues in a community sample is examined. A contributor to this section also discusses various approaches in mental health care and some causes of mental suffering.

Section 6 covers chapters' 26 to 28 and presents psychological issues in general medical conditions. Contributors to this section highlights the higher prevalence of depression in people with chronic medical conditions and the association of depression with poor adherence to medical treatment regimes, poor quality of life, greater morbidity and mortality. Mental fatigue which occurs after meningitis or encephalitis is discussed in this section. A contributor also discusses the evidence on how different physiological responses may be used as potential biomarkers of adverse psychosocial working environment which may be very useful in identifying people at risk of developing physical or psychological disorders.

Finally, I will like to state that this book is well organized, easy to use, and contains very useful topics in psychiatry for mental health students and professionals. It would be a welcome addition to the library of any clinician who treats psychiatric patients.

Dr. Victor Olisah
Department of Psychiatry,
Ahmadu Bello University Teaching Hospital,
Nigeria

Section 1

Organizational Stress and Mental Health

1

Mobbing at Workplaces and the Mental Health Effects on Employees

Hülya Gül
Istanbul University, Istanbul Medical Faculty,
Public Health Department, Capa-Istanbul
Turkey

1. Introduction

Nowadays, rapid technological changes in the workplace, heavy workloads, role conflicts, problems relating to career development, senior–subordinate relations, undefined borders of the working area, etc. lead to a number of problems in the work environment. Such changes may be reflected in the mental health of an individual either positively or negatively. Any situation perceived by the brain and evaluated to be a danger triggers the stress reaction. WHO (Leka et al., 2003) mentioned that stress is the leading cause adversely affecting the mental health of individuals in business life. Stress in the workplace may affect individuals differently. This effect may be witnessed either as psychological violence or in other ways (e.g., smoking, alcohol, sexual abuse, etc.).

A safe, peaceful work environment increases the productivity of the employees and the efficiency of the establishment. Although, nowadays, work provides men and women a place, status, economic power in the society, it also brings certain negative physiological and psychosocial factors, among which mobbing can create undesired results with the heavy individual, organizational and social damages it creates. The fact that discouragement creates more intense and destructive effects than all the stress sources requires considering the process with a special sensitivity (Gül, 2009; Agervold, 2009; Lawa, R., et al., 2011).
Discussions on whether the basic factor in the case of mobbing is the "person with bad personality" or the organizational and social structure, what feeds mobbing must be made. It is very important to determine the reasons behind this social exclusion process leading people to resignation, depressive and obsessive behavior, loss of their health and even suicides, and to understand this psycho-violence spiral, to determine the factors affecting the process. Research must be focused on the conditions leading to the occurrence of mobbing and the determination of the organization's social structure.

In this section, the effects of mobbing on mental health, the personality characteristics of persons faced with mobbing and those who apply mobbing will be analyzed. In short, through discussions on the eventual factors providing a basis for mobbing, the aim is to ensure the development of awareness in workplaces and contribute to the reduction of the risk of realization of such behavior and its frequency.

2. Mobbing

2.1 Frequency

Psychological intimidation leads to a number of inconveniences both for the victim and the entity (Nielsen, M. B. et al., 2010; Ortega, A. et al; 2009). Problems suffered by the employer are essentially of an economic nature. Besides economic losses, severe social outcomes in organizational terms become inevitable as well. The victims, on the other hand, suffer physical or psychological disorders. It should be taken into consideration that attitudes of psychological intimidation in workplaces may increase atrociously day by day particularly nowadays when the effects of the global crisis are being experienced more severely. This situation highlights the importance of the issue once again. In this context, 73.3% of the respondents in a study conducted among finance sector employees in Istanbul/Turkey by Gül (Gül et al., 2010) reported that they had been exposed to psychological intimidation. The high rate of psychological intimidation in this research may be attributed to the respondents comprised of private banking employees and mid-level executives. Rates obtained in other research that has been conducted in Turkey are as follows: 55% of 877 respondents in the research conducted among public sector employees working in health, education and safety fields in Bursa by Bilgel (Bilgel et al., 2006) reported that they had been exposed to psychological intimidation while 47% reported that they witnessed their workmates being exposed to the same. In similar research conducted by Yıldız (Yıldız et al., 2008) among private sector employees working in the education and health fields, 47.5% of the respondents defined themselves as having been exposed to psychological intimidation, and no meaningful difference was observed between males and females in terms of exposure to psychological intimidation. Yılmaz (Yılmaz et al., 2008), reported after a study conducted in state hospitals that 29.8% of 121 respondents had become victims of psychological intimidation. Kök (Kök, 2006) discovered in a survey conducted among 189 employees working in the private and public banking sectors that the rate of exposure to psychological intimidation was higher in private banks than public banks. A research conducted by Yıldırım (Yıldırım &Yıldırım, 2007) among 505 payroll nurses revealed that the rate of exposure to psychological intimidation was higher among the nurses working in private hospitals than those working in public hospitals, where the overall rate was found to be 86.5%. In a study conducted in Portugal (Ferrinho et al., 2003) on the health sector, on average 60% of 218 respondents working in a health center were found to have been exposed to psychological intimidation, whereas it was 38% among those 1100 employed person in a healthcare foundation (Quine, 1999).

2.2 Conceptual framework

Mobbing can be defined as a systematic creation of opposition to an individual, exercise of pressure, suffocation, frightening, emotional attack (Leka & Jain, et al., 2010). Moral and material losses in this process containing a torture which begins insidiously and develops rapidly are very high. The fact that mobbing activities, which spread all over the world, targets honest, reliable, devoted and hard-working persons, and time and productivity costs reach incredible dimensions. Creative persons in particular are more prone to be subject to mobbing, as the new ideas they develop disturb others. In most cases, victims are chosen due to the fact that they create a threat for persons at higher positions. If we make a classification, those who resort to mobbing are:

Antipathic persons: They are excessively controlling, afraid and nervous. They always want to be powerful. They do not refrain from malicious and fraudulent actions.

Narcissist persons: They are considered as social-handicapped clinically and they are persons who use power to keep persons they fear under their control, who always see themselves as superior to other persons, which is a defect of behavior.

Egocentric under threat: If the discouragement actor has an inflated ego, he/she can display a strong reaction when faced with an undesirable situation, because his/her inflated ego conception bears the potential to increase his/her reaction coefficient.

Attempt to make its own norms organization policies: Those who take on psycho-terror and conceive discouragement as a policy, opt for obedience instead of initiative, in order to take others under control, discipline instead of autonomous behavior, fear instead of motivation. They continuously remind rules, establish new rules.

Prejudiced and emotional: The behavior of discouragement actors has no rational basis and explanation.

Those who exposed to mobbing are:

The victim can be subject to violence due to a religious, ethnic reason, or the fact that he/she displays a high performance, acquires an opportunity, promotion or reward may be sufficient to set the "mobbing" actors into motion. According to the findings obtained from researches on discouragement, discouragement victims have no distinctive particularity, discouragement can happen to anyone. However, some researchers indicate that the victim's character and psychological status are efficient on the appearance of discouragement. Clinic psychologists in particular underline that the victims have a high level of fear and anxiety. In this context, it is observed that persons who cannot seek their rights and defend themselves and who fear conflicts that are honest and have good will are subject to discouragement. The fact that victims have good will, are introverted makes the discouragement actors act. After the interviews with the victims of discouragement, it appears that those persons are intelligent, skillful, creative, success-focused, honest, reliable, and non-political. They attract the attention for being persons who do their work well, have solid working principles and values and do not sacrifice them, are honest, reliable and devoted to their work. Some researches made on victims of mobbing consider as responsible for this unfavorable process the behavior of the victims. Characteristics which increase the probability to be subject to discouragement disturb the others by way of creative and independent thinking and putting forth new ideas and methods. In certain cases, the reason may be that the target is of another type. As is known, a person has characteristics which he/she cannot change. For example, his/her color, sex, accent, the class he/she represents, the fact that he/she is less or more well-educated compared to his/her friends. Such characteristics increase the probability to get under the control of those who intend to discourage that person.

Findings of the research conducted by Gül (Gül et al., 2010) revealed that it was mostly the mid-level executives stuck between the expectations of over-performance and tolerance of seniors and subordinates who had been exposed to psychological intimidation. More than half of those (55.1%) who reported to have been exposed to psychological intimidation were mid-level executives. In this research, respondents prioritized the probable reasons for psychological intimidation to be inadequate management skills, and disguising their own failure and jealousy. Individuals exposed to psychological intimidation who suggested that the personality of the victim was the reason for psychological intimidation specified this reason more frequently than those who were not exposed to psychological intimidation at all. It is worth noting that most of the respondents, particularly those who were exposed to psychological intimidation, specified the personality of the victim. This evidence, although not supported by other research, requires further development of this dimension of the issue. In their research on 363 employees working in the private education and health sectors, Yıldız (Yıldız et al., 2008) have stressed that psychological intimidation originates from the job rather than personality in Turkey. Similarly, Aydın and Özkul (Aydın et al., 2007) have concluded, on the basis of comments made by 427 hotel employees that psychological intimidation originates from the work environment to a great extent. Results of the research conducted by Zapf (Zapt et al., 2001) on 149 victims of psychological intimidation and 81 controls reveal that the act of psychological intimidation affects professionals specialized on their respective fields rather than unskilled workers.

2.3 Health effects

Mobbing, as an attenuated form of violence, attracts the attention more with its psycho-social aspects. Therefore, mobbing can create more durable psychosomatic effects than violence. According to the results of the research conducted by Gül (Gül et al., 2010), the main psychological intimidation act disturbing the victims of mobbing most is assaults on their quality of life and career status (43.5%), followed by self-assertion and affecting formation of communication (33%). Other acts of psychological intimidation include assaults on social relations (16.3%), personal esteem (6.2%) and the direct personal health of individuals (1.0%).

Mobbing is a behavior which can create such unfavorable consequences that we speak of persons on whom it is applied, as "victims" (Gökçe, 2009; Rodríguez-Carballeira et al., 2010; Helkavaara, M. et al., 2011). At the beginning, there is a dispute between the two parties. As the victim refuses to obey, displays resistance to being under control, he/she is faced with a person who is getting angry, rude. Sometimes, when the competency at work of the victim is higher than that of the tyrant, if this threatens his/her position, jealousy can initiate the tyranny. "The aim of mobbing is to exercise superiority on the victim, to take him/her under his/her control. The most important is that it ensures that the victim quits work, loses his/her personality and identity. For this reason, certain means of communication without words (Such as whispering, fleeing the eye, inconvenient laughing, tears, the sudden dispersion of a group upon his/her approach, or sudden interruption of the conversion) are applied. The harassment can turn into an agreement of the harasser with the other employees and an isolation of the target. The behavior of those who are aggrieved and observe this can deteriorate; they may start escaping from the organization. Harassment can lead to the deterioration of peace at work. The person who is faced with harassment gets away from social communication networks which play an important role in promotion and advancement. The fear to be misunderstood by others, to be accused, to lose his/her job leads the victims to silence. Persons who are the target of harassment have the feeling of humiliation, shame and faultiness, insecurity, anger and anxiety. Related with this, victims can also be faced with important problems in their private life. Harassment can cause the person feel like a stranger to his/her work and lose his/her will to succeed. It is argued that persons faced with mobbing are more inclined to be involved in accidents and are more frequently on sick leave. In the majority of the cases, this ends up with the victim of harassment changing his/her job where he/she worked for years or being transferred to a more passive job. It is evident that such a result affects persons' careers and opportunity to be promoted. The person, who is harassed for the first time, starts crying alone, suffers from insomnia from time to time, susceptibility and lack of concentration. As long as the effect lasts, the person loses his/her power of resistance, cannot escape, suffers from mental/physical troubles and does not want to go to work. He/she suffers from high blood pressure, permanent insomnia, tummy and intestinal problems, gains or losses weight, suffers from depression. Alcohol or drug addiction begins requests permission to leave work very often. The requirement for medical help is inevitable. At the last stage, he/she becomes unable to work, cannot return to active life. His/her physical and spiritual harm cannot be even cured with rehabilitation. The person lives in great anxiety as if he/she suffered from a great traumatism due to an earthquake or an important traffic accident, violent depression, panic attacks, cardiac attacks, serious diseases, accidents, tentative of suicide and violence against third persons. Medical and psychological aid is required (Virtanen M et al., 2007; Niedhammer I et al., 2009; 2011). Even if storms of feelings are attenuated in time with the treatment applied, such an event causes deep traces in the person. Many feelings, such as the feeling of defeat, anger, vengeance, lack of confidence to people, leads the person to new behavior. To work is now much more difficult for this person. If the person cannot risk leaving his/her work, he/she suffers physically and mentally and continues to be harmed every day. Now, he/she lives with anxiety, lack of self-esteem, pains, difficulty to breath, high blood pressure, depression. The point to be emphasized is that harassment is a process which causes more pain in time. It is observed that the majority of mobbing victims lose their health due to the Post-Trauma-Stress Deficiency, and become unable to work.

If the targeted individual succeeds in resisting and gets away from the environment or re-accommodates the situation, the damage from harassment decreases. Otherwise, the individual frays mentally, psychologically, and physically, and suffers difficulty in focusing on his/her job. As long as mobbing continues, professional integrity and the sense of self of the individual is damaged, their level of self-suspicion rises, paranoid attitudes and confusion emerge, self-confidence is lost, the individual isolates himself/herself from the outer world, or feelings of restlessness, fear, shame, rage or anxiety are experienced. The individual who cannot cope with such stresses either needs some special therapy or loses the chance to return to his/her job or may even commit suicide.

There are various opinions on the reasons of mobbing acts (Keim, J & Cynthia McDermott,C. 2010; Laaksonen E. et al., 2009; Lahelma E, et al., 2011). One of these is the lack of social skills in persons performing discouraging acts. Another reason is the structure of tyrants. The main problem with tyrants is observed to be a lower self-esteem and personal incompetence in realizing itself, compared to the victim. On the other hand, they are observed to be persons inclined to conflicts, who have no love, who grew up in an austere environment, who have been disciplined with physical punishment. Mobbing is generally applied to well-educated, promising persons who have a high emotional intelligence (McKay,R& Fratz, J. 2011; Niedhammer I et al., 2007). In this context, discouragement actors are generally persons striving for interest, compliments, have a conception of exaggerated ego and resort to discouragement in order to compensate his/her own deficiencies, who are weak, unsecure and coward. Mobbing is one of the methods enabling the powerful person to take control of the weak person. In the case of harassment, formal power differences are observed more clearly when the harasser is a superior. If harassment is made by a superior, due to the position of the superior, the consequences of the harassment are more efficient and harmful for both the victim and the establishment. It has been shown that informal power differences between men and women in similar positions can create an environment for harassment. The relationship between the gender of victims and psychological intimidation in the research conducted by Gül (Gül et al., 2010) reveals that females are more exposed to psychological intimidation than males. 43.5% of the respondents reported that they had been exposed to psychological intimidation by males and 39.7% by females, whereas 13.6% reported to have been exposed to psychological intimidation by both genders. Males are exposed to psychological intimidation mostly by their seniors and females by their workmates with similar jobs ($p= 0.026$). Females are more exposed to permanent criticism of their performance, the people around them not speaking to them, or judgment of their emotional situation or efforts than males. The literature contains conflicting results on this issue. Cemaloğlu and Ertürk (Cemaloğlu and Ertürk 2007), found out in their research conducted among 347 teachers that there existed a meaningful relationship between psychological intimidation experienced at the sub-dimensions of "self-assertion and communication," "social relations," "respect to self-esteem," and "life quality and career status" and gender, and that males apply more psychological intimidation on both genders than females. In his research conducted on 189 bank employees, Kök reported that a significant portion of victims of psychological intimidation was constituted by females and employees below the age of 25. On the other hand, Bilgel et al., did not find any meaningful relationship in statistical terms between age, gender, marital status and working hours and psychological intimidation reported in their research conducted among 877 public sector employees working in health, education and security fields. Except for the gender factor, Gül et al., did not report any relationship between marital status and age and psychological intimidation in their research. Einarsen and Skogstad (Einarsen & Skogstad, 1996) reported no difference between males and females in frequency of exposure to psychological intimidation in their research conducted among 7968 employees from 14 private and public entities. And in the research conducted among 377 white collar employees, Salin (Salin, 2003), concluded that females were more exposed to psychological intimidation in their workplaces than males.

Victims in the research conducted by Gül et al. reported anxiety, unworthiness and lack of motivation, respectively, after being exposed to psychological intimidation. It was further reported that those victims most frequently suffered nervousness and tension (58.4%), followed by lack of motivation and feelings of unworthiness (54.2%). The health complaint most frequently reported was headaches by females (70.1%) and high blood pressure by males (53.85). While there was a meaningful difference between the genders in the frequency of suffering headaches only ($p=0.011$), no difference was found in terms of other complaints. No meaningful difference was observed in health-related variables according to positions at the workplaces. There was some statistically meaningful difference among headache ($p=0.005$), lack of motivation to work ($p=0.042$), decrease in work efficiency ($p=0.004$), emotional fluctuations ($p=0.015$) and the term of career presenting health problems after psychological intimidation. 9.8% of the respondents reported that they received professional help after psychological intimidation and 71.5% reported to have received psychological help from immediate relatives and friends, whereas 18.7% reported no help received from anyone or anything done for this purpose. No difference was found between the genders in terms of psychological support received (p=0.646). A brief examination of the findings of that research reveals that assaults on an individual's quality of life and career status represent the acts of psychological intimidation they most frequently faced. Almost half of the victims reported that opportunities for self-assertion were restricted while other half reported hindered means of communication. Yıldırım et al., (Yıldırım & Yıldırım 2007) discovered that feelings of tiredness and stress (75%) and headache (69%) were the most common health problems reported by victims of psychological intimidation in a study conducted on 210 lecturers. Yıldız & Yıldız, determined what level health person is subject to bullying and what level victims face depression. They determined that victims to bullying experience more level of depression. Especially, 33.7% of bullying person appeared to be medium level, 5.1 % severe depression. In total 66.1% of victims reached the depression level.

International literature contains a number of studies evidencing severe psychological and physical problems that have arisen after psychological intimidation, even reaching the alarming degree of suicide (Dikmetaş et al., 2011; Girardi,P., et al., 2007 ; Meseguer de Pedro et al.,2007; Rossi,& D'Andrea., 2001; Monaco et al., 2004; Kreiner, 2008). In the research conducted by Gül et al., approximately three-fourths of the victims reported that the acts of psychological intimidation they faced affected their job efficiency adversely, whereas approximately one-fifth of all respondents did not perceive psychological intimidation to be a problem denigrating the work environment. 45.8% of the victims of psychological intimidation said that they reported these attitudes to senior executives, while 54.2% ignored the situation and did not make any complaint thereof. 15.3% of those who reported these acts to senior executives said that those causing psychological intimidation were slightly punished (reprimanded, etc.), 2% said that they were dismissed and 82.7% said that nothing was done with them. When the reason(s) of no report was (were) asked, 78.8% of the respondents said that no result could have been attained even if they had been reported, 21.6% expressed their concern about losing their jobs, 45.5% stated their fear of negative criticism, 26.8% said that they would give no evidence, 55.5% said that they ignored the situation and 27.9% expressed their belief of accomplishing no legal result - all of which indicates that psychological intimidation is not a well-adopted and clear concept which is considered adequately important yet. Although there is no clear reason, when the employee's motivation decreases, managers must be careful. When sudden performance decrease is observed in the most creative employees, who display the highest performance, and when these employees quit the establishment after a while, the reasons behind must be investigated.

3. Conclusion

Mobbing in the workplaces is one of the preventable public health problems. When it comes to mobbing, the necessity of enlightenment and raising awareness is great, in addition to applicable legislation. This malignancy cannot be prevented unless it is given a name. Describing and description of mobbing is essential. Individuals and entities should assume prevention of mobbing to be one of their primary tasks.

Getting aware of mobbing-psychological intimidation which may result in severely adverse outcomes at individual, organizational or even social level and defining the causes as well as developing appropriate actions are essential for public health. An individual victim of psychological intimidation should be aware that what she/he has experienced is an occupational health and safety issue already defined and scientifically denominated and that being exposed to such an act is not his/her own fault. The victim should refrain from responding against acts of mobbing, inform the senior executives about the situation, collect evidence, be aware of the sanctions set forth in labor legislation and defend his/her rights. It should be remembered, however, that the key factor is the organizational and social structure rather than personality of the individual which encourages psychological intimidation. Assuring a healthy and safe working environment by adopting a holistic approach is an indispensable element of the social policy. Carrying out descriptive and evaluative studies which also aim developing an awareness of the problem shall bring along favorable results for the health of the individual and the community. And those studies may also contribute to making an efficient comparison of findings coming from different cultures and professions.

4. Acknowledgement

I would like to thank Zahide Ceren Atlı for her valuable contributions in the process of the writing the book chapter.

5. References

Agervold M. (2009). The significance of organizational factors for the incidence of bullying. *Scand J Psychol;* 50:267-276.

Aydın, Ş., Özkul, E (2007). The nature and dimensions of mobbing at work: 4-5 star hotel establishment case, *Anadolu Üniversitesi Sosyal Bilimler Dergisi,* 7(2):169–186.

Bilgel, N., Aytac, S., Bayram, N. (2006). Bullying in Turkish White-Collar Workers. *Occupational Medicine,* 56 (4): 226–231.

Cemaloğlu, N., Ertürk, A. (2007). A study on acts of mobbing suffered by teachers in terms of their gender. *Türk Eğitim Bilimleri Dergisi;* 5(2): 345–362.

Dikmetaş, E., Top, M., Ergin, G. (2011).An examination of mobbing and burnout of residents. *Turk Psikiyatri Derg.* 22(3):137-49.

Einarsen, S, Skogstad, A. (1996). Bullying at work: epidemiological findings in public and private organizations. *Eur Work Organ Psychol* 5 (2): 185–201.

Ferrinho, P., Biscaia, A., Fronteira, I et al. (2003). Patterns of perceptions of workplace violence in the Portuguese health care sector. *Hum Resources Health* 1(1):1–11.

Girardi,P., Monaco, E., Prestigiacomo, C., Talamo, A., Ruberto, A., Tatarelli, R. (2007). Personality and psychopathological profiles in individuals exposed to *mobbing,Violence Vict.;*22(2):172-88.

Gökçe, A. (2009). Mobbing in the workplace The conceptual framework, *Universite ve Toplum* 9(2):1-9.

Gül, H. (2009). An Important Psychosocial Risk in Occupational Health: Mobbing *TAF Prev Med Bull* 8(6):515-520

Gül, H., Alçalar, N., Kayı, İ., Özel, S., Özgülnar, N. (2010). Mobbing in working life and its effects on health: A cross-sectional study among privately -owned bank workers, *Türkiye Klinikleri Journal of Medical Sciences 30 (6):1917-1927.*

Helkavaara, M. Peppiina, S.; Lahelma;E. Psychosocial work environment and emotional exhaustion among middle-aged employees, *BMC Research Notes 2011, 4:101.*

Keim, J., Cynthia McDermott. (2010): Mobbing: Workplace Violence in the Academy, *The Educational Forum*, 74:2, 167-173.

Kök, SB. (2006). Mobbing phenomenon in business life as a psychological violence package and its reasons. *Selçuk Üniversitesi, Sosyal Bilimler Enstitüsü Dergisi* 16 (1): 433–449.

Kreiner, B., Sulyok, C., Rothenhäusler, HB (2008). Does mobbing cause posttraumatic stress disorder? Impact of coping and personality, *Neuropsychiatr.* 22(2):112-23.

Laaksonen E, Martikainen P, Lallukka T, et al. (2009). Economic difficulties and common mental disorders among Finnish and British white-collar employees: the contribution of social and behavioral factors. *J Epidemiol Community Health*, 63:439-446.

Lahelma E, Lallukka T, Laaksonen M, et al. (2011). Workplace bullying and common mental disorders: a follow-up study. J Epidemiol Community Health.

Lawa, R., Dollarda, MF.,Michelle R. Dormannb, TC. (2011) Psychosocial safety climate as a lead indicator of workplace bullying and harassment, job resources, psychological health and employee engagement. *Accident Analysis and Prevention 43: 1782–1793.*

Leka S. et al. (2003). Work organization and stress. Geneva, *World Health Organization,*(Protecting workers health series, No. 3.

Leka, S., Jain, A. (2010). Health impact of psychosocial hazards at work: An overview. World Health Organization, Geneva, Switzerland

McKay, R., Fratz, J. (2011). A Cause of Failure in Addressing Workplace Bullying: Trauma and the Employee. *International Journal of Business and Social Science Vol. 2 No. 7, 13.*

Meseguer de Pedro M., Soler Sánchez MI., García-Izquierdo M., Sáez Navarro MC., Sánchez Meca J. (2007).Psychosocial risk factors at work as predictors of mobbing, *Psicothema.* May; 19(2):225-30.

Monaco, E., Bianco, G., Di Simone Di Giuseppe, B., Prestigiacomo, C. (2004). Emergent pathology in occupational medicine: the mobbing.*G Ital Med Lav Ergon.* Jan-Mar;26(1):28-32.

Niedhammer I, David S, Degioanni S et al. 143 occupational physicians. (2009) Workplace bullying and sleep disturbances: findings from a large scale cross-sectional survey in the French working population. *Sleep;* 32: 1211-9.

Niedhammer I, David S, Degioanni S. 143 occupational physicians. (2007) .Economic activities and occupations at high risk for workplace bullying: results from a large-scale cross-sectional survey in the general working population in France. *Int Arch Occup Environ Health;* 80: 346–53.

Niedhammer, I., David, S., Degioanni, P., Drummond, A. Ph,lip, P. and143 occupational physician. (2011). Workplace Bullying and Psychotropic Drug Use: The Mediating Role of Physical and Mental Health Status *Ann. Occup. Hyg.*, Vol. 55, No. 2, pp. 152–163.

Nielsen, M. B., Matthiesen, S. B. and Einarsen, S. (2010). The impact of methodological moderators on prevalence rates of workplace bullying. A meta-analysis. *Journal of Occupational and Organizational Psychology,* 83: 955–979.

Ortega, A., Høgh, A., Pejtersen, JH., et al. (2009).Prevalence of workplace bullying and risk groups: a representative population study. *Int Arch Occup Environ Health,* 82:417-426.

Quine, L (1999). Workplace bullying in NHS community trust: staff questionnaire survey *BMJ* 318 (7178): 228–232.

Rodríguez-Carballeira A, Escartín Solanelles J, Visauta Vinacua B, Porrúa García C, Martín-Peña J. (2010). Categorization and hierarchy of workplace bullying strategies: a Delphi survey, *Span J Psychol.* May;13(1):297-308.

Rossi, M., D'Andrea, R. (2001). Mobbing: a problem in occupational health.*Recenti Prog Med.* Jan;92(1):49-51.

Salin, D. (2003). Bullying and organizational politics in competitive and rapidly changing work environments. International Journal of Management and Decision Maing, 4 (1), 35-46.

Virtanen M, Honkonen T, Kivimaki M et al. (2007) Work stress, mental health and antidepressant medication findings from the Health 2000 Study. *J Affect Disord;* 98: 189–97.

Yıldırım, A., Yıldırım, D. (2007). Mobbing in the workplace by peers and managers: mobbing experienced by nurses working in healthcare facilities in Turkey and its effect on nurses. *Journal of Clinical Nursing* 16 (8): 1444–1453.

Yildiz, S., Tuzunturk, S., Giorgi, G (2008). Workplace bullying in Turkey: Prevalence among private sector employees. *Risorsa Uoma* 14(2):157–170.

Yılmaz, A., Özler, D.E., Mercan, N. (2008).An empirical study of the relationship between mobbing and organizational climate. *Elektronik Sosyal Bilimler Dergisi,* 7 (26):334–357.

Zapf, D., Gross, C. (2001). Conflict escalation and coping with workplace bullying: A replication and extension. *European Journal of Work and Organizational Psychology,* 10 (4): 497–522.

2

The Relationship Between Workplace Civility Level and the Experience of Burnout Syndrome Among Helping Professionals

Zuzana Havrdová[1] and Iva Šolcová[2]
[1]*Faculty of Humanities, Charles University of Prague,*
[2]*Institute of Psychology, Academy of Sciences of the Czech Republic, Prague*
Czech Republic

1. Introduction

The most important stimuli for our experience and behaviour arise in the psychosocial sphere. An increased psychosocial load - related to work and non-work problems - can bring about serious health problems. Beehr (1995:11) defined job stress as "a situation in which some characteristics of the work situation are thought to cause poor psychological or physical health or to cause risk factors making poor health more likely". According to Maslach (2011), stressful jobs are as bad for people's health as smoking and obesity.

However, similar stress triggers different consequences in different individuals and different work settings. What largely explains the difference in outcomes is the moderating effect of risk and support factors. In the case of work stress, the primary moderating factors are social support, psychological safety and organizational civility, as perceived by the worker.

In this chapter we will summarize the most important findings relating to these three factors from the literature, and their impact on mental health risk factors known as burnout syndrome. Then we will present research on a sample of Czech helping professionals to examine whether there are any cultural differences in the way workplace civility levels predict early signs of burnout. Suggestions for workplace management and further research will conclude the chapter.

2. Job strain

Helping professionals typically engage in highly demanding jobs with heavy workloads and high levels of responsibility. The demands placed on these individuals have long been thought to be a major reason for the development of distress. As demands increase, stress also increases. If the level of stress increases beyond an individual's ability to cope, the person will likely develop distress (Karasek & Theorell, 1990). When the state of stress is prolonged, chronic stress results, with burnout syndrome as a possible outcome.

Control over one's job duties ("decision latitude" according to Karasek, 1979, or "autonomy of work" according to Beehr, 1995) and the way these duties are completed is another factor closely linked to the development of distress. Decision latitude refers to employee control over their tasks and how their tasks are executed. It describes the possibility to influence the pace of work, its character and conditions (Karasek, 1979). Perceptions regarding the amount of control in the work setting and whether these perceptions meet individual needs for a degree of autonomy have an immediate effect on the experience of stress (Karasek & Theorell, 1990).

This model is called the demand–control model, and describes the combination of high demand and low control (decision latitude) typical of high strain jobs (Karasek, 1979).

Stress in the helping professions stems mostly from time pressure, shift work, night shifts, prolonged shifts (12 hours), work overload, contact with ill and disabled people and death, helplessness in fatal cases, insufficient sleep and insomnia, the grief of family and relatives, and responsibility in serious situations. A stressful situation can also be caused by clients who can act inadequately because of their fear and inability to cope with a difficult situation; they can be agitated, anxious, arrogant and undisciplined, and may disturb communication. Maturity and experience are necessary for helping professionals, especially when dealing with child clients and with their accompanying persons (Drozdová & Kebza, 2011).

A further frequent source of stress is the accumulation of work tasks with an inadequate number of personnel in an unstable and badly coordinated work team with unclear and undefined work competencies, under suddenly changing work conditions or tensions resulting from difficult interpersonal relationships in the workplace. Another negative factor is dissatisfaction with low financial and social assessment (Drozdová & Kebza, 2011). According to Jones (1987), nursing is the profession with the lowest life expectancy, which can be explained by the corresponding stressfulness of the work.

3. Burnout and its measurement

Burnout syndrome is defined in the literature as negative personal changes that occur over time in persons engaged in a helping profession whose jobs are demanding or frustrating (Cherniss, 1980, 1989, 1990).

According to Maslach and Jackson (1986:1), "burnout is a syndrome of emotional exhaustion, depersonalization and reduced personal accomplishment that can occur among individuals who do 'people work' of some kind". Maslach and colleagues further argued that burnout is characterized by emotional exhaustion (a manifestation of individual stress), cynicism (a job response), and professional inefficacy (a self-evaluation). Emotional exhaustion is considered the core element of burnout, resulting in cynicism toward one's work and colleagues and low efficacy levels (Leiter & Maslach, 2004).

Shirom (2003) particularly emphasized the mental component of exhaustion, which comprises elements of resignation and frustration, ensuing from the disproportion between the effort and energy invested in performing what is categorized as "working with people" and the relatively small manifest results of this effort. The experienced pointlessness of the effort also leads to inhibition of spontaneity and creativity. In the activities of the affected individual, routine procedures, stereotyped phrases and clichés begin to predominate. The inhibition of empathy and loss of positive attitude towards people who should be provided a certain service (e.g. patients, clients and citizens) is also marked. In this context, some authors (e.g. Maslach, Schaufeli & Leiter, 2001) speak of a "dehumanized perception of environment".

Burnout syndrome was first studied from the psychological point of view, with researchers showing interest in psychological reactions to stress and describing its psychological impact. In the 1990s, however, the organizational context of burnout became a topic of study as the concept of organizational culture - as a common environment created by shared beliefs, perceptions, and expectations of individuals (Schein, 1990) - was raised in relations to job satisfaction. Burnout syndrome emerges especially in certain professions as a result of a combination of factors, including chronic stress and a marked drop in motivation, interest in work and sense of satisfaction (Maslach & Leiter, 1997; Kebza & Šolcová, 1998, 2008). This occurs when the job demands exceed the ability of individuals to cope, and they become overwhelmed by the stress of the activity. However, as stress involves subjective as well as objective aspects, how the employee perceives the load and the meaning of the activity is of great significance, as well as the person's perception of management and the entire work environment. The outcomes of burnout (Maslach, 2011) are poor quality work, low morale, absenteeism, turnover, health problems and family problems. Maslach & Jackson (1981) developed the Maslach Burnout Inventory (MBI), a burnout questionnaire for human service organizations, which has been used extensively for 30 years. On the basis of research results, the MBI was modified to create the MBI General Survey (MBI-GS), a measure of burnout for all occupations, which has been used ever since (Schaufeli et al., 1996). According to Maslach (2011), a score above the median in any dimension of the MBI or MBI-GS is an early sign of burnout.

As early as the 1980s, the professional literature worldwide began to indicate a possible relationship between burnout and cardiovascular disease (CVD) risk factors, CVD being the most common cause of death worldwide. In this context, one has to realize that up to 80% of premature cardiovascular deaths are identified as preventable (WHO, 2009). Many findings (Appels, Otten, 1992; Melamed, Kushnir, Shirom, 1992; Melamed et al., 2006; Shirom, 2007) indicate a very likely relationship between burnout syndrome and acute myocardial infarction, ischaemic heart disease, cerebral apoplexy and sudden cardiac death. The overwhelming majority of cases suggest that burnout syndrome is more likely to precede CVD rather than result from it (Hallman et al., 2003).

In one of the most recent studies of this issue, a longitudinal Japanese study examined the impact of burnout syndrome on the emergence of atherosclerosis, using the Japanese version of the MBI-GS. The authors concluded that burnout resulting from chronic stress, for example, can be related to risk factors for atherosclerosis (Kitaoka-Higashiguchi et al., 2009).

To prevent job strain leading to burnout and/or ill health, job conditions as moderating factors are crucially important, especially social support, psychological safety and workplace civility.

4. Social support as a protection against stress

Social aspects assume a pivotal position in the understanding of overall individual functioning. The functioning of the individual, however, cannot be understood without taking into account the conditions of the individual's environment and social context.

One of the first factors identified as a moderator of the influence of unfavourable life events is social support. Although the protective effect of this factor is mentioned in the majority of published studies to date, there is as yet no complete agreement as to the structure of this social support or the essence of its effect.

Sarason (1988) conceives social support as a stress moderator. The basis of social support, obviously, is not so much the general availability of basic social ties but rather their adequacy when unfavourable (stressful) situations develop. Sarason assumes that the perception of social support is particularly important, even more so than the actual support received. Further studies have shown the protective potential of anticipated social support.

Anticipated support is the belief that important persons close to the individual are prepared to help should the need arise (Krause, 1997); it includes the general feeling of being loved, and of having others who take an interest and will help in case of need. It can be best characterized as a feeling of acceptance which contributes to the perception of social support, quite apart from what the social environment actually offers (Sarason et al., 1987). Anticipated social support is usually listed as a resource for coping with stress. The mobilization of social support may be conceived as a strategy for coping with stress (Folkman & Lazarus, 1988).

Received support, on the other hand, means helpful transactions actually provided to the individual; these may be emotional, instrumental or material. Received support is a social or transactional variable determined by a specific pattern of social interaction. Received social support comprises mobilization, receipt and evaluation of received assistance, as part of the process of coping with stress.

Awareness that others are prepared to help creates a sensation of psychological safety, which facilitates risk taking and stimulates people to attempt to resolve problems themselves (Krause, 1997).

5. Psychological safety in the work setting

An important factor in perceiving a work setting as psychologically safe is the extent to which employees are confident that colleagues and supervisors will react constructively towards them (Edmondson, 2003).

The construct of psychological safety has its roots in early research on organizational change, in which Schein and Bennis (1965, cited by Edmondson, 2003) discussed the need to create psychological safety for individuals if they are to feel secure and capable of changing. Psychological safety describes a climate in which people can focus on productive discussion to enable early prevention of problems and the accomplishment of shared goals, because people are less likely to be focused on self-protection (Edmondson, 1999). In psychologically safe environments, according to Edmondson (1999, 2003), people believe that others will not penalize or think less of them if they make a mistake or ask for help, information or feedback. This belief fosters the confidence to take the abovementioned risks and thereby gain from the associated benefits of learning.

Psychological safety reflects the employee's evaluation of a workplace as a supportive environment in which it is safe to raise difficult issues and take risks. An important aspect of safety is the amount of care and support the employee perceives as provided by the organization as well as by the direct supervisor (Kahn, 1990).

Data collected by Kahn (1990) indicated that four factors influence psychological safety most directly: interpersonal relationships, group and intergroup dynamics, management style, and organizational norms.

Psychological safety is connected to engagement. Leiter and Laschinger (2006) found that psychological safety was positively and significant related to work engagement (the opposite of burnout). They examined the determinants of psychological safety within organizational culture and climate and, using data from Canadian healthcare providers, produced a model in which workplace civility and congruence between personal and organizational value predicts perceptions of psychological safety.

6. Organizational civility as an aspect of organizational culture

Contemporary organizations require energetic and dedicated employees who engage with their work. A mismatch between people and their work environment reduces work satisfaction, whereas a match enhances satisfaction. Workplace civility and personal-organizational value congruence represent potent predictors of work satisfaction and perceived psychological safety (Leiter & Laschinger, 2006).

Organizational civility is that aspect of an organization's culture that embraces the norm of mutual respect and responsibility (Kimmel, 2001). Fostering civility in the workplace can increase morale, encourage effective communication, decrease turnover, boost service orientation and significantly impact the bottom line. Thus civility can function as a moderator of the stress–stress consequences relationship among employees.

According to Leiter, "civility goes to the heart of quality of work life, empowering employee to fulfil their potential as members of a community through positive working relationships that are a critical resource for providing excellent healthcare" (2008).

Workplace incivility, on the contrary, is defined as "low-intensity deviant behaviour with ambiguous intent to harm the target, in violation of workplace norms for mutual respect" (Andersson & Pearson, 1999: 457, cited by Gill & Sypher, 2009). Incivility in the workplace (e.g. emotional abuse or rudeness) reflects employees' lack of regard for one another. Besides being a stressor itself, incivility exacerbates the relationship between existing job stressors and its consequences among employees.

7. Six aspects of the work place and workplace civility

Burnout is a serious problem. According to Leiter (2008), 20 years of research has shown that burnout is not an individual problem. A shared work environment can make the difference between burnout and engagement with work (Leiter, 2008). Maslach and Leiter concluded that burnout is not a problem of people but mostly of the places in which they work. When the work place does not recognize the human side of work or demands superhuman effort, people feel overloaded, frustrated and burnt out. Intervention on the side of an individual does not eliminate the problem without an intervention on the side of organization. Self-improvement alone cannot overcome the problem.

Maslach and Leiter (1997) identified six areas of the work environment that are most relevant to the relationships people develop with their work.

The above mentioned authors propose that the greater the perceived gap between the person and the job, the greater the likelihood of burnout; conversely, the greater the consistency, the greater the likelihood of engagement with work. Disharmony between the job and the person can result in increased exhaustion, cynicism and inefficacy, whereas harmony can improve employee engagement and work satisfaction. Leiter and Maslach's research (1997) points to six key areas that are pivotal in the job-person match: a manageable workload and a sense of control correspond to Karasek's demand-control model; the other four components are opportunity for reward, a feeling of community, faith in the fairness of the workplace and shared values. The quality of work-life issues in terms of these six factors can be assessed using a tool called the Areas of Worklife Survey.

The *Areas of Worklife Survey* (AWS) was created to assess employee perceptions of the abovementioned qualities of the work setting. In Maslach and Leiter's programme, AWS is used in conjunction with the MBI-GS. The AWS produces a profile of scores that permits users to identify key areas of strength or weakness in their organizational setting.

AWS became part of a Canadian programme known as Civility, Respect and Engagement in the Workplace (CREW), designed to reduce burnout and increase engagement in organizations. The tipping point, according to Maslach (2011) is a mismatch in at least one area of worklife.

8. Czech study on workplace civility and burnout

Objectives

Burnout syndrome and engagement in work are two poles of one dimension, and should not be neglected, as Tanner (2011) points out. Managers, supervisors and coaches are important figures in health organizations who can contribute to a resilient work setting and civility in the work place for healthcare staff, thus building staff engagement and preventing burnout (Leiter & Maslach, 2000). Measuring those traits of organizational culture that either contribute to or hinder employee wellbeing can provide information to managers in larger organizations, contribute to their understanding of how employees perceive their working environment, and be fine tuned by simple testing.

This study aimed to find out whether the correlation between burnout and workplace civility is also applicable in the unique culture of the Czech environment, and if the measures developed by Maslach and Leiter mirror the hypothetical differences between various Czech healthcare and social care settings. If so, use of these two combined methods should be suitable for students of management and supervision in health and social organizations to practise and as a basis for future communication with their employees.

The concrete objective of applying both instruments was to establish the level of organizational civility in Czech healthcare and social care organizations, its influence on signs of burnout according to Leiter and Maslach's model, and how this is influenced by additional factors.

Procedure

The researchers used a snow-ball method to distribute two paper or electronic version of questionnaires, the MBI-GS and the AWS, together with the instructions and a goal description ("to study the relation of your exhaustion and engagement in work and how you perceive characteristics of your workplace ").. Participants had to be nurses or midwives working in the hospital or social workers working in the NGO non-residential social service. The starting group was participants, who were at the same time mature students at the masters programme management and supervision department. They were then asked to distribute the questionnaires on their own wards and to other relevant helping professionals in their field. Participants filled in the questionnaires anonymously. Depending on circumstances, some questionnaires were returned via boxes in the hospital wards, while others were returned directly to the researchers in envelopes. Some of the questionnaires were also sent by students to their colleagues by e-mail and returned by e-mail to the assistant of the school department. The chief motivation for respondents was that they would receive the research results. They were also directly motivated by their colleagues who studied at the above mentioned masters programme.

Measures

As mentioned above, we used two instruments in this study: the Areas of Worklife Survey (AWS, Maslach & Leiter, 1997) and Maslach's Burnout Inventory-General Survey (MBI-GS, Schaufeli, Leiter, Maslach & Jackson, 1996).

Burnout dimensions

The MBI-GS measures the three dimensions considered crucial by the authors: (1) exhaustion, which is related to depletion of energy and emotional and physical fatigue, (2) cynicism, which is conceptually related to lack of involvement, and (3) withdrawal from work and professional efficacy, which is related to the feeling of competence, achievement and accomplishment at work or its opposite - inefficacy.

The questionnaire has 16 items formulated as statements of job-related feelings (e.g. I feel burned out by my work). These are rated on a 6-point Likert scale (ranging from 0=never to 6=daily). The concept of burnout comprises higher scores on exhaustion and cynicism and lower scores on efficacy.

Areas of worklife

The Areas of Worklife Survey (AWS, Leiter & Maslach, 2004) has 29 items divided into 6 sections, namely workload, reward, control, community, fairness, and values, each with three to six items. The items are statements that express an opinion about the work circumstances (e.g. I have enough time to do what is important in my job). Respondents indicate their degree of agreement with these statements on a 5-point Likert's scale (ranging from 1=strongly disagree through 3=hard to decide to 5=strongly agree). Some items are negatively worded and their scores are thus reversed.

Demographic questions included gender, age, level of education, number of years working in this organization, and number of years in the same position. Another question concerned whether the person worked in a small team, a large collective or individually.

Czech sample description

Our sample consisted of healthcare staff (N=169; 71.6%) working in various wards of five different regional and Prague hospitals and social workers working in the NGO fieldwork (N=44; 18.8%). The total number of respondents (N) was 236. 9.7% of the answers on the type of professions were missing. Of the participants, 71 (30.1%) were 29 years or younger, 96 (40.7%) were 30–39 years, 40 (16.9 %) were 40–49 years, and 27 (11.4%) were over 50 years of age. Women made up 83% and men only 15.5% of the sample. Education levels were 34.3% with middle school, 31.4% with high school and 33.9% with a university degree. Additional questions concerned type of contract and team participation, as shown in Table 1. No significant relationships were shown with the type of contract, so this data was not used for further analysis.

		Frequency	Percent	Valid Percent	Cumulative Percent
Valid	1 Individual	49	20.8	20.9	20.9
	2 Small team	131	55.5	56.0	76.9
	3 Large collective	54	22.9	23.1	100.0
	Total	234	99.2	100.0	
Missing		2	00.8		
Total		236	100.0		

Table 1. Teamwork type.

Goals and outcomes

As our aim was to find out if the correlation between burnout and workplace civility could be replicated in the Czech environment, we started with a descriptive analysis of our data and compared this with data from other studies. We present the results of the psychometric analysis of both instruments within the Czech sample, and also analyse the relationship between the two instruments in the Czech sample.

We were also interested in any differences in perception of the work environment between Czech and Canadian nurses. Lastly, we compared the Czech nurses with a group of social workers to see how the instrument reacted to the differences in their work settings.

Statistical analysis

The following analyses of the Czech data were performed:

- Descriptive statistics of the AWS and MBI-GS scales and their reliability
- Comparison with Canadian samples (AWS and MBI-GS by Leiter)
- Correlation within the AWS and MBI-GS scales
- Correlations between AWS and MBI-GS
- Analysis of difference in scales according to demographic characteristics (age, education, individual/team work)
- Comparison between health workers and social workers

Results

Reliability as measured by the Cronbach alpha test is shown in Tables 2 (a) and (b).

	Workload	Control	Reward	Community	Fairness	Values
Cronbach alfa	0.724	0.495	0.845	0.809	0.818	0.777
Items	6	3	4	5	6	5
Average correlation between items	0.393	0.248	0.582	0.471	0.523	0.423

Table 2(a). AWS reliability.

All scales achieved good item reliability (Cronbach alfa>0.7) except for the item control, which had very low consistency. This was not reported by other researchers in other countries. However in an earlier Czech study low reliability in Control was reported as well (Cronbach alfa=0.53 in Havrdova et al. 2010)

	Exhaustion	Cynicism	Professional efficacy
Cronbach alfa	0.710	0.768	0.794
Items	5	5	6
Average correlation between items	0.465	0.551	0.494

Table 2 (b). MBI-GS reliability.

All MBI-GS scales showed very good reliability in our sample (Cronbach alfa>0.7).

A comparison of Canadian nurses (Leiter, 2003) and the Czech sample (N=234) is shown in Table 3 (a) AWS and Table 3 (b) MBI-GS cut-off values for burnout.

	Canadian sample			**Czech sample**			
	mean	SD	N	mean	SD	N	*p*
Workload	**2.87**	0.84	8609	**3.04**	0.666	230	0.0023
Control	**3.36**	0.89	8609	**3.47**	0.660	229	0.0634
Reward	**3.20**	0.93	8609	**3.21**	0.783	229	0.8719
Community	**3.46**	0.84	8609	**3.71**	0.659	230	0.0001
Fairness	**2.84**	0.83	8609	**2.88**	0.723	230	0.4693
Values	**3.42**	0.74	8609	**3.29**	0.683	228	0.9859

Note: unpaired, two-tailed t-test

Table 3 (a). AWS descriptive statistics.

There is a small but statistically significant (p>0.05) difference between the Czech (CR) sample and the Canadian 2003 sample perceptions of workload and community, which are higher in CR. The other scales are similar. With the Canadian sample, which Leiter refers to in 2009, we find another significant difference in control, which is lower than in the 2003 sample (3.08).

	N	Min	Max	Mean	SD
Exhaustion (MBI-GS)	226	1	6	**2.90**	0.940
Cynicism (MBI-GS)	225	0	6	**1.46**	1.101
Professional efficacy (MBI-GS)	221	1	6	**3.62**	0.994
Valid N (listwise)	221				

Note: according to Leiter (1998), N=1257, exhaustion=2.98 (SD 1.38), cynicism=1.80 (SD 1.24), professional efficacy = 4.41(SD 0.99). According to Leiter (2009:335), N=709, exhaustion=2.65 (SD 1.47), cynicism=1.82 (SD 1.42), and efficacy=4.45 (SD 0.98).

Table 3 (b). MBI-GS descriptive statistics.

We see therefore that the scores for the Canadian population have not changed much over time. The greatest difference was in the scale professional efficacy, where the Czech nurses reported lower levels than the Canadian nurses. Czech nurses were also somewhat lower on cynicism, although their perceptions of exhaustion were similar.

Correlation of scales within the AWS and MBI-GS are shown in Tables 4 (a) and 4 (b), respectively.

		Workload (AWS)	Control (AWS)	Reward (AWS)	Community (AWS)	Fairness (AWS)	Values (AWS)
Workload (AWS)	Pearson correlation	1					
	Sig. (2-tailed)						
	N	230					
Control (AWS)	Pearson correlation	0.242	1				
	Sig. (2-tailed)	0.000					
	N	229	229				
Reward (AWS)	Pearson correlation	**0.369**	**0.498**	1			
	Sig. (2-tailed)	0.000	0.000				
	N	229	228	229			
Community (AWS)	Pearson correlation	0.224	**0.348**	0.264	1		
	Sig. (2-tailed)	0.001	0.000	0.000			
	N	230	229	229	230		

Fairness (AWS)	Pearson correlation	0.230	**0.353**	**0.535**	**0.324**	1	
	Sig. (2-tailed)	0.000	0.000	0.000	0.000		
	N	230	229	229	230	230	
Values (AWS)	Pearson correlation	0.256	**0.494**	**0.571**	0.201	**0.637**	1
	Sig. (2-tailed)	0.000	0.000	0.000	0.002	0.000	
	N	228	227	227	228	228	228

Note: boldface means correlations R>0.3

Table 4 (a). AWS scale correlations.

Correlations between values and fairness (0.64) and values and reward (0.57) are very high, and higher than in Leiter (2009) (which were 0.55 and 0.40, respectively). Reward and fairness also have very high correlation (0.54) as do reward and control (0.50), but do not differ from the cited sample. On the other hand, the correlation between fairness and control is substantially lower than for Canadian nurses (Czech=0.35, Canada=0.51).

		Exhaustion (MBI-GS)	Cynicism (MBI-GS)	Professional efficacy (MBI-GS)
Exhaustion (MBI-GS)	Pearson correlation	1		
	Sig. (2-tailed)			
	N	226		
Cynicism (MBI-GS)	Pearson correlation	**0.548**	1	
	Sig. (2-tailed)	0.000		
	N	224	225	
Professional efficacy (MBI-GS)	Pearson correlation	0.031	**-0.321**	1
	Sig. (2-tailed)	0.643	0.000	
	N	221	221	221

Note: boldface means correlations R>0.3

Table 4 (b). MBI-GS scale correlations.

The strong relationship between cynicism and exhaustion (0.55) is similar to earlier results by Leiter (0.60). The same is true of a weaker negative correlation between efficacy and cynicism (–0.32) as compared to Leiter's result (–0.40). Our sample shows no correlation between exhaustion and professional efficacy, while Leiter's result was –0.27.

Table 5 (a) shows the model of relations between the three MBI-GS scales and perceptions of the work environment as predictors of burnout. Correlations between AWS and MBI-GS scales are shown in Tables 5 (a), (b) and (c).

	Exhaustion (MBI-GS)		
	Pearson correlation	Sig. (2-tailed)	N
Workload (AWS)	**-0.563**	0.000	226
Control (AWS)	-0.172	0.010	225
Reward (AWS)	**-0.361**	0.000	225
Community (AWS)	-0.203	0.002	226
Fairness (AWS)	-0.284	0.000	226
Values (AWS)	**-0.301**	0.000	224

Note: boldface means correlations R>0.3

Table 5 (a). Correlations of MBI-GS exhaustion and AWS scales.

The strong relationship between exhaustion and workload suggest a straightforward relationship between workload as a stressor and exhaustion as a reaction to it, which has already been acknowledged by many authors (Leiter & Maslach, 2004; Leiter & Shaugnessy, 2006, Lasalvia et al., 2009; Leiter & Maslach, 2009). The negative correlation between exhaustion and reward and values was also expected. Surprisingly, there was a very low correlation between exhaustion and perceived lack of control over own work (0.36 for Canadian nurses in Leiter & Maslach, 2009). Perceived lack of reward also had a lower correlation with exhaustion than for Canadian nurses (–0.47). Perceived unfairness is nearly as influential in relation to exhaustion as the assessment of value fit with the organization; however, unfairness had a slightly weaker relationship in the Czech sample than in Leiter's sample (–0.38).

	Cynicism (MBI-GS)		
	Pearson correlation	Sig. (2-tailed)	N
Workload (AWS)	**-0.309**	0.000	225
Control (AWS)	-0.283	0.000	224
Reward (AWS)	**-0.396**	0.000	224
Community (AWS)	-0.192	0.004	225
Fairness (AWS)	**-0.422**	0.000	225
Values (AWS)	**-0.464**	0.000	223

Note: boldface means correlations R>0.3

Table 5 (b). Correlations of MBI-GS cynicism and AWS scales.

There is a high negative correlation between cynicism and perceived value fit and fairness, and a weaker correlation with reward and workload. In comparison to the Canadian nurses, cynicism is more strongly associated with perceived values of the organization than rewards (for Canadian nurses, reward to cynicism=0.54 and values to cynicism=0.42). This also corresponds to the central role of value fit as a predictor of burnout and turnover intention among nurses, as Leiter found (Leiter & Maslach, 2009). In his model, value congruence predicted all three dimensions of burnout, while workload was linked to exhaustion. We found the same in our data. This seems to be the best empirically substantiated and theoretically explained part of the burnout and Areas of Worklife relationships model, which has been proven across various populations. On the contrary, the aspect of control over one's own work, as measured by AWS in the translated Czech version, is rather weaker here. Leiter gives it an important predictive position in his model, although control is not directly predictive of cynicism (Leiter & Maslach, 2009:336).

	Professional efficacy (MBI-GS)		
	Pearson correlation	Sig. (2-tailed)	N
Workload (AWS)	0.098	0.148	221
Control (AWS)	0.297	0.000	220
Reward (AWS)	0.258	0.000	220
Community (AWS)	0.142	0.034	221
Fairness (AWS)	0.239	0.000	221
Values (AWS)	0.282	0.000	219

Table 5 (c). Correlations of MBI-GS professional efficacy and AWS scales.

According to Leiter's model, professional efficacy is mediated by value congruence (0.38), reward (0.35) and control (0.40). Here the same tendency is at least visible, together with fairness; however, all scores are below 0.3. Control has the highest correlation. Comparisons were done according to characteristics of the sample (age, education, type of work in team, type of contract (full-time, part-time).

Here we present only the significant results. Concerning age and type of contract, there were no significant differences between the results of both instruments.

Figure 1 presents an analysis of variance (ANOVA) for educational level (middle school, high school, university) with the AWS scales. Higher education shows higher congruence with control, reward and value.

Here we see that people working independently perceive more control and much higher rewards but also higher workloads. They perceive more congruence in values with their organization and slightly less fairness than those who work in a small team. People working in large collectives score lowest in all AWS scales.

The results of the t-test (not presented here) show statistically significant differences in all AWS scales. In the one-way ANOVA, nurses showed lower scores on all AWS scales (Figure 3).

The greatest differences between healthcare and social workers were found to be values, fairness and reward, but there are significant differences in all AWS scales. Our sample consisted mainly of two professional groups with contrasting working conditions. The

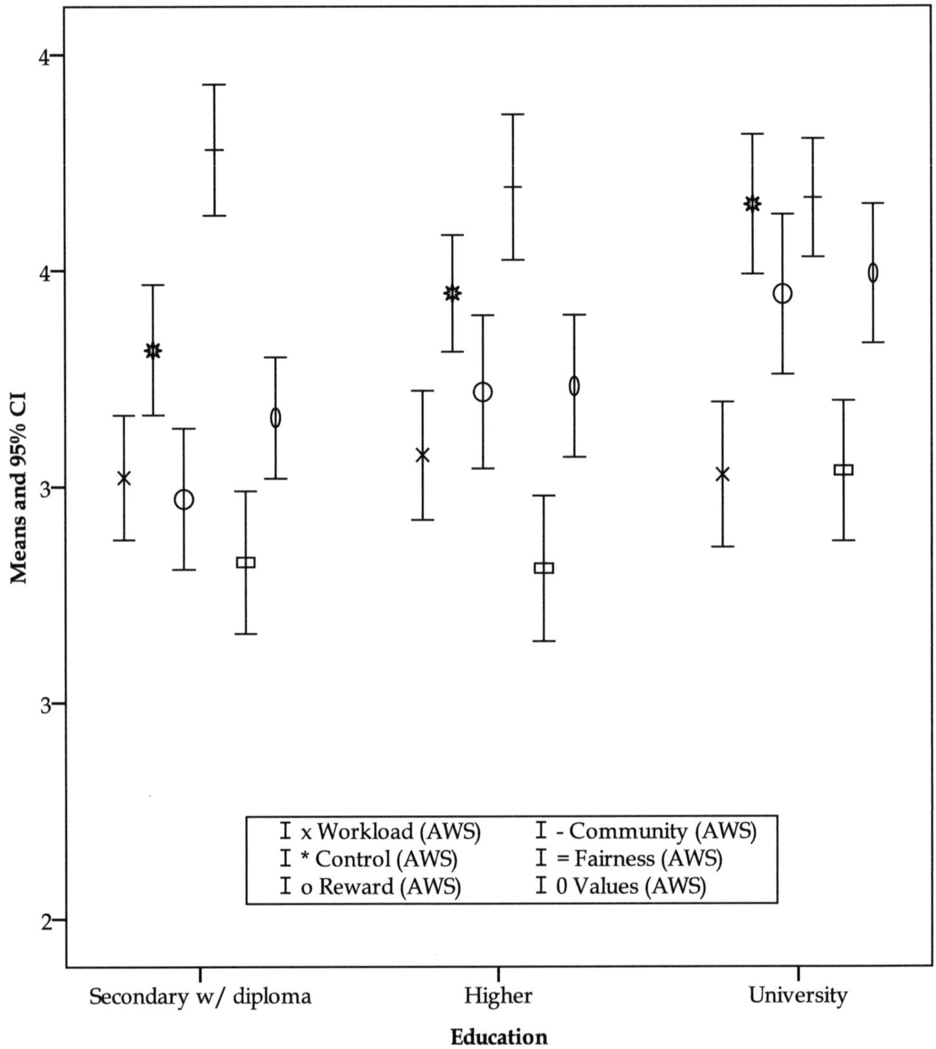

Fig. 1. Education and AWS scales, one-way ANOVA.

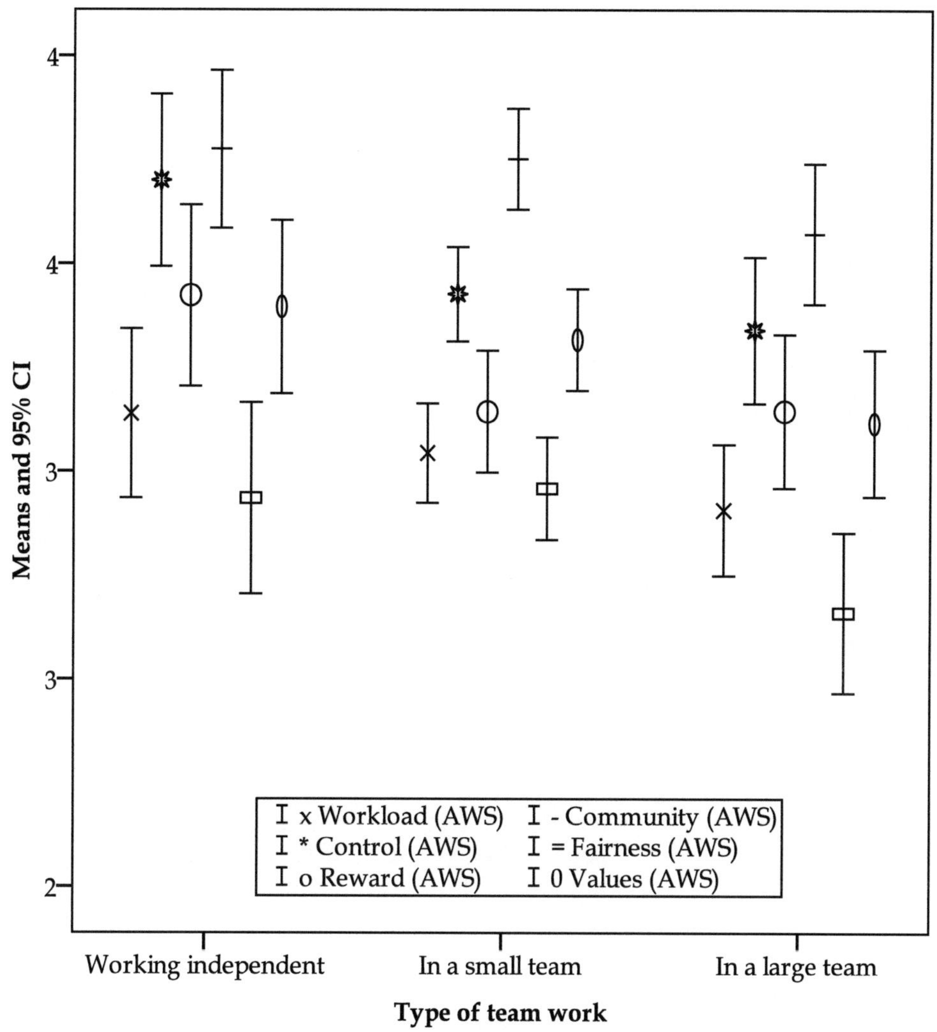

Fig. 2. Type of teamwork (independent, small team, large team) one-way ANOVA, AWS scales.

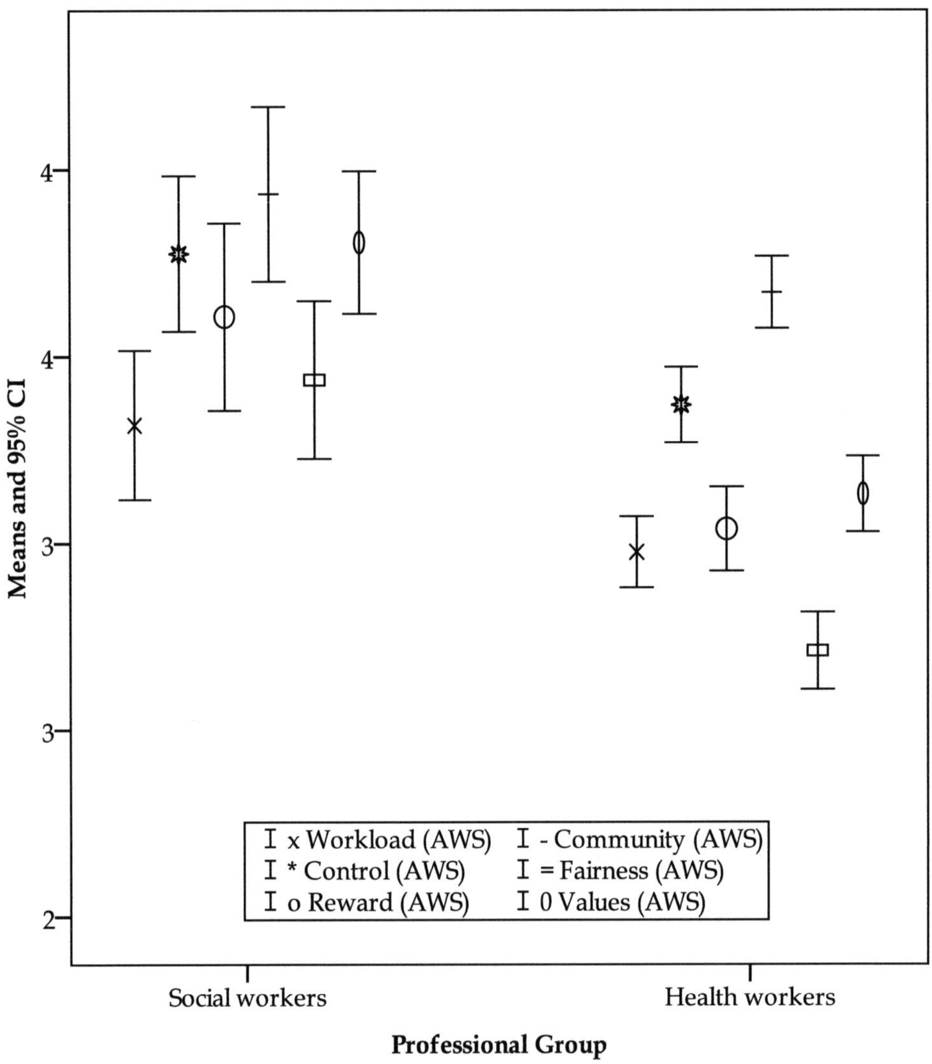

Note: social workers N=44, health (nurses) N=169

Fig. 3. Comparison between health and social workers AWS.

"health" group consisted of nurses and midwifes working in hospitals where management is mostly hierarchical, the culture can be briefly described as outcomes focused, and fiscal restrictions in healthcare are a politically prominent topic. There is generally rather low personal support from the organization, although a shortage of nurses is seen as an important issue.

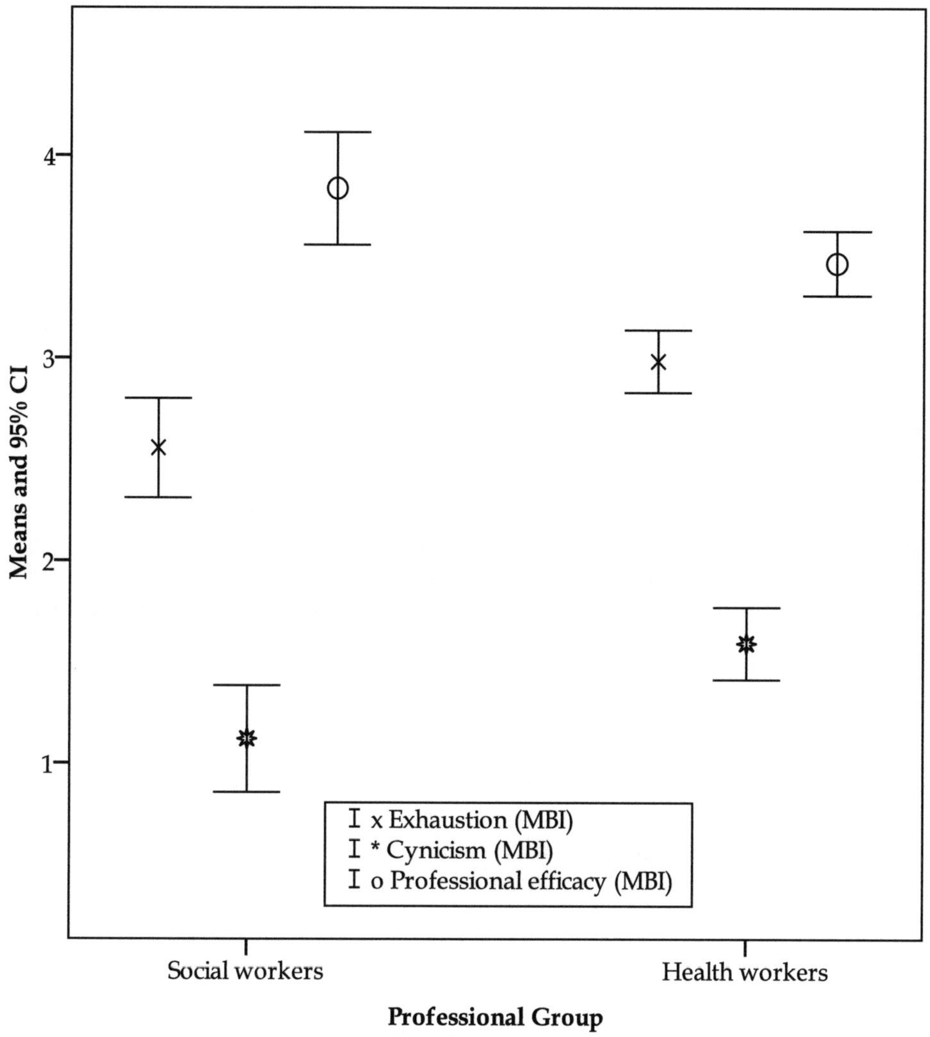

Fig. 4. Comparison between health and social workers MBI-GS.

The "social" group consisted of social workers working in communities in the non-profit sector. In this segment of services, support for employees is some of the best in the field. Most organizations have external team supervision where common issues around social cases and teamwork can be raised and discussed. There is also high participation of organizational members in decision making. These factors influence the attitude of respondents towards their organization, as mirrored in the AWS reports. This is in contrast with the results of an Italian research team (Lasalvia et al., 2009), where social workers had the higher risk of burnout among mental health professionals, including nurses. Figure 4 compares the Czech nurses and social workers on the MBI-GS scale.

We can see that the health group is at higher risk of burnout than the social group, as mean scores on exhaustion and cynicism are higher (above 3) and professional efficacy is lower. The differences are significant for exhaustion ($\chi 2 = 5.662$, df=1, p=0.023, Contingency coefficient CC=0.164) and cynicism ($\chi 2 = 3.69$, df=1, p=0.077, CC= 0.134). No difference was found for professional efficacy.

The high score for exhaustion and cynicism and low score on efficacy corresponds to the Maslach's burnout model.

Discussion

There was good correspondence between the Leiter and Maslach model measuring burnout together with the traits of organizational civility as perceived by employees and the Czech data. Both measures have high reliability in all scales except for control. The measures seem to mirror subtle differences between social and health settings, such as democratic versus hierarchical management styles, which demonstrated significant differences between the contrasting Czech samples from the healthcare and social care settings.

A limitation of this study is its lack of representativity - the sample is not representative of the whole population of Czech nurses or social workers, therefore findings have limiting generalizability. Both AWS and MBI-GS questionnaires in the Czech version showed good reliability. One problem seems to be the dimension of control, where the principal component analysis (not presented here) also showed some problems. Low reliability for this scale was also shown in a previous study (Havrdová et al., 2010). The AWS questionnaire therefore requires further changes in the formulation of control items. Its factor structure needs further analysis based on more data from different respondents.

Another limitation is a lack of qualitative information which would help with a deeper understanding of the cultural differences measured by the AWS. These can be observed not only between Canadian and Czech nurses, with regard to self-perception of professional efficacy, but also in particular between the different workplaces. Nurses often work in large institutions with more hierarchical leadership and less control over their jobs, and are therefore much more prone to burnout and turnover, as predicted by Leiter's model (Leiter & Maslach, 2009) due to lower levels of control, value congruence, perceived fairness and reward, and higher workload.

Tanner (2011) mentions that cynicism can be regarded as an ineffective strategy for coping with workplace stressors, and suggests the introduction of interventions at the organizational level, combined with individual interventions to prevent cynicism. Beddoe (2010) summarizes the central components of so-called resilient cultures as follows: promoting participation, recognizing the emotional impact of work stresses, reviewing mistakes to provide opportunities for learning, reviewing effectiveness and providing mutual feedback, and facilitative and supportive supervision at all level of the organization. This last point contributes substantially to all previous ones, and corresponds to the concept of social support and psychological safety as necessary protective factors (Folkman &

Lazarus, 1989; Kahn, 1990; Edmondson, 2003; and others). In our comparison of level of workplace civility in social versus health settings, one of the main differences can be seen in the regular supportive supervision which the social workers receive. The impact of clinical supervision on the level of burnout by nurses has been recognized earlier (Butterwoth et al., 1999; Brunero, 2008; and others). Supportive and reflective supervision can provide both team and individual support, which can contribute to the development of better coping strategies at both levels.

Gender, age and number of years in the organization did not change the predictive pattern of AWS for burnout or the correlations between scales within the instruments. A higher educational level among nurses also led to higher perceived control, reward and value congruence, but also to a higher workload. That also means that with higher education, the nurse is going to be more flexible on the labour market and can move to an organization where there is higher value congruence. This corresponds to our perception that students who develop their careers to the master's level move to organizations where they are able to implement the ideas and vision they develop during their studies. Similarly, we found that the nature of work - either in a small team, a larger collective, or individually - had an important impact on burnout as mediated by control, reward and values. Individual work often means that the nurse acts as an expert in the field, for example in quality management, which means a higher control over the work and recognition as an expert (high reward).

In a previous study based on AWS (Havrdová & Šafr, 2010) we came to conclusion that the value fit with the social organization depends even at the lower employee level on how the organization realizes its mission to support its clients instead of supporting just itself. The high influence of values in the Czech sample might also be a cultural difference from the Canadian and Italian research samples. In the Italian sample (Lasalvia et al., 2009:542) values were totally absent in the model of predictors of burnout.

In Leiter's model, value fit is predicted by rewards, community and fairness. Leiter admits that community has a weaker impact on value congruence and burnout. We would argue, however, that the perception of common values is much more dependent on the behaviour of leaders in the organization than on the community, and that it can be built by various means, one being reward and fairness, and another being trust based on appropriate decisions and the fulfilment of the organizational mission by management. The relationship of trust to shared values and its impact on employee identification with the organization has already been proven (Edwards & Cable, 2009). Although such information is lacking in the present study, this relationship to AWS and burnout requires further study.

The potential value for Czech managers and supervisors of using both instruments as a fast screening device has been proven, and this can be used for further communication with employees to achieve an optimal strategy for their support.

9. Conclusion

Previous studies over the past 35 years have proven that burnout, as a negative pole of employee engagement, has serious consequences for mental and physical health. Situational and organizational factors such as civility in the workplace play a more important role than individual factors in the development of this syndrome.

Nurses belong to the professional group at highest risk of burnout. Early signs of burnout in nurses are predictive of turnover. This has important consequences for leaders, managers and supervisors, particularly in the healthcare sector, who are perceived as important sources of support for organizational civility.

Interventions at the organizational level combined with individual interventions should be used to support the building of a resilient culture that promotes participation, recognizes the emotional impact of work stress, reviews mistakes in a safe environment, provides time to review effectiveness, and provides mutual feedback and social support. Clinical supervision has been proven as an important means of building such a culture in the helping organizations and thus contributing to the development of better coping strategies for stress at all levels of the organization.

The burnout–workplace civility model, as researched by AWS and MBI-GS questionnaires, has face validity in the Czech environment. The psychometric analysis of the data shows high reliability on all scales except control, which requires some modification in the formulation of its items or the number of items (currently only three) in future Czech research. The mutual relationships between scales showed higher correlations for values and fairness and values and reward than in the Canadian sample. Fairness and control showed much lower correlations and exhaustion did not correlate with professional efficacy at all, which differed from the Canadian sample. However, the Czech sample is not representative of all Czech nurses, therefore these findings have limited generalizability.

Our data fully supports Leiter's model of the predictive strength of value congruence for all three dimensions of burnout. In our case we suggest taking into consideration the role of trust of an organization's management, which seems more important than just reward and community. These two correlated more weakly with value fit than fairness. Organizational behaviour that is more orientated towards client welfare than the organization's welfare also seems to be important.

The factors of age and length of work in the organization did not influence the data. However, the nursing profession and working in larger collectives in hospitals increased the indicators for burnout. With higher education levels, and thus the ability of nurses to move to organizations that better correspond with their own values and where they are more in control of their work, there is a diminished risk of ineffective coping strategies such as cynicism, which is mediated by lower rewards and lower perception of fairness from the employer.

The level of organizational civility and burnout in our data was similar to levels in Leiter's 2009 Canadian sample. However, we found that Czech nurses scored much lower on self-evaluation of professional efficacy than the Canadian and Italian (Lasalvia et al., 2009) samples. This may reflect sociocultural factors, and be a sign of lower self-esteem leading to higher aspirations which can contribute to a higher risk of burnout. On the contrary, the cynicism score was lower in relation to both samples. Another significant difference was the higher workload perception and higher satisfaction with the community at the workplace among Czech nurses. These differences may be due to the small and non-representative sample.

The analysis has shown that AWS and MBI-GS questionnaires and their underlying models of organizational and individual factors, as contributors to the burnout–engagement dimension of employee behaviour, mirror differences in organizational settings, and can be useful measures for further communication with employees and development of organizational support systems in the Czech environment. Further research should focus on modification of the AWS control dimension and measurement of trust in management as a special item. Better validation through use of qualitative sources of data is also recommended.

10. Acknowledgments

The authors thank Jiri Safr and Magdalena Gorcikova for the psychometric analysis and graphics. Thanks also to the management and supervision students of UK FHS who participated in the collection of data in the Czech health and social organizations.

11. References

Aiken, L.H., Clarke, S.P., Sloane, D.M., Sochalski, J. & Silber, J.H. (2002). Hospital nurse staffing and patient mortality, nurse burnout, and job dissatisfaction. *Journal of the American Medical Association*, 288, 16: 1987–93.

Andersson, L.M. & Pearson, C.M. (1999). Tit for tat? The spiraling effect of incivility in the workplace. *The Academy of Management Review*, 24, 3: 452–471.

Appels, A., & Otten, F. (1992). Exhaustion as a precursor of cardiac death. *British Journal of Clinical Psychology*, 31, 351-356.

Beddoe, L. (2010). *Best practice in professional supervision: a guide for the helping professions.* London: Jessica Kingsley.

Beehr, T.A. (1995). *Psychological stress in the workplace*. London, New York: Routledge.

Brunero, S. & Stein-Parbury, J. (2008). The effectiveness of clinical supervision in nursing: an evidence based literature review. *Austr. J. Adv. Nurs.*, 25, 3: 86–94.

Butterworth, T., Carson, J., Jeacock, J., White, E. & Clements, A. (1999). Stress, coping, burnout and job satisfaction in British nurses: findings from the clinical supervision evaluation project. *Stress Med.* 15: 27–33.

Cherniss, C. (1980). *Professional burnout in human service organizations*. New York: Praeger.

Cherniss, C. (1989). Burnout in new professionals: a long-term follow-up study. *Journal of Health and Human Resources Administration*, 12: 11–24.

Cherniss, C. (1990). Natural recovery from burnout: results of a 10-year follow-up study. *Journal of Health and Human Resources Administration*, 13: 132–154.

Edmondson, A.C. (1999). Psychological safety and learning behavior in work teams. *Administrative Science Quarterly*, 44: 350–383.

Edmondson, A.C. (2003). Managing the risk of learning: psychological safety in work teams. In: M. West, D. Tjosvold & K. Smith (eds.), *International Handbook of Organizational Teamwork and Co-operative Working*. Chichester: Wiley and Sons.

Edwards, J.R. & Cable, D.M. (2009) The value of value congruence. *Journal of Applied Psychology*, 94, 3: 654677.

Folkman, S., & Lazarus, R.S. (1988). *Manual for the ways of coping questionnaire: Research edition.* Palo Alto, CA: Consulting Psychologists Press.

Gill, M.J. & Sypher, B.D. (2009). Workplace incivility and organizational trust. In P. Lutgen-Sandvik & B.D. Sypher (eds.), *Destructive organizational communication: processes, consequences, and constructive ways of organizing*. New York: Routlege, pp. 53–74.

Hallman, T., Thomsson, H., Burell, G., Lisspers, J. & Setterlind, S. (2003). Stress, burnout and coping: differences between women with coronary heart disease and healthy matched women. *Journal of Health Psychology*, 8: 433–445.

Havrdová, Z. & Šafr, J. (2010). Kongruence v hodnotách jako ukazatel vztahů v péči o seniory. In Havrdová, Z. et al., *Hodnoty v prostředí sociálních služeb*. FHS UK v Praze, Praha, pp. 85–108.

Havrdová, Z., Šolcová, I., Hradcová, D. & Rohanová, E. (2010). Kultura organizace a syndrom vyhoření. *Československá psychologie*, 64, 3: 235–248.

Jones, J.G. (1987). Stress in psychiatric nursing. In: Payne, R. & Firth-Cozens, J. (eds.), *Stress in health professionals*. Chichester: Wiley.

Kahn, W.A. (1990). Psychological conditions of personal engagement and disengagement at work. *The Academy of Management Journal*, 33: 692–724.

Karasek, R.A. (1979). Job demands, job decision latitude, and mental strain: implications for job redesign. *Administrative Science Quarterly*, 24: 285–308.

Karasek, R.A. & Theorell, T. (1990). *Healthy work: stress, productivity, and the reconstruction of the working life*. New York: Basic Books.

Kebza, V. & Šolcová, I. (1998). Burnout syndrom: teoretická východiska, diagnostické a intervenční možnosti. [Burnout syndrome: theoretical sources, diagnostic and treatment possibilities.] *Československá psychologie*, 42: 429–448. [In Czech.]

Kebza, V. & Šolcová, I. (2008). Syndrom vyhoření: rekapitulace současného stavu poznání a perspektivy do budoucna. [Burnout syndrome - review of contemporary state of knowledge and perspectives for the future.] *Československá psychologie*, 52: 351-365. [In Czech.]

Kebza, V. & Šolcová, I. (2010). Syndrom vyhoření, vybrané psychologické proměnné a rizikové faktory kardiovaskulárních onemocnění. [Burnout syndrome, selected psychological variables, and risk factors of cardiovascular diseases.] *Československá psychologie*, 54: 1-16. [In Czech.]

Kimmel, D.C. (2010). Organizational civility. Available at: http://faculty-staff.ou.edu/K/David.C.Kimmel-1/civility.htm.

Kitaoka-Higashiguchi, K., Morikawa, Y., Miura, K., Sakurai, M, Ishizaki, M., Kido, T., Naruse, Y., & Nakagawa, H. (2009). Burnout and Risk Factors for Arteriosclerotic Disease: Follow-up Study. *Journal of Occupational Health*, 51: 123-131.

Krause, N. (1997). Perceived support, anticipated support, social class, and mortality. *Research on Aging*, 19: 387 - 422.

Lasalvia, A., Bonetto, C., Bertani, M., Bissoli, S., Cristofalo, D., Marrella, G., et al. (2009). Influence of perceived organizational factors on job burnout: survey of community mental health staff. *Br J Psychiatry*, 195: 537–544.

Leiter, M.P. (2008). *Civility, respect and engagement at work*. Available at http://www.workengagement.com/crew.

Leiter, M.P. & Laschinger, H.K.S. (2006). Relationships of work and practice environment to professional burnout: testing a causal model. *NursingResearch, 55*, 2: 137–146.

Leiter, M.P. & Maslach, C. (1999). Six areas of worklife: a model of the organizational context of burnout. *Journal of Health and Human Services Administration*, 21: 472–489.

Leiter, M.P. & Maslach, C. (2000). *Preventing burnout and building engagement.* San Francisco, CA: Josey Bass Inc.

Leiter, M.P. & Maslach, C. (2004). Areas of worklife: a structured approach to organizational predictors of job burnout. In P. Perrewe & D.C. Ganster (eds). *Research in Occupational Stress and Well Being* (Vol. 3.): emotional and physiological processes and positive intervention strategies. Oxford, UK: JAI Press/Elsevier, pp. 91–134.

Leiter, M.P. & Maslach, C. (2009). Nurse turnover: the mediating role of burnout. *Journal of Nursing Management*, 17: 331–339.

Leiter, M.P. & Shaughnessy, K. (2006). The areas of worklife model of burnout: tests of mediation relationships. *Ergonomia: An International Journal*, 28: 327–341.

Lepore, S.J., Evans, G.W. & Schneider, M. (1991). Dynamic role of social support in the link between chronic stress and psychological distress. *Journal of Personality Social Psychol*, 61: 899–909.

Maslach, C. (2011). Burnout and engagement in the workplace: new perspectives. *The European Health Psychologist*, 13, 3: 44–47.

Maslach, C. & Jackson, S.E. (1986). *The Maslach Burnout Inventory* (2nd ed.). Palo Alto, CA: Consulting Psychologists Press.

Maslach, C. & Leiter, M.P. (1997). *The truth about burnout: how organizations cause personal stress and what to do about it.* San Francisco: Jossey-Bass.

Maslach, C., Schaufeli, W. & Leiter, M.P. (2001). Job burnout. *Annual Review of Psychology*, 52: 397–422.

Melamed, S., Kushnir, T., & Shirom, A. (1992). Burnout and risk factors for cardiovascular disease. *Behavioral Medicine*, 18: 53-60.

Melamed, S., Shirom, A., Toker, S., Berliner, S., & Shapira, I. (2006). Burnout and risk of cardiovascular disease: Evidence, possible causal paths, and promising research directions. *Psychological Bulletin*, 132: 327-353.

Sarason, I.G. (1988). Social support, personality, and health. In M.P Janisse (Ed.), *Individual differences, stress, and health psychology*. New York: Springer Verlag.

Sarason, B.R., Shearin, E.N., Pierce, G.R., & Sarason, I.G. (1987). Interrelationship between social support measures: Theoretical and practical implications. *Journal of Personality & Social Psychology*, 52: 813-832.

Schaufeli, W.B., Leiter, M.P., Maslach, C. & Jackson, S.E. (1996).The Maslach Burnout Inventory - General Survey. In MBI Manual (3rd ed) (C. Maslach, S.E. Jackson & M.P. Leiter (eds)Palo Alto, CA: Consulting Psychologists Press, pp. 22–26.

Schein, E. (1990). *Organizational culture and leadership.* San Francisco: Jossey-Bass.

Shirom, A. (2003). The effects of work-related stress on health. In M. J. Schabracq, J. A. M. Winnbust, & C. L. Cooper (Eds.) Handbook of work and health psychology. (2nd Edition; pp. 63-83). New York, New York: Wiley.

Shirom, A. (2007). Burnout and physical health. Evidence, possible causal paths, and promising research directions. State-of-the art lecture. 10th European Congress of Psychology, Prague, July 3-6 2007.

Šolcová, I. & Kebza, V. (1999). Sociální opora jako významný protektivní faktor. [Social support as an important protective factor.] *Československá psychologie*, 43: 19-38. [In Czech.]

Tanner, S. (2011). *People and work*. Tampere: Finnish Institute of Occupational Health. Doctoral dissertation.

3

Reducing Stress in Mental Health Practitioners - Becoming Change Agents in Practice Through Action Research

Eileen Petrie
La Trobe University
Australia

1. Introduction

The social phenomenon of stress and workplace burnout has spanned over five decades. Despite a plethora of literature that exists, there still remain problematic issues that neither scientific investigation or government legislation has been able to resolve. The literature examined throughout this chapter reflects this 50-year period. It demonstrates that studies into this phenomenon have attempted to define stress, identify causal factors of workplace stress, workplace burnout and environmental congruence; and discusses strategies (focused on both the individual and organizational levels) that have been implemented to effect beneficial outcomes for individuals affected by any one of these.

As this chapter continues, the more recent literature gives a greater recognition to violence in the workplace and legislative enactments as preventative measures to reduce the heavy burden of costs, both physical and financial, to organizations. This review indicates no answer to the problem has been identified to date and that this phenomenon remains, giving a clear indication that further scientific investigation is required to find a solution to what was described as the most serious health issue of the 20th century. Whilst there is a formal literature review presented in this chapter, there is a significant amount of literature support embedded into the various stages of the research study.

This chapter will discuss the issues of stress in a rural remote Community Mental Health Team (CMHT)'s realm of practice and examine a research study that led to a conceptual model of practice in changing praxis. The contribution of this study to the nursing profession is demonstrated through its potential to enhance community nursing practice to deliver effective holistic nursing care to consumers with mental health issues whilst maintaining their own psychological and physical wellness. The specified learnings from this research were envisaged to be processes and strategies for employees to overcome the debilitating effects of stress leading to workplace burnout.

2. Literature review

It is well established that CMHT's in rural and remote areas of Australia face issues and constraints specific to their locations relating to distance, population size and recruitment and retention of appropriately experienced and skilled staff (Bushy, 2004; Gibb, 2003). The rural remote CMHT nurse's work is influenced not only by the reduced resources but by the diverse and demanding role of first line managers of care for mental health consumers in the geographically challenging setting (Francis & Chapman, 2008). Further contributing to their workloads, CMHTs extend their case management by maintaining mental health services to the general community. These teams are required to provide flexible and innovative programme development in preventing illnesses and planning of treatment approaches for a comprehensive network of services to meet the ever-changing needs of the general population (Croll, 1997; Gibb, 2003; King, 2001). Lack of resources requires the community nurse to become extremely innovative and creative, with improvisation an important learned skill (Lauder, Reynolds, Reilly & Angus, 2001). These issues are coupled with an increased demand for their services due to an agricultural crisis that, according to some researchers, Australia has been facing for some decades (Bryant, 1992; Fraser at al., 2002). This agricultural crisis has resulted from the decline in wealth in the agricultural sector (following several years of low rainfall and declining produce and stock prices), and the rationalization of government and private sector services that has led to a decline in the financial well-being of rural towns.

The provision of appropriate mental health services is hindered considerably in rural and remote regions. Isolation is a contributing factor in poor recruitment and retention of qualified staff. Health professionals without mental health qualifications, limited or no access to local mental health services and, scarce and scattered resources inhibit the provision of adequate mental health services to the mental health consumer. Changes in the provision of psychiatric care have occurred on a global scale; many countries have trialled various models of care. In recent years, there has been a shift to providing support for these clinicians through the introduction of mental health nurses and other mental health professionals into general health care teams as supporters, educators and advisors.

However, these initiatives are rarely feasible in rural and remote health care settings due to low staff numbers, large distances involved in accessing specialists, and the time taken to transfer patients from rural regions to regional centres. Therefore, nurses in the rural remote setting are more likely to be exposed to stress, as they may be required to work—without substantive education and training and with limited access to specialist services—with patients with mental health issues. Population models for mental health across Australia proposing links between population or public health and integration with personal health care have, to date, become the chief focus in many community mental health settings (Judd & Humphreys, 2001). One model proposes assessments, formulation of interventions from prevention to treatment and maintenance at both population and individual levels. It addresses the issues across the lifespan applying to special populations, culturally and linguistically diverse backgrounds, and Aboriginal and Torres Strait Islander peoples. This model serves to provide for a comprehensive, evidence based and cohesive approach toward the provision of optimum mental health care, lessening the extent and burdens of mental disorders affecting populations (Bushy, 2004).

The model is conceptualized at different levels of care incorporating primary, secondary and tertiary mental health care, applying these across the population matrices of the various groups. Implementation of this model requires the identification of input outcomes (treatment outcome is the effect on a patient's health attributable to an intervention), data and information system infrastructure, workforce, education and training, research and development, quality processes, resource frameworks and review and change processes (Bushy, 2004).

To achieve the improvement in mental health services that lessens the disease burden, proactive interventions must be implemented to impact effectively on relevant factors at both population and individual levels. These programmes open to the community, total accountability in mental health service provision (Judd & Humphreys, 2001). However, in attempting to achieve this idealistic approach in maintaining mental health, a time constraint dilemma exists. It becomes imperative for members of CMHTs to allocate a time frame to provide the mental health intervention while maintaining best practice (Pinikahana & Happell, 2004). The flow-on from this is seen in the detraction from face to face contact and implementation of strategies and interventions to the clients they serve. This has seen an over-extension of personal resources creating a state of constant and unresolved stress for these team members (Pinikahana & Happell, 2004).

The social phenomenon of stress and workplace burnout has spanned over several decades. Despite a plethora of literature that exists, there still remain problematic issues that neither scientific investigation or government legislation has been able to resolve. The more recent literature gives a greater recognition to violence in the workplace and legislative enactments as preventative measures to reduce the heavy burden of costs, both physical and financial, to organizations. An extensive literature review indicated no answer to the problem has been identified to date and that this phenomenon remains, giving a clear indication that further scientific investigation is required to find a solution to what was described as the most serious health issue of the 20th century. Based on the literature examined this health issue has now gone well beyond the 20th century, giving relevance to the research study.

The study of stress has become an important area of study, as suggested in literature, due to its heavy costs in terms of the damage it has caused within society; to individuals, to relationships and to organizations (Snow, 2006). For the individual physical symptoms associated with work-related stress can include depression, anxiety, feelings of being overwhelmed and inability to cope, decreased work performance, increased sick days and absenteeism, sleeping difficulties such as insomnia, cognitive difficulties such as reduced ability to concentrate or make decisions, fatigue, headaches, heart palpitations, gastrointestinal upsets, such as diarrhoea or constipation, and increased aggression (Caufield et al., 2004; Constantini et al. 1997; Duquette et al., 1994; Johnson & Preston, 2001).

3. The impact of stress

Stress exists in all human beings and is evident in all human beings in varying degrees. Thought to be a strong motivating force, stress is required to produce optimum functioning levels. It stimulates individuals into a response to define and cope with any given situation or problem (stressor) (Lazarus & Folkman, 1984). This is known as eustress (healthy stress). Excessive and unrelenting stress becomes distress (unhealthy stress) impacting on and reducing work performances. The level of stress felt by an individual is determined by his/her response to a particular situation. If an individual recognizes that he/she is vulnerable when faced with situations perceived to be stressful, the basic human instinct is fight or flight (Seyle, 1956; 1974; 1976). The effects of stress may vary from one individual to another with different degrees of intensity. This will impact on the homeostasis of each individual, and the adaptation to this stress will be determined by the effectiveness of his/her own coping mechanisms. Distress results when the demands of the situation exceed the person's ability to cope, or become an unconscious threat to his/her psyche. This phenomenon has been the subject of scrutiny for several decades, with Selye (1956) first proposing a link between stress and health problems in his General Adaptation Syndrome (Kenny, 2000). At times, stressors may become excessive and effective coping mechanisms that may have previously worked are no longer adequate to reduce the stress experienced (Bushy, 2004; Gibb, 2003; Hugo, 2001; Melamed et al., 2006; Scopelliti et al., 2004). Relating this to the psychosocial perspective, job-related demands identified as being excessive can lead to burnout (Maslach, 1976; Cherniss, 1982).

The change in eustress to distress is very individualistic and may impact on the person's interpersonal skills, contributing to the reduction of self-esteem and outwardly affecting his/her relationships with work colleagues and family (Melamed et al., 2006). This deterioration can be insidious; individuals may not recognize when a fatigue factor originates, nor may they identify that there is a gradual deterioration within their own psychological wellness. It may take only a simple trigger to cause a downward spiralling of functioning and stress management, leading to the inability to cope with the simplest of tasks within the workplace. This poor interaction can lead to resentment from social networks and co-workers, without recognition from anyone that the individual is actually experiencing a decline in functioning (Melamed et al., 2006). It can be considered at this point that workplace burnout is being experienced. Subject to the severity of this deterioration, this may indicate the need for employees to move away from their chosen profession or take extensive leave in an attempt to come to terms with their inability to cope with the stress of the workplace (Heard & Harris, 2004; Malach-Pines, 2000).

Cohen, McGowen, Fookskas and Rose (1984) contend that it is the notion that others will be available to provide support when needed that acts as a stress-buffering agent. The authors suggest different studies indicating that if there is a perceived support available for the health professional, it is negligible as to whether this support is received or not. The fact remains that it is this belief that support is available which impacts on the health and adjustment of the staff member and the eventual outcome for the individual.

4. Stressful work environments

There is vast literature that supports the notion that the health workplace can be a very stressful situation, particularly in the rural sector of the nursing field (Bushy, 2004; Gibb, 2003; Hugo, 2001; Melamed, Shirom, Toker, Berliner & Shapira, 2006; Scopelliti et al., 2004). Rural and remote areas face unique issues and constraints relating to distances, population sizes and recruitment of appropriately experienced and skilled staff especially within community mental health teams. Many of these areas have seen significant withdrawal of resources with government economic rationalisation across all Australian States (Bushy, 2004; Carlin and Farnell 1985; Gibb, 2003; Hugo, 2001; Melamed et al., 2006; Pompili et al., 2006; Scopelliti et al., 2004).

The impact of stress can not only be derived from organizational, societal, personal and professional sectors but also environmental impacts must be considered in regard to maintaining employees' well-being. Workers at times may be in conflict with any or all of these factors in their work situation (Gillespie & Melby, 2003). There is vast literature on rural health with much focus being placed on the detrimental effects rural and remote areas exert on individuals (Halcomb et al., 2005). These areas face unique issues and constraints relating to distance, isolation, poor technological support, population size and recruitment of appropriately experienced and skilled staff (Productivity Commission, 2005).

The workplace has a profound impact on employees' morale, physical and mental health, and personal identity. Many work demands create stress simply because they do not satisfy basic human needs. The intense nature of nurse-patient interactions and the stress associated with confronting difficult and challenging patient behaviours on a regular basis compound the physical and psychological demands on nurses in an already hostile work environment (Pompili et al., 2006). The working environment and the effectiveness of organizational structure were examined by Carlin and Farnell (1985) with organizational structures being identified as a major origin of workplace stressors, along with poor physical working environments. Lambert (1995) described unhealthy workplaces and work habits as causing stress, lowering productivity and creating physical and psychological difficulties for individuals. Workers suffering prolonged stress and ill-feeling towards their employing organization are more likely to suffer from poor self-esteem, burnout and violent outbursts (Lambert, 1995). Work environment evaluations and changes can minimize these problems and promote health and safety for employees. Workplaces and work habits that fail to allow for periodic unwinding create stress, erode physical and mental health and lower productivity. Lambert discusses the growing concern in Japan about work-related deaths. Karoshi, 'death from overwork', is a major occupational health problem and involves too many hours on the job, producing high blood pressure and high stress levels (Melamed et al. 2006). It is the second highest cause of death after cancer amongst workers in Japan.

5. Unrelenting stress and burnout

Melamed et al. (2006) present evidence to suggest that the literature regards burnout as continuous and prolonged exposure to stress, particularly related to the workplace. The authors acknowledge that there are facets in the coping process such as psychological withdrawal and that there is the concept of a recovery from this state of fatigue that passes after a resting period. Burnout, however, is conceptually distinct from Melamed's concept. The burnout phenomenon is multidimensional in construct, consisting of emotional exhaustion, physical fatigue and cognitive weariness. In a study undertaken by Melamed et al (2006), the results suggested there was a remarkable stability of the burnout syndrome regardless of the sample composition, attesting to chronicity. This study also revealed that a job environment in which there is chronic workload stress was more strongly related than personality factors and age. The authors report that this has led to an increase in workers' compensation claims across the United States of America, United Kingdom and the Netherlands, with Sweden having burnout as a diagnosis on medical certificates. Branco, Chambers, Fallon, Fraser and Howlett (1981) identify burnout as being a common experience in practitioners of the helping professions, regardless of the time spent working within their profession. The authors recognize the physical manifestations of burnout, with symptomatology occurring in the physical, cognitive, attitudinal, affective and social levels of functioning. Branco et al. (1981) recommend that professional training within the helping professions should include education about the signs and symptoms of burnout and its management.

6. Preparing the nursing workforce

In the last 20 years, there has been a marked change in the education of nurses, from the apprenticeship model to the academic model. It is argued that a section of this workforce from either model do not have the comprehensiveness in education when entering the workplace to meet adequately the needs associated with the various cultures and values of today's Australian society and the radically changing requirements of the Australian health system beyond 2000 (Clinton & Hazelton, 2000; Happell & Platania-Phung, 2005). This deficit is significant in the specialty field of mental health nursing. The impact of the change from psychiatric deinstitutionalization to community-based care has required implementation of a diverse community care framework, providing a range of community and hospital-based services. Sharrock and Happell (2002) purport there is increasing evidence to suggest nurses working in general hospital settings consider themselves as inadequately prepared, skilled or experienced to care for consumers with mental health issues. Campbell (1985) contended that the changes in work practices have led to decreases in job satisfaction. Stresses within the work environment, along with personal stresses, have contributed to feelings of the job becoming increasingly undesirable. Current literature suggests this argument is supported and continues to apply in current practice (Clinton & Hazelton, 2000; Happell & Platania-Phung, 2005).

For rural Australia, access to and provision of health-related services have been continuing factors in poorer health outcomes and have been greatly influenced by the economic downturn and changing rural demographics (Mahnken, 2001). Rural communities now require health services involving a more diverse range of health promotion, preventive, chronic and social care. Shifts in health policies during the 1990s reflected this changing need. Hegney et al. (1997) identified the geographical implications for health care in rural Australia. These authors contended that rural areas in general had fewer facilities with shortages of health professionals. They identified significant inter- and intra-State differences in the availability of ease of access to health care services. Major rural towns and regional centres were well provided with primary and specialist services whilst many smaller and rural communities failed to attract the most basic of health care services. Attention was drawn to the fact that accessing basic health care services for many rural Australians presented a major difficulty due to reduced services associated with decreasing population and demographics.

Humphreys and Rolley (1991) identified three themes that exist in any discussion of rural health care needs. The first of these was the specific difficulty associated with the provision of any health intervention, including staffing and hospital availability in remote and rural areas. The second of these themes identified the necessity for flexibility in the delivery of services, providing accessibility whilst considering the monetary cost involved to the health regions. The final theme these authors identified was related to the appropriateness of service models designed for metropolitan areas when utilized in rural regions. Many of these had proved to be unsuccessful in application. Referring to a study conducted in the Hunter Valley, NSW, the authors identified that rural residents expected complete competence from their health care provider, placing an additional stress on rural health personnel. Compounding this issue, and increasing the stress levels for the practitioner, was the considerable distance from acute care facilities, accompanied at times by 'fragile and erratic means of communication' (Humphreys and Rolley, 1991, p.69).

Health professionals working in the health sector make up 6.7% of the employed workforce in Australia (Duckett, 2005). Community Mental Health Teams (CMHT) providing illness treatment/rehabilitation based on the recovery model and preventative services of education, health promotion and prevention programmes are part of this cohort. The expectation placed upon this service is proving to be an increasingly difficult, if not near impossible, task to achieve and maintain in light of the socio-economic situation of rural communities (Bushy, 2004; Fraser et al., 2002). Effective delivery of health care in community nursing practice within rural areas encounters a range of barriers, such as the remoteness of some communities and the vast distances of travel required, and the isolation and fragmentation of supportive health service providers (Hays & Beaton, 2004).

Since deinstitutionalization, mental health care in the community is now provided through collaboration between representatives from several disciplines (Cook & Fontaine, 1991; Gibb, 2003; King, 2001; Murray & Huelskoetter, 1991). The role of psychiatric nurses is significantly different to that of their equally qualified and skilled counterparts in other specialty areas of nursing. Cutcliffe and Goward (2000) contend that psychiatric nurses have a relationship with their clients that are qualitatively different to their counterparts in other disciplines. In psychiatric nursing, the role is based on the development of a mutually influenced relationship between the mental health consumer and the nurse. Pivotal to this relationship are the use of the self as a tool by the nurse and the closeness of the relationship that is formed (Maude & Warelow, 2011; Young, 2011). A significant amount of trust in oneself is required by the psychiatric nurse, as this relationship can be problematic or unpredictable.

7. Community mental health teams and unique issues

Community mental health teams in rural and remote areas face issues and constraints specific to their locations relating to distance, population size and recruitment and retention of appropriately experienced and skilled staff (Bushy, 2004; Gibb, 2003). The rural remote community mental health nurse's work is influenced not only by the reduced resources but by the diverse and demanding role of first line managers of care for mental health consumers in the geographically challenging setting (Francis & Chapman, 2008). Further contributing to their workloads, the community mental health teams extend their case management by maintaining mental health services to the general community. These teams are required to provide flexible and innovative programme development in preventing illnesses and planning of treatment approaches for a comprehensive network of services to meet the ever-changing needs of the general population (Croll, 1997; Gibb, 2003; King, 2001).

Lack of resources requires the community nurse to become extremely innovative and creative, with improvisation an important learned skill (Lauder, Reynolds, Reilly & Angus, 2001). These issues are coupled with an increased demand for their services due to an agricultural crisis that, according to some researchers, Australia has been facing for some decades (Bryant, 1992; Fraser at al., 2002). This agricultural crisis has resulted from the decline in wealth in the agricultural sector (following several years of low rainfall and declining produce and stock prices), and the rationalization of government and private sector services that has led to a decline in the financial well-being of rural towns.

Strong et al. (1998) suggest that the major challenges facing health service provision in rural Australia can be identified according to four categories. These are:

- Health status: (generally lower in the rural sector), a rapidly ageing population (with a higher rate of illness chronicity), and higher incidence of lifestyle related diseases;
- Community expectations: self sufficiency in health, and skewed perceptions of government agendas to reduce costs and services;
- Infrastructure: logistical considerations in accessing specialist health services, poor transport between services with many consumers requiring escorting, disparity in the physical condition of the infrastructure of health facilities with many lacking appropriate security, and difficulty in the recruitment and retention of appropriately qualified staff;
- Service delivery: areas of low population fall below the level required to maintain a viable and quality service, service duplication in an adjoining community, and the unsuitability/rigidity of Commonwealth and State funding for the specific requirements of each community.

8. The research study

Although there have been attempts to investigate nursing science through the reductionist approach invented in a laboratory, it is not always possible to apply such approaches to nursing research or practice (Gerber, 1999; Whitehead, 2007; Tolley, 1995). Consequently, much nursing research has moved away from the traditional medical science model to the social science model of investigation grounded in the qualitative research paradigm (Ezzy, 2006; Owens et al., 1999; Walter, 2006; Wright, 1991). Qualitative methodologies involve exploring participants' perspectives and experiences and locating these within a wider social context. Data collection, which involves the interactions of the researcher and respondents, is recognized as being based on a subjective process (Simmons, 1995). Qualitative research permits data analysis within the research as it progresses in the identification of patterns of meanings and interpretations. The aim of this is to develop sociological theory that contributes to the understanding of the social world (Willis, 2006). New knowledge that is socially constructed must be understood in its political and cultural context (Taylor, 1993) expanding nursing knowledge with the developed new theories to be applied in practice.

From a theoretical viewpoint action research can be deemed to be both action learning theory and critical social theory (Carr & Kemmis, 1990; Owens et al., 1999). Critical social theory allows for a collective inquiry into social reality with the potential for change in practice through collective analysis and action. This theory emerged after shortcomings were identified in both positivist and interpretive approaches to social science (Carr & Kemmis, 1990; Owens et al., 1999). A direct correlation between knowledge and practice forms critical social theory, which results from the 'outcome of human activity' (Tolley, 1995, p.185). The separation of the ideal world from the real world may contribute to the theory-practice gap (Tolley, 1995; Owens et al., 1999). Action research is a methodology that facilitates a greater union between researchers and clinicians and thus is in a better position to address the theory–practice gap (Owens et al., 1999; Whitehead & Elliott, 2007). It provides an ecological perspective in viewing social problems and individuals' behaviours, encompassing a focus on organizational, community, and cultural factors. In collaboration with participants, this form of research develops natural helping resources in communities rather than limiting the focus to professional resources only. This includes the change and development of new social policies and work environments. Action research can be described as a holistic social process facilitating change; organizational change is effected as this methodology marries the change process to the research findings (Owens et al, 1999; Whitehead & Elliott, 2007). It provides a way to work with people in the research field in a non-hierarchical and non-exploitative manner, enabling participants to reclaim the authority to identify their own roles and to establish conditions within their work practices (Kemmis & McTaggart, 1982).

Observation is a technique that facilitates description of actions, behaviours and interactions. It allows for individuals to be observed utilizing all their senses, including their verbal and non-verbal communication. Their perceptions, beliefs and assumptions can also be noted. The researcher examines within the practice context while not being dependent on categories of established theory and techniques, and constructs new theories defining means and ends interactively (Rolfe, 1996; Whitehead & Elliott, 2007). Reason (1988) viewed expression as a mode that allowed the meaning of experience to be verbalized and to take form. This requires the use of a creative medium. Human inquiry facilitates this medium. Language is expressed in various forms and can be identified through words, actions, art forms and silence, and can be 'analogical and symbolic' (p.82).

As in all social research, action research involves people as key stakeholders/co-researchers who determine the appropriateness of both the action and the research. Wallis (1998) and Owens et al. (1999) identify that the collaboration and participation processes of action research are essential to facilitate the knowledge, skills and confidence needed to change practice and to maximize the link between research and practice. Participants in the research are known as the critical group and they work collaboratively with the researcher as co-researchers (Whitehead & Elliott, 2007). Participation by all members of the critical group is the predominant factor giving rise to the emancipatory process, by allowing each member to become a co-researcher and to be given a voice (Whitehead & Elliott, 2007). Collaborative reflection and action among those with shared concerns can implement social change through this method of research, which is conceptualized as a spiral of collective, self-reflective inquiry (Kemmis and McTaggart, 1988; Whitehead & Elliott, 2007).

Susman and Evered (1978, p.587) describe the characteristics of action research as providing a 'corrective to the deficiencies' of positivist science. These characteristics are explained by these authors as being 'future orientated' by creating a more desirable future for people when dealing with their practical concerns. The authors describe an interdependent relationship involving collaboration between the researcher and the participant.

9. The cyclic nature of action research

The action research method includes a wide range of variations on a theme, including participatory research, collaborative inquiry, emancipatory research, action learning and contextual action research (Sheehan, 1996; Susman & Evered, 1978; Whitehead & Elliott, 2007). The cyclic or spiral process first introduced in the previous section involves the four steps of planning, acting, observing and reflecting (Kemmis & McTaggart, 1982). The aim of the planning phase is to develop an exact description of what changes should be implemented into practice (Kemmis & McTaggart, 1982). The critical group involved in the research carefully considers what is believed to be the most effective intervention to effect change of practice in order to resolve an identified problem (Kemmis & McTaggart, 1982). Critical communication practice (the formation of abstract generalizations and concepts then testing and applying these in a new situation) facilitates a reflection-in-action and a reflection-on-action and provides the basis for subsequent cycles. It is designed to create change in practice and develop and refine theory within its local setting (Kemmis & McTaggart, 1982; Owens et al., 1999).

The action step provides a rationale for strategic interventions aimed at an improvement in practice and greater understanding of the practice situation (Kemmis & McTaggart, 1982; Owens et al., 1999; Whitehead & Elliot, 2007). The second step, the planning step, is deliberate where controlled variations are implemented into practice and used as a platform for further actions in subsequent cycles. This step is guided by the critical group and takes place in real time. It may encounter variables and constraints such as the political climate and availability of resources (Kemmis & McTaggart, 1982; Whitehead & Elliot, 2007). It is described as fluid and dynamic, which requires instant decision-making by the critical group and the exercise of practical judgment (Kemmis & McTaggart, 1982; Whitehead & Elliot, 2007). The third step of action research, observation, serves to document and reflect on the effects of the action step, providing reflection for possible changes and thus being prospective to future cycles. With actions having constraints of reality, the observation step must be carefully reviewed, allowing for responsive and expanded views on the subject under consideration. Observing and reflecting on the action process allows identification of the implementation's constraints and benefits and any changes to circumstances, and provides a basis for subsequent reflection (Kemmis & McTaggart, 1982; Owens et al., 1999; Whitehead & Elliot, 2007). The final step, reflection, is retrospective, recalling action previously recorded in the observation step (Kemmis & McTaggart, 1982; Owens et al., 1999; Whitehead & Elliot, 2007). All of the identified material relevant to the action process is assimilated and related to the varying perspectives and circumstances observed. This step involves discussion amongst the critical group leading to evaluation of data and reconstruction of a subsequent action. Evaluation is an integral part of this step, assessing the effects of the action in terms of its impact on the thematic concern and the potential theoretical implications arising from the action research cycles (McCaugherty, 1991; Rolfe, 1996; Owens et al., 1999; Whitehead & Elliot, 2007). The reflective step is descriptive, identifying progress for proceeding into any subsequent cycles, eventually establishing a final outcome to the research while allowing for reflection on what has happened and providing a basis for future planning (Kemmis & McTaggart, 1982; McCaugherty, 1991; Rolfe, 1996; Owens et al., 1999; Whitehead & Elliot, 2007).

By implying a system development, action research facilitates the maintenance and regulation of a cyclic process of diagnosing, action planning and taking, evaluating and learning generating theory. Theory grounded in action provides a guide for diagnosing problems and evaluating their consequences. The generation of theory is a deliberate process in action research. Theory generation provides for emancipation of practitioners from constraints and ideal practices, providing the means to create democratic conditions through collaborative practical discourse (Carr & Kemmis, 1994; Whitehead & Elliott, 2007). Implementation of the findings is built into the research process circumventing the possible situation of research findings not being put into practice, which may occur when using other research methodologies (Annells & Whitehead, 2007; Carr & Kemmis, 1994). Action research can provide both the flexibility and responsiveness required for effective change and a check on the adequacy of data and conclusions (Adami & Kiger, 2005; Whitehead & Elliot, 2007).

One of the main characteristics separating action research from other forms of research is that researchers have limited control over the environment in which it is conducted. Although traditional scientific approaches seek to produce an objective body of knowledge that can be generalized to a larger population, action research collaboratively constructs a descriptive and interpretive brief of events that facilitates a mutually accepted resolution to a problem identified by a group of people.

10. Implementing an action research study

Action research is a form of research that empowers participants to change their practice and gives ownership of this change to participants. It is designed to create change in practice, and to develop and refine theory within its local setting. Theory is developed from the bottom up and is generated by an interactive process within the cycles of the research (Kemmis & McTaggart, 1988). Participatory action research facilitates implementation of research findings by empowering the individual with autonomy, decision-making processes, and programme design. Implementation of the findings is built into the research itself, thus circumventing the situation of research findings not being put into practice (Wadsworth, 1997; Whitehead, 2007).

An action research study undertaken was in a rural remote area health service in Australia which identified several deficits in policies that impacted on the wellbeing of staff and influenced the outcome for mental health consumers. Key outcomes from this research identified an inability to adequately meet quality care for consumers and carers, and ineffective frontline responses for people with mental health issues across a range of sectors in the rural setting. Through this research the participants identified an inadequately trained and sustainable supply of skilled mental health workers, lack of a valued and respected mental health workforce and inefficient organisational protocols contributed to the concerns in practice.

The objectives of this research was to work collaboratively with a rural Community Mental Health Team (CMHT) to examine the issue of workplace stress and, address issues specified by that group by empowering them to become active change agents through AR.

Two overarching themes drove the research cycles: staff safety, and, inadequate education of nursing staff to appropriately assess and manage a consumer with mental health issues. Through this a collaborative social process, action research, empowered participants to identify and change stressful factors identified within their practice indicative to rural remote community mental health teams. Critical social theory arose from identified problems within the context of the research setting permitting a new model of praxis to be established within the research study which should ensure a positive patient outcome and staff safety.

11. Research questions

The questions that were addressed in this research were:

- 'What stressor(s) does a community mental health team in a rural and remote region identify as critical in the creation of occupational stress that may lead to workplace burnout, and
- How can the team overcome this particular issue/s in their setting?'

These types of questions are ideally suited to the Participatory Action Research methodology because it allows a group to be involved in the diagnosis of a problem and permits action to be taken that is conducive to establishing solutions that best suit the group's area of practice.

12. Study aims and objectives

Broadly, the objectives of the study were to work collaboratively with a community mental health team practising in the rural setting to examine the issue of workplace stress and address issues specified by the group. The specific aims of the study were:

a. To identify distinctive factors that impact on occupational stress associated with workplace burnout;
b. To identify what processes are currently utilized by the team to minimize occupational stress and the potential for workplace burnout;
c. To identify problems that lead to occupational stress and the potential for workplace burnout and strategies to overcome these problems;
d. To develop an Action Plan to address the problems identified;
e. To implement the Action Plan;
f. To evaluate the impact, if any, of the engagement of Action Research;
g. To evaluate and specify learnings from the implemented Action Plan and develop a theoretical basis for understanding the issue of workplace stress and burnout in community mental health teams in rural remote Australia.

13. Ethical considerations

Approval for this study was sought and obtained from the University of Adelaide Human Ethics Committee and the health service ethics committee where this research study was conducted. The research did not commence until ethics approval was gained from both ethics committees, with the research following all human research ethics guidelines. Each letter of approval was provided to the other ethics committee. Once completed, the CEO of the Area Health Service received an explanatory letter detailing the proposed research.

14. Sampling

Qualitative research uses human subjects to examine human experiences who then become known as participants. It is a non-statistical approach in understanding the depth and subtleties of the human experience (Jackson & Borbasi, 2008; Llewellyn, Sullivan & Minichiello, 2004; Whitehead & Annells, 2007). Tending to be small in sample size, qualitative research uses various sampling techniques that result in the selected sample being 'information rich or experienced in the phenomenon of interest' (Jackson & Borbasi, 2008, p. 167). This study adopted the purposive sampling technique.

15. Sample population

The population of interest in this study refers to the health care workers working within this health area (Llewellyn, Sullivan & Minichiello, 2004). The selection of participants in the sample population reflected the key characteristics of a representative sample (Whitehead & Annells, 2007). These included Community Mental Health Team (CMHT) members, Registered Nurses registered with the State nurses' registration body, Clinical Nurse Specialists, Clinical Nurse Consultants, Health Promotion Officers, social workers, occupational therapists and psychologists.

16. Purposive sampling

Based on the limited number of staff within this specific isolated CMHT this sampling technique was deemed to be the most suitable for this study. This form of sampling (deemed to be judgmental sampling) enabled the researcher to select participants best suited to address the issue under study and to target a representative selection of participants (Jackson & Borbasi, 2008; Mugo, 2003; Patton, 1990; Walter, 2006; Whitehead & Annells, 2007). Experts in this specialty field of mental health service provision were selected on this basis. Despite the sample size being limited, Jones (2002) argues that the focus of qualitative research is on the depth and richness of text rather than on participant numbers.

17. Inclusion criteria

Suitability for participant inclusion in this study required characteristics that represent health staff that have sufficient experience in the phenomena under examination. It was determined that staff with a minimal work history in a rural remote region would not have had sufficient exposure to this and therefore health staff who have practised nursing and health care in a rural remote area for a period of not less than twelve (12) months would be accepted into the study. These also ensured participants were selected to give a cross-section of years of experience.

18. Limitations of sampling method

The limitations of this method of sampling must be identified. Through the sampling method the researcher attempted to achieve a representative cross-section of the target population in order to increase the efficiency of the research study (Jackson & Borbasi, 2008; Whitehead & Annells, 2007), despite the fact that the Area Health Service was quite small. The risk of conscious sampling bias may exist and this method did not allow for the precision of the researcher's judgment to be measurable. It did not provide any external objective method for assessing the representativeness of the selected group. Despite these limitations, the majority of nursing researchers and qualitative researchers use non-probability sampling (Polit & Hungler, 1991; Whitehead & Annells, 2007).

19. Critique of the research study

A researcher strives to do justice to the research being undertaken without subjective dogmatic theoretical viewpoints. Openness in a research methodology permits the researcher to appreciate biases and perspectives that may influence the interpretation of data (Gerber & Moyle, 2004; Silverman, 2006; Willis, 2006). Qualitative research methodologies provide the opportunity to undertake research within the social context and allow the researcher to become closer to the study (Whitehead & Elliot, 2007). The reciprocal relationship between the researcher and the participant facilitates recognition of backgrounds that may influence how the research is conducted (Gerber & Moyle, 2004). In doing this, there are certain strengths and limitations whatever methodology is adopted. For this study, both the strengths and limitations of action research are listed as key points.

20. Strengths

The strengths of this study must be acknowledged as contributing to the success of the research. These are identified as:

i. It was focused on a specific problem in a defined context, not on obtaining generalized information
ii. the application of fact finding to practical problem solving
iii. generation and validation of theories through practice
iv. individual input guided the course of the research
v. participants were empowered to shift the parameters in which they practised
vi. participants had ownership of the project
vii. individuals took responsibility for change within the organization and,
viii. enhancement of practice skills flowed through to patient care (Greenwood, 1994; Hart & Bond, 1995; Holter & Schwartz-Barcott, 1993; Whitehead & Elliot, 2007).

21. Limitations

Equally as important to be recognized in this study are the limitations that may have impacted and/or influenced the outcome of the research. These are listed as:

i. Research conducted within the scientific realm must conform to the canons of the scientific method to be granted legitimacy. It is questionable whether this qualitative research method could generate evidence that is recognized as truly scientific
ii. qualitative forms of research reflect the humanistic perspective thus this study required a different type of study design
iii. underlying democratic and civil discourses guided the process of investigation that then provided a greater chance of researcher bias
iv. action research may have facilitated a forum that allowed the researcher and participants to have an agenda that gave priority to meeting their own goals. It did however facilitate social change
v. the method of sampling did not allow for the evaluation of the precision of the researcher's judgment
vi. difficulties and dilemmas arose over the availability of persons within the group to attend critical group meetings. This was due to demands such as shift work and patient emergencies and the remoteness of the setting, and

vii. co-workers' acceptance of the research process in the local environment may have had an impact on the expected workload of those not involved in the research (Greenwood, 1994; Hart & Bond, 1995; Holter & Schwartz-Barcott, 1993; Whitehead & Elliot, 2007).

22. The study plan

Following the Susman and Evered (1978) model with the Pearson (1989) adaptation, the critical group in this study was selected in the contracting stage. Similar to other action research approaches previously identified, this model involves a cyclic process.

The Development Phase provides for the client-system infrastructure to be established. This client-system infrastructure is the social system under study in which the participant members exist. In this phase, understanding and general consensus is developed between all parties. Each participant is given a speaker position, thus addressing the issue of participant bias agenda. Common power comes from a shared understanding permitting democratic contribution to the critical group and providing respect to each contributor without judgment.

The Diagnosing Phase involves problem identification and determines what is happening within the setting. It involves the collaborative analysis of the social situation by the researcher and the participants of the research. Theories are formulated concerning the nature of the research domain. A collective postulation of several possible solutions is examined from which a single plan of action emerges and is implemented. In this phase, a problem is identified and data is collected for a more detailed diagnosis.

The Action Planning Phase gives an exact description of what changes will be implemented into practice. Through a collaborative process, the researcher and the co-participants collate the information discussed in the previous phase and determine an appropriate action towards resolving the identified problem.

The Action Taking Phase implements mutually agreed changes in practice. A defined course of action is undertaken, directed at an area of practice perceived in previous phases to warrant amending. Deliberate and controlled variations are implemented into practice and used as a platform for further action in subsequent cycles.

The Evaluation Phase reports the findings and data generated by the action taken. Data analysis is undertaken based on the results of the interventions and the findings are interpreted to determine how successful the action has been. This phase serves as documentation of the effects of action, providing reflection, and thus being prospective to future cycles.

The Learning Phase provides critical reflection, theorizing and analysis of identified themes. Retrospectively it recalls previously recorded actions, reviewing the effectiveness of any actions taken guided by the evaluation phase. The emergence of new knowledge is identified taking the research to a new level. Gaps in knowledge can be identified and theories can be deduced with the potential aim of informing new policies.

23. Becoming change agents

The concept of a change agent can be related to those within an organization who provide 'technical, specialised or consulting assistance in the management of a change effort'

(Pearson, 1992, p.25). The deliberate process to change the status quo and reduce the stressors experienced in the Area Health Service within the research study required a deliberative and collaborative partnership between this client system and the researcher (Holter & Schwartz-Barcott, 1993; Whitehead & Elliott, 2007). The participants, who were eager to bring about change, turned actions within their practice into research strategies (Bond, Barker, Pearson & Proctor, 1996) by adopting the role of co-researchers. This process of becoming change agents can be said to be a characteristic of action research (Baskerville, 1999; Holter & Schwartz-Barcott, 1993; Street, 2004). The team considered for this research was comprised of the CNC, three Registered Nurses (RNs), a RN (Child and Maternal Health) who held a Postgraduate Diploma of Mental Health Nursing, and a RN undertaking a Postgraduate Diploma of Child and Adolescent Mental Health.

This team is employed as the Mental Health Support Team and it receives services from the Community Mental Health Team located in the regional centre of the Area Health Service. This regional centre is located approximately 150 kilometres from the site and provides limited visits once a fortnight to the site if the regional team deems there is a client need. All mental health consumer consultations are carried out by the MHST at the site, with a variety of interventions undertaken by this team to address any specific needs. Consultations and assessments are undertaken by the CNC, who is frequently called at any time and regardless of whether or not she is on duty. She is also responsible for assisting GPs who have patients with mental health issues/referrals; providing outreach for Aged Psychiatric services, Adult Mental Health services and Child and Adolescent Mental Health services; supporting clients and carers; assessment and early intervention in mental health; mental health promotion and generalist counselling.

While not all participants within this study had continuous practice in the region under study, each individual had experienced the stressors found in rural regions. Several similarities and themes became obvious during these discussions. These ranged through:

- isolation from regional support services during critical incidents;
- very poor access to a contact person for debriefing after a critical incident;
- absence of technological support (no mobile phone service or pager system was operational in the region);
- long distances involving extensive travel when accessing clients;
- the remote location of farm properties, each with several closed gates that visitors had to pass through to gain access (the golden rule of farmers—each closed gate must be closed again after passing through it);
- seasonal climatic conditions producing ice and snow on roads, hampering access to clients;
- political dilemmas when involved in interdisciplinary discussions;
- difficulties with anomalies associated with different Mental Health Acts and hospitalisation procedures between the two States;
- the delay in accessing specialist care/interventions (lengthy periods of up to eleven hours);
- difficulties with transporting clients after hours due to the challenges of driving large distances (for example, a two-hour delay on the road after hitting a kangaroo);
- poor access to emergency transport resulting in excessive delays for client assessment/hospitalization (the ambulance may not be available for a number of reasons);

- limited professional supervision;
- limits to assistance from the police when they were required elsewhere.

24. Diagnosing phases

These phases of the research provided the opportunity for the critical group to speak openly about issues that caused the greatest amount of stress for each of them. The enormity of the issues that concerned them was notable. On several occasions, these clinicians had limited support and recognized that the geographical isolation factor contributed to feelings of uncertainty and doubt in the provision of effective and safe practice. Lengthy discourse occurred within the critical group and it was decided preference should be given to a few significant issues then narrowed down to reflect the most imperative stressors to be addressed, rather than attempting to address all stressors. It became evident there was consensus that the danger of being alone or with limited support presented the most concern for all participants, particularly with the unpredictability of consumers with mental health issues. There was a level of despair amongst the members of the group as to how big this issue was, with no idea as to how it could be resolved. After careful consideration, staff safety became a predominant theme that the group decided should be considered in the first instance. There was a degree of relief when this was proposed despite the fact that no decision had been made as to how it would be addressed.

There was significant discussion amongst the group that their levels of distress were not necessarily debilitating as a direct result of the contact with consumers in crisis, but they agreed that such incidents did cause them concern due to their uncertainty of practice and knowledge in these matters. There is a widely held belief that the nursing profession is inherently one of the most stressful occupations within the workplace (Rees & Cooper, 1992). Some of these stressors include dealing with death and dying, severe and emergency illnesses, aggressive and abusive patients and relatives, long working hours, shift and weekend work (Descamp & Thomas, 1993; Kennedy & Grey, 1997; Schaefer & Moos, 1996).

The nature of mental health nursing, in which emotional clients seek help by imparting information to nurses (Gladding, 1992; Maslach, 1982), can lead to the phenomenon of workplace burnout (Freudenberger, 1989; Maslach, 1986). Patients expressing very strong, direct and negative emotions to the health professional during the course of therapy can at times direct this towards the health professional (transference). Maslach and Jackson (1981) identified that mental health professionals scored lowest on personal accomplishment and highest on emotional exhaustion on the Maslach Burnout Inventory when compared with other professionals. For the critical group the combination of insufficient education in mental health nursing and the nursing skills required to deal with the demands of such intensity proved to be of significant concern. Greater expansion of their concerns led the group to the impact of the unrelenting stressors particularly experienced by the MHST leader.

The critical group identified that patients frequently accessed the ED with mental health issues as first point of contact under the guise of general health concerns. The ED staff lacked the skills and knowledge to assess and treat these consumers appropriately prior to any access to the CMHT. The ramifications of this are twofold. First, the consumer may have the appropriate treatment withheld, as statistics show waiting times for treatment in EDs have been problematic for many years. Secondly, the professional and personal safety of nursing staff may be compromised. In Australia a major responsibility of the employer is to ensure the well-being of the employee (NSW Occupational Health and Safety Act, 2004; Victoria Occupational Health and Safety Act, 2004). These laws provide for a general duty of care by employers to provide a safe and healthy workplace and one that is free from psychological and physical hazards. Occupational health and safety legislation throughout Australia has now been implemented in an attempt to reduce workplace injuries and reduce workers' compensation claims.

The helplessness of the situation in the ED as perceived by one group member was clearly articulated. This group member felt that despite several strategies having been implemented to provide nursing care to these clients in an effective and positive manner, there was little support within the health sector, including the emergency services. Because of the emphasis in mental health legislation across Australian States of nursing people in the least restrictive environment, a wide range of crisis intervention models is being developed that incorporate a multidisciplinary approach to the management of people with a mental illness. These were discussed at length by the critical group.

These models provide interventions as a solution to treating the exacerbation of psychiatric symptoms that may have resulted from poor medication compliance, physical illness and exposure to environmental stressors. In a relapse into a psychotic episode, sufferers may experience symptoms resulting in disturbed and difficult behaviour. This may be exhibited in aggressive and threatening outbursts either vented towards themselves or others. Crisis intervention at this stage becomes imperative to prevent further deterioration of an uncontrolled situation. The flow-on effects of continuing this type of management of mental illness, however, become time-consuming and stressful to implement for community mental health teams, with staff burnout becoming an increasing concern (Joy, Adams & Rice, 1999).

Staff safety became a central focus during these discussions within the critical group. Complacency due to the location of the town led some critical group members to admit that they had not, at times, considered safety factors when dealing with unknown clients. Others acknowledged that, due to a transient population, they had been concerned about unknown persons accessing the health service regardless of the nature of their illnesses.

Benveniste, Hibbert and Runciman (2005) discuss the issue of critical incidents in Australia involving mental health patients. In reports from twelve EDs, 16 per cent of all reported incidents (190 of 1214 incidents) involved violence (p.348). Mental health problems were patient-related contributing factors for over half of the violent incidents, with alcohol or drug intoxication contributing to more than 25 per cent of violent outbursts. The Australian Patient Safety Foundation has developed systems to collect, aggregate, monitor and analyse incidents related to patient safety since its formation in 1988. The Foundation created a taxonomy and software which became the Australian Incident Monitoring System to re-analyse data from the Quality in Australian Health Care Study in 1998. A classification of health care incidents including adverse events and near misses was developed.

The incidence of psychological and psychiatric work-related injuries tends to indicate that employers may not have taken reasonable care of employees. The progressive disillusionment and loss of idealism within the workplace is deemed to result in detachment and decreased workplace effectiveness with increased absenteeism. Stress injuries are as liable as any other injury to lead to prosecution of employers under the law (NSW Occupational Health and Safety Act, 2000, Sec.3c; Victoria Occupational Health and Safety Act, 2004, Sec. 21).

25. The action planning stages

These stages involved consideration of alternative courses of actions to achieve improvement or resolve the problems identified by the critical group. Mental health treatment involves nursing staff interacting in many aspects of clients' lives. It is imperative that all interactions are well planned and have continuity across all staff members to ensure both clients and staff remain safe. Once the group had agreed that there was a clear need for interventions to overcome their safety need and the level of staffing in crisis periods, several action plans were discussed. This section outlines the development of these action plans, which would be later refined and implemented and adopted by the health service in providing an appropriate service. Discussion around these action plans centred on regaining control over the health care environment and maintaining staff safety.

In the work situation a stressor can be deemed to be either resolvable (short duration) or prolonged according to how it is viewed and the context in which nurses may find themselves (Pines & Aronson, 1981; Pines & Maslach, 1978). Individuals have different responses to stressors, ranging from slight psychological arousal with minimal performance deterioration to an intense arousal with psychological distress (Lazarus & Folkman, 1984; Light, 1981; Turnipseed, 1994). When examining this situation, an initial distinction can be made between the problems that are experienced as challenges requiring innovative problem-solving ideas to bring about a resolution and ongoing problems causing distress. This could be due to personal needs not being met, with expectations or demands being beyond the control or exceeding the limitations of the nurses involved which requires extra energy resources when confronting the situation. Associated with stress from this level and linked to the burnout syndrome is reduced organizational efficiency and work-related problems such as staff turnover, low morale, poor quality of patient care, absenteeism and, interpersonal problems (Jackson and Maslach, 1982; Maslach, 1979; 1981; Turnipseed, 1988).

26. The action taking stages

These phases saw the courses of action considered in the previous stages implemented into practice. The critical group continued to examine a range of emergency triage tools from various Australian States and develop ideas that could be useful to include in a tool specific to their organization. Limitations were identified in many tools but modifications were suggested that could be adopted. The mental health initiative undertaken by the Victorian Government involved 41 teams on a national basis and was the first major initiative of the Emergency Care Community of Practice (Department of Human Services, Victoria, 2007). Teams of mental health and ED clinicians collaborated to improve the care of mental health presentations to EDs. The focus of the project was on the ED triage and assessment of patients with mental health issues, and sedation of acute emergencies involving agitation or behavioural difficulties. A literature search undertaken by Broadbent, Jarman and Berk (2004) identified scant literature addressing the provision of triage and management guidelines to assist nurses in making objective clinical decisions to ensure appropriate care for clients with mental illness. The authors examined the need for such guidelines and reviewed several mental health triage scales that had been evaluated for use in EDs. The results indicated that the effective implementation of triage scales had seen improvements in staff confidence and attitudes when dealing with clients with mental health problems. This resulted in improved outcomes for clients.

The suggestion from various group members was that the identified existing triage tools be disseminated among hospital and community staff to gain feedback on what could be included into the tools to become locally relevant. The critical group recognized the value of the input from this staff which would give a cross representation of what the various needs would be from varying perspectives.

The ensuing discussion led the group to identify existing emergency triage tools that could be used as guidelines in developing a triage tool specific to the area under study. It was acknowledged that the existing tools were based on well-resourced medium-sized hospitals and did not adequately address the issues inherent in this region. The group recognized that it was not a matter of adopting a suitable tool but of creating tools that complemented each other and became user friendly. The Action Plan developed from this would involve input from all staff within the hospital for inclusion into the creation of these tools to ensure it would also be a suitable and workable solution for the MHST whilst remaining a workable document for hospital staff.

Ongoing discussions led the group to choose several aspects from a range of existing emergency triage tools from various Australian States. Although they did not cover the exact needs of the Area Health Service involved in the study, they provided a guide as to how the critical group could develop the tools needed for the specific needs of this organization. An investigation into triage tools by Hegney et al. (2003) found that there has been considerable variation in the application of the Australasian Triage Scale (ATS) since its introduction. The authors identified a need for improved uniformity in the application of the ATS by triage nurses. A reproducible, reliable and valid method to classify the illness acuity of ED patients is required regardless of which hospital is being accessed. Their impressions were that a standardized tool would be of considerable value to emergency nurses. It would support nurses working in this challenging area by promoting standardization and decreasing subjectivity in the triage process. A study undertaken by Shaban (2006) revealed that problems of routine mental status examinations (MSEs) and mental health assessments (MHAs) by psychiatrists, physicians and nurses were well documented, however were too lengthy and complicated. This indicated such assessments were unsuitable for use in emergency situations. Shaban (2006) referred to an American study (Kaufman and Zun, 1995) which examined the use of a quantifiable Brief Mental Status Examination (BMSE) for emergency patients. The study comprised a six-item BMSE and was administered to 100 ED patients who warranted an assessment of their mental status. The results of this study indicated examiners rated the BMSE as useful in 98% of cases. The study concluded that the BMSE may prove to be a valid and useful tool for assessing the mental status of emergency patients in both pre-hospital and ED settings. This supported the critical group's decision to design a framework that was user friendly and simple to implement.

27. The evaluation phases

Following the completion of the action taking phases a collaborative approach was used to evaluate the outcomes. These phases determined whether the theoretical effects of the action were realized and whether these effects provided a suitable outcome. The final two cycles of the four cycles undertaken in the action research model used in this research reflected the final development of the 'Emergency Flowchart, Triage Tools and the Risk Monitoring Chart' based on the two overarching themes of staff safety and limited knowledge of mental health nursing. Personal safety was indicated as being crucial for staff given the unpredictability of mental health consumers and the limited resources for assistance in violent situations. Literature reported violence in the workplace is often unreported with attempts by nursing staff to de-escalate a situation to preserve the safety of other staff and patients. Various occupational health and safety controls were considered in attempting to reduce the potential of violence and injuries. However, it was recognized that rural and remote areas presented unique situations where many of these controls could not be facilitated.

28. Specify learning phases

These phases were undertaken as the last formal phase of the action cycle. The knowledge gained from the previous action research phases was used to resolve the staff safety issue by restructuring organizational norms to reflect the new knowledge gained in the research. This additional knowledge provided the foundations for the critical group to maintain focus on the identified stressor leading to the diagnosing phase of the next action research cycle. The theoretical framework provided relevant knowledge for future research settings (Baskerville, 1999). In this study, the specific learning revealed that stress from the workplace impacted on the functioning levels of nursing staff. Despite a nurse's feeling of how he or she is able to cope, if there is a perceived loss of control in one's practice the stress levels increase. In general, it appeared that a simpler approach to reducing the stress within the ED and for the MHST leader should be adopted in keeping with organizational economic constraints. Having determined that the original action plan was not a suitable option for the organization, the critical group examined alternative strategies to change practice. Some of these alternatives were identified in feedback from hospital staff. The specific learning indicated that the group believed through the action research process they had implemented a strategy that would significantly reduce their workplace stress. It reflected the collaborative and cohesive process required to initiate new programmes into the workforce. Staff and client safety should be a priority and staff should feel comfortable and supported in decision-making to determine clinical assessment and treatment without prejudice. The critical group had achieved this with the introduction of the emergency flowchart and triage tools.

29. A nursing model of practice

From the initial theoretical concept the reduction of stress and an increase in occupational health safety and wellness was well discussed. The critical group was able to assert their need to address such significant issues and design a change in praxis to reflect this. Several factors contributed to this requirement for a variation to practice norms. This became central to a new nursing model. The theory generated from the research cycles saw the critical group being enabled to identify circles that intersected allowing a complete interaction of all concepts whilst maintaining the core circle of reduced stress. These are identified as:

- An increased occupational health, safety and wellness, and, improved positive patient outcomes.
- Issues relevant to rural and remote nursing practice
- A change to a positive cultural influence within the workplace would provide the nurses with a relationship of mutual respect.
- Education and up-skilling in nursing knowledge and best practice.
- Support and acceptance of change between management and themselves.
- The amelioration of knowledge deficit through ongoing education to all nursing staff would provide the knowledge and skills required to effect a therapeutic practice when dealing with consumers with mental health issues.
- Safe practice environment and support in decision making.

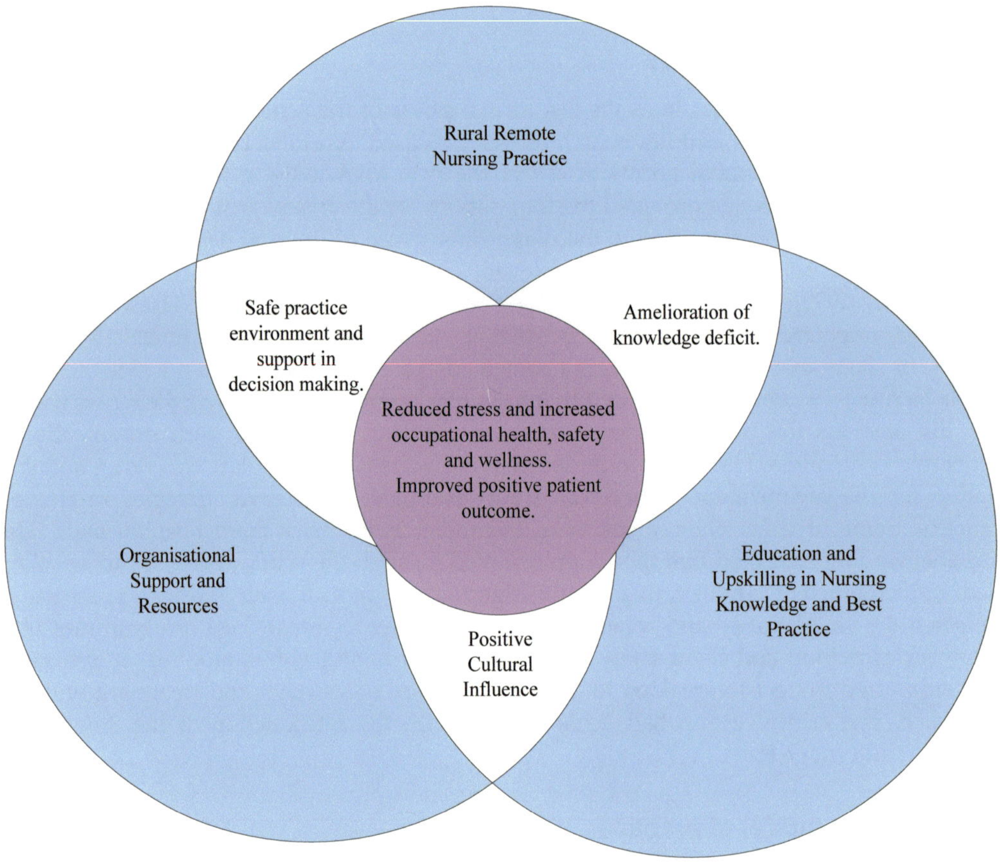

Fig. 1. Conceptual Model of Praxis.

30. Educating the nursing workforce

Many community mental health workers in Australia were practitioners in the psychiatric realm prior to the various Mental Health Acts (e.g. Victoria 1986 and New South Wales [NSW] 1990) and were required to undertake service provision for consumers of mental health services at a time when limited rehabilitative education had been afforded to the clinician. Prior to deinstitutionalization in Australia in the early 1990s it was recognized that custodial care was no longer an acceptable practice; however, there was only a decade or so (1985–1994) where rehabilitative care education was afforded to psychiatric nurses. This has meant that many of nursing staff who had been educated in psychiatric nursing practice under custodial care practices left the stand-alone institutions ill-prepared to work in the community or general hospital psychiatric wards (Clinton & Hazelton, 2000; Croll, 1997; Glasson, 1996; Kenny & Duckett, 2003). Their primary role had been to address and care for patients who had a diagnosis of mental illness with the necessary support and safety from within an institution. The new concept from a community mental health focus saw the nurse having to deal with the needs and requirements of clients from a primary care perspective within community settings. This may have occurred without the consumer necessarily having a formal diagnosis of a mental illness.

Concurrent with the shifting of education from hospital training (an apprenticeship model) to university training in a comprehensive nursing degree (an academic model) there was a significant depletion of the workforce within the psychiatric nursing industry. In one Australian State, the nursing workforce recruitment in rural regions is predominantly from nursing students graduating from regional universities (Kenny & Duckett, 2003). Preference for nursing students wanting to pursue career paths in the more glamorous areas of nursing creates a deficit in the potential recruitment pool. This has led to a history of poor recruitment and retention in the psychiatric nursing workforce, particularly evident in rural and remote contexts (Gibb, 2003).

Clark, Brown, Hughes and Motluk (2006) discuss education in improving triage of mental health patients in general hospital EDs. The authors contend there is a distinct lack of knowledge, expertise and confidence in undertaking psychiatric assessments by generalist nurses which leads to less accurate assessments for these patients. This is supported by Kerrison and Chapman (2007) who discuss what general emergency nurses want to know about mental health patients presenting to ED. In their investigation, set in a Western Australian hospital ED, the authors refer to non-mental health trained nurses as ill-equipped in psychiatric knowledge, assessment and communication skills.

31. Reflection on action research methodology

This study employed the Susman and Evered (1978) model of action research and the use of critical social theory based on Habermas' (1971) assumption that people have a basic need to act independently and are capable of self-reflection. This study permitted the participants to effect change to their practice through embracing the research study with the belief they could contribute to the well-being of the organization and the body of nursing knowledge. The Susman and Evered (1978) model of action research proposes sequential phases of diagnosing, action planning, action taking, evaluation and specify learning. Within the diagnosing and action planning phases an opportunity existed for the participants to respond to an existing stressor, giving rise to rich data. An informal process was adopted to implement an action taking phase that had been designed to incorporate ideas from the expanded stakeholders and the critical group. Extensive evaluation of this action taking phase led the group to carry out a review of best practice in other Australian States. The purpose of this review was based on recommendations from the stakeholders and provided an opportunity for the group to meet the needs of the 'nurses at the coal face' in reducing a major stressor.

The prominent involvement of the critical group to examine the thematic concern and develop the tools to guide staff in clinical pathways in ED is characteristic of action research. The premise that the purpose of action research is to solve practical problems through direct contact with practical problem situations (Lauri, 1982) was validated in this study. Throughout the research the critical group contributed by sharing, suggesting, advising, debating, accepting each others' ideas and recognizing and valuing experiences. Through this process the group effected changes within their practice by developing tools to assist nursing practice and reduce significant stress within the workplace. Responsibility was a shared role, with the group taking control of how the research progressed. This emancipatory process is characteristic of action research, allowing the group to address their own concerns relevant to the thematic concern. Participant validation provided a process for checking accuracy and completeness of researcher interpretation. This reflection allowed each participant to ensure their voice was accurately reported without researcher bias tainting their perspectives (Titchen & Binnie, 1993). Limitations existed for this method of validity as not all participants were at every meeting to obtain consensus.

32. The concept of change

The critical group worked well within this study to effect changes to their practice to eliminate the two significant stressors identified. Their development of clinical pathways for managing clients in the ED and the acknowledgement of the need for education indicated the staff's commitment to shape and mould their nursing practice in an effort to strive for best practice and maintain their own wellness. Change and its effectiveness are difficult to measure and are not always apparent for some time (Meyer, 1995). The change proposed in this study aimed to solve problems associated with occupational stress. An understanding of the basic nature of change influences the effectiveness of change techniques (Lancaster, 1982) with success depending largely on organizational and individual qualities of participants (Lancaster and Lancaster, 1982). The qualities of a change agent include accessibility, trustworthiness, honesty, being goal focused while assisting others to do so, and facilitating openness in discussion and listening (Lancaster, 1982). Trust is the key element among participants involved in change (Lancaster, 1982) with change being effectively achieved by academically prepared, practising nurses introducing a systematic and reasoning approach to change (Pearson, 1992). The critical group members became change generators (leading conversion of issues into felt needs) and change implementers (agents implementing the change after the felt need was identified) (Pearson, 1992).

33. Conclusion

Change and its effectiveness are difficult to measure and are not always apparent for some time. The change proposed in this study aimed to solve problems associated with occupational stress. An understanding of the basic nature of change influences the effectiveness of change techniques with success depending largely on organizational and individual qualities of participants. The qualities of a change agent include accessibility, trustworthiness, honesty, being goal focused while assisting others to do so, and facilitating openness in discussion and listening. Trust is the key element among participants involved in change with change being effectively achieved by academically prepared, practising nurses introducing a systematic and reasoning approach to change. The critical group members became change generators (leading conversion of issues into felt needs) and change implementers (agents implementing the change after the felt need was identified).

Nursing literature has previously examined occupational stressors and burnout as separate identities but has not considered these factors jointly in relation to the impact of a hostile work environment within rural, remote and isolated community mental health teams. The contribution of this study to the nursing profession is demonstrated through its potential to enhance community nursing practice to deliver effective holistic nursing care to consumers with mental health issues whilst maintaining their own psychological and physical wellness.

The impact of stress can be both advantageous and detrimental to an individual depending on his or her vulnerability at any given time. The degree of intensity of stress impacts on homeostasis for the individual and the degree of effectiveness of that individual's coping mechanisms. This results in the level of wellness for the person and the ability to cope with workplace demands.

Occupational stress and workplace burnout are significant issues affecting modern day workplaces. Occupational stress has been linked to a decrease in physiological well-being of individuals. This results from a combination of low job control, high job demands and low work-related support. It is apparent that the helping professions have endured a significant shift in praxis with the changing profile of the health system, cost-control measures, working conditions and societal expectations, and that these changes have likely added to stresses experienced by health practitioners, particularly in the rural remote setting.

The preparation of the workforce in today's society, particularly in nursing, may have impacted on the individual in coping with workloads. The change in nurse education from exposure to the rigorous demands on nurses under the apprenticeship model to the academic model has seen the nursing students less workplace ready. This is particularly evident in the psychiatric nursing field.

The action research process, being a holistic process, facilitated this change in practice, developed and refined theory as it proceeded in a cyclic fashion within this local setting. It concerned actual not abstract practices in the social world in which these participants practice. This methodology facilitated examining the significant stressors identified by the CMHT that caused distress, allowing them to implement changes in their practice.

A combination of factors, the appraisal and interpretation of the situation, responses to stressors and coping mechanisms and appraisals of outcomes determine whether a potential stressor is perceived as a threat to the individual. Based on this assumption it was proposed that individuals working in a collaborative process could influence changes in their practice using an action research methodology to reduce the physical and psychological impact to the employee from a significant stressor.

This study set out to examine which stressors a CMHT in a rural and remote region identify as critical in the creation of occupational stress and, potentially, workplace burnout and how they can overcome these particular issues in their setting. Unrelenting exposure to workplace stress is suggested by literature as being significant in the burnout phenomenon that has seen an increase in workers' compensation claims around the world. Burnout, common among the helping professions, impacts across the biopsychosocial perspectives of peoples' lives.

The aim of the study was to work collaboratively with a community mental health team to identify the distinctive factors that increase and reduce occupational stress associated with workplace burnout. An examination of the processes that were currently utilized by the team to minimize occupational stress and workplace burnout was undertaken; and which of the problems that led to occupational stress and workplace burnout were to be explored. In exploring what strategies could be developed to overcome these problems, an Action Plan to address the problems identified would be introduced. The implementation of the Action Plan would: evaluate the impact, if any, of the engagement of action research and evaluate and specify the learning from the implemented Action Plan. The underlying assumption in this study was that occupational stress could have deleterious consequences for employees and may lead to workplace burnout. This stress could be from any internal (within an organization) or external (from outside the organization) source.

The forum provided an avenue that could reduce stressors significantly and prevent ongoing occupational stress that contributes to workplace burnout. It offered an opportunity to work with a group of participants in a non-hierarchical and non-exploitative manner and enabled members of this group to identify their roles as effective practitioners, empowering them to effect the changes they deemed as essential criteria to reduce the stress they were experiencing indicative to their remoteness.

Critical reviewing throughout the data collection attempted to understand and redefine these significant issues. It aimed to acknowledge the way things were relative to how things could be improved from organizational, personal and wider community perspectives. Simple principles and guidelines of action research were followed potentiating acceptance as a rigorous research approach from a positivist perspective whilst retaining the attributes that characterise action research.

Organizational factors causing stress typically consist of poor positive feedback in reference to job performance, lack of autonomy and control, lack of participation in organizational decisions, ambiguity in job description, and conflicting role demands. Organizational factors that impact on individuals can cause frustration and disillusionment resulting from the differences between job realities and job expectations. Other organizational constraints include communication problems within interdisciplinary teams, role ambiguity, conflicting goals of the clinical staff and administration and the perceived lack of institutional support. High job turnover and absenteeism are also evident. For the critical group the response from the Aged Care Review Committee indicated to them that the expectation for nursing staff to be autonomous in their decision-making when assessing clients did not reflect true autonomy.

The specified learnings from this research were envisaged to be processes and strategies for employees to overcome the debilitating effects of stress leading to workplace burnout. Examining the nursing profession from a social perspective provides alternatives to medicalising workplace injuries and illnesses. The concerns for staff safety and wellness remain paramount as the States across Australia continue to amend legislation and develop best practice policies and procedures to safeguard employees. The study results will contribute to the knowledge base of the mental health discipline and extend the scientific body of nursing and midwifery knowledge. It will also inform future research priorities regarding mental health care provision utilizing an action research methodology.

The research study led to the development of a new understanding of the phenomena of interest in the study. Dealing with people who have serious mental health issues and/or illnesses is difficult and stressful for those who have no experience or training in the process of developing a therapeutic relationship and adequate assessment. The resulting stress may impact negatively on work satisfaction, perceptions of safety within the workplace and team functioning. Exploring the knowledge and skill deficits and other factors that contribute to the stress and identifying and implementing agreed actions helped to generate a "new" practice environment.

The new model of praxis resultant from this study can now be applied by the nurses when nursing consumers with mental health issues (Figure 1). The interpretation reflects the three main circles to represent the critical group (top), the training and education provided (right) and the flowcharts accepted by the organization (left). At the core of the model, these shared domains contribute to a reduction on the stress of the nurse participants, improvements in the occupational health, safety and wellness of staff, and improved patient outcomes.

There are solutions to the dilemma of the employee overcoming the debilitating effects of stress leading to workplace burnout. This includes the cooperation of managers, policy makers, academic researchers and government officials working collaboratively to reduce the impact of occupational stress. Through this collaborative process, changes can be effected to ensure the health of the nation improves and that relevant recognition is given to the fact that there is a significant threat to a healthy workforce. Examining the nursing profession from a social perspective provides alternatives to medicalising workplace injuries and illnesses.

34. References

Adami, M. F., & Kiger. A. (2005). The use of triangulation for completeness purposes. Nurse Researcher, 12(4), 19-29.

Allen, D. (1990). Critical social theory and nursing education. In N. Greenleaf (Ed.), Curriculum revolution: Redefining the student-teacher relationship, (pp. 67-86). New York: National League for Nursing Press.

Annells, M., & Whitehead, D. (2007). Analysing data in qualitative research. In Z. Schneider, D. Whitehead, D. Elliott, G. Lobiondo-Wood & J. Haber (Eds.), Nursing & midwifery research. Methods and appraisal for evidence-based practice, (3rd ed., pp. 138-155). Sydney: Elsevier.

Armstrong, P., & Schulman, M. (1990). Financial strain and depression among farm operators: The role of perceived economic hardship and personal control. Rural Sociology, 55, 475-493.

Australian Institute of Health and Welfare (2005). (Catalogue No. HSE 40). Mental health services in Australia 2003-04. Canberra: AIHW.

Bailey, S. (1998). An exploration of critical care nurses' and doctors' attitudes towards psychiatric patients. Australian Journal of Advanced Nursing, 15, 8-14.

Baskerville, R. (1999). Investigating information systems with action research. Communications of the Association for Information Systems, 2(19), 1-23. Accessed 7 November 2007 from http://www.cis.gsu.edu/~rbaskerv/CAIS_2_19/CAIS_2_19.html

Baskerville, R., & Lee, A. S. (1999). Distinctions among different types of generalizing in information systems research. In L. Ngwenyama, M. Introna, M. Myers & J. I. DeGross (Eds.), New information technologies in organizational processes: field studies and theoretical reflections on the future of work. (pp. 49-65). New York: Kluwer.

Beeson, P., & Johnson, D. (1987). A panel study of change (1981-1986) in rural mental health status. Effects of the rural crisis. Paper presented at the National Institute of Mental Health Conference on Mental Health Statistics, Denver, CO.

Benveniste, K. A., Hibbert, P. D., & Runciman, W. B. (2005). Violence in health care: The contribution of the Australian Patient Safety Foundation to incident monitoring and analysis. Medical Journal of Australia, 183(7), 348-351.

Bond, S., Barker, P., Pearson, P., & Proctor, S. (1996). Forging links between academe and practice through research. Nursing Standard, 10(27), 43-45.

Borland, M. (2000). Australia's most wanted: the remote area nurse. Nursing Review, 5(3), 18.

Branco, E., Chambers, I., Fallon, A., Fraser, J., & Howlett, S. (1981). Management of burnout in the helping professions, Australian Social Work, 34(3), 27-31.

Brent, K. (1993). Perspectives on critical and feminist theory in developing nursing praxis. Journal of Professional Nursing, 9(5), 296-303.

Broadbent, M., Jarman, H., & Berk, M. (2004). Emergency department mental health triage scales improve outcomes. Journal of Evaluation in Clinical Practice, 10(1), 57-62.

Bryant, L. (1992). Social aspects of the farm financial crisis. In F. M. Vanclay, G.A. Lawrence, & B. Furze (Eds.), Agriculture, environment & society: Contemporary issues for Australia, (pp. 157-171). South Melbourne: MacMillan.

Burns, N., & Grove, S. (1993). The practice of nursing research. Conduct, critique & utilization. (2nd ed.). Philadelphia: W. B.Saunders Company.

Bushy, A. (2004). Creating nursing research opportunities in rural healthcare facilities. Journal of Nursing Care Quality Assurance, 19(2), 162-168.

Buunk, B. P., & Schaufeli, W. B. (1993). Burnout: A perspective from social comparison theory. In W. B. Schaufeli, C. Maslach & T. Marek (Eds.), Professional burnout: Recent developments in theory and research, (pp. 53-69). Washington, DC: Taylor & Francis.

Campbell, J. E. (1985). A role for nurse psychotherapists: Primary prevention counselling for general hospital staffs. Perspectives in Psychiatric Care, 23(3), 85-90.

Carlin, L., & Farnell, L. (1985). The stress audit—An avenue for individual and organizational change. Work and People, 11(1), 21-27.

Carr, W., & Kemmis, S. (1986). Becoming critical: Knowing through action research. London: Falmer Press.

Carr, W. & Kemmis, S. (1990). Becoming critical: Education, knowledge and action research, Deakin University.

Carr, W. & Kemmis, S. (1994). Becoming Critical: Education, knowledge and action research, Waurn Ponds: Deakin University.

Caufield, N., Chang, D., Dollard, F., & Elshaug, C. (2004). A review of occupational stress interventions in Australia. International Journal of Stress Management, 11(2), 149-166.

Cherniss, C. (1982). Staff burnout. Job stress in the human services. Sage Studies in Community Mental Health 2. London: Sage Publications.

Clark, D. E., Brown, A.M., Hughes, L., & Motluk, L. (2006). Education to improve the triage of mental health patients in general hospital emergency departments. Accident and Emergency Nursing, 14(4), 210-218.

Cleary, M., & Walter, G. (2006). Educating mental health nurses in clinical settings. Contemporary Nurse, 21(1), 153-159.

Clinton, M., & Hazelton, M. (2000). Scoping the prospects of Australian mental health nursing. Australian and New Zealand Journal of Mental Health Nursing, 9(4), 159-165.

Cohen, L. H., McGowen, J., Fookskas, S., & Rose, S. (1984). Positive life events and social supports and the relationship between life stress and psychological disorder. American Journal of Community Psychology, 12, 564-587.

Cook, S., & Fontaine, K. (1991). Essentials of mental health nursing. (2nd ed.).Redwood City: Addison-Wesley Nursing.

Constantini, A., Solano, I., DiNapoli, R., & Bosco, A. (1997). Relationship between hardiness and risk of burnout in a sample of 92 nurses working in oncology and AIDS wards. Psychotherapy and Psychosomatics, 66, 78-82.

Cotton, P., & Hart, P.M. (2003). Occupational wellbeing and performance: A review of organisational health research. Australian Psychologist, 38(2), 118-127.

Coup, A., & Schneider, Z. (2007). Ethical and legal issues in research. In Z. Schneider, D. Whitehead, D. Elliott, G. Lobiondo-Wood & J. Haber (Eds.), Nursing & midwifery research. Methods and appraisal for evidence-based practice, (3rd ed., pp. 80-101). Sydney. Elsevier.

Croll, N. (1997). Community mental health policy. In H. Gardner (Ed.), The politics of health: The Australian experience, (2nd ed., pp. 292-299). Melbourne: Churchill Livingstone.

Cronenwett, L. R., & Redman, R. (2003). Partners in action. Nursing education and nursing practice. Nurse Educator, 28(4), 153-155.

Cutcliffe, J. R., & Goward, P. (2000). Mental health nurses and qualitative research methods: a mutual attraction? Journal of Advanced Nursing, 31, 590-598.

Department of Human Services, Victoria. (2007). Mental health and Victoria's Emergency Departments [online]. Accessed 6 October 2007 from http://www.health.vic.gov.au/emergency/mental.htm

Descamp, K., & Thomas, C. (1993). Buffering nursing stress through play at work. Western Journal of Nursing Research, 15, 619-627.

Drury, V., Francis, K., & Delhunty, G. (2005). The lived experience of rural mental health nurses. Online Journal of Rural Nursing and Health Care, 5(1), 19-27. Accessed 4 May 2008 from http://www.rno.org/journal/index.php/online-journal/issue/view/15

Duckett, S. (2005). Health workforce design for the 21st century. Australian Health Review, 29(2), 201-210.

Duquette, A., Kerouac, S., Sandhu, B. K., & Beaudet, L. (1994). Burnout: a review of empirical knowledge. Issues in Mental Health Nursing, 15, 337–358.

Ellis, N. (1995). The organizational approach to stress management. In P. Cotton (Ed.), Psychological health in the workplace: Understanding and managing occupational stress, (pp. 31–50). Melbourne: Australian Psychological Society.

Ezzy, D. (2006). The research process. In M. Walter (Ed.), Social research methods an Australian perspective, (pp. 29–52). South Melbourne: Oxford University Press.

Falk-Rafael, A. (2005). Advanced nursing theory through theory-guided practice. The emergence of a critical caring perspective. Advances in Nursing Science, 28(1), 49–56.

Francis, K., & Chapman, Y. (2008). Rural and remote community nursing. In D. Kralik & A. van Loon (Eds.), Community nursing in Australia, (pp. 148–158). Oxford: Blackwell Publishing.

Fraser, C., Judd, F., Jackson, H., Murray, G., Humphreys, J., & Hodgins, G. A. (2002). Does one size really fit all? Why the mental health of rural Australians requires further research. Australian Journal of Rural Health, 10(6), 288–295.

Freire, P. (1990). Education for critical consciousness.(Trans. M. Ramos). New York: Continuum.

Freudenberger, H. J. (1989). Burnout: Past, present and future concern. Loss and Grief Care, 3(1–2), 1–10.

Gerber, R. (1999). The role of theory in social and health research. In V. Minichiello, G. Sullivan, K. Greenwood & R. Axford, (Eds.), Handbook for research methods in health sciences, (pp. 16–33). South Melbourne: Addison Wesley Longman.

Gerber, R, & Moyle, W. (2004). The role of theory in health research. In V. Minichiello, G. Sullivan, K. Greenwood & R. Axford (Eds.), Handbook of research methods for nursing and health science, (2nd ed., pp. 34–58). Frenchs Forest: Pearson Education Australia.

Gibb, H. (2003). Rural community mental health nursing: A grounded theory account of sole practice. International Journal of Mental Health Nursing, 12(4), 243–250.

Gillespie, M. & Melby, V. (2003). Burnout among nursing staff in accident and emergency and acute medicine: a comparative study. Journal of Clinical Nursing, 12, 842–851.

Gladding, S.T. (1992). Counselling: A comprehensive profession. New York: Merrill.

Glasberg, A-L., Norberg, A., & Söderberg, A. (2007). Sources of burnout among healthcare employees as perceived by managers. Journal of Advanced Nursing, 60, pp. 10–19.

Glasson, J. (1996). The public image and the mentally ill and community care. British Journal of Nursing, 5(10), 615–617.

Greenwood, J. (1994). Action research: a few details, a caution and something new. Journal of Advanced Nursing, 20, 13–18.

Habermas, J. (1971). Knowledge and human interests. (Trans. J. J. Shapiro). Boston: Beacon Press.

Habermas, J. (1984).The theory of communicative action. Vol. 1. Reason and rationalization of society. (Trans. T. McCarthy). Boston: Beacon Press.

Halcomb, E., Davidson, P., Daly, J., Griffiths, R., Yallop, J., & Tofler, G. (2005). Nursing in Australian general practice: directions and perspectives. Australian Health Review, 29(2), 156–166.

Happell, B., & Plantania-Phung, C. (2005). Mental health issues within the general health care system: the challenge for nursing education in Australia. Nurse Education Today, 25(6), 465–471.

Hart, E. & Bond, M. (1995). Action research for health and social care. A guide to practice. Buckingham: Open University Press.

Hays, R., & Beaton, N. (2004). Rural hospital medicine. In D. Wilkinson, R. Hays, R. Strasser & P. Worley (Eds.), The handbook of rural medicine in Australia, (pp. 128–135). South Melbourne: Oxford University Press.

Heard, R., & Harris, L. M. (2004). Experimental, quasi-experimental and correlational quantitative research designs. In V. Minichiello, G. Sullivan, K. Greenwood & R. Axford (Eds.), Handbook of research methods for nursing and health science, (2nd ed., pp.124–150). Frenchs Forest: Pearson Education Australia.

Heath, P., Duncan, J., Lowe, E., Macri, S., Ramsay, J., Selby Smith, C., & Watts, R. (2002). Our duty of care: National review of nursing education. (Catalogue No. DEST6880 HERCO 2A). Canberra: Commonwealth Department of Education, Science & Training. Accessed 24 April 2007 from http://www.dest.gov.au/archive/highered/nursing/pubs/duty_of_care/default.html

Hegney, D., Pearson, A., & McCarthy, A. (1997). The role and function of the rural nurse in Australia. Canberra: Royal College of Nursing Australia.

Hehir, B. (2006). Is it all in the mind? [Reflections]. Nursing Standard, 21(7), 28–29.

Holter, I. M., & Schwartz-Barcott, D. (1993). Action research: what is it? How has it been used and how can it be used in nursing? Journal of Advanced Nursing, 18, 298–304.

Hugo, G. (2001). What is really happening in regional and rural populations? In M. F. Rogers & Y. M. J. Collins (Eds.), The future of Australia's country towns, (pp. 57–71). Bendigo: La Trobe University.

Humphreys, J., & Rolley, F. (1991). Health and health care in rural Australia. Armidale: University of New England.

Jackson, D., & Borbasi, S. (2008). Qualitative research: the whole picture. In S. Borbasi, D. Jackson & R. Langford (Eds.), Navigating the maze of nursing research. An interactive learning adventure, (2nd ed., pp.151–177). Sydney: Elsevier.

Johnson, D., & Preston, B. (2001). (Catalogue No. DETYA 6761HERCO1A).An overview of issues in nursing education. Canberra: Department of Education, Training and Youth Affairs. Accessed 23 June, 2007 from http://www.dest.gov.au/archive/highered/eippubs/eip01_12/default.htm

Jones, S. R. (2002). (Re)writing the word: Methodological strategies and issues in qualitative research. Journal of College Student Development, 43, 461–473.

Joy, C. B., Adams, C. E., & Rice, K. (1999, reprinted 2008). Crisis intervention for people with severe mental illnesses. Cochrane Database of Systematic Reviews 2008, (4). Article CD001087.

Judd, F., & Humphreys, J. (2001). Mental health issues for rural and remote Australia. Australian Journal of Rural Health, 9(5), 254–258.

Kemmis, S., & McTaggart, R. (1982). The action research planner. (2nd ed.). Deakin University.

Kemmis, S. & McTaggart, R. (Eds.). (1988). The action research planner (3rd ed.). Deakin University.

Kennedy, P., & Grey, N. (1997). High pressure areas. Nursing Times, 93(29), 26-27.
Kenny, J. W. (2000). Women's 'inner-balance'; a comparison of stressors, personality traits and health problems by age groups. Journal of Advanced Nursing, 31, 639-650.
Kenny, A., & Duckett, S. (2003). Educating for rural nursing practice. Journal of Advanced Nursing, 44, 613-622.
Kenny, A. & Duckett, S. (2005). An online study of Australian enrolled nurse conversion. Journal of Advanced Nursing, 49, 423-431.
Kerrison, S. A., & Chapman, R. (2007). What general emergency nurses want to know about mental health patients presenting to their emergency department. Accident and Emergency Nursing, 15(1), 48-55.
King, C. (2001). Severe mental illness: Managing the boundary of a CMHT. Journal of Mental Health, 10(1), 75-86.
Lachman, V. (1996). Stress and self-care revisited. A literature review. Holistic Nursing Practice, 10(2), 1-12.
Lambert, B, (1995). Give your company a check-up. Personnel Journal, 74(9), 143-145.
Lancaster, J. (1982). Change theory: An essential aspect of nursing practice. In J. Lancaster & W. Lancaster (Eds.), Concepts for advanced nursing practice: The nurse as change agent, (pp. 5-23). St.Louis: C.V. Mosby Company.
Lancaster, J., & Lancaster, W. (1982). Theoretical foundations for change. In J. Lancaster & W. Lancaster (Eds.), Concepts for advanced nursing practice: The nurse as change agent, (pp. 1-4). St.Louis: C.V. Mosby Company.
Lauder, W., Reynolds, W., Reilly, V., & Angus, N. (2001). The role of the district nurses in caring for people with mental health problems who live in rural settings. Journal of Clinical Nursing, 10(3), 337-344.
Lauri, S. (1982). Development of nursing process through action research. Journal of Advanced Nursing, 7, 301-307.
Lawrence, G. (1987). Capitalism and the countryside: the rural crisis in Australia. Sydney: Pluto.
Lazarus, R. S., & Folkman, S. (1984). Stress, appraisal and coping. New York: Springer.
Lewis, D. J., & Robinson, J. A. (1992). ICU nurses' coping measures: Response to work related stressors. Critical Care Nurse, 12(2), 18-23.
Light, K. (1981). Cardiovascular responses to effortful active coping: Implications for the role of stress in hypertension development. Psychophysiology, 18, 216-225.
Lindsey, E., Stajduhar, K., & McGuinness, L. (2001). Examining the process of community development. Journal of Advanced Nursing, 33, 828-835.
Llewellyn, G. Sullivan, G., & Minichiello, V. (2004). Sampling in qualitative research. In V. Minichiello, G. Sullivan, K. Greenwood & R. Axford (Eds.), Handbook of research methods for nursing and health science, (2nd ed., pp. 210-241). Frenchs Forest: Pearson Education Australia.
Mahnken, J. E. (2001). Rural nursing and health care reforms: building a social model of health. Rural and Remote Health, 1. Accessed 15 May 2008 from http://www.regional.org.au/au/rrh/2001/011214_104.htm
Malach-Pines, A. (2000). Nurses' burnout, an existential psychodynamic perspective. Journal of Psychosocial Nursing & Mental Health Services, 38(2), 23-31.
Maslach, C. (1976). Burnout, anxiety, stress and coping. Human Behavior, 5(9), 16-22.

Maslach, C. (1979). The burnout syndrome in patient care. In C. Garfield (Ed.), Stress and survival: The emotional realities of life-threatening illness, (pp. 111-120). St. Louis: Mosby.

Maslach, C. (1981). Burnout: A social psychological analysis. In J. W. Jones (Ed.), The burnout syndrome, (pp. 30-50). Park Ridge: London House Press.

Maslach, C. (1982). Burnout: the cost of caring. New York: Prentice Hall.

Maslach, C. (1986). Stress, burnout and alcoholism. In R. R. Kilburg, P. E. Nathan & R. W. Thoreson (Eds.), Professionals in distress: Issues, syndromes and solutions in psychology, (pp. 53-76). Washington, DC: American Psychological Association.

Maslach, C., & Jackson, S. E. (1981). Maslach Burnout Inventory. Palo Alto: Consulting Psychologists Press.

Maslach, C., & Jackson, S. E. (1982). Burnout in health professionals: A social psychological analysis. In G. Sanders & J. Suls (Eds.), Social psychology of health and illness, (pp. 227-231). Hillsdale: Erlbaum.

Maude, P., & Warelow, P. (2011). 'Wise Men, Devils and fools': The History of Mental Illness and its Treatment. In Edward, K-L., Munro, I., Robins, A., Welch, A. (Eds). Mental Health Nursing Dimensions of Praxis. Melbourne, Oxford.

McCaugherty, D. (1991). The use of a teaching model to promote reflection and the experiential integration of theory and practice in first-year student nurses: an action research study. Journal of Advanced Nursing, 16, 534-543.

McLaren, S., Jude, B., Hopes, L., & Sherritt, T. (2001). Sense of belonging, stress and depression in rural-urban communities. International Journal of Rural Psychology, 2(7). Accessed 21 September 2007 from http://www.ruralpsych.com/Members/RefereedArticles/RR-McLaren-Jude-Hopes-Sherritt.htm

Melamed, S., Shirom, A., Toker, S., Berliner, S., & Shapira, I. (2006). Burnout and risk of cardiovascular disease: Evidence, possible causal paths, and promising research directions. Psychological Bulletin, 132(3), 327-353.

Meyer, J. (1995). Stages in the process: a personal account. Nurse Researcher, 2(3), 24-37.

Mugo, F.W. (2003). Sampling in research. [online] Accessed 21 July 2007 from http://trochim.human.cornell.edu/tutorial/mugo/tutorial.htm

Murphy, L. R. (1996). Stress management in work settings: A critical review of the health effects. American Journal of Health Promotion, 11(2), 112-135.

Murray, R. B., & Huelskoetter, M. M. W. (1991). Psychiatric mental health nursing. (3rd ed.). Norwalk, Conn.: Appleton & Lange.

National Health and Medical Research Council. (2007). National statement on ethical conduct in human research [online]. Accessed 22 October 2007 from http://www.nhmrc.gov.au/publications/synopses/e72syn.htm

New South Wales Mental Health Act. (1990). Accessed 23 October 2011 from http://www.health.wa.gov.au/mhareview/resources/legislation/nsw_mental_health_act_1990.pdf

New South Wales Occupational Health and Safety Act. (2004). Accessed 23 October 2007 from http://www.legislation.nsw.gov.au/fullhtml/inforce/act+40+2000+FIRST+0+N

Owens, J., Stein, I., & Chenoweth, L. (1999). Action research. In V. Minichiello, G. Sullivan, K. Greenwood & R. Axford (Eds.), Handbook for research methods in health sciences, (pp. 247-270). Frenchs Forest: Addison Wesley Longman.

Pante, M. (1999). Thrown in at the deep end: Psychiatric nurses' attitudes to educational preparation for clinical practice. Melbourne: Health and Community Services Union.

Patton, M. Q. (1990). Qualitative evaluation and research methods. Newbury Park: Sage.

Pearce, J. (1981). Bringing some clarity to role ambiguity research. Academy of Management Review, 6, 665–674.

Pearson, A. (1989). Action research methodology. Paper presented at the Quantitative and Qualitative Methods Workshop, Melbourne University, 13-15 July.

Pearson, A. (1992). Nursing at Burford. A story of change. Harrow: Scutari Press.

Perkin, R., Young, T., Freier, M., Allen, J., & Orr, D. (1997). Stress and distress in paediatric nurses: Lessons from Baby K. American Journal of Critical Care, 6(3), 225-232.

Pines, A. M., & Aronson, E. (1981). Burnout. New York: Free Press.

Pines, A. M., & Maslach, C. (1978). Characteristics of staff burnout in a mental health setting. Hospital and Community Psychiatry, 29, 233-237.

Pinikahana, J., & Happell, B. (2004). Stress, burnout and job satisfaction in rural psychiatric nurses: A Victorian study. Australian Journal of Rural Health, 12(3), 120-125.

Polit, D. & Hungler, B. (1991). Nursing research. Principles and methods. (4th ed.). Philadelphia: J. B. Lippincott Company.

Pompili, M., Rinaldi, G., Lester, D., Girardi, P., Ruberto, A., & Tatarelli, R. (2006). Hopelessness and suicide risk emerge in psychiatric nurses suffering burnout and using specific defence mechanisms. Archives of Psychiatric Nursing, 20(3), 135-143.

Productivity Commission. (2005). Australia's health workforce. Research report. Melbourne: Productivity Commission.

Quevillon, R. P., & Trenerry, M. R. (1983) Research on rural depression: implications of social networks for theory and treatment. International Journal of Mental Health, 12, 45-61.

Reason, P. (1988). Human inquiry in action: Developments in new paradigm research. London: Sage Publications.

Rees, D., & Cooper, C. (1992). The occupational stress indicator locus of control scale: Should this be regarded as a state rather than a trait measure? Work and Stress, 6, 45-48.

Rolfe, G. (1996). Going to extremes: action research, grounded practice and the theory-practice gap in nursing. Journal of Advanced Nursing, 24, 1315-1320.

Saines, J. C. (1999). Violence and aggression in A&E: Recommendations for action. Accident and Emergency Nursing, 7(1), 8-12.

Schaefer, J. A., & Moos, R. H. (1996). Effects of work stressors and work climate on long-term care staff's job morale and functioning. Research in Nursing and Health, 19, 63-73.

Schmitz, N., Neumann, W., & Oppermann, R. (2000). Stress, burnout and locus of control in German nurses. International Journal of Nursing Studies, 37(2), 95-99.

Scopelliti, J., Judd, F., Grigg, M., Hodgins, G., Fraser, C., Hulbert, C., Endacott, R., & Wood, A. (2004). Dual relationships in mental health practice: Issues for clinicians in rural settings. Australian and New Zealand Journal of Psychiatry, 38, (11-12), 953-959.

Senate Community Affairs Reference Committee [SCARC]. (2002) The patient profession, time for action report on the inquiry into nursing. Canberra: Senate Community Affairs Reference Committee Secretariat.

Seng, J. S. (1998). Praxis as a conceptual framework for participatory research in nursing. Advances in Nursing Science, 20(4), 37–41.

Selye, H. (1956). The stress of life. New York: McGraw Hill.

Selye, H. (1974). Stress without distress. Philadelphia: Lippincott.

Selye, H. (1976). Further thoughts on "stress without distress." Medical Times, 104, 124-132.

Shaban, R. (2006). Paramedics' clinical judgment and mental health assessments in emergency contexts: Research, practice, and tools of the trade. Journal of Emergency Primary Health Care, 4(2), paper no. 990177. Accessed 21 October 2007 from http://www.jephc.com/full_article.cfm?content_id=375

Sharrock, J., & Happell, B. (2002). The role of a psychiatric consultation liaison nurse in a general hospital: A case study approach. Australian Journal of Advanced Nursing, 20(1), 39–44.

Sheehan, J. (1996). Aspects of research methodology. Nurse Education Today, 6, 193–203.

Silverman, D. (2006). Interpreting qualitative data. (3rd Ed.). London: Sage Publications Ltd.

Simmons, S. (1995). From paradigm to method in interpretive action research. Journal of Advanced Nursing, 21, 837–844.

Simoni, P. S., & Paterson, J. J. (1997). Hardiness, coping and burnout in the nursing workplace. Journal of Professional Nursing, 13(3), 178–185.

Snow, T. (2006).Taking the strain. Nursing Standard, 20(46), 16–17.

Stevens, P. (1989). A critical social reconceptualization of environment in nursing: implications for methodology. Advances in Nursing Science, 11(4), 56–58.

Stewart, E., McKenery, P., Rudd, N., & Gavazzi, S. M. (1994). Family processes as mediators of depressive symptomatology among rural adolescents. Family Relations, 43, 38–45.

Street, A. F. (2004). Action research. In V. Minichiello, G. Sullivan, K. Greenwood & R. Axford (Eds.), Handbook of research methods for nursing and health science, (2nd ed., pp. 278–294). Frenchs Forest: Pearson Education Australia.

Stringer, E. T. (1996). Action research: A handbook for practitioners. Newbury Park: Sage Publications Inc.

Strong, K., Trickett, P., Titulaer, I., & Bhatia, K. (1998). (Catalogue No. PHE 6). Health in rural and remote Australia. The first report of the Australian Institute of Health and Welfare on rural health.. Canberra: Australian Institute of Health and Welfare.

Susman, G. I., & Evered, R.D. (1978). An assessment of the scientific merits of action research. Administrative Science Quarterly, 23, 582-603.

Taylor, C. (1993). Intershift report: oral communication using a quality assurance approach. Journal of Clinical Nursing, 2(5), 266–267.

The health Services Advisory committee. (1997). Violence in the education sector (Education Service Advisory Committee, HSE Books, 1997, ISBN 0 7176 1293 7

Titchen, A., & Binnie, A. (1993). Research partnerships: Collaborative action research in nursing. Journal of Advanced Nursing, 18, 858–865.

Tolley, K. (1995). Theory from practice: is this a reality? Journal of Advanced Nursing, 21, 184–190.

Turnipseed, D. L. (1988). An integrated, interactive model of organizational climate, culture, and effectiveness. Leadership and Organizational Journal, 9, 17-21.

Turnipseed, D. (1994). An analysis of the influence of work environment variables and moderators on the burnout syndrome. Journal of Applied Psychology, 24(9), 782-800.

Vanclay, F. (1994). A crisis in agricultural extension? Rural Society, 4(1). Accessed 20 September 2007 from http://www.csu.edu.au/research/crsr/ruralsoc/v4n1p10.htm.

Victoria Mental Health Act. (1986).

Victoria Occupational Health and Safety Act. (2004).

Wadsworth, Y. (1997). Do it yourself social research. (2nd ed.). St Leonards: Allen and Unwin.

Wallis, S. (1998). Changing practice through action research. Nurse Researcher, 6(2), 5-15.

Walter, M. (2006). Surveys and sampling. In M. Walter (Ed.), Social research methods an Australian perspective, (pp. 187-222). South Melbourne: Oxford University Press.

Whitehead, D. (2007). An overview of research theory and process. In Z. Schneider, D. Whitehead, D. Elliott, G. Lobiondo-Wood & J. Haber (Eds.), Nursing & midwifery research. Methods and appraisal for evidence-based practice, (3rd ed., pp. 20-32). Sydney: Elsevier.

Whitehead, D., & Annells, M. (2007). Sampling data and data collection in qualitative research. In Z. Schneider, D. Whitehead, D. Elliott, G. Lobiondo-Wood & J. Haber (Eds.), Nursing & midwifery research. Methods and appraisal for evidence-based practice, (3rd ed., pp. 122-137). Sydney: Elsevier.

Whitehead, D., & Elliott, D. (2007). Mixed methods research. In Z. Schneider, D. Whitehead, D. Elliott, G. Lobiondo-Wood & J. Haber (Eds.), Nursing & midwifery research. Methods and appraisal for evidence-based practice, (3rd ed., pp. 248-267). Sydney: Elsevier.

Willis, K. (2006). Analysing qualitative data. In M. Walter (Ed.), Social research methods an Australian perspective, (pp. 256-279). South Melbourne: Oxford University Press.

Wright, S. (1991). Tameside Nursing Development Unit: a decade of success. Nursing Standard, 6(7), 49-56.

Wynaden, D., O'Connell, B., McGowan, S., & Popescu, A. (2000). The educational needs of nurses' [sic] in the area of mental health. The Australian Electronic Journal of Nursing Education, 6(2), no pagination. Accessed 24 April 2006 from http://www.scu.edu.au/schools/nhcp/aejne/archive/vol6-1/wynadend.html

Young, K. (2011). Child and Adolescent Mental Health. In Edward, K-L., Munro, I., Robins, A., Welch, A. (Eds). Mental Health Nursing Dimensions of Praxis. Melbourne, Oxford.

4

Effort-Reward Imbalance and Quality of Life Among Female Nurses at a General Hospital in Japan

Yoko Kikuchi[1], Makoto Nakaya[1,2], Miki Ikeda[1], Kyoko Narita[1], Mihoko Takeda[1] and Miyoko Nishi[3]
[1]*Department of Psychiatry, Musashino Red Cross Hospital*
[2]*Faculty of Medicine, Tokyo Medical and Dental University*
[3]*Department of Nursing, Musashino Red Cross Hospital*
Japan

1. Introduction

An effort-reward imbalance (ERI) model is a measurement of psychosocial work stress. The ERI model with both the effort-reward ratios and the concept of overcommitment (OC) indicates that work stress is related to high effort with low reward. Effort is evaluated by measuring work demands. Reward includes money, esteem, status, and control over promotion prospects, and job security. Overcommitment is a set of attitudes, behaviors, and emotions that reflect excessive work effort[13,14,18)]. This model has been used to study psychosocial work stress in various occupational groups. It has been suggested that the ERI model has a predictive power for poor physical or mental health[2-3,6-8,10,12,14-16,18-21)]. Concerning overcommitment, according to Siegrist and Tsutumi et al., overcommitment causes emotional exhaustion and exacerbates the negative effects of the effort-reward imbalance[14,18)]. Weyers et al. found that nurses who report higher ERI with high overcommitment scores were twice as likely to suffer from poor psychological health compared to those who report higher ERI with low overcommitment scores[21)]. Aust et al. and Ire et al. found that overcommitment was significantly reduced in an intervention group through stress management programs or counseling[1,4)].

Quality of life measures were developed mainly to reflect consequences of health problems. Health-related quality of life indicators usually encompass a person's ability to effectively perform in physical, emotional, and social domains and to maintain a sense of well-being [9,11)]. Therefore, quality of life is an important measurement of health-related outcomes. To our knowledge, 10 studies have examined the relationships between ERI and health-related quality of life among working and healthy populations using the Short-Form Health Survey or the World Health Organization Quality of Life (WHOQOL-26)[3,6-8,10,12,15-16,20-21)]. Only three studies were conducted among hospital staff members, one of which was conducted among physicians in China[10)]; the others were among nurses in Denmark[21)] and Brazil[15)]. Li et al. used the SF-8 to investigate the relationship between ERI, physical health, and mental health among physicians in China. Their findings suggested that poor physical and mental health were significantly related to higher effort-reward imbalance[10]. Weyers et al. examined the relationship between ERI, physical health, and mental health among nurses in Denmark and found that risks for poor health functioning were elevated among nurses who were experiencing high effort and low reward[21]. All previous studies suggested a significant relationship between ERI and health-related quality of life, and higher ERI is likely to be a risk factor for poor health. In Japan, Watanabe et al. investigated the relationship between ERI and health-related quality of life among Japanese employees of a manufacturing plant, and suggested that ERI was associated with health-related quality of life[20]. However, no research has been conducted among Japanese nurses to examine the relationship between ERI and health-related quality of life.

Nurses are exposed to high-stress work environments, including irregular work schedules, shift work, and interaction with patients and other hospital staff members. Tsutsumi found that the level of ERI in nurses and dental technicians in Japan was almost twice that of workers in production companies[18]. The research investigating the relationship between ERI and health-related quality of life among nurses is necessary to elevate their quality of life or to prevent physical or mental impairments or disease.

We had already investigated the relationship between the ERI and depressive state in the same sample[5]. In the previous study, depressive state was measured by one item of the quality of life (WHOQOL-26), i.e., item 26, which questioned how often the subject feels despair, anxiety or depressed mood. And we found that effort-money (effort-job promotion) imbalance and overcommitment had significantly influenced on depressive state. However, depressive state is an important problem for mental health but only a part of health functioning. In the present study, we investigated the relationship between the ERI and health functioning as a whole.

The aim of the present study was to investigate the effects of ERI on quality of life among nurses at a Japanese general hospital.

2. Subjects and methods

2.1 Subjects and procedure

A part of the present study was described elsewhere[5]. Subjects consisted of all the nurses (n=682) at a general hospital in Japan, which is located in urban and has 611 beds. We conducted the present study in November 2007. The questionnaire was distributed by supervisors and was returned by 465 nurses (response rate, 68.2%). Male nurses were excluded from the sample because there were so few (n = 13). Subjects with missing ERI values were also excluded (n = 46). The final sample consisted of 406 female nurses (59.5%).

Participants were asked to fill out a questionnaire explaining the voluntary of the survey, and we assumed that participants consented to the survey with answering the questionnaire. This self-report survey was approved by the Committee for the Prevention of Physical Disease and Mental Illness among Health Care Workers in the general hospital.

3. Measured variables

3.1 Work environment

The survey included demographic variables such as age and work-related variables (work style, occupational status, overtime hours, and shift work). Age was coded into a four-category classification and ranged from 20s to 50s or over (<30, 30 to <40, 40 to <50, and ≥50). Work style was either full-time or part-time. Occupational status responses included: manager, middle manager or subordinate. Overtime work responses were in hours per week. Shift work categories included: no shift work, shift work with night shift, or shift work without night shift. Table 1 shows the characteristics of the subjects.

3.2 Effort-reward imbalance

Work stress was measured using the Japanese version of the ERI (23 items) translated by Tsutsumi [19]. The ERI consists of three subscales: efforts (6items, e.g., quantitative and qualitative load), rewards(11items) and overcommitment(6items). The rewards subscale is further divided into three subgroups: esteem (5items, e.g., "I receive the respect I deserve from my superiors."), job security (2 items, e.g., "My job security is poor.") and job promotion (4 items, e.g., "My job promotion prospects are poor."). Overcommitment is measured by six items which refer to respondent's inability to withdraw from work obligations and to develop a more distant attitude towards job requirements. The validity of this questionnaire has been confirmed [18]. Higher ERI ratio and overcommitment scores indicate high-risk conditions. Means and standard deviations of ERI subscales and overcommitment are presented in Table 1.

3.3 Health-related quality of life

Quality of life was measured by the Japanese version of WHOQOL-BREF (WHOQOL-26) [17]. The WHOQOL-26 contains 26 items divided into the following domains: Physical Health (7 items), Psychological (6 items) Social Relationships (3 items), and Environment (8 items). The four domain scores denote an individual's perception of their quality of life in each particular domain. Higher scores represent better quality of life. The WHOQOL has been applied to assess health functioning [9,11].

3.4 Statistical analysis

Four kinds of ERI ratios (effort-reward imbalance, effort-esteem imbalance, effort-job security imbalance and effort-job promotion imbalance) were calculated according to Tsutsumi[19]. The effort-reward imbalance was calculated as effort × 11/reward × 6. The effort-esteem imbalance was calculated as effort × 5/esteem × 6. The effort-job security imbalance was calculated as effort × 2/security × 6. The effort-job promotion imbalance was calculated as effort × 4/job promotion × 6. Higher scores of the three imbalances and overcommitment were defined as high-risk conditions. The lower tertile of the four domain scores of QOL were each assigned to the poor health functioning group (n =117, 111, 183, 120 for Physical Health, Psychological, Social Relationship, and Environment, respectively). The upper tertile of each of the four domain scores of QOL was assigned to the good health functioning group (n =114, 116, 128, 121 for Physical Health, Psychological, Social Relationship, and Environment, respectively). The medium scores (n =175, 179, 95, 165 for

Physical Health, Psychological, Social Relationship, and Environment, respectively) were all excluded from further analyses. Mean and standard deviation of the four domain scores of QOL are presented in Table 1.

		Nurses (n = 406)
		n (%)
Age, years	<30	272 (67)
	30 to <40	91 (22)
	40 to <50	25 (6)
	≥50	13 (3)
Work style	Full-time	368 (91)
	Part-time	21 (5)
Occupational status	Manager	18 (4)
	Middle manager	21 (5)
	Subordinate	367 (90)
Overtime work, h/wk	<50	353 (87)
	≥50	1 (0)
Quality of life*	Poor Physical Health	117
	Good Physical Health	114
	Poor Psychological	111
	Good Psychological	116
	Poor Social Relationship	183
	Good Social Relationship	128
	Poor Environment	120
	Good Environment	121
Scale	Mean	SD
ERI		
Effort	18.65	5.31
Reward	42.66	8.06
Esteem	20.36	4.12
Job security	8.05	1.8
Money	14.25	3.26
Effort-reward ratio	0.86	0.42
Effort-esteem ratio	0.83	0.44
Effort-security ratio	0.86	0.55
Effort-job promotion ratio	0.97	0.55
Overcommitment	15.8	3.54
Quality of life		
Physical Health	20.98	4.51
Psychological	17.6	3.79
Social Relationship	9.77	1.71
Environment	23.62	4.17

*Poor group, lower tertile; good group, upper tertile

Table 1. Characteristics of study subjects.

In order to investigate the influence of age and work-related variables on quality of life, these variables were compared between the poor health functioning group and the good health group using chi-square tests (Table 2~Table 5). In addition, we compared the means of overtime work hours, the four ERI ratios and overcommitment scores between the two groups using *t*- tests (Table 2~Table 5).

	Poor Physical Health group n=117	Good Physical Health group n=114	
	n (%)	n (%)	$\chi 2$ (Chi-square value)
Age, years			2.41 n.s
<30	82 (70.0)	74 (64.9)	
30 to <40	22 (18.8)	27 (23.7)	
40 to <50	8 (6.8)	5 (4.4)	
≥50	4 (3.4)	6 (5.3)	
Work style			4.29 n.s
Full-time	110 (94.0)	103 (90.4)	
Part-time	2 (1.7)	8 (7.0)	
Occupational status			0.88 n.s
Manager	7 (6.0)	4 (3.5)	
Middle manager	5 (4.3)	6 (5.3)	
Subordinate	105 (89.7)	104 (91.2)	
Shift work			6.12 *
without night shift	8(6.8)	2(1.8)	
with night shift	90(76.9)	83(72.8)	
no shift work	17(14.5)	27(23.7)	
	Mean (SD)	Mean (SD)	t value
Overtime work, h/wk	9.01(8.4)	6.09(4.8)	3.01 **
Effort-reward ratio	1.13 (0.53)	0.64 (0.28)	8.41 ***
Effort-esteem ratio	1.08 (0.57)	0.64 (0.28)	7.56 ***
Effort-job security ratio	1.19 (0.82)	0.64 (0.27)	6.72 ***
Effort-job promotion ratio	1.31 (0.75)	0.74 (0.34)	7.41 ***
Overcommitment	18.10 (3.42)	13.55 (3.09)	10.60 ***
		* **p ＜ 0.01	***p ＜ 0.001

Table 2. Comparison between Poor and Good Physical Health groups.

	Poor Psychological group n=111	Good Psychological group n=116		
	n (%)	n (%)	χ2 (Chi-square value)	
Age, years			6.12	n.s
<30	77 (69.4)	71 (61.2)		
30 to <40	24 (21.6)	28 (24.1)		
40 to <50	7 (6.3)	9 (7.8)		
≥50	2 (1.8)	6 (51.7)		
Work style			8.40	*
Full-time	106 (95.5)	105 (90.5)		
Part-time	0 (0)	8 (6.9)		
Occupational status			0.60	n.s
Manager	4 (3.6)	4 (3.4)		
Middle manager	5 (4.5)	8 (6.9)		
Subordinate	102 (91.9)	104 (89.7)		
Shift work			6.5	*
without night shift	5(4.5)	1(0.9)		
with night shift	86(77.5)	84(72.4)		
no shift work	17(15.3)	31(26.7)		
	Mean (SD)	Mean (SD)	t value	
Overtime work, h/wk	8.64(7.08)	6.27(5.46)	2.67	**
Effort-reward ratio	1.09 (0.51)	0.67 (0.29)	7.74	***
Effort-esteem ratio	1.04 (0.52)	0.65 (0.33)	6.91	***
Effort-job security ratio	1.12 (0.78)	0.65 (0.27)	6.20	***
Effort-job promotion ratio	1.27 (0.75)	0.74 (0.35)	6.89	***
Overcommitment	17.88 (3.38)	13.38 (3.07)	10.51	***
			*p < 0.05	***p < 0.001

Table 3. Comparison between Poor and Good Psychological groups.

	Poor social Relationship group n=183	Good social relationship group n=128		
	n (%)	n (%)	χ2 (Chi-square value)	
Age, years			8.40	n.s
<30	117 (63.9)	92 (71.9)		
30 to <40	43 (23.5)	25 (19.5)		
40 to <50	15 (8.2)	4 (3.1)		
≥50	5 (2.7)	5 (3.9)		
Work style			3.26	n.s
Full-time	166 (90.7)	116 (90.6)		
Part-time	7 (3.8)	9 (7.0)		
Occupational status			3.43	n.s
Manager	10 (5.5)	5 (3.9)		
Middle manager	12 (6.6)	3 (2.3)		
Subordinate	161 (88.0)	120 (93.8)		
Shift work			0.82	n.s
without night shift	6(3.3)	6(4.7)		
with night shift	142(77.6)	95(74.2)		
no shift work	32(17.5)	26(20.3)		
	Mean (SD)	Mean (SD)	t value	
Overtime work, h/wk	8.13(7.39)	6.68(5.04)	1.78	n.s
Effort-reward ratio	0.98 (0.48)	0.71 (0.31)	5.66	***
Effort-esteem ratio	0.96 (0.51)	0.68 (0.35)	5.32	***
Effort-job security ratio	0.99 (0.69)	0.68 (0.29)	4.70	***
Effort-job promotion ratio	1.09 (0.60)	0.81 (0.39)	4.72	***
Overcommitment	17.87 (3.41)	14.35 (3.25)	6.38	***
				***p < 0.001

Table 4. Comparison between Poor and Good Social Relationship groups.

	Poor Environment group n=120	Good Environment group n=121		
	n (%)	n (%)	χ2 (Chi-square value)	
Age, years			7.28	n.s
<30	87 (72.5)	76 (62.8)		
30 to <40	25 (20.8)	27 (22.3)		
40 to <50	5 (4.2)	9 (7.4)		
≥50	2 (1.7)	7 (5.8)		
Work style			7.90	*
Full-time	111 (92.5)	107 (88.4)		
Part-time	2 (1.7)	11 (9.1)		
Occupational status			1.10	n.s
Manager	5 (4.2)	7 (5.8)		
Middle manager	5 (4.2)	8 (6.6)		
Subordinate	110 (91.7)	106 (87.6)		
Shift work			9.62	**
without night shift	7(5.8)	3(2.5)		
with night shift	95(79.2)	82(67.8)		
no shift work	16(13.3)	35(28.9)		
	Mean (SD)	Mean (SD)	t value	
Overtime work, h/wk	8.46(7.80)	6.65(5.76)	1.92	n.s
Effort-reward ratio	1.04 (0.46)	0.70 (0.31)	6.73	***
Effort-esteem ratio	0.99 (0.48)	0.68 (0.34)	5.79	***
Effort-job security ratio	1.06 (0.68)	0.67 (0.28)	5.79	***
Effort-job promotion ratio	1.21 (0.70)	0.76 (0.35)	6.29	***
Overcommitment	17.43 (3.61)	14.18 (3.36)	7.23	***
	*p < 0.05, **p < 0.01, ***p < 0.001			

Table 5. Comparison between Poor and Good Environment groups.

In the next step, the relationships between health functioning and work-related or ERI variables were examined using stepwise logistic regression. We used the tertile of the four domain scores as dependent variables and the ERI ratios, overcommitment scores, and the work-related scores as independent variables. The results are shown as odds ratios (ORs) with 95% confidence intervals (CIs). All analyses were conducted using SPSS 11 (SPSS Inc., Chicago, IL, USA).

4. Results

The four effort-reward ratios and overcommitment scores significantly correlated with poor health functioning in the four domains (Table 2~Table 5).

4.1 ERI and physical health domain

Shift work and overtime hours per week also significantly correlated with poor physical health functioning (Table 2). According to the stepwise logistic regression analyses between Physical Health and the work-related variables (shift work and overtime hours per week), the three imbalances (effort-esteem imbalance, effort-job security imbalance and effort-job promotion imbalance), and overcommitment, significant correlations were found with Poor Physical Health: a higher effort-job promotion ratio (OR, 0.24; 95% CI, 0.09-0.64) and higher overcommitment (OR, 0.64; 95% CI, 0.64-0.83) (Table 6).

4.2 ERI and psychological domain

We found significant differences for work style, shift work and overtime hours per week between the two groups (Table 3). According to the stepwise logistic regression analyses between Psychological and the work-related variables (shift work and overtime hours per week), the three imbalances, and overcommitment, significant correlations were found with Poor Psychological Health: a higher effort-job promotion ratio (OR, 0.25; 95% CI, 0.09-0.70) and higher overcommitment (OR, 0.71; 95% CI, 0.62-0.81) (Table 6).

4.3 ERI and social relationship domain

We found no significant differences for age or work-related variables (work style, occupational status, shift work, and overtime hours per week) (Table 4). According to the stepwise logistic regression analyses between Social Relationship and the three imbalances and overcommitment, significant correlations were found with Poor Social Relationship: a higher effort-esteem ratio (OR, 0.31; 95% CI, 0.13-0.71) and higher overcommitment (OR, 0.86; 95% CI, 0.79-0.94) (Table 6).

4.4 ERI and environment domain

We found significant differences for work style and shift work between the two groups (Table 5). According to the subsequent stepwise logistic regression analyses between Environment and the work-related variables (work style and shift work), the three imbalances and overcommitment, significant correlations were found with Poor Environment: a higher effort-job promotion ratio (OR, 0.27; 95% CI, 0.11-0.64), higher overcommitment (OR, 0.85; 95% CI, 0.77-0.94), and shift work (OR, 1.99; 95% CI, 1.04-3.80) (Table 6).

5. Discussion

The four effort-reward ratios and overcommitment scores of the poor health functioning group were significantly higher than those of the good health group in the four domains of the WHOQOL (Table 2~5). Moreover, all the effort-reward ratios of the poor health functioning group were above 1, and therefore were defined as a high-risk condition for poor physical and mental health [19)].

The significant association between Physical Health or Psychological domains of the WHOQOL and the ERI was similar to previous findings among hospital staff members, including nurses in other countries[10,15,21)].

The strength of our study is also that we investigated in detail the independent contribution of the three ratios of effort-reward imbalance (effort-esteem imbalance, effort-job security imbalance and effort-job promotion imbalance) and overcommitment to health functioning measured by the WHOQOL. Physical Health, Psychological, and Environment domains of the WHOQOL were each significantly associated with a higher effort-job promotion ratio and higher scores of overcommitment (Table 6). Social Relationship domain was significantly associated with a higher effort-esteem ratio and higher scores of overcommitment (Table 6). According to Chandola et al., the ERI has been extended to include general and close social relationships, and lack of close social relationships was

	Poor Physical Health		Poor Psychological		Poor Social Relationship		Poor Environment	
	B	OR (95% CI)	B	OR (95% CI)	B	OR (95% CI)	B	OR (95% CI)
Effort–job promotion ratic	−1.42	0.24 (0.09–0.64)**	−1.40	0.25(0.09–0.70)**			−1.32	0.27(0.11–0.64)**
Effort–esteem ratio					−1.18	0.31(0.13–0.71)**		
Overcommitment	−0.32	0.64 (0.64–0.83)***	−0.34	0.71(0.62–0.81)***	−0.15	0.86(0.79–0.94)***	−0.17	0.85(0.77–0.94)**
Shift work							0.69	1.99(1.04–3.80)*
R2		0.47		0.46		0.19		0.32

Note: OR, odds ratio; 95% confidence intervals are shown in parentheses
*p < 0.05, **p < 0.01, ***p < 0.001

Table 6. Odds ratios of QOL domains by effort-reward imbalance and overcommitment.

associated with poorer health [2]. Social Relationship domain of the WHOQOL included three items: satisfaction with human relations, support from friends, and satisfaction with sex life. For our results, the association between effort-esteem imbalance and Social Relationship partially agreed with the findings of Chandola et al., possibly indicating that nurses with higher effort-esteem imbalance tend to be dissatisfied with their social relationships.

For work-related variables and the WHOQOL, only shift work was significantly associated with the Environment domain.

The present findings suggest that nurses must reduce subjective feelings of overcommitment. In addition, improving the work situation—for example, better promotion prospects, higher salaries, respect from supervisors, or reducing the burden of shift work—may improve the physical and mental health of nurses.

In this study, overcommitment was associated with all four domains of the WHOQOL. In accordance with previous studies[1,4,14,18], overcommitment is a set of attitudes, behaviors and emotions that reflect excessive work effort, and is combined with a strong desire for approval. Therefore, the overcommitment that many nurses experience may be reduced through mental health services such as group cognitive psychotherapy. Such interventions may improve immediate and long-term health functioning. In the future, investigations should be done to determine whether such mental health services actually improve health functioning among nurses through a reduction of overcommitment.

From the position of occupational health practitioners, it is possible to improve working conditions such as shift work, or respect from superiors. Concerning shift work, planning shift duty in an orderly manner (ie. morning shift → afternoon shift → night shift → morning shift) will reduce the burden of work shift. We may be able to educate the supervisors and administrators about issues related to mental health of nurses; the stressors or burden for nurses, respect to their skill or the adequate support in difficult situations.

Nevertheless, the present study has some limitations. First, the sample size was small and only one general hospital was surveyed. A larger sample should be examined in the future. Second, our results were inconclusive about the impact of ERI on health-related quality of life. We should conduct follow-up studies to investigate the change of health functioning through reduction of nurses' overcommitment or improvement of the effort-job promotion imbalance and effort-esteem imbalance.

In spite of the limitations, our findings provide insight into the factors influencing health functioning among nurses in the general hospital. From a practical point of view, our suggestion to reduce feelings of overcommitment among nurses may be valuable for professionals who care for hospital nurses, such as occupational health practitioners.

6. References

[1] Aust B, Peter R, Siegrist J. (1997) Stress Management in Bus Drivers: A Pilot Study Based on the Model of Effort-Reward Imbalance. Int J Stress Management 4(4), 297-305.

[2] Chandola T, Marmot M, Siegrist J (2007) Failed reciprocity in close social relationships and health: findings from the Whitehall II study. J Psychosom Res 63(4), 403-11.

[3] Eum KD, Li J, Lee HE, Kim SS, Paek D, Siegrist J, Cho SI. (2007) Psychometric properties of the Korean version of the effort-reward imbalance questionnaire: a study in a petrochemical company. Int Arch Occup Environ Health 80(8), 653-61.

[4] Irie M, Tsutsumi A, Kobayashi A. (2003) Effort-reward imbalance and workers' health in a period of structural economic change. Sangyo Igaku Journal 26, 69-74 (in Japanese).

[5] Kikuchi Y, Nakaya M, Ikeda M, Narita K., Takeda M, Nishi M. (2010) Effort-reward imbalance and depressive state in nurses. Occup.Med. 60, 231-233.

[6] Krause N, Rugulies R, Maslach C. (2010) Effort-reward imbalance at work and self-rated health of Las Vegas hotel room cleaners. Am J Ind Med 53(4), 372-86.

[7] Kudielka BM, Hanebuth D, von Kanel R, Gander ML, Grande G, Fischer JE (2005) Health related quality of life measured by the SF12 in working populations: associations with psychosocial work characteristics. J Occup Health Psychol 10, 429-40.

[8] Kuper H, Singh-Manoux A, Siegrst J, Marmot M (2002) When reciprocity fails: effort-reward imbalance in relation to coronary heart disease and health functioning within the Whitehall II study. Occup Environ Med. 59, 777-84

[9] Levine S, Croog SH. (1984) What constitutes quality of life? A conceptualization of the dimensions of life quality in healthy populations and patients with cardiovascular diease. In: Assessment of quality of life in clinical trials of cardivovascular therapies. Eds. by Wenger NK, Mattson ME, Furberg CD, Elinson J, 46-66, Lejacq Publications, New York, NY.

[10] Li J, Yong, W, & Cho, SI (2006) Gender differences in job strain, effort-reward imbalance, and health functioning among Chinese physicians. Soc Sci Med 62, 1066-77.

[11] Nasermoaddeli.A, Sekine.M, Hamanishi.S, and Kagamimori.S (2003) Associations between Sense of Coherence and Psychological Work Characteristics with Changes in Quality of Life in Japanese Civil Servants: A 1-Year Follow-Up Study. Industrial Health. 41,236-241

[12] Neril, Rocca Rey LA, Gallieni M, Brancaccio D, Cozzolono M, Colombi A, Burroughs TE. (2009) Occupational stress is associated with impaired work ability and reduced quality of life in patients with chronic kidney failure. Int J Artif Organs 32(5), 291-8

[13] Siegrist J, Starke D, Chandolo T, Godin I, Marmot M, Niedhammer I, Peter R. The measurement of effort-reward imbalance at work: European comparisons Soc Sci Med, 2004, 58(8):1483-1499

[14] Siegrist J (1996) Adverse health effects of high -effort/low-reward conditions. J Occup Health Psychol 1, 27-41.

[15] Silva AA, Souza JM, Borges FN, Fischer FM. (2010) Health-related quality of life and working conditions among nursing providers. Rev Saude Publica 44(4), 718-25.

[16] Stansfeld SA, Bosma H, Hemingway H, Marmot MG (1998) Psychosocial work characteristics and social support as predictors of SF-36 health functioning: the Whitehall II study. Psychosom Med. 60, 247-55.

[17] Tazaki M, Nakane Y (1997) WHOQOL-26 information. Kk. Kaneko Shobou, Tokyo (in Japanese).

[18] Tsutsumi A, Kayaba K, Nagami M, Miki A, Kawano Y, Ohya Y, Odagiri Y, & Shimomitsu T (2002) The Effort-Reward Imbalance Model: Experience in Japanese working population. J Occup Health 44, 398-407.

[19] Tsutsumi A, Ishitake T, Peter R, Siegrist J, & Matoba T (2001) The Japanese version of the Effort-Reward Imbalance Questionnaire: a study in dental technicians. Work Stress 15, 86-96.

[20] Watanabe M, Tanaka K, Aratake Y, Kato N, Sakata Y. (2008) The impact of effort-reward imbalance on quality of life among Japanese working men. Ind Health 46(3), 217-22.

[21] Weyers S, Peter R, Boggild H, Jeppesen HJ, & Sigtrist J. (2006) Psychosocial work stress is associated with poor self-rated health in Danish nurses: a test of the effort-reward imbalance model. Scand J Caring Sci 20, 26-34.

Section 2

Emotional and Trauma Related Conditions

5

Anxiety Disorder and Its Types

M. Shiri, S. Akhavan and N. Geramian
Vice-Chancellery for Health, Isfahan University of Medical Sciences, Isfahan, Iran

1. Introduction

As we know mind, body, and sprit are seen as equal parts of the whole. As we know the unity of the body, mind and spirit is quite complex. Mental imagery, entrainment theory, divinity theory, split- brain research, and beta-endorphins all approach the same unity, each from a different vantage point, and each supporting the ancient axiom that "all points connect". As the global village knock on your doorstep, insights from all over the world offer a multicultural approach to seeking and maintaining balance in our lives. As planetary citizens, we are not immune from change. Moreover, with change comes stress, humans are not immune from stress either. The importance of anxiety stems from the need to get a handle on this condition- to deal with anxiety effectively on so as to lead a "normal" and happy life. Many people's attitudes, influenced by their rushed lifestyles and expectations of immediate gratification, reflect the need to eradicate stress rather than to manage, reduce or control their perceptions of it. As a result, stress never really goes away; it just reappears with a new face.

Anxiety Disorders affect about 40 million American adults age 18 years and older (about 18%) in a given year, causing them to be filled with fearfulness and uncertainty. Neurotic disorders with anxiety as a prominent symptom are common: a recent British survey found that 16% of the population suffered from some form of pathological anxiety. Anxiety is one of a handful of core, negative affective states.

Anxiety represents a core phenomenon around which considerable psychiatric theory has been organized. Fear and anxiety can be conceptualizes as two key core negative emotions.

Unlike "fear", "anxiety" refers to brain states elicited by signals that predict impending but not immediately present danger. Thus unlike "fear", "anxiety" involves a more sustained change in the brain, manifest when a threat is still relatively removed from the organism in a spatial or temporal context. Anxiety" is considered an analogue of pathological reactions to danger in humans. On the other hand when an acute, proximal threat is particularly dangerous, the emotional state elicited in the organism might better be characterized as "panic" as opposed to" fear". In both the clinical and the community setting, the prevalence of anxiety disorders is among the most common of all mental disorders. Unlike the relatively mild, brief anxiety caused by a stressful event (such as speaking in public), anxiety disorders last at least 6 months and can get worse if they are not treated. Anxiety disorders commonly occur along with other mental or physical illnesses, including alcohol or substance abuse, which may mask anxiety symptoms or make them worse. In some cases, these other illnesses need to be treated before a person will respond to treatment for the anxiety disorder.

A preexisting anxiety disorder could be an independent risk factor for subsequent onset of suicidal ideation and attempts. Moreover, the data clearly demonstrate that comorbid anxiety disorders amplify the risk of suicide attempts in persons with mood disorders. Clinicians and policymakers need to be aware of these findings, and further research is required to delineate whether treatment of anxiety disorders reduces the risk of subsequent suicidal behavior.

Anxiety disorders are the most common of all mental health problems. It is estimated that they affect approximately 1 in 10 people. They are more prevalent among women than among men, and they affect children as well as adults. Anxiety disorders are illnesses. They can be diagnosed; they can be treated.

Individuals with childhood symptoms of anxiety and depression may have an increased tendency to use MDMA in adolescence or young adulthood. (MDMA 3,4-methylenedioxymethamphetamine- Ecstasy- is a synthetic, psychoactive drug that is chemically similar to the stimulant methamphetamine and the hallucinogen mescaline). Its effects are supposed to include enhanced feelings of bonding with other people, euphoria, or relaxation. Especially individuals with symptoms of anxiety or depression may be susceptible to these positive effects. Effective therapies for anxiety disorders are available, and research is uncovering new treatments that can help most people with anxiety disorders lead productive, fulfilling lives.

This chapter will describe the etiology, symptoms and effective treatments of anxiety disorders. The following anxiety disorders which are classified in DSM-IV-TR are discussed in this chapter:

- Panic disorder with and without agoraphobia,
- Agoraphobia with and without panic disorder
- Specific phobia
- Social phobia
- Obsessive-compulsive disorder
- Posttraumatic stress disorder
- Acute stress disorder and
- Generalized anxiety disorder

The purpose of this chapter is to provide an overview of the" anxiety disorder" and its types with emphasis on a psychological approach to these disorders.

2. Definitions

Definitions of anxiety in humans rest on the presence of impairment, a disruption in normal functioning, or the presence of "clinically significant" distress.

Stress: The experience of a perceived threat (real or imagined) to one's mental, physical, or spiritual well-being, resulting from a series of physiological responses and adaptations.

"Fear": It refers to the specific set of emotions or brain states that are elicited in an organism when it confronts danger. **Basic Human fears:**

Virtually anything can trigger fear. However, events or situations that elicit anxiety tend to fall into one of six categories:

Fear of failure: it is a conditioned response from a past experience wherein one's performance did not meet one's own expectations.

Fear of rejection: Anxious feelings of not meeting the expectations of others.

Fear of the unknown: Anxious feelings about uncertainty and future events.

Fear of death: Anxious feelings about death and the dying process.

Fear of isolation: Anxious feelings of being left alone.

Fear of the loss of self-dominance: Anxious feelings of losing control of life.

The "emotion" refers to the brain state associated with the perception of a motivationally salient stimulus, a stimulus that creates a need for the organism to act. **"Fear"** refers to the specific set of emotions or brain states that are elicited in an organism when it confronts danger. Different forms of danger elicit different neural responses and associated differences in information processing and behavior. The term **"danger"** refers to any stimulus or situation that is capable of producing harm to the organism. The act of encountering a specifically dangerous object, such as a predator, can be conceptualized as a threat. **"Threats"** and "dangerous scenarios" can also be conceptualized as **"punishments".**

Despite the importance of self-reported feeling states in research, self reported feeling states must not be confused with emotions per se. The term **"emotion"** does not refer to a self-report but rather to a stimulus -evoked brain state, along with changes in behavior or physiology.

3. Clinical features of anxiety disorders

The history of anxiety, increased anxiety sensitivity (the fear of anxiety related sensations), and increased neuroticism are significant predictors. The trend level support for assertiveness is a predictor of anxiety onset. However, history of anxiety and anxiety sensitivity provides unique prediction.

Each anxiety disorder has different symptoms, but all the symptoms cluster around excessive, irrational fear and dread.

Anxiety is a universal and generally adaptive response to a threat, but in certain circumstances it can become maladaptive. Characteristics that distinguish abnormal from adaptive anxiety include:

- Anxiety out of proportion to the level of threat
- Persistence or deterioration without intervention (> 3 weeks)
- Symptoms that are unacceptable regardless of the level of threat, including
- Recurrent panic attacks
- Severe physical symptoms

- Abnormal believes such as thoughts of sudden death
- Disruption of usual or desirable functioning

Anxiety disorders should be differentiated from stress reactions, in which anxiety may be a prominent feature. These include acute stress reactions–a rapid response (in minutes or hours) to sudden stressful life events, leading to anxiety with autonomic arousal and some disorientation–and adjustment reactions–slower responses to life events (such as divorce) that occur days or weeks later as symptoms of anxiety, irritability, and depression (without biological symptoms). These are generally self limiting and are helped by reassurance, ventilation, and problem solving. Although there is considerable overlap between the various anxiety disorders, it is important to make a diagnosis as they have different optimal treatments. Extreme fear or apprehension can be considered "clinical anxiety" if it is developmentally inappropriate to an individual's life circumstances (e.g. fear of separation in a 12-year-old child) or if it is inappropriate to an individual's life circumstances' (e.g. worries about supporting one's family in a successful businessman). The clinical decision making rests heavily on clinical judgments about impairment and distress. Panic disorder is associated with reductions in total occipital cortex GABA levels. (Gamma-Amino Butyric acid -GABA-is an amino acid which acts as a neurotransmitter in the central nervous system). This abnormality might contribute to the pathophysiology of panic disorder. Patients with Panic disorder (PD) or generalized anxiety disorder (GAD) are more sensitive to bodily changes than nonanxious individuals, and patients with PD are more sensitive than those with GAD. Patients with PD experience more frequent distress than those with GAD, but their physiologic responses are comparable in intensity. The findings suggest that the perception of panic attacks reflects central rather than peripheral responses. The diminished autonomic flexibility observed in both anxiety conditions may result from dysfunctional information processing during heightened anxiety that fails to discriminate between anxiety-related and neutral inputs. The current versions of both the Diagnostic and Statistical Manual of Mental Disorders (DSM) and the World Health Organization's International Statistical Classification of Diseases and Related Health Problems (ICD-10) recognize similar groups of anxiety-related syndromes as discrete diagnostic entities. Doctors often consider anxiety to be a normal response to physical illness. Yet, anxiety afflicts only a minority of patients and tends not to be prolonged. Any severe or persistent anxious response to physical illness merits further assessment.

4. Panic disorder and agoraphobia

Recurrent "panic attacks" represent the hallmark feature of panic disorder. Classically, panic attacks are characterized by rapid onset-within minutes - and short duration -usually less than 10 to 15 minutes. The presence of lifetime panic spectrum symptoms in some patients with BPI (Bipolar type I) disorder is associated with greater levels of depression, more suicidal ideation, and a marked (6-month) delay in time to remission with acute treatment. Alternate treatment strategies are needed for patients with BPI disorder who endorse lifetime panic spectrum features. Although the major societal burden of panic is caused by PD and Panic attack without agoraphobia (PA-AG), isolated PAs also have high prevalence and meaningful role impairment.

Panic attack is an episode of abrupt intense fear accompanied by at least four of the autonomic or cognitive symptoms such as palpitations, pounding heart, or accelerated heart rate, sweating, trembling or shaking, sensations of shortness of breath or smothering, feeling of choking, chest pain or discomfort, nausea or abdominal distress, feeling dizzy, unsteady, lightheaded, or faint, derealization (feelings of unreality) or depersonalization (being detached from oneself), fear of losing control or going crazy, fear of dying, paresthesias and chills or hot flashes.

Whole-body and regional sympathetic nervous activity are not elevated at rest in patients with panic disorder. Contrary to popular belief, the sympathetic nervous system is not globally activated during panic attacks.

DSM-IV-TR recognizes three types of panic attacks:

a) Spontaneous or unexpected panic attacks occur without cue or warning. b) Situationally bound attacks occur in the presence of a situational trigger, such as a spider. And c) Situationally predisposed panic attacks both occur on exposure to or in anticipation of exposure to a feared stimulus, and increases by an environmental cue, but does not inevitably precipitate one.

In some young adults with low levels of lead exposure, higher blood lead levels were associated with increased odds of major depression and panic disorders. Exposure to lead at levels generally considered safe could result in adverse mental health outcomes.

A panic disorder diagnosis requires the presence of at least two spontaneous panic attacks at some point. At least one of these attacks must be associated with concern about additional attacks, worry about attacks, or changes in behavior. Agoraphobia is comorbid condition of panic disorder. Agoraphobia refers to fear of or anxiety regarding places from which escape might be difficult in the event of a panic attack or panic symptoms. Agoraphobia can occur independent of a history of panic. Like most anxiety disorders, panic disorder often co-occurs with mental conditions beside agoraphobia, particularly other anxiety and depressive disorders. These include specific and social phobias, generalized anxiety disorder, and major depressive disorder. The comorbid mental conditions frequently compound panic disorder as it occurs in the community. The current edition of the ICD (ICD-10) de-emphasizes the relationship between panic disorder and agoraphobia, instead classifying agoraphobia as one of many panic disorders.

Differential Diagnosis: This condition must be differentiated from a number of medical conditions that produce similar symptomatology such as: Hypothyroid state, Hyperthyroid state, Hyperparathyroidism, Pheochromocytomas, Hypoglycemia associated with insulinomas, Primary neuropathlogical processes such as seizure disorders, vestibular dysfunction, neoplasms, and effects of substances on CNS, and some disorders of the cardiac and pulmonary systems such as asthma. The key to correctly diagnosing panic disorder and differentiating the condition from other anxiety disorders involves documenting recurrent spontaneous panic attacks at some point in the illness.

Epidemiology: The lifetime prevalence of panic disorder is in the 1 to 4 percent range, with 6-month prevalence approximately 0.5 to 1 percent. Estimates of agoraphobia prevalence vary from 2 to 6 percent across studies.

Course: Panic disorder typically has its onset in late adolescence or early adulthood, panic disorder tends to exhibit a fluctuating course.

5. Phobias

The term "phobia" refers to an excessive fear of a specific object circumstance, or situation. They are classified based on the nature of the feared object or situation, and DSM-IV -TR recognizes three distinct classes of phobia: Agoraphia (which is considered to relate closely to panic disorder), specific phobia and social phobia. Both specific and social phobia require the development of intense anxiety.

Specific phobia: There are four primary subtypes of specific phobias (animal type, natural environment type, bleed - injury type, and situational type) along with a residual category for phobias that do not clearly fit any of these four categories. The key feature of each type of phobia is that fear symptoms occur only in the presence of a specific object.

Specific phobia often involves fears of multiple objects, particularly objects that cluster within a specific subcategory.

In the clinical setting, specific phobia often co- occur with other anxiety or mood disorder. Impairment associated with specific phobia typically manifests as restricted social or professional activities.

Social Phobia: According to DSM -IV- TR criteria, social phobia or "social anxiety disorder" involves the fear of social situation, including situations that involve scrutiny or contact with strangers. In social anxiety disorder, social phobia represents a distinct condition, in terms of course, treatment, and patterns of comorbidity, from specific phobias. Individuals with social phobia typically fear embarrassing themselves in social situations, such as at social new gathering, during oral presentations, or when meeting new people. They may have specific fears about performing certain activities, such as speaking or eating in front of others. The anxiety which appears in social situations becomes social phobia when the anxiety either prevents an individual from participating in desired activities or causes marked distress during such activities. The ICD has a similar approach to categorizing phobias as in DSM-IV-TR.

Approximately 10 percent of individuals in the United States meet criteria for specific phobia. The condition is more commonly diagnosed in females than males. Prevalence estimates of social phobia vary widely, from 2 to 15 percent.

Social phobia tends to have its onset in late childhood or early adolescence. Social phobia is typically chronic.

6. Obsessive-Compulsive Disorder (OCD)

Obsessive-compulsive disorder can occur at any age but most often presents for the first time in adolescence. Long delays in diagnosis often occur. Practitioners should ask specific screening questions if obsessive-compulsive disorder is suspected. The prevalence of OCD is 2 to 3 percent and is equal for males and females.

Symptomatology

Obsessions and compulsions are the essential features of OCD, and an individual must exhibit either or both of them to meet the criteria. DSM-IV-TR recognizes obsessions as "persistent ideas, thoughts, impulses, or images that are experienced as intrusive and inappropriate" and cause distress. Neuropsychological deficits were observed in patients with OCD that were not observed in matched patients with panic disorder or unipolar depression. As such, the cognitive dysfunction in OCD appears to be related to the specific illness processes associated with the disorder. Obsessions are anxiety provoking, which is why OCD is classified as an anxiety disorder. But they differ qualitatively from excessive worries about real-life problems. Typical obsessions associated with OCD include thoughts about contamination or doubts. In addition, anxiety- provoking thoughts must be associated with efforts to either ignore or suppress them.

Compulsions are defined as repetitive acts, behaviors, or thoughts that are designed to counteract the anxiety associated with an obsession. The key characteristic of a compulsion is that it reduces the anxiety associated with the obsession. Many compulsions are acts associated with specific obsessions, such as hand washing to counteract thoughts of contamination. Compulsions can also manifest as thoughts. Obsessions and compulsions must cause an individual marked distress, consume **at least 1 hour/day** of time, or interfere with functioning to be considered as OCD. During at least some point in the illness, adult patients must recognize symptoms of OCD as unreasonable, although there is great variability in the degree to which this is true, both across individuals and in a given individual over time. DSM-IV-TR recognizes a " poor insight" subtype of OCD in which individuals fail to recognize the irrational or unreasonable nature of their obsessions. OCD frequently co-occurs with other disorders such as major depression, panic disorder, phobias, attention -deficit/hyperactivity disorder (ADHD), eating disorders, and Tourette,s syndrome.

ICD-10 emphasizes that a compulsive act must not be pleasurable. ICD-10 also stipulates that obsessions or compulsions must be present on most days for 2 weeks.

Inflated responsibility is increasingly regarded a pathogenetic mechanism in obsessive-compulsive disorder. In seeming contrast, there is mounting evidence that latent aggression is also elevated in OCD. Building upon psychodynamic theories that an altruistic facade including exaggerated concerns for others is partly a defense against latent aggression. Evidence was recently obtained for high interpersonal ambivalence in (OCD) patients relative to psychiatric and healthy controls. Psychotic symptoms often lead to obsessive thoughts and compulsive behaviors.

Differential Diagnosis: some primary medical disorders can produce syndromes with resemblance to OCD. Some of the diseases of basal ganglia produce OCD like disorders, diseases such as Sydenham,s chorea and Huntington,s disease. OCD exhibits a superficial resemblance to obsessive -compulsive personality disorder, which is associated with an obsessive concern for details, perfectionism, and similar personality traits. Only OCD is associated with a true syndrome of obsessions and compulsions. Sometimes OCD can be difficult to differentiate from depression. The two conditions are best distinguished by their courses.

OCD typically begins in late adolescence. Small minorities of patients exhibit either complete remission of their disorder or a progressive, deteriorating course.

7. Posttraumatic stress and acute stress disorders

The prevalence of posttraumatic stress disorder (PTSD) is 2 to 15 percent in the community. It is persistent or chronic in 10 to 25 percent of patients with the disorder.

Symptomatology

Both PTSD and acute stress disorder are characterized by the onset of psychiatric symptoms immediately following exposure to a traumatic event. DSM-IV-TR explicitly notes that such a traumatic event must involve experiencing or witnessing events that involve actual or threatened death or injury or threats to the physical integrity of oneself or others. The response to the traumatic event must involve intense fear or horror. Such traumatic events include a violent accident or crime, military combat, or assault, being kidnapped, being involved in natural disasters and so on. The greater the proximity and intensity of the trauma, the greater is the probability that an individual will develop symptoms. Symptoms are in three domains: Reexperiencing the trauma, avoiding stimuli associated with the trauma, and experiencing symptoms of increased autonomic arousal, such as an enhanced startle. Flashbacks, in which the individual may act and feel as if the trauma is recurring, represent the classic form of reexperiencing. Symptoms of avoidance include: efforts to avoid thoughts or activities related to the trauma, anhedonia, reduced capacity to remember events related to the trauma, blunted affect, feelings of detachment or de-realization, and a sense of a foreshortened future. A patient must exhibit at least three such symptoms. Symptoms of increased arousal include insomnia, irritability, hypervigilance, and exaggerated startle. A patient must exhibit at least two such symptoms. The diagnosis of PTSD is only made when symptoms persist for at least 1 month; the diagnosis of acute stress disorder is made in the interim. Acute PTSD refers to an episode that lasts less than 3 months. Chronic PTSD refers to an episode lasting 3 months or longer. PTSD with delayed onset refers to an episode that develops 6 months or more after exposure to the traumatic event. The diagnosis of acute stress disorder is applied to syndromes that resemble PTSD but last less that 1 month after a trauma. Acute stress disorder is characterized by re-experiencing, avoidance, and increased arousal, much like PTSD.

Acute stress disorder is also associated with at least three of the dissociative symptoms such as:

1. A subjective sense of numbing, detachment, or absence of emotional responsiveness.
2. A reduction in awareness of his /her surroundings.
3. Derealization
4. Depersonalization and
5. Dissociative amnesia (i.e. inability to recall an important aspect of the trauma).

ICD-10 groups PTSD and acute stress reaction in a distinct category -"stress-related disorders" –rather than group them with other anxiety disorders.

Differential Diagnosis: Neurological injury following head trauma, psychoactive substance use disorders or withdrawal syndromes can contribute to clinical presentation of PTSD. Symptoms of panic disorder or generalized anxiety disorder could be similar to those of PTSD. PTSD must be differentiated from major depression, borderline personality disorder, dissociative disorders, and factitious disorders.

8. Generalized anxiety disorder

Generalized anxiety disorder (GAD) is a syndrome of ongoing anxiety and worry about many events or thoughts that the patient generally recognizes as excessive and inappropriate. Most people with GAD also have other mood and anxiety disorders. About 1%-5% of the general population report having GAD. Many of these people also have other disorders, and those with GAD report a considerable level of disability. Long term follow-up studies suggest that GAD is a condition that worsens the prognosis for any other condition, and that people who have only GAD are likely to develop further conditions. People with symptoms of generalized anxiety disorder tend to always expect disaster and can't stop worrying about health, money, family, work, or school. In people with GAD, the worry often is unrealistic or out of proportion for the situation. Daily life becomes a constant state of worry, fear, and dread. Eventually, the anxiety so dominates the person's thinking that it interferes with daily functioning, including work, school, social activities, and relationship.

Symptomatology: GAD is characterized by a pattern of frequent, persistent worry and anxiety that is disproportionate to the impact of the events or circumstances on which the worry focuses. These patients must be bothered by their degree of worry. This pattern must occur "more days than not" for at least 6 months. They find it difficult to control their worry and must report three or more of six somatic or cognitive symptoms, which include: feelings of restlessness, fatigue, muscle tension, or insomnia. Worry is a common characteristic of a variety of anxiety disorders: patients with panic disorder worry about panic attacks, patients with OCD worry about their obsessions. The worries in GAD must exceed in breath or scope the worries that characterize these other anxiety disorders. Children with marked and persistent worry can also be diagnosed with GAD; unlike adults, however, they must only meet one of the six somatic/ cognitive symptom criteria.

Prior to DSM-III, panic disorder and GAD were both subsumed under the broader category of anxiety neurosis.

GAD can be seen in all clinical settings, and in primary care. Practitioners are usually good at identifying GAD patients.

More work is needed to elucidate the potentially unique aspects of pathways and mechanisms involved in the etiopathogenesis of GAD.

Differential Diagnosis: Panic disorder, phobias, OCD and PTSD should be differentiated from GAD. Criteria for GAD include pervasive and lasting worry and associated symptoms. Patients with GAD frequently develop major depressive disorder. The prevalence of GAD ranges from 2 to 5 percent and is more common in men than women. Survival analyses reveal that the factors associated with GAD overlap more strongly with those specific to anxiety disorders than those specific to depressive disorders. In addition, GAD differs from anxiety and depressive disorders with regard to family climate and personality profiles. Hence anxiety and depressive disorders appear to differ with regard to risk constellations and temporal longitudinal patterns, and GAD is a heterogeneous disorder that is, overall, more closely related to other anxiety disorders than to depressive disorders.

9. Other anxiety disorders

I) Anxiety Disorder Not Otherwise Specified (NOS).

It is relatively common to encounter patients who do not meet criteria for any of the disorders discussing in this chapter. These patients are classified as suffering from Anxiety Disorder NOS. Two clinical Features of this disorder are:

1. The anxiety described by the patients must be distressing and interfere with some aspect of functioning.
2. The anxiety must not be attributable to another psychiatric condition.

II) Substance- Induced Anxiety and Anxiety Due to a General Medical Condition.

These conditions are characterized by prominent anxiety that arises as the direct result of some underlying physiological perturbation. For patients with substance– induced anxiety, clinically significant symptoms of panic, worry, phobia or obsessions emerge in the context of the use of either prescribed or illicit substances. The first step in identifying an anxiety disorder due to either a medical condition or substance is to confirm the presence of one or the other complicating factor.

10. Treatment

10.1 Obsessive-Compulsive Disorder (OCD)

10.1.1 Pharmacotherapy

The efficacy of pharmacotherapy in OCD has been proved in many clinical trials and is enhanced by the observation that the studies find a placebo response rate of only about 5 percent.

The drugs, some of which are used to treat depressive disorders or mental disorders, can be given in their usual dosage ranges. Initial effects are generally seen after 4 to 6 weeks of treatment, although 8 to 16 weeks are usually needed to obtain maximal therapeutic benefit. Treatment with antidepressant drugs is still controversial and significant proportion of patients with OCD who respond to treatment with antidepressant drugs seem to relapse if the drug therapy is discontinued.

The standard approach is to start treatment with an SSRI or Clomipramine and then move to other pharmacological strategies if the serotonin- specific drugs are not effective. The serotonergic drugs have increased the percentage of patients with OCD who are likely to respond to treatment to the range of 50 to 70 percent.

Serotonin- Specific Reuptake Inhibitors (SSRIs)- The usual SSRIs available are: - Fluoxetine (Prozac), Fluvoxamine (Luvox), Paroxetine (Paxil) and Sertraline (Zoloft). Citalopram (Celexa) has been approved by the US Food and Drug Administration (FDA) for the treatment of OCD. Higher dosages have often been necessary for a beneficial effect, such as 80 mg a day of fluoxetine. Although the SSRIs can cause sleep disturbance, nausea and diarrhea, headache, anxiety, and restlessness, these adverse effects are often transient and are generally less troubling than the adverse effects associated with tricyclic drugs, such as Clomipramine. The best clinical outcomes occur when SSRIs are used in combination with **behavioral therapy**.

Clomipramine- Of all the tricyclic drugs, clomipramine is the most selective for serotonin reuptake versus norepinephrine reuptake and is exceeded in this respect only by the SSRIs. The potency of serotonin reuptake of clomipramine is exceeded only by sertraline and paroxetine. Clomipramine was the first drug to be FAD approved for the treatment of OCD. Its dosing must be titrated upward over 2 to 3 weeks to avoid gastrointestinal adverse effects and orthostatic hypotension, and as with other tricyclic drugs, it causes significant sedation and anticholinergic effects, including dry mouth.

If treatment with Clomipramine or an SSRI is unsuccessful, many therapists augment the first drug by the addition of Valproate (Depakene), lithium (Eskalith), or carbamazepine (Tegretol). Other drugs that can be tried in the treatment of OCD are venlafaxine (Effexor), pindolol (Visken), and the monoamine oxidase inhibitors (MAOIs) especially phenelzine (Nardil). Other pharmacological agents for treatment of unresponsive patients include buspirone (BuSpar), l-tryptophan,

5-hydroxyptamine (5-HT) and clonazepam (Klonopin). Adding an atypical antipsychotic such as risperidol has helped in some cases.

10.1.2 Cognitive-behavioral therapy

This form of therapy for obsessive-compulsive disorder involves some components:

Exposure and response prevention

It involves repeated exposure of patient to the source of obsession. Then is asked to refrain from the compulsive behavior usually perform to reduce his/her anxiety. For example, if he/she is a compulsive hand washer, might be asked to touch the door handle in a public restroom and then be prevented from washing. As he/she sits with the anxiety, the urge to wash hands will gradually begin to go away on its own. In this way, he/she learns that he/she does not need the ritual to get rid of anxiety—that he/she has some control over his/her obsessive thoughts and compulsive behaviors.

Cognitive therapy focuses on the catastrophic thoughts and exaggerated sense of responsibility. A big part of cognitive therapy for OCD is teaching healthy and effective ways of responding to obsessive thoughts, without resorting to compulsive behavior.

Four Steps for Conquering Symptoms of Obsessive-Compulsive Disorder:

Relabel - Recognize that the intrusive obsessive thoughts and urges are the result of OCD. For example, train yourself to say, "I don't think or feel that my hands are dirty. I'm having an obsession that my hands are dirty." Or, "I don't feel that I have the need to wash my hands. I'm having a compulsive urge to perform the compulsion of washing my hands."

Reattribute - Realize that the intensity and intrusiveness of the thought or urge is caused by OCD; it is probably related to a biochemical imbalance in the brain. Tell yourself, "It's not me—it's my OCD," to remind you that OCD thoughts and urges are not meaningful, but are false messages from the brain.

Refocus - Work around the OCD thoughts by focusing your attention on something else, at least for a few minutes. Do another behavior. Say to yourself, "I'm experiencing a symptom of OCD. I need to do another behavior."

Revalue – Do not take the OCD thought at face value. It is not significant in itself. Tell yourself, "That's just my stupid obsession. It has no meaning. That's just my brain. There's no need to pay attention to it." Remember: You can't make the thought go away, but neither do you need to pay attention to it. You can learn to go on to the next behavior.

Family therapy for OCD treatment- Because OCD often causes problems in family life and social adjustment, family therapy can often be beneficial.

Group therapy for OCD treatment- Through interaction with fellow OCD sufferers, group therapy provides support and encouragement and decreases feelings of isolation.

Self-help for OCD:

1. Challenge obsessive thoughts and compulsive behaviors

- **Learn to recognize and reduce stress-** If you have OCD, there are many ways you can help yourself in addition to seeking therapy.
- **Refocus your attention-** When you're experiencing OCD thoughts and urges, try shifting your attention to something else.

You could exercise, jog, walk, listen to music, read, surf the web, play a video game, make a phone call, or knit. The important thing is to do something you enjoy for at least 15 minutes, in order to delay your response to the obsessive thought or compulsion.

At the end of the delaying period, reassess the urge. In many cases, the urge will no longer be quite as intense.

Try delaying for a longer period. The longer you can delay the urge, the more it will likely change.

- **Write down your obsessive thoughts or worries-** Keep a pad and pencil on you, or type on a laptop, Smartphone, or tablet. When you begin to obsess, write down all your thoughts or compulsions.

Keep writing as the OCD urges continue, aiming to record exactly what you're thinking, even if you're repeating the same phrases or the same urges over and over.

Writing it all down will help you see just how repetitive your obsessions are.

Writing down the same phrase or urge hundreds of times will help it lose its power.

Writing thoughts down is much harder work than simply thinking them, so your obsessive thoughts are likely to disappear sooner.

- **Anticipate OCD urges-** By anticipating your compulsive urges before they arise, you can help to ease them. For example, if your compulsive behavior involves checking that doors are locked, windows closed, or appliances turned off, try to lock the door or turn off the appliance with extra attention the first time.

Create a solid mental picture and then make a mental note. Tell yourself, "The window is now closed," or "I can see that the oven is turned off."

When the urge to check arises later, you will find it easier to relabel it as "just an obsessive thought."

- **Create an OCD worry period-** Rather than trying to suppress obsessions or compulsions, develop the habit of rescheduling them.

Choose one or two 10 minute "worry periods" each day, time you can devote to obsessing.

During your worry period, focus only on negative thoughts or urges. Don't try to correct them. At the end of the worry period, take a few calming breaths, let the obsessive thoughts or urges go, and return to your normal activities. The rest of the day, however, is to be designated free of obsessions and compulsions.

When thoughts or urges come into your head during the day, write them down and "postpone" them to your worry period. Save it for later and continue to go about your day.

Go over your "worry list" during the worry period. Reflect on the thoughts or urges you wrote down during the day. If the thoughts are still bothering you, allow yourself to obsess about them, but only for the amount of time you've allotted for your worry period.

- **Create a tape of your OCD obsessions-** Focus on one specific worry or obsession and record it to a tape recorder, laptop, or smartphone.

Recount the obsessive phrase, sentence, or story exactly as it comes into your mind.

Play the tape back to yourself, over and over for a 45-minute period each day, until listening to the obsession no longer causes you to feel highly distressed.

By continuously confronting your worry or obsession you will gradually become less anxious. You can then repeat the exercise for a different obsession.

2. **Take care of yourself-** A healthy, balanced lifestyle plays a big role in keeping OCD behavior, fears, and worry at bay.

Practice relaxation techniques- While stress doesn't cause OCD, a stressful event can trigger the onset of obsessive and compulsive behavior, and stress can often make obsessive-compulsive behavior worse.

Mindful meditation, yoga, deep breathing, and other stress-relief techniques may help reduce the symptoms of anxiety brought on by OCD. Try to practice a relaxation technique for at least 30 minutes a day.

Adopt healthy eating habits- Start the day right with breakfast, and continue with frequent small meals throughout the day. Going too long without eating leads to low blood sugar, which can make you feel more anxious.

Eat plenty of complex carbohydrates such as whole grains, fruits, and vegetables. Not only do complex carbs stabilize blood sugar, they also boost serotonin, a neurotransmitter with calming effects.

Exercise regularly- Exercise is a natural and effective anti-anxiety treatment that helps to control OCD symptoms by refocusing your mind when obsessive thoughts and compulsions arise.

For maximum benefit, try to get 30 minutes or more of aerobic activity on most days. Aerobic exercise relieves tension and stress, boosts physical and mental energy, and enhances well-being through the release of endorphins, the brain's feel-good chemicals.

Also Exercise training reduces anxiety symptoms among sedentary patients who have a chronic illness.

Avoid alcohol and nicotine- Alcohol temporarily reduces anxiety and worry, but it actually causes anxiety symptoms as it wears off. Similarly, while it may seem that cigarettes are calming, nicotine is actually a powerful stimulant. Smoking leads to higher, not lower, levels of anxiety and OCD symptoms.

Get enough sleep- Not only can anxiety and worry cause insomnia, but a lack of sleep can also exacerbate anxious thoughts and feelings. When you're well rested, it's much easier to keep your emotional balance, a key factor in coping with anxiety disorders such as OCD.

3. **Reach out for support-** OCD can get worse when you feel powerless and alone, so it's important to build a strong support system. The more connected you are to other people, the less vulnerable you'll feel. Just talking about your worries and urges can make them seem less threatening.

Stay connected to family and friends- Obsessions and compulsions can consume your life to the point of social isolation. In turn, social isolation can aggravate your OCD symptoms. It's important to have a network of family and friends you can turn to for help and support. Involving others in your treatment can help guard against setbacks and keep you motivated.

Join an OCD support group- You're not alone in your struggle with OCD, and participating in a support group can be an effective reminder of that. OCD support groups enable you to both share your own experiences and learn from others who are facing the same problems.

Helping a loved one with OCD- If a friend or family member has OCD, your most important job is to educate yourself about the disorder. Share what you've learned with your loved one and let them know that there is help available. Simply knowing that OCD is treatable can sometimes provide enough motivation for your loved one to seek help.

11. Generalized anxiety disorder (GAD) treatment

11.1 Pharmacotherapy

The decision to prescribe an anxiolytic to patients with GAD should rarely be made on the first visit. Because of the long-term nature of the disorder, a treatment plan must be carefully thought out. The major drugs to be considered for the treatment of GAD are benzodiazepines, the serotoand the nin-specific reuptake inhibitors (SSRIs) , buspirone (BuSpar), and venlafaxine (Effexor). Other drugs that may be useful are the tricyclic drugs(e.g., imipramine [Tofranil]), antihistamines, ß-adrenergic antagonists (e.g., propranolol [Inderal]).

Although drug treatment of GAD is sometimes seen as a 6-to 12-month treatment. Some evidence indicates that treatment should be long term, perhaps lifelong. About 25 percent of patients in the first month after the discontinuation of therapy, and 60 to 80 percent relapse over the course of the next year. Although some patients become dependent on the benzodiazepines, tolerance rarely develops to the therapeutic effects of the benzodiazepines, buspirone, venlafaxine, or the SSRIs.

Benzodiazepines- Benzodiazepines have been the drugs of choice for GAD. They can be prescribed on as- needed basis, so that patients take a rapidly acting benzodiazepine when they feel particularly anxious. The alternative approach is to prescribe benzodiazepines for a limited period, during which psychosocial therapeutic approaches are implemented.

Several problems are associated with the use of benzodiazepines in GAD. About 25 to 30 percent of all patients fail to respond, and tolerance and dependence can occur. Some patients also experience impaired alertness while taking the drugs and, therefore, are at risk for accidents involving automobiles and machinery.

The clinical decision to initiate treatment with a benzodiazepine should be considered and specific. The patient's diagnosis, the specific target symptoms, and the duration of treatment should all be defined, and the information should be shared with the patient. Treatment for most anxiety conditions lasts for 2 to 6 weeks, followed by 1 or 2 weeks of tapering drug use before it is discontinued. The most common clinical mistake with benzodiazepine treatment is routinely to continue treatment indefinitely.

For the treatment of anxiety, it is usual to begin giving a drug at the low end of its therapeutic range and to increase the dosage to achieve a therapeutic response. The use of a benzodiazepine with an intermediate half-life (8 to 18 hours) will likely avoid some of the adverse effects associated with the use of benzodiazepines with long half-lives, and the use of divided doses prevents the development of adverse effects associated with high peak plasma levels. The improvement produced by benzodiazepines may go beyond a simple anti-anxiety effect. For example, the drugs may cause patients to regard various occurrences in a positive light. The drugs can also have a mild dis-inhibiting action, similar to that observed after ingesting modest amounts of alcohol.

Buspirone- Buspirone is a 5-HT1A receptor partial agonist and is most likely effective in 60 to 80 percent of patients with GAD. Data indicate that buspirone is more effective in reducing the cognitive symptoms of generalized anxiety disorder than in reducing the somatic symptoms. Evidence also indicates that patients who have previously had treatment with benzodiazepines are not likely to respond to treatment with buspirone. The lack of response may be caused by the absence, with buspirone treatment, of some of the nonanxietyolytic effects of benzodiazepines. The major disadvantage of buspirone is that its effects take 2 t0 3 weeks to become evident, in contrast to the almost immediate anxietyolytic effects of the benzodiazepines. One approach is to initiate benzodiazepine and buspirone use simultaneously, then taper off the buspirone use after2 to 3 weeks, at which point the buspirone should have reached its maximal effects. Some studies have also reported that long-term in combined treatment with benzodiazepine and buspirone may be more effective than either drug alone. Buspirone is not an effective treatment for benzodiazepine withdrawal.

Venlafaxine- Venlafaxine is effective in treating the insomnia, poor concentration, restlessness, irritability, and excessive muscle tension associated with GAD. Venlafaxine is a nonselective inhibitor of the reuptake of three biogenic amines - serotonin, and, to a lesser extent, dopamine.

Selective Serotonin Reuptake Inhibitors -SSRIs may be effective, especially for patients with comorbid depression. The prominent Disadvantage of SSRIs, especially fluoxetine (Prozac), is that they can transiently increase anxiety and cause agitated states. For this reason, the SSRIs sertraline (Zoloft), citalopram (Celexa), or paroxetine (Paxil) are better choices in patients with high anxiety disorder. It is reasonable to begin treatment with sertraline, citalopram, or paroxetine plus a benzodiazepine, then to taper benzodiazepine use after 2 to 3 weeks. Further studies are needed to determine whether SSRIs are as effective for GAD as they are for panic disorder and OCD.

Other Drugs- If conventional pharmacological treatment (e.g., with buspirone or a benzodiazepine) is ineffective or not completely effective , then a clinical reassessment is indicated to rule comorbid conditions, such as depression, or to better understand patient's environmental stresses. Other drugs that have proved useful for generalizes anxiety disorder include the tricyclic and tetracyclic drugs. The ß-adrenergic receptor antagonists may reduce the somatic manifestations of anxiety, but not the underlying condition, and their use usually limited to situational anxieties, such as performance anxiety.

Treatment of GAD with an antidepressant should be continued for at least 12 months. Preliminary data demonstrate that improved patients who relapse while off their anti-anxiety medication after at least 6 months of treatment will again most likely respond to a second course of treatment with the same medication.

11.2 Psychotherapy

1. **Look at your worries in new ways-** The core symptom of GAD is chronic worrying. It's important to understand what worrying is, since the belief you hold about worrying play a huge role in triggering and maintaining GAD.

Understanding worrying- You may feel like your worries come from the outside—from other people, events that stress you out, or difficult situations you're facing. But, in fact, worrying is self-generated. The trigger comes from the outside, but an internal running dialogue maintains the anxiety itself.

When you're worrying, you're talking to yourself about things you're afraid of or negative events that might happen. You run over the feared situation in your mind and think about all the ways you might deal with it. In essence, you're trying to solve problems that haven't happened yet, or worse, simply obsessing on worst-case scenarios. All this worrying may give you the impression that you're protecting yourself by preparing for the worst or avoiding bad situations. But more often than not, worrying is unproductive, sapping your mental and emotional energy without resulting in any concrete problem-solving strategies or actions.

How to distinguish between productive and unproductive worrying? If you're focusing on **"what if"** scenarios, your worrying is unproductive. Once you've given up the idea that your worrying somehow helps you, you can start to deal with your worry and anxiety in more productive ways. This may involve challenging irrational worrisome thoughts, learning how to postpone worrying, and learning to accept uncertainty in your life.

Self-help strategies for chronic worriers- Have fears and "what ifs" taken over your life? Is your worrying out of control? The good news is that chronic worrying is a mental habit you can learn how to break. You can teach yourself to stay calm and collected and to look at your fears from a more balanced perspective.

2. **Practice relaxation techniques-** Anxiety is more than just a feeling. It's the body's physical "fight or flight" reaction to a perceived threat. Your heart pounds, you breathe

faster, your muscles tense up, and you feel light-headed. When you're relaxed, the complete opposite happens. Your heart rate slows down, you breathe slower and more deeply, your muscles relax, and your blood pressure stabilizes. Since it's impossible to be anxious and relaxed at the same time, strengthening your body's relaxation response is a powerful anxiety-relieving tactic.

If you struggle with GAD, relaxation techniques such as progressive muscle relaxation, deep breathing, and meditation can teach you how to relax.

The key is regular practice. Try to set aside at least 30 minutes a day. As you strengthen your ability to relax, your nervous system will become less reactive and you'll be less vulnerable to anxiety and stress. Over time, the relaxation response will come easier and easier, until it feels natural.

Progressive muscle relaxation- When anxiety takes hold, progressive muscle relaxation can help you release muscle tension and take a "time out" from your worries. The technique involves systematically tensing and then releasing different muscle groups in your body. As your body relaxes, your mind will follow.

Deep breathing- When you're anxious, you breathe faster. This hyperventilation causes symptoms such as dizziness, breathlessness, lightheadedness, and tingly hands and feet. These physical symptoms are frightening, leading to further anxiety and panic. But by breathing deeply from the diaphragm, you can reverse these symptoms and calm yourself down. **Meditation-** Many types of meditation have been shown to reduce anxiety. Mindfulness meditation, in particular, shows promise for anxiety relief. Research shows that mindfulness meditation can actually change your brain. With regular practice, meditation boosts activity on the left side of the prefrontal cortex, the area of the brain responsible for feelings of serenity and joy.

3. **Learn to calm down quickly**

Learn to recognize and reduce hidden stress - Many people with GAD don't know how to calm and soothe themselves. But it's a simple, easy technique to learn, and it can make a drastic difference in your anxiety symptoms. The best methods for self-soothing incorporate one or more of the physical senses: vision, hearing, smell, taste, and touch. Try the following sensory-based, self-soothing suggestions when your generalized anxiety disorder (GAD) symptoms are acting up:

Sight (Take in a beautiful view). **Sound** (Listen to soothing music. Enjoy the sounds of nature)**. Smell** (Light scented candles. **Taste (**Cook a delicious meal. Slowly eat a favorite treat, savoring each bite). **Touch (**Take a warm bubble bath. Wrap yourself in a soft blanket and so on).

4. **Connect with others**

GAD gets worse when you feel powerless and alone, but there is strength in numbers. The more connected you are to other people, the less vulnerable you'll feel. **Identify unhealthy relationship patterns.** Once you're aware of any anxiety-driven relationship patterns, you can look for better ways to deal with any fears or insecurities you're feeling. **Build a strong support system.** Connecting to others is vital to your emotional health. A strong support system doesn't necessarily mean a vast network of friends. **Talk it out when your worries**

start spiraling. It's helpful to bounce your worries off someone who can give you a balanced, objective perspective. **Know who to avoid when you're feeling anxious.** No matter how close you are.

5. **Change your lifestyle**

A healthy, balanced lifestyle plays a big role in keeping the symptoms of GAD at bay. **Adopt healthy eating habits-** Start the day right with breakfast. Eat plenty of complex carbohydrates such as whole grains, fruits, and vegetables. Not only do complex carbs stabilize blood sugar, they also boost serotonin, a neurotransmitter with calming effects. **Limit caffeine and sugar-** Stop drinking or cut back on caffeinated beverages, including soda, coffee, and tea. Caffeine can increase anxiety, interfere with sleep, and even provoke panic attacks. Reduce the amount of refined sugar you eat, too. Sugary snacks and desserts cause blood sugar to spike and then crash, leaving you feeling emotionally and physically drained. **Exercise regularly-** For maximum relief for GAD, try to get at least 30 minutes of aerobic activity on most days. Aerobic exercise boosts physical and mental energy, and enhances well-being through the release of endorphins, the brain's feel-good chemicals. **Avoid alcohol and nicotine-** Alcohol temporarily reduces anxiety and worry, but it actually causes anxiety symptoms as it wears off. Drinking for GAD relief also starts you on a path that can lead to alcohol abuse and dependence. Lighting up when you're feeling anxious is also a bad idea. While it may seem like cigarettes are calming, nicotine is actually a powerful stimulant. Smoking leads to higher, not lower, levels of anxiety. And finally **get enough sleep.**

12. Panic

With treatment, most patients exhibit dramatic improvement the symptoms of panic disorder and agoraphobia. The two most effective treatments are pharmacotherapy and cognitive-behavioral therapy. Family and group therapy may help affected patients and their families adjust to the patient's disorder and to the psychosocial difficulties that the disorder may have precipitated.

12.1 Pharmacotherapy

Overview. Alprazolam (Xanax) and paroxetine (Paxil) are the two drugs approved by the FDA for the treatment of panic disorder. In general, experience is showing superiority of the selective serotonin reuptake inhibitors (SSRIs) and clomipramine (Anafranil) over the benzodiazepines, Monoamine oxidase inhibitors (MAOIs), and tricyclic and tetracyclic drugs in terms of effectiveness and tolerance of adverse effects. A few reports have suggested a role for venlafaxine (Effexor), and buspirone (BuSpar) has been suggested as an additive medication in some cases. Venlafaxine is approved by the FDA for treatment of GAD and it may be useful in panic disorder combined with depression. Badrenergic receptor antagonists have not been found to be particularly useful for panic disorder. A conservative approach is to begin treatment with paroxetine, sertraline (Zoloft), citalopram (celexa), or fluvoxamine (Luvox) in isolated panic disorder. If rapid control of severe symptoms is desired, a brief course of alprazolam should be initiated concurrently with the SSRI, followed by slowly tapering use of the benzodiazepines in long-term use. Fluoxetine (prozac) is an effective drug for panic with comorbid depression, although its initial activating properties may mimic panic symptoms for the first several weeks, and it may be poorly tolerated on this basis.

Clonazepam (klonopin) can be prescribed for patients who anticipate a situation in which panic may occur (0.5to 1 mg as required). Common dosages for antipanic drugs are listed in the table below.

DRUG	Starting (mg)	Maintenance(mg)
SSRIs		
Paroxetine	5-10	20-60
Paroxetine CR	12.5-25	62.5
Fluoxetine	2-5	20-60
Sertraline	12.5-25	50-200
Fluvoxamine	12.5	100-150
Citalopram	10	20-40
Escitalopram	10	20
Tricyclic Antidepressants		
Clomipramine	5-12.5	50-125
Imipramine	10-25	150-500
Desipramine	10-25	150-200
Benzodiazepines		
Alprazolam	0.25-0.5 tid	0.5-2 tid
Clonazepam	0.25-0.5 bid	0.5-2 bid
Diazepam	2-5 bid	5-30 bid
Lorazepam	0.25-0.5 bid	0.5-2 bid
MAOIs		
Phenelzine	15 bid	15-45 bid
Tranylcypromine	10 bid	10-30 bid
RIMAs		
Moclobemide	50	300-600
Brofaromine	50	150-200
Atypical Antidepressants		
Venlafaxine	6.25-25	50-150
Venlafaxine XR	37.5	150-225
Other Agents		
Valproic acid	125 bid	500-750 bid
Inositol	6'000 bid	6'000 bid

SSRIs': selective serotonin reuptake inhibitors, MAOIs: monoamine oxidase Inhibitors,
RIMAs: reversible inhibitors of monoamine oxidase type-A, Bid: twice a day, Tid: three times a day

Table 1. Recommended daily dosages for antipanic drugs.

Selective Serotonin reuptake Inhibitors (SSRIs) - All SSRIs are effective for panic disorder. Paroxetine and paroxetine CR have sedative effects and to calm patients immediately, which leads to greater compliance and less discontinuation. Citalopram, escitalopram (Lexapro), fluvoxamine, and sertraline are the next best tolerated. Anecdotal reports suggest that patients with panic disorder are particularly sensitive to the activating effects of SSRIs, particularly fluoxetine, so they should be given initially at small dosages and titrated up slowly. Once at therapeutic dosages- for example, 20 mg a day of paroxetine–some patients may experience increased sedation. One approach for patients with panic disorder is to give 5 or 10 mg a day of paroxetine or 12.5 to25 mg of paroxetine CR for 1 to 2 weeks, then increase the dosage by 10mg of paroxetine or 12.5 mg of paroxetine CR a day every 1 to 2weeks to a maximum of 60 mg of paroxetine or 62.5 mg of paroxetine CR. If sedation becomes intolerable, then taper the paroxetine dosage down to 10 mg a day of paroxetine or 12.5 mg of paroxetine CR and switch to fluoxetine at 10 mg a day and titrate upward slowly. Other strategies can be used, based on the experience of clinician.

Benzodiazepines- Benzodiazepines have the most rapid onset of action against panic, often within the first week, and they can be used for long periods without the development of tolerance to the antipanic effects. Alprazolam has been the most widely used benzodiazepine for panic disorder, but controlled studies have demonstrated equal efficacy for lorazepam (Ativan), and case reports have also indicated that clonazpam may be effective. Some patients use Benzodiazepines as needed when faced with a phobic stimulus. Benzodiazepines can reasonably be used as the first agent for treatment of panic disorder, while a serotonergic drug is being slowly titrated to a therapeutic dost. After 4 to 12 weeks, benzodiazepine use can be slowly tapered (over 4 to 10 weeks) while the serotonergic drug is continued. The major reservation among clinicians regarding the use of benzodiazepines for panic disorder is the potential for dependence, cognitive impairment, and abuse, especially after long-term use. Patients should be instructed not to drive, abstain from alcohol or other CNS depressant medications or operate dangerous equipment while taking benzodiazepines. Benzodiazepines elicit a sense of well- being, whereas discontinuation of benzodiazepines produces a well- documented and unpleasant withdrawal syndrome. Anecdotal reports and small case series have indicated that addiction to alprazolam is one of the most difficult to overcome, and it may require a comprehensive program of detoxification. Benzodiazepines dosage should be tapered slowly, and all anticipated withdrawal effects should be thoroughly explained to the patient.

Tricyclic and Tetracyclic Drugs- At the present time SSRIs are considered the first line agents for the treatment of panic disorder. Data however, show that among tricylic drugs, clomipramine and imipramine (Tofranil) are the most effective in the treatment of panic disorder. Clinical experience indicates that the dosages must be titrated slowly upward to avoid overstimulation and that the full clinical benefit requires full dosages and may not be achieved for 8 to 12 weeks. Some data support the efficacy of desipramine (Norpramin), and less evidence suggests a role for maprotiline (Ludiomil), trazodone (Desyrel), nortriptyline (Pamelor), amitriptylin (Elavil), and doxepin (Adapin). Tricyclic drugs are less widely used that SSRIs because the Tricyclic drugs generally have more severe adverse effects at the higher dosages required for effective treatment of panic disorder.

Monoamine Oxidase Inhibitors (MAOIs) - The most robust data support the effectiveness of phenelzine (Nardil) , and some data also support the use of tranylcypromine (Parnate). MAOIs appear less likely to cause overstimulation that either SSRIs of tricyclic drugs, but they may require full dosages for at least 8 to 12 weeks to be effective. The need for dietary restrictions has limited the use of MAOIs, particularly since the appearance of the SSRIs.

12.2 Treatment nonresponse

If patients fail to respond to one class of drugs, another should tried. Recent data support the effectiveness of venlafaxine. The combination of a SSRIs or a tricyclic drug and a benzodiazepines or of a SSRIs and lithium or a tricyclic drug can be tried. Case reports have suggested the effectiveness of carbamazepine (Tegretol), valproate (Depakene) and calcium channel inhibitors. Buspirone may have a role in the augmentation of other medications but has little effectiveness by itself. Clinicians should reassess the patient, particularly to establish the presence of comorbid conditions such depression, alcohol use or other substance use.

12.3 Duration of pharmacotherapy

Once it becomes effective pharmacological treatment should generally continue for 8 to 12 months. Data indicate that panic disorder is a chronic, perhaps lifelong condition that recurs when treatment is discontinued. Studies have reported that 30 to 90 percent of patients with panic disorder who have had successful treatment have a relapse when their medication is discontinued. Patients may be likely to relapse if they have been given benzodiazepines and the benzodiazepine therapy is terminated in that causes withdrawal symptoms.

13. Cognitive behavioral therapy

Cognitive behavioral therapy focuses on the thinking patterns and behaviors that are sustaining or triggering the panic attacks. It helps you look at your fears in a more realistic light. For example, if you had a panic attack while driving, what is the worst thing that would really happen? While you might have to pull over to the side of the road, you are not likely to crash your car or have a heart attack. Once you learn that nothing truly disastrous is going to happen, the experience of panic becomes less terrifying.

Exposure therapy for panic attacks and panic disorder - In exposure therapy for panic disorder, you are exposed to the physical sensations of panic in a safe and controlled environment, giving you the opportunity to learn healthier ways of coping. You may be asked to hyperventilate, shake your head from side to side, or hold your breath. These different exercises cause sensations similar to the symptoms of panic.

If you have agoraphobia, exposure to the situations you fear and avoid is also included in treatment. You face the feared situation until the panic begins to go away. You learn that the situation isn't harmful and that you have control over your emotions.

Self-help tips for panic attacks and panic disorder:

Learn to recognize and reduce hidden stress

Learn about panic- Simply knowing more about panic can help relieving your distress. Read about anxiety, panic disorder, and the fight-or-flight response experienced during a panic attack. You'll learn that the sensations and feelings you have when you panic are normal and that you aren't going crazy.

Avoid smoking and caffeine- Smoking and caffeine can provoke panic attacks in people who are susceptible. As a result, it's wise to avoid cigarettes, coffee, and other caffeinated beverages. Also be careful with medications that contain stimulants, such as diet pills and non-drowsy cold medications.

Learn how to control your breathing - Hyperventilation brings on many sensations (such as lightheadedness and tightness of the chest) that occur during a panic attack. Deep breathing, can relieve the symptoms of panic.

Practice relaxation techniques - When practiced regularly, activities such as yoga, meditation, and progressive muscle relaxation strengthen the body's relaxation response.

Telephone-based collaborative care for panic disorder and generalized anxiety disorder is more effective than usual care at improving anxiety symptoms, health-related quality of life, and work-related outcomes.

14. Phobia

14.1 Treatment of phobia

Although phobias are common, they don't always cause considerable distress or significantly disrupt life. For example, if somebody has a snake phobia, it may cause no problems in his/her everyday activities if he/she lives in a city. On the other hand, if he/she has a severe phobia of crowded spaces, living in a big city would pose a problem. If phobia doesn't really impact life that much, it's probably nothing to be concerned about.

Consider treatment for your phobia if:

It causes intense and disabling fear, anxiety, and panic. You recognize that your fear is excessive and unreasonable.

You avoid certain situations and places because of your phobia. Your avoidance interferes with your normal routine or causes significant distress. You've had the phobia for at least six months.

Self-help or therapy for phobias: which treatment is best?

When it comes to treating phobias, self-help strategies and therapy can both be effective. What's best for you depends on a number of factors, including the severity of your phobia, finances and the amount of support you need. The more you can do for yourself, the more is control you'll feel, which goes a long way when it comes to phobias and fears. If your phobia is so severe that it triggers panic attacks or uncontrollable anxiety, you may need more help. Therapy for phobias not only does work extremely well, but you tend to see results very quickly. However, support doesn't have to come in the guise of a professional therapist. Just having someone to hold your hand or stand by your side.

What you can do:

1. **Face your fears, one step at a time.**

When it comes to conquering phobias, facing your fears is the key. While avoidance may make you feel better in the short-term, it prevents you from learning that your phobia may not be as frightening or overwhelming as you think.

Exposure: Gradually and repeatedly facing your fears - The most effective way to overcome a phobia is by gradually and repeatedly exposing yourself to what you fear in a safe and controlled way. You'll learn to ride out the anxiety and fear until it inevitably passes. Through repeated experiences facing your fear, you'll begin to realize that the worst isn't going to happen. Successfully facing your fears takes planning, practice, and patience.

The following tips will help you get the most out of the exposure process:

Climbing up the "fear ladder" - If you've tried exposure in the past and it didn't work, you may have started with something too scary or overwhelming. It's important to begin with a situation that you can handle, and work your way up from there, building your confidence and coping skills as you move up the "fear ladder."

- **Facing a fear of dogs:**

A sample fear ladder- Look at pictures of dogs. - Watch a video with dogs in it. - Look at a dog through a window. - Stand 10 feet away from a dog on a leash. - Stand 5 feet away from a dog on a leash. - Stand beside a dog on a leash. **-** Pet a small dog that someone is holding. - Pet a larger dog on a leash. - Pet a larger dog off leash.

Make a list- Make a list of the frightening situations related to your phobia. If you're afraid of flying, your list (in addition to the obvious matters, such as taking a flight or getting through takeoff) might include booking your ticket, packing your suitcase, driving to the airport, watching planes take off and land, going through security, boarding the plane, and listening to the flight attendant present the safety instructions.

Build your fear ladder- Arrange the items on your list from the least scary to the scariest. When creating the ladder, it can be helpful to think about your end goal (for example, to be able to be near dogs without panicking) and then break down the steps needed to reach that goal.

Work your way up the ladder-Start with the first step (in this example, looking at pictures of dogs) and don't move on until you start to feel more comfortable doing it. If at all possible, stay in the situation long enough for your anxiety to decrease. Once you've done a step on several separate occasions without feeling too much anxiety, you can move on to the next step. **Practice-** It's important to practice regularly. The more often you practice, the quicker your progress will be. However, don't rush. Your fears won't hurt you.

2. **Learn relaxation techniques.**

By learning and practicing relaxation techniques, you can become more confident in your ability to tolerate uncomfortable sensations and calm yourself down quickly. Relaxation techniques such as deep breathing, meditation, and muscle relaxation are powerful antidotes to anxiety, panic, and fear.

3. **Challenge negative thoughts.**

Learning to challenge unhelpful thoughts is an important step in overcoming your phobia. You may underestimate your ability to cope. The anxious thoughts that trigger and fuel phobias are usually negative and unrealistic. Begin by writing down any negative thoughts you have when confronted with your phobia. Many times, these thoughts fall into the following categories (with examples):

Fortune telling- I'll make a fool of myself for sure.

Overgeneralization - All dogs are dangerous.

Catastrophizing- The person next to me coughed. Maybe it's the swine flu. I'm going to get very sick!

15. Social anxiety disorder treatment

1. **Challenging negative thoughts**

The one with social anxiety disorder, or social phobia, may find himself/herself overwhelmed by thoughts like:

People will think I'm stupid. I won't have anything to say. I'll seem boring.

Challenging these negative thoughts is one effective way to reduce the symptoms of social anxiety disorder. The first step is to identify the automatic negative thoughts that underlie fear of social situations. The next step is to analyze and challenge them. It helps to ask questions about the negative thoughts: "Even if I'm nervous, will people necessarily think I'm incompetent?" Through this logical evaluation of negative thoughts, he/she can gradually replace them with more realistic and positive ways of looking at social situations that trigger anxiety.

15.1 Unhelpful thinking styles involved in social phobia

Mind reading - Assuming you know what other people are thinking, and that they see you in the same negative way that you see yourself.

Fortune telling- Predicting the future, usually while assuming the worst will happen. You just "know" that things will go horribly, so you're already anxious before you're even in the situation.

Catastrophizing -Blowing things out of proportion. If people notice that you're nervous, it will be "awful," "terrible," or "disastrous."

Personalizing -Assuming that people are focusing on you in a negative way or that what's going on with other people has to do with you.

2. **Breathing control**

Learning to slow your breathing down can help you bring your physical symptoms of anxiety back under control.

3. **Facing fears**

Avoidance leads to more problems- While avoiding nerve-wracking situations may help you feel better in the short term. In fact, the more you avoid a feared social situation, the more frightening it becomes.

Challenging social anxiety one step at a time- While it may seem impossible to overcome a feared social situation, you can do it by taking it one small step at a time. The key is to start with a situation that you can handle and gradually work your way up to more challenging situations.

Working your way up the social phobia "anxiety ladder"- Don't try to face your biggest fear right away. This will backfire and reinforce your anxiety.

Be patient- Overcoming social anxiety takes time and practice.

Use the skills you've learned to stay calm, such as focusing on your breathing and challenging negative assumptions.

4. **Building better relationships**

The following suggestions are good ways to start interacting with others in positive ways:

Take a social skills class or an assertiveness training class. Volunteer doing something you enjoy, such as stuffing envelopes for a campaign. Work on your communication skills. Clear and emotionally-intelligent communication.

5. **Changing the lifestyle**

Avoid or limit caffeine- Coffee, tea, caffeinated soda, energy drinks, and chocolate act as stimulants that increase anxiety symptoms.

Avoid drinking- alcohol increases your risk of having an anxiety attack.

Quit smoking- Nicotine is a powerful stimulant. Smoking leads to higher, not lower, levels of anxiety.

Get adequate sleep- Being well rested will help you stay calm in social situations.

Group therapy for social anxiety disorder / social phobia would help a lot.

Other cognitive-behavioral techniques for social anxiety disorder include **role-playing and social skills training**, often as part of a therapy group.

Group therapy for social anxiety disorder uses acting, videotaping and observing, mock interviews, and other exercises to work on situations that make you anxious in the real world.

15.2 Medication for social anxiety disorder/social phobia

Medication is sometimes used to relieve the symptoms of social anxiety, but it's not a cure for social anxiety disorder or social phobia. After stopping the medication, symptoms will probably return full force. Medication is considered most helpful when used in addition to therapy and other self-help techniques that address the root cause of social anxiety disorder.

Cognitive therapy and Interpersonal psychotherapy (IPT) led to considerable improvements that were maintained 1 year after treatment .Cognitive therapy (CT) is more efficacious than is IPT in reducing social phobia symptoms.

15.3 Medical treatment of social disorder

Three types of medication are used in the treatment of social anxiety disorder / social phobia:

Beta blockers - Beta blockers are used for relieving performance anxiety. They work by blocking the flow of adrenaline that occurs when you're anxious. While beta blockers don't affect the emotional symptoms of anxiety, they can control physical symptoms such as shaking hands or voice, sweating, and rapid heartbeat.

Antidepressants - Antidepressants can be helpful when social anxiety disorder is severe and debilitating. Three specific antidepressants- paroxetine (Paxil), venlafaxine (Effexor), and sertraline (Zoloft) -have been approved by the FDA for the treatment of social phobia.

Benzodiazepines – Benzodiazepines are fast-acting anti-anxiety medications. However, they are sedating and addictive, so they are typically prescribed only when other medications for social phobia have not worked.

15.4 Medication alone is not enough

Remember, anxiety medications aren't a cure. Medication may treat some symptoms of anxiety, but can't change the underlying issues and situations in your life that are making you anxious. Anxiety medication won't solve your problems if you're anxious because of mounting bills, a tendency to jump to "worst-case scenarios", or an unhealthy relationship. That's where therapy and other lifestyle changes come in. Alternatives to medication include: cognitive-behavioral therapy, which is widely accepted to be more effective for anxiety than drugs. To overcome anxiety for good, you may also need to make major changes in your life. Lifestyle changes that can make a difference in anxiety levels include regular exercise, adequate sleep, and a healthy diet. Other effective treatments for anxiety include talk therapy, meditation, biofeedback, hypnosis, and acupuncture.

The advantage of non-drug treatments for anxiety is that they produce lasting changes and long-term relief. If your anxiety is so severe that it interferes with therapy, medication may be useful in the short-term to get your symptoms under control. Once your anxiety is at a manageable level, other forms of behavior and talk therapy can be successfully pursued.

15.5 Anti-anxiety drug dependence and withdrawal

Anti-anxiety medications including popular benzodiazepines such as alprazolam (Xanax) , clonazepam (klonopin), diazepam (Valium), and lorazepam (Ativan) are meant for short-term use. However, many people take anti-anxiety drugs for long periods of time. This is risky because, when taken regularly, benzodiazepines quickly lead to physical dependence. Drug tolerance is also common, with increasingly larger doses needed to get the same anxiety relief as before.

According to the American Academy of Family Physicians, benzodiazepines lose their therapeutic anti-anxiety effect after 4 to 6 months of regular use.

Most people become addicted to their anti-anxiety drug within a couple of months, but problems may arise sooner. For some, drug dependency develops after a few short weeks. The body is used to the medication, so withdrawal symptoms occur if the dose is decreased or discontinued.

Psychological dependence can be an issue, too. If the patient has been relying on an anti-anxiety drug to keep his/her anxiety in check, he/she may lose confidence in his/her abilities to deal with life's difficulties and start to think he/she "needs" the medication to survive.

To quit anti-anxiety medication, it's important to do so under the guidance of a medical health professional. The key is to slowly decrease the dose over a period of time. If it stops abruptly, the patient may experience severe withdrawal symptoms such as: Increased anxiety, Insomnia, Confusion, Pounding heart, Sweating and Shaking.

Gradually tapering off the drug will help minimize the withdrawal reaction. However, if the patient has taken anti-anxiety medication for a few months, he/she may still experience some withdrawal symptoms. Anxiety, insomnia, and depression may last for months after he/she has quit. Unfortunately, these persistent withdrawal symptoms are frequently mistaken for a return of the original problem, causing some people to restart the medication.

16. References

[1] Sadok B J, Sadok V A, Ruiz P. Pine D S. Comprehensive Textbook of Psychiatry, Anxiety Disorders. 9th ed USA:Lippincott Williams & Wilkins;2009:1839-1900

[2] Seaward B L, Managing Stress. Sixth ed Jones and Bartlett; 2009:125-127

[3] Anxiety Disorders. U.S. Department of Health and Human Services. National Institute of Mental Health. Available at: http://www.nimh.nih.gov/health/publications/anxiety-disorders/complete-index.shtml . accessed 15 June 2011 .

[4] Anxiety Disorders. Canadian Mental Health association. . Available at : http://www.cmha.ca . accessed 16June 2011 .

[5] Treichel j a. Anxiety Disorder. American Psychiatric Association. WebMD Network.2009 Available at: http://www.medicinenet.com/anxiety/article.Htm#tocb.accessed 13 June 2011

[6] Beesdo K, Pine D S, Lieb R, Wittchen H U. Incidence and Risk Patterns of Anxiety and Depressive Disorders and Categorization of Generalized Anxiety Disorder. Arch Gen Psychiatry. 2010;67(1):47-57.

[7] Anxiety Disorders, National Institute of Mental Health; 2009 Available at: http://www.nimh.nih.gov/health/publications/anxiety-disorders/complete-index.shtml, accessed Oct 2011

[8] Sareen J, Cox B J, Afifi T O, Graaf R, Asmundson G G, Have M T, Stein M B. Anxiety Disorders and Risk for Suicidal Ideation and Suicide Attempts, A Population-Based Longitudinal Study of Adults . Arch Gen Psych. Iatry. Nov. 2005;62:1249-1257. disturbance;146(4):412-417Vol. 62 No.11 available at: htttp://pubs.ama-assn.org(Jama&Archives Journals), accessed Oct 2011.

[9] Bouchard M F, Bellinger D C, Weuve J, Bellinger J M, Gilman S E, Wright R O, et al. Blood Lead Levels and Major Depressive Disorder, Panic Disorder, and Generalized Anxiety Disorder in US Young Adults. Arch Gen Psychiatry. Dec 2009,Vol. 66 No. 12;66(12):1313-131910.

[10] Arehart-Treichel J, Several Strategies Successful for Treating Anxiety Disorders. psychiatric News Oct 2009 Vol. 44 No.19 page 33, American Psychiatric Association Vol. 59 No. 10, 2002;59:905-911

[11] Frank E, Cyranowski J M, Rucci P, Shear M K, Fagiolini A, Michael E, et al. Clinical Significance of Lifetime Panic Spectrum Symptoms in the Treatment of Patients With Bipolar I Disorder. Arch Gen Psychiatry. Oct. 2002 Vol. 59 No. 10;59:905-911 available at: htttp://pubs.ama-assn.org(Jama&Archives Journals), accessed Oct 2011.

[12] Goddard A W, Mason G F, Almai A, Rothman D L, Behar K L, Petroff O C, et al. Reductions in Occipital Cortex GABA Levels in Panic Disorder Detected With 1H-

Magnetic Resonance Spectroscopy. Arch Gen Psychiatry. June 2001 Vol. 58 No. 6,58:556-561 available at: htttp://pubs.ama-assn.org(Jama&Archives Journals), accessed Oct 2011.

[13] Wilkinson D C, Thompson J M, Lambert G W, Jennings G L, Schwarz R G, Jefferys D, et al. Sympathetic Activity in Patients With Panic Disorder at Rest, Under Laboratory Mental Stress, and During Panic Attacks. Arch Gen Psychiatry. June 1998 Vol. 55 No. 6, 55:511-520 available at: htttp://pubs.ama-assn.org(Jama&Archives Journals), accessed Oct 2011.

[14] Hoehn-Saric R, McLeod D R, Funderburk F, Kowalski P. Somatic Symptoms and Physiologic Responses in Generalized Anxiety Disorder and Panic Disorder An Ambulatory Monitor Study .Arch Gen Psychiatry. Sep 2004 Vol. 61 No. 9, 61:913-92

[15] Purcell R, Maruff P, Kyrios M, Pantelis C. Clinical Significance of Lifetime Panic Spectrum Symptoms in the Treatment of Patients With Bipolar I Disorder. Arch Gen Psychiatry .May 1998 Vol. 55 No. 5, 55:415-423 available at: htttp://pubs.ama-assn.org(Jama&Archives Journals), accessed Oct 2011.

[16] Frank E, Cyranowski J M, Rucci P, M. Shear K, Fagiolini A, Thase M E, et al.clinical Significance of Lifetime Panic Spectrum Symptoms in the Treatment of Patients With Bipolar I Disorder. Arch Gen Psychiatry. Oct 2002 Vol. 59 No. 10, 59:905-911.

[17] Kessler R C, Chiu W T, Jin R, Ruscio A M, Shear K, Ellen E. Walters E E .The Epidemiology of Panic Attacks, Panic Disorder, and Agoraphobia in the National Comorbidity Survey Replication. Arch Gen Psychiatry. April 2006 Vol. 63 No. 4, 63:415-424

[18] Hale A S. Obsessive-compulsive disorder Anxiety, ABC of mental health, Clinical Review, 28 June 1997, BMJ, 10.1136/bmj.314.7098.1886,available at: www.bmj.com, accessed Sep 2011.

[19] Heyman I, Mataix-Cols D, Fineberg N A. Obsessive-compulsive disorder, Clinical review. Aug 2006, BMJ; 333 doi: 10.1136/bmj.333.7565.424 , available at: www.bmj.com, accessed Oct 2011.

[20. House A, Stark D. Anxiety in medical patients, ABC of psychological medicine, Clinical Review, July 2002 , BMJ; 325 : 207 doi: 10.1136/bmj.325.7357.207. available at: www.bmj.com, accessed Sep 2011.

[21] Huizink A C, Ferdinand R F, Ende J, Verhulst F C. Symptoms of anxiety and depression in childhood and use of MDMA: prospective, population based study, Research, Feb 2006, BMJ 332 : 825 doi: 10.1136/bmj.38743.539398.3A. available at: www.bmj.com, accessed Oct 2011.

[22] Gale C, Davidson O, Generalised anxiety disorder, Generalised anxiety disorder, Clinical Review. March 2007, BMJ 334 : 579 doi: 10.1136/bmj.39133.559282. . available at: www.bmj.com, accessed Sep 2011.

[23] Moritz S, Kempke S, Luyten P, Randjbar S, Jelinek L. Was Freud partly right on obsessive–compulsive disorder (OCD)? Investigation of latent aggression in OCD. May 2011, Psychiatry Research, Volume 187, Issues 1-2, 180-184, Available online 14 October 2010

[24] Calkins A W, Otto M W, Cohen L S, Soares C N, Vitonis A F, Hearon B A, et al. Psychosocial predictors of the onset of anxiety disorders in women: Results from a prospective 3-year longitudinal study. Dec 2009, Journal of Anxiety Disorders, Volume 23, Issue 8,1165-1169 available at: www.bmj.com, accessed Sep 2011.

[25] Robinson L. Smith M. M.A. Segal J. Find a Support Group: September 2011. available at: WWW.HELPGUIDE.ORG.

[26] Richards T A, Anxiety Therapy. Cognitive-Behavioral Therapy (CBT) - Outlines the cognitive, behavioral, and emotional aspects of cognitive behavioral therapy for anxiety. (The Anxiety Network) available at: http://www.anxietynetwork.com/hcbt.html ,accessed Oct 2011

[27] Smith M, M.A., Robinson l L, Segal J. Anxiety Medication, July 2011, available at: http://www.helpguide.org/mental/anxiety_medication_drugs_treatment.htm, accessed Oct 2011

[28] Herring M P, O'Connor P J, Rodney K. Dishman R K.The Effect of Exercise Training on Anxiety Symptoms Among Patients. *Arch Intern Med.* 2010;170(4):321-331. February 22, 2010 No. 4, available at: archinte.ama-assn.org/cgi/content/abstract/, accessed Sep 2011

[29] Stangier U, Schramm E, Heidenreich T, Berger M, Clark D M. Cognitive Therapy vs Interpersonal Psychotherapy in Social Anxiety Disorder . Arch Gen Psychiatry, Vol. 68 No. 7, July 2011;68(7):692-700. doi:10.1001/ available at: www.ncbi.nlm.nih.gov/pubmed , accessed Oct 2011

[30] Davidson JR. Trauma: the impact of post-traumatic stress disorder. Journal of Psychopharmacology, 2000; 14(2 Suppl 1): S5-S12.

[31] Hyman S E, Rudorfer M V. Anxiety disorders. In: Dale DC, Federman DD, eds. Scientific American® Medicine. Volume 3. New York: Healtheon/WebMD Corp., 2000, Sect. 13, Subsect. VIII. available at: books.google.com/books , accessed Oct 2011

[32] Healy D, Psychiatric Drugs Explained, Section 5: Management of Anxiety, Elsevier Health Sciences, 2008, pp. 136–137

[33] Post-Traumatic Stress Disorder and the Family. Veterans Affairs Canada. 2006. ISBN 0-662-42627-4. available at: http://www.vac-acc.gc.ca/clients. accessed Oct 2011

[34] "What Causes Anxiety Disorders?" available at: http://www.mhawestchester.org/diagnosechild/canxiety.asp. Retrieved 2010-05-19, accessed Sep 2011

[35] Dunlop BW, Davis PG. "Combination treatment with benzodiazepines and SSRIs for comorbid anxiety and depression: a review".2008, available at: http://www.pubmedcentral.nih.gov . accessed Jun 2011

[36] Radua, Joaquim; van den Heuvel, Odile A.; Surguladze, Simon; Mataix-Cols, David). "Meta-analytical comparison of voxel-based morphometry studies in obsessive-compulsive disorder vs other anxiety disorders". Archives of General Psychiatry 67، 2010. 701–711

[37] McLaughlin K, Behar E, Borkovec T. "Family history of psychological problems in generalized anxiety disorder". Journal of Clinical Psychology ,Aug 2005, available at: http://www3.interscience.wiley.com , accessed Jun 2011

[38] Davidson J T, Foa E B, Hupper J D, Keefe F J, Franklin M E, Compton J S, et al. Fluoxetine, Comprehensive Cognitive Behavioral Therapy, and Placebo in Generalized Social Phobia. Archives of General Psychiatry (2004),Volume: 61, Issue: 10, Publisher: American Medical Assn, Pages: 1005-1013,Available from archpsyc.ama-assn.org, accessed Jun 2011

[39] Stein, D J. Clinical Manual of Anxiety Disorders (1st ed.). USA: American Psychiatric Press Inc. (16 February 2004).. http://books.google.com. accessed July 2011

[40] Stein MB, Liebowitz M R, Lydiard R B, Pitts C D, Bushnell W, Gergel I. "Paroxetine treatment of generalized social phobia (social anxiety disorder): a randomized controlled trial".(August 1998) JAMA 280 (8): 708–713. available at: http://jama.ama-assn.org/cgi/content/full/280/8/708.: htttp://pubs.ama-assn.org(Jama&Archives Journals), accessed Oct 2011.

[41] Hollon S; Stewart O, Strunk D. "Enduring effects for Cognitive Behavior Therapy in the Treatment of Depression and Anxiety". Annual Review of Psychology(August 25, 2005) 57: 285–315. available at: http://faculty.psy.ohio-state.edu/strunk/personal/Hollon . accessed Jun 2011

[42] Simon H, Zieve D, Anxiety disorders - Psychotherapy and Other Treatments – Overview of therapies and complementary treatments for anxiety, University of Maryland Medical Center. Jan. 2009, available at: http://www.umm.edu/patiented/articles/ , accessed July 2011

[43] MDMA(Ecstasy), The National Institute on Drug Abuse (NIDA), part of the National Institutes of Health (NIH). Dec.2010, available at: http://www.drugabuse.gov/infofacts/ecstasy. html, accessed Nov. 2011

[44] GABA: Gamma-Amino Butyric Acid. Denver Naturopathic Clinic, available at: http://www.denvernaturopathic.com/news/GABA.html, accessed Nov. 2011

6

Mental Health, Trauma and Trauma Related Disorders

Sevgi Guney
Ankara University, Ankara
Turkey

1. Introduction

Mental health is a complex phenomena including life satisfaction and subjective well-being. Satisfaction with life reflects the degree to which external living-conditions 'fit' with inner life-abilities. Subjective well-being refers to how people evaluate their lives, and include variables such as life satisfaction, marital satisfaction, positive moods and emotions, lack of depression, lack of anxiety (Diener, 2004). The investigations on people suffering from mood and anxiety disorders abound in psychology and psychiatry literatures (Seligman & Diener, 2002). The interaction between individuals and their environment generates both happiness and psychopathology. Traumas may easily influence negatively the interaction. In other words, psychological traumas as one of the crucial dimension of mental health may cause some impairment in the intra and interpersonal adaptive process of human functioning (Guney, et. al., 2010).

2. What is "mental health"?

It is good to mention about what mental disorder is to answer the question? There is no any single reason causing mental disorders. That's why mental health may be seen as a continuum where an individual's mental health may have many different possible aspects. In this continuum, mental health can be defined as "a state of well-being in which the individual realizes his or her own abilities, can cope with the normal stresses of life, can work productively and fruitfully and is able to make a contribution to his or her community". While a healthy individual can remain focused, flexible and creative in bad times as well as good the individual suffering from a mental disorder can not. The people suffering from mental disorder have problems in everday functioning in their life with some degrees. Research has shown that a combination of existing factors and triggers may cause mental health problems and disorders (Ozer and Weiss, 2004; Linden, 2003; Linley, 2003). These existing factors are traumatic life events, family history, social and individual environment, hormonal changes, drugs, and alcohol etc. Some mental disorders have some aspects of conditions. Most common of these are anxiety disorders including post-traumatic stress disorder, eating disorders, clinical depression, bipolar disorder and schizophrenia. These disorders are a different form of "an overdose" of "normal" fears and concerns. The disorders are particularly amenable to modification through existing evidence-based mental health treatment procedures and preventive interventions.

3. Psychosocial trauma

A psychosocial trauma is a type of damage to the psyche that occurs as a result of a traumatic event experienced by individuals in their psychosocial environment. Psychological trauma can be caused by natural disasters including earthquakes, floating, bush fires, and man-made events including war, rape, abuse, violence, mechanized accidents such as car, train or plane crashes etc. or medical emergencies. The trauma responses potentially are normal responses to an unusual, an extreme traumatic event. They also involve the creation of emotional memories about the distressful event that are stored in structures deep within the brain. Moreover a traumatic event involves a single experience, or an enduring or repeating event or events that completely overwhelm the individual's ability to cope the emotions involved with that experience. There are several behavioral responses common towards stressors including the proactive, reactive and passive responses. Proactive responses include attempts to correct a stressor before it has a noticeable effect on lifestyle. The individuals who are able to be proactive can often overcome stressors. They are more likely to be able to cope well with unexpected situations. Reactive responses occur after the stress and possible trauma has occurred and is aimed more at minimizing the damage of a stressful event. The individuals who are more reactive will often experience more noticeable effects from an unexpected stressor. The individuals who are passive, victims of a traumatic event are more likely to suffer from long term traumatic effects. They often enact no intentional coping actions. However there is no available research outcome showing that these reactions are always true for the trauma victims. By the way, the clinical study outcomes suggest that a passive response is often characterized by an emotional numbness or ignorance of a stressor (Ozer and Weiss, 2004; Street et.al., 2005). The only evidence based outcome we have on the effect of the psychological traumas indicated that they may lead to serious, long-term negative mental health consequences. This ambiguity comes from the differences in the perception of the trauma at individual level.

Different individuals react differently to similar events. One may experience an event as traumatic while another person would not suffer trauma as a result of the same event. This unique characteristic of the perception of traumatic events makes the explore of the traumatic experience of the individual much more complex. Post traumatic reactions such as flashback memories, heightened anxiety, feeling depressed, feeling overwhelmed, strained family reactions, social withdrawal required to work with the biological, cognitive, emotional and behavioural areas of the individual suffered as a back ground factors of the reactions precisely. For example, the maladaptive cognitions of the individual such as self-talks "I don't think I can manage seeing what's left of our home, because there won't be much. I'll probably get so upset I won't handle it well and he'll think I'm a wimp.", self-rules ("I must never show signs of weakness"), schemas ("I deserve to feel bad for letting my family down") are examined and treated precisely by the trauma professionals. Therefore working with psychosocial trauma is essentially difficult not only for the individual suffered but also the professional dealt with them. There is increasing theoretical, clinical and research evidence for the role of perceived trauma and personal characteristics in trauma related disorders. There are many studies examining intra and interpersonal process investigating the role of cognitive variables such as anxiety, depression, life satisfaction, negative attributional style, and dysfunctional attitudes of the traumatized individuals (Ozer and Weiss, 2004; Ehring and Ehlers, 2010, Ehring, et.al., 2008 and Guney, et. al., 2010). The studies represent these process are the serving moderator variables of the trauma - psychopathology - post traumatic growth association and interaction (Tedeshi and Calhoun, 2004; Zoellner and Maercher, 2005; Seligman, 2002; Rashid and Anjum, 2007, Guney, 2009). The perception of the trauma experienced and the attributions to the trauma are another crucial factor in the road of understanding of the effect of the trauma. There has been little research done on the perceived attribution of traumatic events and the effect of this on posttraumatic growth. A literature review done by Linley and Joseph (2006) suggests that posttraumatic growth scores are affected by the subjective experience of a traumatic event and not just the event itself. This result shows a relationship between perceived attribution of the traumatic event experienced and posttraumatic growth but does not explain if these two concepts are negatively or positively related. There has been little research done about the perceived traumatic life events and their influences into individual's daily life. Guney (2011) in her study asked university students to review their traumatic experiences last two years. In the study the students sorted out their negative and traumatic memories and then they labeled their experiences as traumatic and non-traumatic in terms of their subjective perception. The main result of the study has showed that there is an association between the reported traumatic events, the strengthspotting characteristics and the scores from posttraumatic embitterment disorder in the well-functioning university students who had suffered a variety of negative and traumatic events. While the ruminated more about negative events, the students also have reported low overall affective intensity in her study. The traumatized students in her study reported a paucity of pleasant for a while, and then highly activated and loving interpersonal emotions in their social environment. Some of them did not even report more anxious mood on a daily basis.

4. The trauma related disorders

Trauma symptoms refer to cognitive, emotional and behavioral difficulties that are directly related to traumatic experiences. These typically correspond to symptoms of post-traumatic stress disorder and also encompass other depressive, anxiety or behavioral symptoms including self-injury, substance abuse, impaired interpersonal trust and affective instability. It is true that individuals with traumatic symptoms may experience a profound change in the way they see themselves, the world and other people. Additionally, there is growing evidence that many of these individuals also experience psychobiological changes that may contribute to the development and maintenance of these psychological and psychiatric symptoms. These symptoms may be divided into several general categories. These symptom categories are with affective, cognitive, behavioral, and psychobiological trauma symptoms, acute stress disorder, the complex PTSD, and the post traumatic embitterment disorder offered as a new traumatic disorder category for DSM-V by Michael Linden (Unal et.al., 2011), a German Psychiatrist. The disorders on mental health including PTSD are a complex psychiatric phenomenon resulting in considerable emotional distress and impaired social functioning and often constitutes a significant treatment challenge. The mental health professionals have pointed out the critical importance of the impact of the negative life events and traumas in people's life time in terms of the occurrence of mental health disorders. From this perspective there are several threats in the traumatic experience: threat to life, to physical integrity, to injury and loss of close and beloved people, threats to self-image and values. The traumatic event shatters survivors' basic assumptions about the world being a safe place, their known self-image and the values on which they based their lives (Street, et.al., 2005; Herman, 1997), disrupting the normal life of the survivors and rupturing their connection with the surrounding normal environment. The consequence of these negative life events may cause some psychological problems because the fear of the unknown and helplessness arise. Even after the event there remains the worry that the physical or mental injury will decrease the quality of life of the injured including their ability to continue and maintain an independent and productive life. Guney, et. al. (2011) found that there are statistically significant relations between the aspect of the mental health such as anxiety and other psychiatric symptoms and the impact of negative and traumatic life events.

Therefore the preventive mental health professionals take into account the interrelations between traumatic life events and the people's psychological states. The DSM IV-R (APA, 1994) delineates two types of disorders which develop in response to traumatic events: acute stress disorder, which develops immediately and resolves within one month, and Post Traumatic Stress Disorder (PTSD), which is considered as a chronic condition. In both disorders the first criteria is exposure to a traumatic event. Both disorders are classified as anxiety disorders and require three central categories of symptoms: intrusive, avoidant and hyper-arousal. In order to merit a diagnosis the symptoms must cause clinically significant distress or impairment. Acute stress disorder also includes symptoms of dissociation. We usually believe in that 'it will never happen to us'. This denial is necessary for normal life. So when something terrible does happen, we are in a state of shock. The experience haunts the survivors, enters their dreams, impacts their lives and changes their perception of reality. Some lose their faith in mankind, distance themselves from people and from close connections, and shut themselves off psychologically, sometimes physically. This is especially true if the traumatic experience was caused by another person or a group of persons, such as in the case of sexual abuse, terror attacks or domestic violence. In such instances the survivors' normal denial of the possibility of human cruelty is fractured, because other human beings inflicted merciless harm upon them. In response, they develop distrust in relationships. They feel helpless and horrified long after the experience has ended, especially if the trauma was continuous and they had no control of its occurrence or recurrence. They develop learned helplessness that occurs whenever organisms learn that their actions have nothing to do with the consequences of their behavior. This helplessness also occurs in cases of natural disaster or other traumas.

The post traumatic responses of the traumatized individual may not lead to a psychiatric disorder such as post traumatic stress disorder, anxiety disorder, and some affective disorders. These responses differ in the level of functioning. Many individuals suffered from some acute stress symptoms diagnosed as acute stress disorder and then they return to their previous level of functioning. Some resists the traumatic event with no traumatic and/or stress responses. Others react to the traumatic event as delayed response. Some others suffered the traumatic event with the chronic states. Therefore it is known by all the mental health professionals working on trauma mental health problems can be manageable for a while, then return previous level of functioning and/or a psychiatric disorder. The overall percentage of the individuals suffering from the psychiatric disorders such as PTSD, anxiety and affective disorders after a traumatic event is very small (e.g. 10 - 15 %). The back ground factors of the traumatic experience may cause some psychiatric disorder. In this context, adversity, life threatening experiences and negative life events may trigger mental disorders and also cause the post traumatic growth. The triggering event may happen over a short or prolonged period of time. As the event triggering, the high levels of personal trauma carry out the potential risk for making the damages of adaptive human functioning. It may be good to say personal trauma has a different meaning and refers to an experience being emotionally painful, distressful, shocking, which often results in lasting mental and physical effects. Dealing with the post traumatic growth, there is a recent approach called as positive psychology.

5. Positive psychology: the recent approach to psychosocial trauma

In general it is believed that the more direct the exposure to the traumatic event, the higher the risk for emotional harm. In some degrees this may be true but the recent research and approaches (Seligman, 2000, 2002,2004; Fazio and Fazio, 2005; Rashid, 2008; Diener and Diener, 2005) on the area show that the traumatic experiences can be converted into successful life experiences in the condition of individuals realized their basic aspects of human functioning. Seligman (2011) in his last book named as flourishing states that "there are two kinds of reality. One kind is not influenced by what human beings think, desire, expect, or wish for. There is an independent reality out there when you are a pilot deciding whether to fly during a thunderstorm. There is an independent reality out there when you are deciding which graduate school to attend: how well you will get along with the professors, whether there is adequate laboratory space, whether you can afford the cost. There is the reality of her rejecting you when you propose marriage. In all of these your thinking and your wishes do not influence the reality, and I am all for keen realism in these circumstances. The other kind of reality called as "reflexive reality", is influenced and sometimes even determined by expectations and perceptions. Reflexive reality is strongly influenced by perception and expectation. I believe "reality" is reflexive and the value of fundamentals is influenced." The science of Positive Psychology (and his book) is entirely about such reflexive realities.

In the line of Seligman words (2000, 2002, 2006, 2011), a new direction within psychology for traumatic life events gains more and more popularity. Thus the effect of trauma can be considered as a "reflexive reality". There are human strengths that act as buffers against mental illness: courage, future-mindedness, optimism, interpersonal skills, faith, work ethic, hope, honesty, perseverance, the capacity for flow and insight, to name several. Positive psychology considers the traumatic events suffered as its pioneering concept, that the trauma psychology should be as concerned with strength as with weakness, be as interested in building the best things in life as in repairing the worst, be as concerned with making the lives of normal people fulfilling as with healing pathology, develop interventions to increase well being, not just to decrease misery. Positive Psychology does not rely on wishful thinking, self-deception or hand-waving; instead it tries to adapt what is best in the scientific method to the unique problems that human behavior presents in all its complexity.

The approach from which Positive Psychotherapy evolves is the scientific study of positive emotions, positive individual traits and strengths (Seligman, et.al., 2006). The goal is to help individuals learn that they can grow as a result of their experiences even if the experience is traumatic. Character strengths serve individuals best not only when life is easy but also when life is difficult (Park, et.al., 2004) . During challenging times, helping people to discover their strengths such as optimism, hope, humor, resilience, and meaning takes added importance for mental health professionals. Thus it is found that individuals who use their strengths more have been shown to have higher levels of self-esteem, self-efficacy, vitality, well-being (Linley, et.al., 2010; Govindji, and Linley, 2007) and also to be more effective in their personal growth (Rashid, 2008) after a traumatic exposure in their daily lives. Focusing on strengths can provide the clinician a powerful perspective to understand individuals' intact repertoires which can be effectively deal with troubles stimulates a very different discussion. Trauma "get under individual's skin" as it's subsequent outcomes can not always recognized and lead to a psychiatric morbidity. In other words it may disrupt the adaptive processing of human funtioning for a while but not for long-term psychological disorder. In a study, the traumatized students in this study reported a paucity of pleasant for a while, highly activated and loving interpersonal emotions. Some of them did not report more anxious mood or a daily basis (Guney, 2011). In the condition of the mechanisms linking traumatic life events and psychopatologycal symptoms and their influences to the adaptive human functioning process are explored, the personal traumatic experiences can be converted into successful life experiences which mean traumatic growth.

Over the last 10 years there has been significant progress in the understanding, diagnosing and the treatment of trauma related disorders. Even their chronic and debilitating states have been extensively documented. By the recent advances in psychotherapeutic research great professional awareness of effective treatment is offered through cognitive, behavioral and positive psychological approaches with post-traumatic growth. More recently applied positive psychological approach has pointed out the prevention strategies emphasizing the avoidance of risk factors, and has promoted aims to enhance the individual's ability to achieve a positive sense of self-esteem, mastery, well-being, and social inclusion.

Positive therapy emphasises the need to understand the positive side of human experience as well as understanding and ameliorating psychopathology and distress (Joseph and linley, 2006). Both of the terms refer to how people evaluate their traumatic experiences and also the terms include lack of anxiety, lack of depression, positive moods and emotions. Therefore it may be said that the application of positive psychology principals into the mental health settings is going to give an opportunity to the professionals in the area to train their patients and clients on how the patients/clients can help themselves and their lives with positive and optimistic thinking style. If so, we teach them the positive psychology principles. They can easily learn how to "not being into depressed/anxiety mood and states". A positive change following the experience of traumatic, negative events and adversity may occur or the return to a higher level of functioning than which existed before the trauma occur. This positive changes include the perception of better relations to others, new possibilities in life, enhanced personal strength and an increased appreciation of life (Tedeshi and Calhoun, 1995; 2004; Tedeshi, 1999; Guney, 2011). Bonanno, Wortman, et. al. (2002) provided strong evidence in support of the idea that many individuals exhibit little or no grief and that these individuals are not cold and unfeeling or lacking in attachment but, rather, are capable of genuine resilience in the face of loss, and adversity.

In this manner, by reminding the fact that the entire well-being can increase the quality of life, the psychologists and all mental health professionals are to meaningfully contribute to the public applications including universities with the positive psychology principals in the way of flourishing communities with happy people even with their traumatic experience (Seligman, 2006; 2011).

6. References

Diener,E., Diener, M. & Diener, C.(1995). Factors predicting the subjective well-being of nations. *Journal of Personality and Social Psychology*, 69, 851-864.

Ehring, T. and Ehlers, A. (2010) Enhanced Priming for Trauma-Related Words Predicts Posttraumatic Stress Disorder, Journal of Abnormal Psychology, DOI: 10.1037/a0021080

Ehring, T., Ehlers, A., & Glucksman, E. (2008). Do cognitive models help in predicting the severity of posttraumatic stress disorder, phobia, and depression after motor vehicle accidents? A prospective longitudinal study. *Journal of Consulting and Clinical Psychology*, 76, 219–230. doi:10.1037/0022-006X.76.2.219

Fazio R. J., & Fazio, L. M. (2005). Growth through loss: Promoting healing and growth in the face of trauma, crisis and loss. *Journal of Loss and Trauma*,10, 221–252.

Guney, S.(2009) *Life satisfaction of university students in Turkey,* poster presentation, 1stWorld Positive Psychology Conference, Pennsylvania, USA, 18-23 June.

Guney, S.(2011) "The Strengthspotting Scale: Reliability and Validity Study in Turkish Population", *Procedia Social and Behavioural Sciences (Elsevier)*, vol. 12, 126-132.

Guney, S., Akca, F. And Gulcilem, S. (2011) "The interrelation between traumatic life events and mental health in Turkish university students", *Procedia Social and Behavioural Sciences (Elsevier)*, vol. 12, 122-125.

Guney,S., Kalafat, T., Boysan, M. (2010) Dimensions of Mental Health: Life Satisfaction, Anxiety and Depression: A Preventive Mental Health Study in Ankara University Students Population, *Procedia Social and Behavioural Sciences(Elsevier)*, vol. 2, issue 2, 1210-1213.

Herman, J. (1997) *Trauma and Recovery: The Aftermath of Violence Domestic Abuse to Political Terror.* New york City. Basic Books.

Joseph, S. & Linley, P.A. (2005). Positive adjustment to threatening events: an organismic valuing theory of growth through adversity. *Review of General Psychology, 9,* 262-280.

Linley, P.A. (2003). Positive adaptations to trauma: wisdom as both process and outcome. *Journal of Traumatic Stress,* 16, 601-610.

Linden M. (2003) Posttraumatic Embitterment Disorder. *Psychother Psychosom*, 72:195-202.

Macnab, F.A. (1991)*The Contextual Modular Therapy: New Directions for Clinical Practice,* spectrum publications, Victoria, Australia.

Macnab, F.A.(1984) *Conflict and stress: The malcolm millar lecture in psychotherapy.* Aberdeen:University Press Aberdeen.

Macnab, F.A. (1999) The doctor's case book: Discovering wisdom and contentment. Melbourne: Information Australia.

Macnab, F.A. (2000) *Traumas of life (volume 1).*Melbourne:Spectrum Publications, Australia.

Macnab, F.A. (2000) *Traumas of life (volume 2).* Melbourne:Spectrum Publications, Australia.

McLaughlin, K., A., Hatzenbuehler, M.,L. (2009) Mechanisms Linking Stressful Life Events and Mental Health Problems in a Prospective, Community-Based Sample of Adolescents. *Journal of Adolescent Health* , 44, 153–160.

Ozer, Emily J. and Weiss, Daniel, S. (2004) Who Develops Posttraumatic Stress Disorder? *Current Directions in psychological Science,* 13, 169.

Park, N., Peterson, C.& Seligman, M.E. (2004b) Strenghts of character and well-being. *Journal of Social & Clinical Psychology,* 23, 603-619

Rashid, T., & Anjum. A (2007). Positive psychotherapy for children and adolescents. In J. R. Z. Abela & B. L. Hankin (Eds.), *Depression in children and adolescents: Causes, treatment and prevention.* New York: Guilford Press.

Seligman, M. E. P. (2002). *Authentic happiness: Using the new Positive Psychology to realize your potential for lasting fulfillment.* New York: Free Press.

Seligman, M. E. P. (2004). Positive interventions: More evidence of effectiveness. *Authentic Happiness Newsletter,* Retrieved January 9, 2007, from http://www.authentichappiness.sas.upenn.edu/newsletter.aspx?id=45

Seligman, M. E. P., & Csikszentmihalyi, M. (2000). Positive psychology: An introduction. *American Psychologist, 55,* 5-14.

Seligman, M.E.P. (2006). *Positive interventions (and other new stuff).* Paper presented at the Fifth International Positive Psychology Summit, October, Washington, DC.

Seligman, M.E.P., Rashid, T. & Parks, A.C. (2006). Positive psychotherapy. *American Psychologist,* 61,774–788.

Street, A.E., Gibson, L.E.& Holohan, D.R. (2005). Impact of childhood traumatic events, trauma-related guilt, and avoidant coping strategies on PTSD symptoms in female survivors of domestic violence. Journal of Traumatic Stress, 18, 245-252.

Tedeschi, R.G., & Calhoun, L.G. (2004). A clinical approach to posttraumatic growth. In P.A., Linley and S. Joseph (Eds.) *Positive Psychology in Practice* (pp.405-419), Hoboken, New Jersey: John Wiley & Sons.

Suheyla Unal, S., Guney, S., Kartalci, S. and Reyhani, İ. (2011) The Study of The Reliability and Validity of The Turkish Version of Post Traumatic Embitterment Disorder Self-Rating Scale (PTED Self-Rating Scale) *Düşünen Adam The Journal of Psychiatry and Neurological Sciences,* 24:32-37.

Valliant, G. (2000). Adaptive mental mechanisms: their role in positive psychology. *American Psychologist,* 55, 89 – 98.

Zoellner, T., & Maercker, A. (2005). Posttraumatic growth in clinical psychology: A critical review and introduction of a two component model. *Clinical Psychology Review,* 26, 626–653.

7

PTSD in Primary Care: A Physician's Guide to Dealing with War-Induced PTSD

Jeffrey S. Yarvis[1] and Grace D. Landers[2]
[1]*Department of Psychiatry*
Uniformed Services University of the Health Sciences
[2]*Family Medicine Resident*
Naval Hospital Camp Lejeune
USA

1. Introduction

Posttraumatic stress disorder (PTSD), as defined in DSM IV-TR, is the most common and conspicuous psychiatric problem associated with the stress experienced by soldiers in combat yet it is often misunderstood even by frontline primary care providers. Diagnosis of PTSD requires exposure to a traumatic event that involves experiencing, witnessing, or being confronted by death or serious injury to self or others; a response of intense fear, helplessness, or horror; and development of a set of symptoms that persist for at least a month and cause significant impairment of functioning (American Psychiatric Association, 2000). Some factor analytic studies have demonstrated four basic dimensions of PTSD symptoms (e.g., King, Leskin, King, & Weathers, 1998): reexperiencing (e.g., nightmares, flashbacks), avoidance (e.g., efforts to avoid thinking about the trauma), numbing of general responsiveness (e.g., restricted range of affect), and hyperarousal (e.g., exaggerated startle response), but some suggest other complex relationships between symptoms (McWilliams, Cox, & Asmundson, 2005). Most individuals who develop chronic PTSD experience immediate distress that then persists over time (Buckley, Blanchard, & Hickling, 1996). However, a small but significant number of individuals reports increases in PTSD symptoms over time (delayed onset PTSD; Gray, Bolton, & Litz, 2004).

Current data suggest that approximately 5-20% of armed forces personnel deployed for combat, peacekeeping, or humanitarian disaster relief will develop PTSD following their tour of duty (Bramsen, Dirkzwager, & van der Ploeg, 2000; Litz et al., 1997; Mehlum & Weisaeth, 2002; Ward, 2002; Dohrenwend, Turner, Turse, Adams, Koenen, & Marshall, 2006; Tanielian & Jaycox, 2008). Current estimates for those serving in Iraq/Afghanistan run as high as 15% and while exposure to specific combat traumas are the single best predictor for the development of PTSD, service members who have experienced more lengthy and more frequent deployments are at the greatest risk (Tanielian & Jaycox, 2008).

In considering the problem of PTSD, it should also be acknowledged that problematic reactions to trauma are not limited to full-blown disorder. A considerable percentage (i.e., 10% - 25%) of those not meeting threshold diagnostic criteria for PTSD experience significant subsyndromal symptoms (e.g., Schlenger et al., 1999) that may require treatment.

Subthreshold or partial PTSD is associated with significant levels of impairment of social, occupational, and family functioning (e.g., Stein, Walker, Hazen, & Forder, 1997; Weiss et al., 1992; Zlotnick et al., 2002; Yarvis et al., 2005), often similar to those reported in individuals with full PTSD (Stein et al., 1997. Those diagnosed with PTSD almost always experience concurrent additional mental health disorders, such as substance use disorder, other anxiety disorders, and major depressive disorder (e.g., Breslau, Davis. Peterson, et al., 2000; Helzer et al., 1987; Kessler, Sonnega, Bromet, Hughes, & Nelson, 1995; Kulka et al.,1990).

Risk factors for development of PTSD include characteristics of the traumatic event itself, pre-trauma factors, and post-trauma factors. Event characteristics that increase the risk for chronic PTSD include type of trauma, greater amount of exposure, injury, involvement in atrocities, and perceived life threat (Engdahl et al., 1997; Green, Grace, Lindy, Gleser, & Leonard, 1990; D. W. King et al., 1996; Kulka et al., 1990; Wolfe, Erickson, Sharkansky, King, & King, 1999). Degree of exposure to potentially traumatic combat events during deployment is strongly associated with development of PTSD (Hoge et al., 2004). Military sexual trauma is more strongly associated with PTSD than premilitary or postmilitary sexual trauma (Himmelfarb, Yaeger, & Mintz, 2006) or other traumas (Yaeger, Himmelfarb, Cammack, & Mintz, 2006). In a sample of women veterans seeking treatment for stress disorders, sexual stress was found to be almost four times as influential in the development of PTSD as duty-related stress (Fontana & Rosenheck, 1998). In veterans, predisposing factors have included non-Caucasian ethnicity, lower intelligence or education, younger age at exposure, lower socioeconomic status, family problems in childhood, pre-trauma psychopathology, and childhood behavior problems (Engdahl, Dikel, Eberly, & Blank, 1997; D. W. King, King, Foy, & Gudanowske, 1996; Kulka et al., 1990; McNally & Shin, 1995). Post-event factors that predict chronic PTSD in veterans include low levels of social support, negative homecoming experiences, poor coping, and adverse life events post-trauma (Boscarino, 1995; Engdahl et al., 1997; Green et al., 1992; L. A. King, King, Fairbank, Keane, & Adams, 1998). While many risk factors exert a similar effect in military and civilian populations, trauma severity and post-trauma social support may be more important in military than in civilian samples (Brewin, Andrews, & Valentine, 2000).

2. Psychological theories of PTSD and treatment

Conceptions of the etiology of PTSD, both psychosocial and biological, have implications for the understanding of treatment. Many such theories have focused on the intense fear often experienced during traumatic experiences and the impact of fear on conditioned emotional reactions and encoding of traumatic memories.

Foa and Kozak (1986) suggest that here are two conditions for change in these problematic fear-related memories once they have been created: the fear structure must be activated, and there must be an incorporation of new information into the memory. Memory activation alone is insufficient for change; in fact, trauma memories are being activated frequently without benefit to the survivor, by nightmares, conversations, or trauma reminders. These experiences often increase fear for the person, or prompt maladaptive escape or avoidance behaviors. Dual Representation Theory (Brewin, Dalgleish, & Joseph, 1996) argues that activation of memories can lead not only to recovery but to chronic emotional processing (permanent preoccupation with consequences of trauma and intrusive memories), or to premature inhibition of processing that results from avoidance and is associated with continued phobic avoidance, somatization, and vulnerability to reactivation later in life. When PTSD symptoms become chronic, this is thought to reflect a failure to engage in successful emotional processing of the traumatic experience. Avoidance limits activation of the memory and access to new, corrective information (Foa & Cahill, 2001).

Following this thinking, it is the job of the treatment provider to encourage conditions for change and reduce emotional avoidance. Deliberate therapeutic activation of traumatic memories is most directly attempted in exposure therapies that require the individual to repetitively talk about the trauma in detail and approach previously-avoided trauma-related stimuli. During effective treatment, therefore, avoidance is limited and new information of many kinds is purposefully incorporated into the memory. The individual learns that it is not dangerous to remember the trauma and experience strong emotions, that the memory can be remembered deliberately with a feeling of personal control and manageable physical reactions, that the trauma memory is not completely accurate and must be updated, and/or that some beliefs or judgments about the experience can be challenged and changed.

While most theories of PTSD emphasize the relationship of fear to the development of PTSD, combat and other deployment-related traumas often activate other intense emotions - including sadness, anger, and guilt - that can be connected with the development of PTSD and other post-trauma problems. In Operation Iraqi Freedom, for example, substantial percentages of Army and Marine Corps personnel reported experiencing potentially traumatic experiences that included not only events likely to be associated with fear (e.g., "being attacked or ambushed"), but also those related to loss (e.g., "knowing someone seriously injured or killed"), moral conflict (e.g., "being responsible for the death of a noncombatant"), horror (e.g., "handling or uncovering human remains"), or helplessness (e.g., "seeing ill or injured women or children whom you were unable to help") (Hoge, Castro, Messer, McGurk, Cotting, & Koffman, 2004). This range of experiences is associated with a range of intense emotions that can continue to trouble trauma survivors. Some of these emotions are fueled by negative interpretations or appraisals (e.g., of personal behavior during the trauma, or the effects of the trauma), so that it may be important to supplement exposure interventions with those explicitly designed to modify appraisals. The cognitive theory of PTSD emphasizes the "idiosyncratic negative appraisals of the traumatic event and/or its sequelae that have the common effect of creating a sense of serious current threat" (Ehlers & Clark, 2000, p. 320) and thus help to maintain acute stress reactions.

Generally, cognitive-behavioral psychological theories of PTSD and its treatment instruct that the trauma memory needs to be actively confronted, elaborated, and integrated into context of an individual's preceding and subsequent experience; that problematic appraisals that maintain sense of threat and other negative emotions need to be modified; and that dysfunctional coping strategies that prevent emotional processing of the trauma and thus recovery need to be reduced.

3. The process of treatment of deployment-related PTSD

Treatment of PTSD must depend upon a careful assessment of the individual and the formulation of a treatment plan that is based on judgments about the factors that may have caused problems for that particular person, those that maintain them, the co-occurring problems of the person, and the priorities for intervention. Generally, however, and regardless of specific interventions, treatment of individuals with PTSD can be conceptualized as a temporal process, starting with engagement with the client and alliance building, and education about the nature of trauma, post-traumatic stress reactions, and the recovery process. This process often gradually moves into coping skills training and/or trauma-focused interventions, aspects of treatment that require greater commitment and involvement of the client. Finally, as treatment intensity is decreased, attention is focused on relapse prevention and maintenance of treatment gains.

Active engagement and alliance building. In order for treatment of PTSD to commence, individuals with PTSD must present for care. However, many are reluctant to seek mental health treatment, and those experiencing higher levels of symptoms may be less likely to seek help and report more barriers to help-seeking (Maguen & Litz, 2006). In an anonymous survey of four U.S. combat infantry units administered three to four months after their return from combat duty in Iraq or Afghanistan (Hoge, Castro, Messer, McGurk, Cotting, & Koffman, 2004), only 38 to 45 percent of individuals whose responses met criteria for a mental health disorder indicated an interest in receiving help, and only 23 to 40 percent reported having received professional help in the past year. Those screening positive for disorder were twice as likely to report concern about being stigmatized and about other barriers to seeking mental health services. In this study, barriers to help-seeking included concern about being seen as weak, feelings of embarrassment, and concern about reactions from leadership. For some, another barrier to seeking treatment for PTSD within a Veterans Healthcare Administration (VHA) or Department of Defense (DoD) setting is fear that documentation of PTSD-related problems in the medical record might have an adverse effect on advancement in a military career or later employment in some occupations (e.g., police).

Initial presentation does not necessarily result in active involvement in the treatment process. The importance of this issue is highlighted by clinical experience with OIF returnees one and two years after their return to the United States. In VHA settings, many veterans come to one or two sessions of treatment but do not begin active participation in counseling services. In fact, once an individual presents for help, clinicians must take steps to maintain attendance and achieve active engagement in the treatment process. It is important to assess for obstacles to participation and make efforts to ensure that treatment makes sense to the individual and is perceived as relevant to his or her needs.

Ongoing assessment and monitoring of treatment effectiveness. Assessment of military-related PTSD requires a multi-method approach in which multiple measures are used to assess different domains of functioning, both to improve diagnostic confidence and identify multiple targets for intervention (e.g., Keane, Street, & Stafford, 2004). Here, a few key issues can be identified. First, it is important for the provider to gather information about the individual's experiences during deployment. Use of self-report questionnaires such as the Deployment Risk and Resilience Inventory (King, King, Vogt, Knight, & Samper, 2006) can make this process more complete and efficient for provider and patient. Second, findings of high rates of lifetime physical and sexual victimization among veterans in treatment for chronic PTSD (Lapp, Bosworth, Strauss, Stechuchak, Horner, Calhoun, Meador, Lipper, & Butterfield, 2005) support the need for routine assessment of history of trauma exposure; adverse childhood experiences are strongly associated with mental health symptoms

(Cabrera, Hoge, & Bliese, 2007) and predict the presence of PTSD and depression among active duty soldiers seeking mental health services (Gahm & Lucenko, 2008). Third, it is important that clinicians engage in ongoing assessment/monitoring of treatment impact. While this is not currently routine practice in many treatment settings, it is important to help provider and survivor evaluate the effectiveness of their work together, and make changes when necessary. The Clinical Practice Guideline for PTSD jointly developed by the Veterans Healthcare Administration and the Department of Defense (VA-DoD Clinical Practice Guideline Working Group, 2003) recommends routine use of validated self-administered checklists (and interviews as appropriate) at intake and to monitor follow-up status (at least every 3 months).

Ongoing interactive education. Patient education comprises a basic component of most forms of psychotherapy for PTSD, and should be introduced early and continued throughout all stages of the treatment process. Although education alone is unlikely to result in remission of PTSD, it is important to build commitment to treatment participation and help the survivor more clearly understand his or her own experience and how to actively participate in treatment (Gray, Elhai, & Frueh, 2004).

Coping skills training. There is a great difference between knowing what to do versus knowing how to do it. Skills training methods are designed to help individuals learn and practice what to do to cope more effectively with the various kinds of situations that challenge them. Skills training methods are commonly used to help those suffering with PTSD to increase their ability to reduce anxiety, communicate with loved ones, manage anger, and respond assertively (not aggressively) to conflict situations. Through a cycle of instruction, demonstration, rehearsal/practice, feedback/coaching, and more practice, survivors learn skills in treatment sessions and practice them in the natural environment. They keep written records of their attempts to apply the skills, which help them learn and provide practitioner and survivor with real-world experiences to review. Clinical experience indicates that survivors are typically attracted to the idea of learning skills ("tools") for coping. The methods of skills training help to actively involve the survivor in treatment, provide him or her with a greater sense of control (and responsibility for active participation in treatment), and strengthen the transfer of what is learned in treatment to the natural environment of the client.

Deliberate, planned confrontation of trauma memories and reminders. The core element of PTSD treatment is active discussion and exploration of traumatic experiences and their implications. The treatments that focus explicitly on traumatic memories and meanings - PE, CT, and EMDR - have received the most empirical support to date, and comprise three of the four "strongly recommended" treatments in the VA-DOD Practice Guideline.

Methods of direct therapeutic exposure involve the most direct confrontation of memories and reminders. Imaginal exposure involves a repeated retelling of the trauma story with emotional activation. *In vivo* exposure adds real-world exposure to stimuli associated with the trauma via confrontation of avoided trauma-related stimuli in the natural environment. These procedures involve multiple repetitions via assignments to listen to a cassette recording of the trauma narrative, write about the experience, or approach real-world trauma reminders systematically in between-session tasks. A combination of imaginal and *in vivo* exposure, to include virtual-reality exposure therapy, is thought to be more effective than either procedure alone (Rizzo, Reger, Gahm, Difede & Rothbaum, 2009) . According to

Foa and Jaycox (1999), PE treatment assists the individual in incorporating new information into the memory, by reducing cognitive avoidance of trauma-related feelings, demonstrating that remembering the experience is not dangerous and that anxiety will diminish via habituation, fostering discrimination between the trauma and similar non-traumatic situations, strengthening ability to tolerate memories and thereby challenging perceptions of personal incompetence, and reviewing details of the experience that provide evidence against disabling beliefs about danger and incompetence.

Exposure to trauma memories is an element of a number of treatments other than PE that are supported in the research literature. For example, individuals being treated with Cognitive Processing Therapy (Resick & Schnicke, 1993) are asked to write out the details of their traumatic experience and to read their account on a regular basis. EMDR includes an exposure component, in that it involves bringing to mind an image of a traumatic event while visually tracking a therapist's finger as it moves back and forth in front of the patient's visual field (or tracking a light moving back and forth, or listening to tones alternating from one ear to the other).

Challenging of negative trauma-related thoughts. Cognitive therapy is a systematic approach that includes education about the role of beliefs in causing distress; identification of distressing beliefs held by the individual; discussion and a review of evidence for and against the beliefs; generation of alternative beliefs; and rehearsal of new, more adaptive beliefs. Thoughts that create significant distress (e.g., trauma-related guilt, exaggerated thoughts about danger) are replaced with more realistic and self-supportive thoughts. For example, if an individual has the thought "I will never be safe again, the world is a very dangerous place," cognitive therapy might focus on helping the individual to consider evidence for and against the belief and move toward a more realistic appraisal (e.g., "I am safe in most situations and the chances of harm coming to me are quite small in the civilian world"). It is often important that trauma-related guilt be made a formal target of PTSD treatment.

Negative thoughts can be challenged through direct review of the belief and consideration of alternatives, and through encouraging real-world experiences that can help to disconfirm them. For example, having a successful experience in disclosing personal information to another person can help challenge the belief that "other people cannot be trusted." Successful implementation of PE can also result in modification of distressing trauma-related cognitions, by disconfirming beliefs ("anxiety stays forever" or "I will go crazy") and helping the survivor differentiate the trauma from similar but safe events (disconfirming "the world is extremely dangerous"). PTSD symptoms themselves may begin to be associated with mastery rather than incompetence (disconfirming "I am incompetent").

Pharmacotherapy. Medication is an important treatment option that should be considered for almost all patients with significant symptoms of PTSD. The use of a medication in patients with PTSD may be directed at PTSD symptoms generally, specific PTSD symptoms, common co-occurring symptoms, or at co-morbid conditions (e.g., depression). Initiating a medication trial may occur at different phases in treatment depending on a variety of the patient-specific factors.

Despite the wide use of a variety of medications for the treatment of PTSD, in fact there is a relative lack of definitive evidence for their efficacy (Institute of Medicine 2007). The most thoroughly investigated agents are the selective serotonin reuptake inhibitors (SSRIs). SSRIs have demonstrated superiority over placebo in large randomized, controlled trials as well as in a number of smaller investigations, and they are now considered the first-line pharmacological treatment option for PTSD (Ballenger et al. 2004).

SSRIs have proven effectiveness for many other anxiety and depressive disorders that are highly co-morbid with PTSD. PTSD and major depression overlap to a considerable degree; both share sleep disturbances, social withdrawal and isolation, decreased pleasure and enjoyment, and impaired concentration. Major depression is the most common co-morbid disorder in patients with PTSD, with close to 50% of PTSD subjects having a history of major depression (Kessler et al., 1995). Although SSRIs improve both PTSD and depression, SSRIs are efficacious for both PTSD patients with and without depression (Stein et al. 2003). Panic disorder and generalized anxiety are also responsive to SSRI treatment and also often co-occur with PTSD (Stein et al. 2000). As with most other disorders treated with antidepressants, a full therapeutic response to SSRIs in PTSD takes 4-6 weeks.

In summary, medications, particularly antidepressants, may reduce the global severity of PTSD symptoms and serve as useful tools in the treatment of PTSD. Psychotropic medications may also be used to treat associated features and/or co-morbid conditions. But the practitioner and the patient must be aware that, with the exception of antidepressants, their use is off-label. Polypharmacy can occur in patients with PTSD in the absence of empirical support (Mellman et al., 2003) and should be avoided.

Maintenance/Relapse prevention. Relatively little is known about rates and processes of relapse after treatment for PTSD. Studies in the civilian section suggest that improvements resulting from use of evidence-based treatments can be maintained for significant periods of time (e.g., Resick, Williams, Orazem, & Gutner, 2005). Some evidence suggests that patients discharging from residential PTSD treatment and referred for outpatient aftercare are more likely to make an outpatient visit within one month of discharge if they receive biweekly telephone calls after discharge (Rosen, Dilandro, Corwin, Drescher, Cooney, & Gusman, 2006). Research also suggests that long-term treatment of PTSD with SSRIs maintains treatment response and quality of life improvements, and that discontinuation of SSRI treatment after 12 weeks results in a greater relapse risk, compared with extended treatment (Davis, Frazier, Williford, & Newell, 2006).

4. Associated problems in PTSD treatment

As noted above, approximately 80% of those diagnosed with PTSD experience concurrent additional mental health disorders (Kessler et al., 1995). In addition, they experience a range of problems in living that are often addressed in treatment. PTSD symptoms are associated with reduced quality of life before treatment and, encouragingly, evidence suggests that change in PTSD is significantly associated with change in quality of life (Schnurr, Hayes, Lunney, McFall, & Uddo, 2006). Most PTSD outcomes research has focused on reduction of PTSD symptoms, so that the impact of treatment on the wider range of quality of life and functional outcomes is less well investigated.

Substance abuse/Addictive behaviors. Co-occurrence of PTSD and substance abuse problems is well documented in populations of civilians and veterans (Ouimette & Brown, 2002; Ruzek, 2002). Some research suggests that veterans with PTSD who also abuse substances will benefit more from substance abuse treatment if they also address PTSD;

patients who received PTSD treatment in the first 3 months following discharge from substance abuse treatment were more likely to be in remission from substance use disorders at follow-up (Ouimette, Moos, & Finney, 2003).

Evidence also suggests that PTSD is associated with increased risk of smoking (Beckham, Kirby, & Feldman, 1997) and that unremitted PTSD is a risk factor for late-onset smoking among individuals who were nonsmokers prior to developing PTSD (Koenen, Hitsman, & Lyons, 2006). Other addictive behaviors may also be associated with PTSD. In civilians seeking treatment for pathological gambling, frequency of PTSD symptoms has been found to predict greater lifetime gambling severity (Ledgerwood & Petry, 2006).

Depression and Suicidality. PTSD is strongly comorbid with depression (Kessler, et al., 1995; Blanchard et al., 1998; Breslau et al., 2000; Yarvis et al., 2005; Yarvis & Schiess, 2008). Presence of PTSD is associated with increased risk of suicide. Sareen, Houlahan, Cox, and Asmundson (2005) used data from the nationally representative National Comorbidity Survey to investigate the relationships between anxiety disorders and suicidal ideation and attempts. PTSD was significantly associated with suicidal ideation and suicide attempts; none of the other anxiety disorders showed such an association. Generally, PTSD in U.S. Army veterans is associated with mortality from external causes, including homicide, suicide, drug overdoses, and unintended injury (Boscarino, 2006). Clinicians treating PTSD should therefore routinely screen for suicidality and remain alert to the need to monitor suicide ideation and provide preventive interventions.

Anxiety. PTSD, itself classified as an anxiety disorder, is highly comorbid with other anxiety disorders, including panic disorder, generalized anxiety disorder, social anxiety disorder, obsessive-compulsive disorder, and phobias.

Anger/Violence. Anger and irritability comprise one of the symptoms of PTSD. Intense anger is commonly part of the presentation of those with PTSD (Novaco & Chemtob, 2002) and is more significant among those whose traumas were experienced during military service (Orth & Wieland, 2006). The volatile anger reactions of their patients can present treatment providers with challenges in establishing therapeutic relationships and in delivering treatment itself. In a study of Australian veterans, anger at intake was the most potent predictor of symptom change (Forbes, Creamer, & Hawthorne, 2003). Anger might interfere with the confrontation with and processing of traumatic memories that can be important in recovery from the disorder (Foa & Rothbaum, 1998); a high level of anger at the beginning of PE treatment interferes with response to treatment (Foa et al., 1995). Anger reduction should often be made an explicit goal of treatment and individuals can be taught skills (e.g., time out/cool down, anger self-monitoring, identifying anger situations, relaxation/breathing, anger discrimination, self-talk, assertion training) to reduce their anger or modify its expression.

Anger problems may also require the provider to assist the veteran in reducing risk of violence. Veterans with PTSD often have ready access to weapons and engage in potentially dangerous firearm-related behaviors (Freeman, Roca, & Kimbrell, 2003), and clinicians should routinely address gun storage and safety issues as part of the treatment process.

Complicated or traumatic bereavement. Many of those deployed to a war zone will be exposed to significant personal losses, and these deaths will often be encountered in traumatic circumstances. Traumatic bereavement can lead to anhedonia and depression and grief about fallen friends can make social interaction and activity seem pointless. Loss of close comrades and friends in battle is associated with post-war distress and social dysfunction. Treatment for traumatic or complicated grief has received relatively little formal evaluation, but most treatments include education about grief, restructuring of cognitive distortions about events, restoration of positive memories of the deceased, acknowledgment of caring feelings toward those lost, retelling of the story of the death, and help in tolerating painful feelings (e.g., Shear & Frank, 2006). Elements of treatment for PTSD can be adapted for treatment of complicated grief (Ehlers, 2006).

Physical health problems. PTSD is associated with poorer perceived health status, greater somatic complaints, greater number of chronic health problems, and increased levels of health care utilization (Schnurr & Green, 2004a; Kulka et al., 1990; Richardson, Elhai, & Pedlar, 2006; Stapleton, Asmundson, & Woods, 2006; Yarvis et al. 2005, Yarvis & Schiess, 2008). Overall, studies suggest that PTSD mediates the relationship between war zone exposure and physical health for both males and females (e.g., Schnurr & Green, 2004b). The majority of veterans seeking PTSD treatment do not engage in preventive health behaviors (e.g., exercise and medical screening) at levels consistent with health care guidelines (Buckley, Mozley, Bedard, Dewulf, & Greif, 2004), and these issues should be assessed and if necessary, addressed in treatment.

The strong relationships between PTSD and health outcomes extends to Operation Iraqi Freedom returnees (Hoge, Terhakopian, Castro, Messer, & Engel, 2007), and for this population, early severity of physical injury is strongly associated with development of later PTSD or depression (Grieger, Cozza, & Ursano, 2006). Such findings support the need for increasing integration of mental health screening and services in primary care and other medical settings.

Traumatic brain injury. The high rate of co-occurring traumatic brain injury (TBI) and PTSD in those deployed to Iraq and Afghanistan poses clinical challenges that are ill-understood at present. Evidence suggests that PTSD can develop following both mild and severe TBI, even in individuals who have lost consciousness during the event or display post-traumatic amnesia (McMillan, Williams, & Bryant, 2003). In one study of military personnel deployed to Iraq, mild TBI (i.e., concussion) was found to be strongly correlated with PTSD and physical health problems 3 to 4 months after return to the United States, and the relationship between mild TBI and health was largely mediated by PTSD and depression (Hoge, McGurk, Thomas, Cox, Engel, & Castro, 2008). PTSD treatment for those with TBI may need to include modifications that address difficulties that may be associated with injury, including difficulty in retrieving the traumatic memory, comprehending and remembering treatment recommendations, and reporting on symptoms and experience. Bryant, Moulds, and Guthrie (2003) found that civilians diagnosed with mild TBI and ASD could be effectively treated with a brief CBT protocol designed to prevent development of PTSD.

Impaired family functioning. The anger, emotional numbing, and social withdrawal often associated with PTSD can isolate the veteran from his or her family. PTSD veterans and their partners report more problems in their relationships and more difficulties with intimacy (and have taken more steps toward separation and divorce) than veterans without PTSD and their partners; degree of relationship distress is correlated with the severity of veterans'

PTSD symptoms, particularly symptoms of emotional numbing (Riggs, Byrne, Weathers, & Litz, 1998). Emotional numbing symptoms are also correlated with perceived relationship quality with children (Ruscio, Weathers, King, & King, 2002), and higher levels of PTSD symptoms (avoidance and emotional numbing symptoms in particular) may lower parent-child relationship satisfaction (Samper et al, 2004). Men reporting combat as their worst trauma are more likely to be divorced and physically abusive to their spouses than men reporting other traumas as their worst experience (Prigerson, Maciejewski, & Rosenheck, 2001).

A treatment focus on improvement of family functioning would suggest that steps should be taken to more systematically involve spouses/partners in care (Devilly, 2002; Sautter, Lyons, & Manguno-Mire, 2006). Significant others can be included in the assessment process, in the setting of treatment goals, and in treatment itself.

Impaired social functioning. Military-related PTSD is often associated with withdrawal from participation in social activities, limited friendships, and reduced emotional intimacy (Riggs, Byrne, Weathers, & Litz, 1998; Jordan, Marmar, Fairbank, Schlenger, Kulka, Hough, & Weiss, 1992). As noted above, some research suggests that veterans with PTSD have greater rates of Social Anxiety Disorder. Poor social support predicts development of PTSD and a more chronic course of the disorder; veterans with PTSD who are more involved in the community are more likely to show remission in PTSD symptoms than those with less community involvement (Koenen et al., 2003) and adjustment to peacekeeping is significantly related to self-disclosure, especially to supportive significant others (Bolton et al., 2003). Overcoming problems in social functioning and promoting social participation may require active, sustained intervention. When indicated, improvements in social functioning must be established as a formal treatment goal.

Impaired workplace functioning. Evidence indicates that PTSD impairs work performance and reduces work productivity (Kessler & Frank, 1997).It has been suggested that even modest reductions in PTSD symptoms may lead to employment gains, even if the overall symptom levels remain severe (Smith et al., 2005).

Although no interventions to date have targeted the workplace functioning of individuals with PTSD, it would seem useful for clinicians to provide assistance to employed patients in applying stress and anger management skills on the job, and problem-solving difficult situations, to help reduce the impact of traumatic stress reactions on this important domain of functioning.

5. Conclusion

Management of deployment-related PTSD has been changing rapidly. Screening for PTSD is widespread, returning personnel are informed about the disorder, and the Veterans Healthcare Administration and Department of Defense have collaborated to establish practice guidelines for responding to the specific needs of those with PTSD. As treatment systems evolve, it is critical that more and better quality evaluation of treatment effectiveness be undertaken. q The necessity for civilian social workers to be attuned to the nuances of PTSD is imperative. As more and more returning service members are seeking care in the private sector, social workers and other non-government mental health care providers will be working with those with PTSD and those close to them. Management poses many challenges and understanding both the challenges and approaches to care will benefit service members to better return to civilian life.

6. References

Ballenger Jc, Davidson Jr, Lecrubier Y, Nutt Dj, Marshall Rd, Nemeroff Cb, Shalev Ay, Yehuda R (2004) Consensus statement update on posttraumatic stress disorder from the international consensus group on depression and anxiety *J Clin Psychiatry* 65 Suppl 1:55-62.

Bartzokis, G., Lu, P. H., Turner, J., Mintz, J., & Saunders, C. S. (2005). Adjunctive risperidone in the treatment of chronic combat-related posttraumatic stress disorder. *Biological Psychiatry, 57*, 474-479.

Beckham, J. C., Crawford, A. L., Feldman, M. E., et al. (1997). Chronic posttraumatic stress disorder and chronic pain in Vietnam veterans. *Journal of Psychosomatic Research, 43*(4), 379-389.

Blanchard, E. B., Buckley, T. C., Hickling, E. J., & Taylor, A. E. (1998). Posttraumatic stress disorder and comorbid depression: Is the correlation an illusion? *Journal of Anxiety Disorders, 12*, 21-37.

Bolton, E. E., Glenn, D. M., Orsillo, S., Roemer, L., & Litz, B. T. (2003). The relationship between self-disclosure and symptoms of posttraumatic stress disorder in peacekeepers deployed to Somalia. *Journal of Traumatic Stress, 16*, 203-210.

Boscarino, J. A. (1995). Post-traumatic stress and associated disorders among Vietnam Veterans: The significance of combat exposure and social support. *Journal of Traumatic Stress, 8*, 317 - 336.

Boscarino, J. A. (2006). External-cause mortality after psychologic trauma: The effects of stress exposure and predisposition. *Comprehensive Psychiatry, 47*, 503-514.

Bramsen, I., Dirkzwager, A. J. E., & van der Ploeg, H. M. (2000). Pre-deployment personality traits and exposure to trauma as predictors of posttraumatic stress symptoms: A prospective study of former peacekeepers. *American Journal of Psychiatry, 157*, 1115-1119.

Breslau, N., Davis, G. C., Peterson, E. L., and Schultz, L. R. (2000). A second look at comorbidity in victims of trauma: The posttraumatic stress disorder - major depression connection. *Biological Psychiatry, 48*, 902-909.

Brewin, C. R., Andrews, B., & Valentine, J. D. (2000). Meta-analysis of risk factors for posttraumatic stress disorder in trauma-exposed adults. *Journal of Consulting and Clinical Psychology, 68*, 748-766.

Brewin, C. R., Dalgleish, T.., & Joseph, S. (1996). A dual representation theory of post-traumatic stress disorder. *Psychological Review, 103*, 670-686.

Bryant, R. A., Moulds, M. L., & Guthrie, R. M. (2003a). Imaginal exposure alone and imaginal exposure with cognitive restructuring in treatment of posttraumatic stress disorder. *Journal of Consulting and Clinical Psychology, 71*, 706-712.

Bryant, R. A., Moulds, M., & Guthrie, R. (2003b). Treating acute stress disorder following mild traumatic brain injury. *American Journal of Psychiatry, 160*, 585-587.

Buckley, T. C., Blanchard, E. B., & Hickling, E. J. (1996). A prospective examination of delayed onset PTSD secondary to motor vehicle accidents. *Journal of Abnormal Psychology, 105*, 617–625.

Buckley, T. C., Mozley, S. L., Bedard, M. A., Dewulf, A. C., & Greif, J. (2004). Preventive health behaviors, health-risk behaviors, physical morbidity, and health-related role functioning impairment in veterans with post-traumatic stress disorder. *Military Medicine, 169*, 536-540.

Cabrera, O. A., Hoge, C. W., & Bliese, P. D. (2007). Childhood adversity and combat as predictors of depression and post-traumatic stress in deployed troops. *American Journal of Preventive Medicine, 33*, 77-82.

Davis Ll, Davidson Jr, Ward Lc, Bartolucci A, Bowden Cl, Petty F (2008) Divalproex in the treatment of posttraumatic stress disorder: a randomized, double-blind, placebo-controlled trial in a veteran population *J Clin Psychopharmacol* 28:84-8

Devilly, G. J. (2002). The psychological effects of a lifestyle management course on war veterans and their spouses. *Journal of Clinical Psychology, 58*, 1119-1134.

Devilly, G. J., Spence, S. H., & Rapee, R. M. (1998). Statistical and reliable change with eye movement desensitization and reprocessing: Treating trauma within a veteran population. *Behavior Therapy, 29*, 435-455.

Dieperink, M., Erbes, C., Leskela, J., Kaloupek, D., Farrer, M.K., Fisher, L., & Wolf, E. (2005). Comparison of treatment for posttraumatic stress disorder among three Department of Veteran Affairs Medical Centers. *Military Medicine, 170*, 305-308..

Dohrenwend, B. P., Turner, J. B., Turse, N. A., Adams, B. G., Koenen, K. C., & Marshall, R. (2006). The psychological risks of Vietnam for U.S. veterans: A revisit with new data and methods. *Science, 313*, 979-982.

Ehlers, A. (2006). Understanding and treating complicated grief: what can we learn from posttraumatic stress disorder? *Clinical Psychology: Science and Practice, 13*, 135-140.

Ehlers, A. & Clark, D. M. (2000). A cognitive model of posttraumatic stress disorder. *Behaviour Research and Therapy, 38*, 319-345.

Engdahl, B., Dikel, T., Eberly, R., & Blank, A. (1997) Posttraumatic stress disorder in a community sample of former prisoners of war: A normative response to severe trauma. *American Journal of Psychiatry, 154(11)*, 1576-1581.

Foa, E. B. & Cahill, S. P. (2001). Psychological therapies: Emotional processing. In N. J. Smelser & P. B. Bates (Eds.), *International encyclopedia of the social and behavioral sciences* (pp. 12,363-12,369). Oxford, UK: Elsevier.

Foa, E. B. & Jaycox, L. H. (1999). Cognitive-behavioral theory and treatment of post-traumatic stress disorder. In D. Spiegel (Ed.), *Efficacy and cost-effectiveness of psychotherapy* (pp. 23-61). Washington, D.C.: American Psychiatric Press.

Foa, E. B. & Kozak, M. J. (1986). Emotional processing of fear: Exposure to corrective information. *Psychological Bulletin, 99*, 20-35.

Foa, E. B., Riggs, D. S., Massie, E. D., & Yarczower, M. (1995). The impact of fear activation and anger on the efficacy of exposure treatment for posttraumatic stress disorder. *Behavior Therapy, 26*, 487–499.

Foa, E.B. & Rothbaum, B.O. (1998). *Treating the trauma of rape: Cognitive-behavioral therapy for PTSD*. New York: Guilford Press.

Fontana, A. & Rosenheck, R. (1998). Duty-related and sexual stress in the etiology of PTSD among women veterans who seek treatment. *Psychiatric Services, 49*, 658-662.

Freeman, T. W., Roca, V., & Kimbrell, T. (2003). A survey of gun collection and use among three groups of Veteran patients admitted to Veterans Affairs hospital treatment programs. Southern Medical Journal, 96, 240-243

Gahm, G. A. & Lucenko, B. A. (2008). Screening soldiers in outpatient care for mental health concerns. *Military Medicine, 173*, 17-24.

Gray, M. J., Bolton, E. E., & Litz, B. T. (2004). Analysis of PTSD symptom course: Delayed-onset PTSD in Somalia peacekeepers. *Journal of Consulting and Clinical Psychology, 72*, 909-913.

Gray, M. J., Elhai, J. D., & Frueh, B. C. (2004). Enhancing patient satisfaction and increasing treatment compliance: Patient education as a fundamental component of PTSD treatment. *Psychiatric Quarterly, 75*, 321-332.

Green, B. L., Lindy, J. D., Grace, M. C., & Leonard, A. C. (1992). Chronic posttraumatic stress disorder and diagnostic comorbidity in a disaster sample. *Journal of Nervous and Mental Disease, 180*, 760-766.

Grieger, T. A., Cozza, S. J., & Ursano, R. J. (2006). Posttraumatic stress disorder and depression in battle-injured soldiers. *American Journal of Psychiatry, 163*, 1777-1783.

Helzer, J. E., Robins, L. N., & McEvoy, L. (1987). Posttraumatic stress disorder in the general population: Findings of the Epidemiologic Catchment Area survey. *New England Journal of Medicine, 317*, 1630-1634.

Himmelfarb, N., Yaeger, D., & Mintz, J. (2006). Posttraumatic stress disorder in female veterans with military and civilian sexual trauma. *Journal of Traumatic Stress, 19*, 837-846.

Hoge, C. W., Castro, C. A., Messer, S. C., McGurk, D., Cotting, D. I., & Koffman, R. L. (2004). Combat duty in Iraq and Afghanistan, mental health problems, and barriers to care. *The New England Journal of Medicine, 351*, 13-22.

Hoge, C. W., McGurk, D., Thomas, J. L., Cox, A. L., Engel, C. C., & Castro, C. A. (2008). Mild traumatic brain injuries in U.S. soldiers returning from Iraq. *New England Journal of Medicine, 358*, 453-463.

Hoge, C.W., Terhakopian, A., Castro, C.A., Messer, S.C., & Engel, C.C. (2007). Association of posttraumatic stress disorder with somatic symptoms, health care visits, and absenteeism among Iraq War veterans. *American Journal of Psychiatry, 164*,150-153.

Institute of Medicine (2007). Treatment of posttraumatic stress disorder: An assessment of the evidence. Washington, DC,. National Academy of the Sciences.

Jordan, B. K., Marmar, C. R., Fairbank, J. A., Schlenger, W. E., Kulka, R. A., Hough, R. L., & Weiss, D. S. (1992). Problems in families of male Vietnam veterans with posttraumatic stress disorder. *Journal of Consulting and Clinical Psychology, 60*, 916-926.

Keane, T. M., Street, A. E., & Stafford, J. (2004). The assessment of military-related PTSD. In J. P. Wilson & T. M. Keane (Eds.), *Assessing psychological trauma and PTSD (2nd edition)* (pp. 262-285). New York: Guilford Press.

Kessler, R. C. & Frank, R. G. (1997). The impact of psychiatric disorders on work loss days. *Psychological Medicine, 27*, 861-873.

Kessler RC, Sonnega A, Bromet E, Hughes M, Nelson CB. Posttraumatic stress disorder in the National Comorbidity Survey. *Arch Gen Psychiatry*. 1995: 52:1048-60.

King, L. A., King, D. W., Fairbank, J. A., Keane, T. M., & Adams, G. A. (1998). Resilience/recovery factors in posttraumatic stress disorder among female and male Vietnam veterans: Hardiness, postwar social support, and additional stressful life events. *Journal of Personality and Social Psychology, 74*, 420-434.

King, L. A., King, D. W., Vogt, D. S., Knight, J., & Samper, R. E. (2006). Deployment Risk and Resilience Inventory: A collection of measures for studying deployment-related experiences of military personnel and veterans. *Military Psychology, 18*, 89-120.

King, D.W., King, L.A., Foy, D.W., & Guadanowski, D.M. (1996). Prewar factors in combat-related posttraumatic stress disorder: Structural equation modeling with a national sample of female and male Vietnam veterans. *Journal of Consulting and Clinical Psychology 64,* 520-531.

Koenen, K. C., Hitsman, B., & Lyons, M. J. (2006). Posttraumatic stress disorder and late-onset smoking in the Vietnam era twin registry. *Journal of Consulting and Clinical Psychology, 74,* 186-190.

Kulka, R. A., Schlenger, W. E., Fairbank, J. A., Hough, R. L., Jordan, B. K., Marmar, C. R., & Weiss, D. S. (1990). *Trauma and the Vietnam War generation: Report of the findings from the National Vietnam Veterans Readjustment Study.* New York: Brunner/Mazel.

Lapp, K. G., Bosworth, H. B., Strauss, J. L., Stechuchak, K. M., Horner, R. D., Calhoun, P. S., Meador, K. G., Lipper, S., & Butterfield, M. I.. (2005). Lifetime sexual and physical victimization among male veterans with combat-related post-traumatic stress disorder. *Military Medicine, 170,* 787-790.

Ledgerwood, D. M. & Petry, N. M. (2006). Posttraumatic stress disorder symptoms in treatment-seeking pathological gamblers. *Journal of Traumatic Stress, 19,* 411-416.

Litz, B., Orsillo, S., Friedman, M., Ehlich, P., & Batres, A. (1997). Posttraumatic stress disorder associated with peacekeeping duty in Somalia for U.S. military personnel. *American Journal of Psychiatry, 154,* 178-184.

Maguen, S. & Litz, B. T. (2006). Predictors of barriers to mental health treatment for Kosovo and Bosnia peacekeepers: A preliminary report. *Military Medicine, 171,* 454-458.

McMillan, T. M., Williams, W. H., & Bryant, R. (2003). Post-traumatic stress disorder and traumatic brain injury: A review of causal mechanisms, assessment, and treatment. *Neuropsychological Rehabilitation, 13,* 149-164.

McNally, R., Shin, L. (1995). Association of intelligence with severity of posttraumatic stress disorder symptoms in Vietnam combat veterans. *American Journal of Psychiatry, 152:* 936-938.

McWilliams, L. A., Cox, B. J., & Asmundson, G. J. G. (2005). Symptom structure of posttraumatic stress disorder in a nationally representative sample. *Journal of Anxiety Disorders, 19,* 626-641.

Mehlum, L., & Weisaeth, L. (2002). Predictors of posttraumatic stress reactions in Norwegian U.N. Peacekeepers 7 years after service. *Journal of Traumatic Stress, 15*(1), 17-26.

Mellman Ta, Clark Re, Peacock Wj (2003) Prescribing patterns for patients with posttraumatic stress disorder *Psychiatr Serv* 54:1618-21

Novaco, R. W. & Chemtob, C. M. (2002). Anger and combat-related posttraumatic stress disorder. *Journal of Traumatic Stress, 15,* 123-132.

Orth, U. & Wieland, E. (2006). Anger, hostility, and posttraumatic stress disorder in trauma-exposed adults: A meta-analysis. *Journal of Consulting and Clinical Psychology, 74,* 698-706.

Ouimette. P. & Brown, P. J. (2002). *Trauma and substance abuse: Causes, consequences, and treatment of comorbid disorders.* Washington, DC: American Psychological Association.

Ouimette, P., Moos, R. H., & Finney, J. W. (2003). PTSD treatment and 5-year remission among patients with substance use and posttraumatic stress disorders. *Journal of Consulting and Clinical Psychology, 71,* 410-414.

Prigerson, H. G., Maciejewski, P. K., & Rosenheck, R. A. (2001). Combat trauma: Trauma with highest risk of delayed onset and unresolved posttraumatic stress disorder symptoms, unemployment, and abuse among men. *Journal of Nervous and Mental Disease, 189,* 99-108.

Resick, P. A., Williams, L., Orazem, R., & Gutner, C. (2005). Can we cure PTSD? Five-year follow-up of a clinical trial comparing Cognitive Processing Therapy and Prolonged Exposure. Paper presented at the annual meeting of the Association for Behavioral and Cognitive Therapies, Washington, DC.

Richardson, J. D., Elhai, J. D., & Pedlar, D. J. (2006). Association of PTSD and depression with medical and specialist care utilization in modern peacekeeping veterans in Canada with health-related disabilities. *Journal of Clinical Psychiatry, 67,* 1240-1245.

Riggs, D. S., Byrne, C. A., Weathers, F. W., & Litz, B. T. (1998). The quality of the intimate relationships of male Vietnam veterans: Problems associated with posttraumatic stress disorder. *Journal of Traumatic Stress, 11,* 87-101.

Riggs, D. S., Cahill, S. P., & Foa, E. B. (2006). Prolonged exposure treatment of PTSD. In V. F. Follette & J. I. Ruzek (Eds.), *Cognitive-behavioral therapies for trauma (2nd Edition,* pp. 65-95). New York: Guilford Press.

Rizzo, A., Reger, G., Gahm, G., Difede, J. and Rothbaum, B.O. (2009) Virtual Reality Exposure Therapy for Combat-Related PTSD. New York: Humana Press.

Ruscio, A. M., Weathers, F. W., King, L. A., & King, D. W. (2002). Male war-zone veterans' perceived relationships with their children: The importance of emotional numbing. *Journal of Traumatic Stress, 15,* 351-357.

Samper, R. E., Taft, C. T., King, D. W., & King, L. A. (2004). Posttraumatic stress disorder symptoms and parenting satisfaction among a national sample of male Vietnam veterans. *Journal of Traumatic Stress, 17,* 311-315.

Sareen, J., Houlahan, T., Cox, B. J., & Asmundson, G. J. G. (2005). Anxiety disorders associated with suicidal ideation and suicide attempts in the National Comorbidity Survey. *Journal of Nervous and Mental Disease, 193,* 450-454.

Sautter, F., Lyons, J. A., & Manguno-Mire, G. (2006). Predictors of partner engagement in PTSD treatment. *Journal of Psychopathology and Behavioral Assessment, 28,* 123-130.

Schlenger, W. E., Fairbank, J. A., Jordan, B. K., et al. (1999). Combat-related posttraumatic stress disorder: Prevalence, risk factors and comorbidity. In P. A. Saigh & J. D. Bremner (Eds.), *Posttraumatic stress disorder: A comprehensive text.* Boston: Allyn & Bacon.

Schnurr, P. P., Hayes, A. F., Lunney, C. A., McFall, M., & Uddo, M. (2006). Longitudinal analysis of the relationship between symptoms and quality of life in veterans treated for posttraumatic stress disorder. *Journal of Clinical Psychology, 74,* 707-713.

Schnurr, P. P. & Green, B. L. (2004). *Trauma and health: physical health consequences of exposure to extreme stress.* Washington: American Psychological Association.

Shear, K. & Frank, E. (2006). Treatment of complicated grief: Integrating cognitive-behavioral methods with other treatment approaches. In V. M. Follette & J. I. Ruzek (Eds.), *Cognitive-behavioral therapies for trauma (2nd Edition,* pp. 290-320), New York: Guilford Press.

Smith, M. W., Schnurr, P. P., & Rosenheck, R. A. (2005). Employment outcomes and PTSD symptom severity. *Mental Health Services Research, 7,* 89-101.

Solomon, Z., Kotler, M., & Milkulincer, M. (1988). Combat-related posttraumatic stress disorders among second generation Holocaust survivors: Preliminary findings. *American Journal of Psychiatry, 145,* 865-868.

Stapleton, J. A., Asmundson, G. J. G., & Woods, M. (2006). Health care utilization by United Nations peacekeeping veterans with co-occurring, self-reported, post-traumatic stress disorder and depression symptoms versus those without. *Military Medicine, 171,* 562-566.

Stein Mb, Mcquaid Jr, Pedrelli P, Lenox R, Mccahill Me. Posttraumatic stress disorder in the primary care medical setting *Gen Hosp Psychiatry*. 2000:22:261-9.

Stein, M. B., Walker, J. R., Hazen, A. L., & Forder, D. R. (1997). Full and partial posttraumatic stress disorder: Findings from a community survey. *American Journal of Psychiatry, 154*(8), 1114-1119.

Tanielian, T. & Jaycox, L. H. (2008). *Invisible wounds of war: Psychological and cognitive injuries, their consequences, and services to assist recovery*. RAND: Santa Monica, Calif.: MG-720-CCF.

VA-DoD Clinical Practice Guideline Working Group, Veterans Health Administration, Department of Veterans Affairs and Health Affairs, Department of Defense (2003). *Management of Post-Traumatic Stress*. Washington, DC: Office of Quality and Performance publication 10Q-CPG/PTSD-04.

Ward, J. (2002). Stress hits 1 in 5 Afghan war vets, ombudsman says: Stigma 'is still very much alive', Marin warns of possible law suits. *Toronto Star*, pp. A06.

Weiss, D. S., Marmar, C. R., Schlenger, W. E., Fairbank, J. A., Jordan, B. K., Hough, R. L., et al. (1992). The prevalence of lifetime and partial post-traumatic stress disorder in Vietnam theater veterans. *Journal of Traumatic Stress, 5*(3), 365-376.

Wolfe, J., Erickson, D., Sharkansky, E., King, D., & King, L. (1999). Course and predictors of posttraumatic stress disorder among Gulf War veterans: A prospective analysis. *Journal of Consulting and Clinical Psychology, 67*, 520–528.

Yaeger, D., Himmelfarb, N., Cammack, A., & Mintz, J. (2006). DSM-IV diagnosed posttraumatic stress disorder in women veterans with and without military sexual trauma. *JGIM: Journal of General Internal Medicine, Mar2006 Supplement, 21*, S65-S69.

Yarvis, J., Bordnick, P., Spivey, C., & Pedlar, D. (2005) Subthreshold PTSD: A comparison of alcohol, depression, and health problems in Canadian Peacekeepers with different levels of traumatic stress. *Stress, Trauma, and Crisis 8*, 195-213.

Yarvis, J. and Schiess, L. (2008) Subthreshold PTSD as a predictor of depression, alcohol use, and health problems in soldiers. Journal of Workplace Behavioral Health 23(4).

Zlotnick, C., Franklin, C. L., & Zimmerman, M. (2002). Does "subthreshold" posttraumatic stress disorder have any clinical relevance? *Comprehensive Psychiatry, 43*(6), 413-419.

Ballenger Jc, Davidson Jr, Lecrubier Y, Nutt Dj, Marshall Rd, Nemeroff Cb, Shalev Ay, Yehuda R (2004) Consensus statement update on posttraumatic stress disorder from the international consensus group on depression and anxiety *J Clin Psychiatry* 65 Suppl 1:55-62

Bartzokis G, Lu Ph, Turner J, Mintz J, Saunders Cs (2005) Adjunctive risperidone in the treatment of chronic combat-related posttraumatic stress disorder *Biol Psychiatry* 57:474-9

Becker Me, Hertzberg Ma, Moore Sd, Dennis Mf, Bukenya Ds, Beckham Jc (2007) A placebo-controlled trial of bupropion SR in the treatment of chronic posttraumatic stress disorder *J Clin Psychopharmacol* 27:193-7

Brady K, Pearlstein T, Asnis Gm, Baker D, Rothbaum B, Sikes Cr, Farfel Gm (2000) Efficacy and safety of sertraline treatment of posttraumatic stress disorder: a randomized controlled trial *Jama* 283:1837-44

Braun P, Greenberg D, Dasberg H, Lerer B (1990) Core symptoms of posttraumatic stress disorder unimproved by alprazolam treatment *J Clin Psychiatry* 51:236-8

Briley M (2004) Clinical experience with dual action antidepressants in different chronic pain syndromes *Hum Psychopharmacol* 19 Suppl 1:S21-5

Cates Me, Bishop Mh, Davis Ll, Lowe Js, Woolley Tw (2004) Clonazepam for treatment of sleep disturbances associated with combat-related posttraumatic stress disorder *Ann Pharmacother* 38:1395-9

Davidson J, Pearlstein T, Londborg P, Brady Kt, Rothbaum B, Bell J, Maddock R, Hegel Mt, Farfel G (2001) Efficacy of sertraline in preventing relapse of posttraumatic stress disorder: results of a 28-week double-blind, placebo-controlled study *Am J Psychiatry* 158:1974-81

Davidson J, Rothbaum Bo, Tucker P, Asnis G, Benattia I, Musgnung Jj (2006) Venlafaxine extended release in posttraumatic stress disorder: a sertraline- and placebo-controlled study *J Clin Psychopharmacol* 26:259-67

Davidson Jr, Brady K, Mellman Ta, Stein Mb, Pollack Mh (2007) The efficacy and tolerability of tiagabine in adult patients with post-traumatic stress disorder *J Clin Psychopharmacol* 27:85-8

Davidson Jr, Weisler Rh, Butterfield Mi, Casat Cd, Connor Km, Barnett S, Van Meter S (2003) Mirtazapine vs. placebo in posttraumatic stress disorder: a pilot trial *Biol Psychiatry* 53:188-91

Davis Ll, Davidson Jr, Ward Lc, Bartolucci A, Bowden Cl, Petty F (2008) Divalproex in the treatment of posttraumatic stress disorder: a randomized, double-blind, placebo-controlled trial in a veteran population *J Clin Psychopharmacol* 28:84-8

Davis Ll, Jewell Me, Ambrose S, Farley J, English B, Bartolucci A, Petty F (2004) A placebo-controlled study of nefazodone for the treatment of chronic posttraumatic stress disorder: a preliminary study *J Clin Psychopharmacol* 24:291-7

Davis Ll, Ward C, Rasmusson A, Newell Jm, Frazier E, Southwick Sm (2008) A placebo-controlled trial of guanfacine for the treatment of posttraumatic stress disorder in veterans *Psychopharmacol Bull* 41:8-18

Gelpin E, Bonne O, Peri T, Brandes D, Shalev Ay (1996) Treatment of recent trauma survivors with benzodiazepines: a prospective study *J Clin Psychiatry* 57:390-4

Hamner Mb, Faldowski Ra, Ulmer Hg, Frueh Bc, Huber Mg, Arana Gw (2003) Adjunctive risperidone treatment in post-traumatic stress disorder: a preliminary controlled trial of effects on comorbid psychotic symptoms *Int Clin Psychopharmacol* 18:1-8

Hermos Ja, Young Mm, Lawler Ev, Rosenbloom D, Fiore Ld (2007) Long-term, high-dose benzodiazepine prescriptions in veteran patients with PTSD: influence of preexisting alcoholism and drug-abuse diagnoses *J Trauma Stress* 20:909-14

Hertzberg Ma, Moore Sd, Feldman Me, Beckham Jc (2001) A preliminary study of bupropion sustained-release for smoking cessation in patients with chronic posttraumatic stress disorder *J Clin Psychopharmacol* 21:94-8

Institute of Medicine (2007). Treatment of posttraumatic stress disorder: An assessment of the evidence. Washington, DC,. National Academy of the Sciences.

Kessler Rc, Sonnega A, Bromet E, Hughes M, Nelson Cb (1995) Posttraumatic stress disorder in the National Comorbidity Survey *Arch Gen Psychiatry* 52:1048-60

Lindley Se, Carlson Eb, Hill K (2007) A randomized, double-blind, placebo-controlled trial of augmentation topiramate for chronic combat-related posttraumatic stress disorder *J Clin Psychopharmacol* 27:677-81

Martenyi F, Brown Eb, Zhang H, Koke Sc, Prakash A (2002) Fluoxetine v. placebo in prevention of relapse in post-traumatic stress disorder *Br J Psychiatry* 181:315-20

Mellman Ta, Clark Re, Peacock Wj (2003) Prescribing patterns for patients with posttraumatic stress disorder *Psychiatr Serv* 54:1618-21

Monnelly Ep, Ciraulo Da, Knapp C, Keane T (2003) Low-dose risperidone as adjunctive therapy for irritable aggression in posttraumatic stress disorder *J Clin Psychopharmacol* 23:193-6

Mullins Cd, Shaya Ft, Meng F, Wang J, Harrison D (2005) Persistence, switching, and discontinuation rates among patients receiving sertraline, paroxetine, and citalopram *Pharmacotherapy* 25:660-7

Neylan Tc, Lenoci M, Samuelson Kw, Metzler Tj, Henn-Haase C, Hierholzer Rw, Lindley Se, Otte C, Schoenfeld Fb, Yesavage Ja, Marmar Cr (2006) No improvement of posttraumatic stress disorder symptoms with guanfacine treatment *Am J Psychiatry* 163:2186-8

Padala Pr, Madison J, Monnahan M, Marcil W, Price P, Ramaswamy S, Din Au, Wilson Dr, Petty F (2006) Risperidone monotherapy for post-traumatic stress disorder related to sexual assault and domestic abuse in women *Int Clin Psychopharmacol* 21:275-80

Pitman Rk, Sanders Km, Zusman Rm, Healy Ar, Cheema F, Lasko Nb, Cahill L, Orr Sp (2002) Pilot study of secondary prevention of posttraumatic stress disorder with propranolol *Biol Psychiatry* 51:189-92

Raskind Ma, Peskind Er, Hoff Dj, Hart Kl, Holmes Ha, Warren D, Shofer J, O'connell J, Taylor F, Gross C, Rohde K, Mcfall Me (2007) A parallel group placebo controlled study of prazosin for trauma nightmares and sleep disturbance in combat veterans with post-traumatic stress disorder *Biol Psychiatry* 61:928-34

Raskind Ma, Peskind Er, Kanter Ed, Petrie Ec, Radant A, Thompson Ce, Dobie Dj, Hoff D, Rein Rj, Straits-Troster K, Thomas Rg, Mcfall Mm (2003) Reduction of nightmares and other PTSD symptoms in combat veterans by prazosin: a placebo-controlled study *Am J Psychiatry* 160:371-3

Reist C, Duffy Jg, Fujimoto K, Cahill L (2001) beta-Adrenergic blockade and emotional memory in PTSD *Int J Neuropsychopharmacol* 4:377-83

Robert S, Hamner Mb, Ulmer Hg, Lorberbaum Jp, Durkalski Vl (2006) Open-label trial of escitalopram in the treatment of posttraumatic stress disorder *J Clin Psychiatry* 67:1522-6

Rothbaum Bo, Killeen Tk, Davidson Jr, Brady Kt, Connor Km, Heekin Mh (2008) Placebo-Controlled Trial of Risperidone Augmentation for Selective Serotonin Reuptake Inhibitor-Resistant Civilian Posttraumatic Stress Disorder *J Clin Psychiatry*e1-e6

Seedat S, Stein Dj, Emsley Ra (2000) Open trial of citalopram in adults with post-traumatic stress disorder *Int J Neuropsychopharmacol* 3:135-140

Southwick Sm, Bremner Jd, Rasmusson A, Morgan Ca, 3rd, Arnsten A, Charney Ds (1999) Role of norepinephrine in the pathophysiology and treatment of posttraumatic stress disorder *Biol Psychiatry* 46:1192-204

Stein Dj, Davidson J, Seedat S, Beebe K (2003) Paroxetine in the treatment of post-traumatic stress disorder: pooled analysis of placebo-controlled studies *Expert Opin Pharmacother* 4:1829-38

Stein Mb, Kerridge C, Dimsdale Je, Hoyt Db (2007) Pharmacotherapy to prevent PTSD: Results from a randomized controlled proof-of-concept trial in physically injured patients *J Trauma Stress* 20:923-32

Stein Mb, Kline Na, Matloff Jl (2002) Adjunctive olanzapine for SSRI-resistant combat-related PTSD: a double-blind, placebo-controlled study *Am J Psychiatry* 159:1777-9

Stein Mb, Mcquaid Jr, Pedrelli P, Lenox R, Mccahill Me (2000) Posttraumatic stress disorder in the primary care medical setting *Gen Hosp Psychiatry* 22:261-9

8

Posttraumatic Growth and Recovery from Post Traumatic Stress Disorder

Megan Walter and Glen Bates
Swinburne University
Australia

1. Introduction

The inclusion of Posttraumatic Stress Disorder in the third edition of the Diagnostic and Statistical Manual of Mental Disorders (DSM-III, American Psychiatric Association [APA], 1980) prompted a plethora of research attempting to categorise the effects of trauma through quantification and statistical procedures. This process has greatly increased our understanding of the destructive effects of traumatic experiences that are reflected in the PTSD core symptom dimensions of hyperarousal, re-experiencing, and avoidance. This research has also led to a belief that traumatic events shatter the individual's core beliefs, leading the person to question their view of themself, the world and the interaction between the two. Thus, traumatic events produce disruptions to the person's sense of self and identity as well as physiological and psychological distress.

As research has progressed, understanding of the impact on the person's sense of self and identity has grown. Contemporary accounts of the impact of trauma now identify beneficial as well as detrimental outcomes on a person's sense of self and world view. This chapter discusses these contemporary views of trauma, outlining the relationship between the disruptive and destructive processes and the constructive processes that can be experienced in the aftermath of a traumatic event. After an initial discussion of the development of PTSD, four questions are addressed: What role does the traumatic event play in the formation of symptoms as well as the recovery process?; what kind of changes to the self occur in the aftermath of trauma?; what cognitive processes determine whether the changes are positive or negative?; and are the changes long lasting?

1.1 What is PTSD and how is it currently defined?

In the contemporary psychometric literature, trauma is defined as an event that involves "actual or threatened death, serious injury, or other threat to one's physical integrity" (APA, 2000, p. 463). Posttraumatic stress disorder (PTSD) is a common psychological and physiological response to a traumatic event. According to the DSM-IV-TR (APA, 2000), the essential feature of this disorder is that symptoms occur as a direct result of exposure to a traumatic event involving either direct personal experience, or witnessing or learning about an event that involves another person (APA, 2000). The person must also feel "intense fear, helplessness, or horror" (APA, 2000, p. 463) in response to the event, as well as persistently re-experiencing the traumatic event, avoiding trauma-related stimuli, demonstrating a numbing of general responsiveness, and experiencing increased arousal and significant distress or impairment for at least one month after trauma (APA, 2000, Full criteria are listed in Table 1). Epidemiological studies have established that PTSD develops for about 55% of rape victims, 35% of childhood sexual or physical abuse survivors, 17% of those experiencing physical and armed assaults, and 7% of individuals following severe accidents (Kessler et al., 1995; Maercker et al., 2004). The DSM-IV-TR (APA, 2000) report that lifetime prevalence rates of Posttraumatic Stress Disorder are approximately 8% of the adult population in the United States. Other studies have reported lower rates in national representative samples in the Netherlands (7.4%, de Vries & Olff, 2009), Australia (5.8%, Gould et al., 2011), and New Zealand (6%, Oakley Browne et al., 2011).

1.2 The history of trauma through the DSM

PTSD was included in the International Classification of Diseases (ICD, World Health Organization, [WHO], 1992) around the same time as it was first cited in the DSM. Both classification systems have adjusted the diagnostic criteria several times and are largely consistent with each other. The current classification of PTSD in both the DSM-IV-TR (APA, 2000) and ICD-10 (WHO, 1992) can be found in Table 1. The focus is on the DSM criteria which have been routinely applied in the majority of the literature on trauma.

The original edition of the Diagnostic and Statistical Manual of Mental Disorders (DSM, APA, 1952), published in 1952, was the first time that trauma-induced psychopathology was systematically defined. In this version, the impact of trauma was recognised as an anxiety disorder known as Traumatic Neurosis (APA, 1952) and stressful events were viewed as having a modifying effect on mental health; stress could worsen or lengthen the presentation of disorders or symptoms, but the effect was brief or transient (O'Brian, 1998). At this time, the term trauma generally referred to a physical trauma, such as brain damage, that resulted in psychological problems. If the trauma was due to combat stress, the appropriate diagnosis was an "adjustment reaction of adult life", which was "fear associated with military combat and manifested by trembling, running and hiding" (APA, 1968). This definition appeared again in the DSM-II (APA, 1968). However, the theoretical views of the effects of trauma shifted between the second and third editions due to discoveries from research into the impact of war on men and sexual assault on women (Hunt, 2010). Trauma was now considered to be an antecedent of symptoms rather than a modifier. This change in view was reflected in the DSM-III, with trauma-induced psychopathology now appearing under the title Posttraumatic Stress Disorder.

Despite the controversy caused by the shift in theoretical perspective at the time, the inclusion of PTSD into the DSM-III (APA, 1980) was an important step. PTSD's inclusion as a diagnosable disorder enabled more rigorous empirical evaluation of the impact of trauma by providing clear diagnostic criteria by which to assess such events. It also provided support for the emerging biopsychosocial premise that an individual and their environment interact and affect one another (Van der Kolk, 1996). Another benefit was that the creation of PTSD criteria recognised and supported the claims of many individuals reporting ongoing or long-term detrimental effects after trauma (Andreasen, 2004). Moreover, clinicians and researchers could now recognise communalities in the core aspects of psychological trauma and its aftermath across seemingly disparate trauma types, such as natural disaster, combat,

Criterion	ICD10-DCR	DSM-IV-TR
Criterion A:	A. Exposure to stressor	A1 . Exposure to stressor
Stressor	*No subjective Stressor Criterion*	A2. Emotional reaction to stressor
Criterion B:	B. Persistent remembering of the stressor in **one** of:	B. Requires **one** or more of:
Re-experiencing	* Intrusive Flashbacks	B1. Intrusive recollections
	* Vivid memories or recurring dreams	B2. Distressing dreams
	* Experiencing distress when reminded of the stressor	B3. Acting/feeling as though event were recurring
		B4. Psychological distress when exposed to reminders
		B5. Physiological reactivity when exposed to reminders
Criterion C:	C. Requires only **one** symptom of actual or preferred	C. Requires **three or more** of: (Includes both
Avoidance	avoidance	numbing and avoidance symptoms)
	Does not specify avoidance symptoms	C1 . avoidance of thoughts, feelings or conversations associated with the stressor
	Does not include numbing symptoms	C2. avoidance of activities, places or people associated with the stressor
		C3. inability to recall
		C4. diminished interest in significant Activities
		C5. detachment from others
		C6. restricted affect
		C7. sense of foreshortened future
Criterion D:	**Either** D1, **or two** of D2:	
Hyperarousal	D1. Inability to recall	
	D2. **Two** or more of:	D. **Two or more** of:
	A. sleep problems	D1. sleep problems
	B. Irritability	D2. Irritability
	C. concentration problems	D3. concentration problems
	D. hypervigilance	D4. Hypervigilance
	E. exaggerated startle response	D5. exaggerated startle response
Criterion E:	E. Onset of symptoms **within 6 months of the stressor**	E. Duration of the disturbance is **at least 1 month**
Criterion F:	*Does not specify level of distress or impairment*	F. Requires significant distress or impairment

Table 1. Diagnostic Criteria for Posttraumatic Stress Disorder: Comparison of the ICD-10 and DSM-IV-TR Criteria.

and sexual assault. Finally, it was in this edition of the DSM that a stressful life event was etiologically related to mental health diagnoses (Long & Elhai, 2009). The perception that PTSD was caused by an external event, rather than an intrinsic weakness or character fault, was a considerable change within models of mental health (Brunner, 2002).

The etiological connection between a traumatic event and PTSD symptomatology makes this diagnosis unique among psychiatric disorders. Criterion A, also known as "The Stressor Criterion", is considered to be the "gatekeeper" of PTSD diagnosis as this disorder cannot be diagnosed without this criterion being satisfied. In the DSM-III, criterion A was defined as "a recognisable stressor that would evoke significant symptoms of distress in almost everyone" (APA, 1980, p.236). This definition referred to events such as war, torture, bombings, rape, natural disasters, and man-made disasters such as airplane crashes; situations that were considered to be distinct from more common life stressors such as bereavement, divorce and chronic illness (Long & Elhai, 2009). Responses to more 'common' stressors were identified as Adjustment Disorders rather than PTSD at this time (APA, 1980). The distinction between 'traumatic' and 'common' stressors was based on the assumption that people were able to adapt to ordinary stressors but their abilities to adapt would be overwhelmed by traumatic stressors.

The PTSD criteria were revised over the subsequent DSM versions. The Stressor Criterion received the most attention due to criticisms suggesting that it lacked specificity and only included traumatic events of great magnitude or severity (Long & Elhai, 2009). The change in view of trauma from a modifier (i.e., could worsen symptoms) to an antecedent of psychiatric symptoms also prompted an ongoing debate regarding the appropriateness of linking PTSD with a limited group of stressors (e.g., Gold et al., 2005; Lasiuk & Hegadoren, 2006b). In response to such criticisms, the Stressor Criterion has been expanded with each DSM edition in an effort to cover a broad range of traumatic experiences.

In the DSM-IV (APA, 1994), the structure of the Stressor Criterion was broken into two parts, both of which must be satisfied to enable a PTSD diagnosis. First, Criterion A1 specifies the type of exposure by outlining situations in which the person "experienced, witnessed, or was confronted with an event or events that involved actual or threatened death or serious injury, or the threat to physical integrity of self or others" or "learning about the unexpected or violent death, serious harm, or threat of death or injury experienced by a family member or other close associate" (APA, 1994, p. 427-428). These statements are accompanied by an extensive list of events believed to result in PTSD symptomatology. Second, Criterion A2 requires that the individual responded to the event with "intense fear, helplessness, or horror" (APA, 1994, p.428). This created further controversy as traumatised individuals report a myriad of emotions but not always fear, helplessness, or horror (e.g., O'Donnell et al., 2010). This two-part structure has remained in the current DSM-IV-TR (APA, 2000). Although the Stressor Criterion has been broadened, the debate is still ongoing.

2. What role does the traumatic event play in the formation of symptoms as well as the recovery process?

The debate around the Stressor Criterion has concentrated on whether it should be broad or restrictive (Kilpatrick et al., 1998). Those that argue for a broad definition believe that Criterion A1 should include any event that prompts the development of PTSD symptoms, including low magnitude events such as divorce or job loss (Anders et al., 2011). It is argued that this will enable those who suffer PTSD symptoms resulting from non-Criterion A1 traumatic events, to obtain treatment or compensation currently available to those who have experienced a qualifying event (Kilpatrick et al., 2009). Conversely, those who argue for a restrictive definition consider that broadening the criterion could prompt "frivolous" use of the diagnosis (Kilpatrick et al., 2009). Finally, others argue the Criterion A is redundant and diagnosis should focus on the core symptoms of Criterion B-F (e.g., Brewin et al., 2009).

Since the release of the DSM-IV (APA, 1994) Criterion A2 has also attracted attention. Criterion A2 states that the person's response to a traumatic event must involve "intense fear, helplessness or horror" (APA, 2000, p. 467). Some argue that this criterion has no impact on the prevalence of PTSD and should be separated from the Stressor Criterion and developed into its own "acute response for the emergence of PTSD" criterion (e.g., Breslau & Kessler, 2001). However, other researchers argue that Criterion A2 works well as a screening measure for early PTSD identification and narrows the definition from previous DSM versions (Weathers & Keane, 2007). The following review discusses both of these arguments, and an argument is made that an individual's response to a potentially traumatic event is of crucial importance in determining its ongoing impact. The source of recovery lies, therefore, in how the person relates the event to the self.

2.1 Criterion A1 – the type of traumatic event

The list of potentially traumatic events has increased across each DSM edition, leading some experts to argue that Criterion A1 has become too broad. In the current DSM-IV-TR (APA, 2000), the mode of exposure has also been expanded to enable individuals to experience, witness or be confronted with a traumatic event to meet diagnostic criteria. Many researchers argue that specifying the mode of exposure has led to misapplication of the construct and inappropriate diagnoses. For example, Spitzer et al. (2007) stated that although experiencing or witnessing a traumatic event is in keeping with the original definition of the construct, the term "confronted with" is vague enough to enable such events as "hearing the news of a loved one being hurt" (First et al., 2002, p. 253) as being considered a qualifying event. The broadening of the Stressor Criterion and misapplication of the construct has been referred to as the "conceptual bracket creep" for the PTSD diagnosis (McNally, 2003).

Conversely, some researchers are advocates for an even broader criterion to allow the inclusion of less severe, but still serious, stressful life events such as childbirth, chronic illness, sexual harassment and bullying as these events are empirically associated with PTSD symptomatology (e.g., Avina & O'Donohue, 2002; Lev-Wiesel et al., 2006; Palmieri & Fitzgerald, 2005). Experts argue that as individuals can develop PTSD after experiencing low magnitude stressors, the strict criterion is preventing many individuals from accessing health services and receiving appropriate treatment and compensation that is available to those who experience a qualifying event. To rectify the dilemma over which events can qualify as 'traumatic' and satisfy the Stressor Criterion, and those that are distressing but below the 'traumatic' threshold, many researchers (e.g., Anders et al., 2011; Kilpatrick et al., 1998), argue that decisions should be based on empirical data.

2.2 Research into frequency and severity of PTSD

After the release of DSM-III (APA, 1980), the debate was prompted by epidemiological data demonstrating that some traumatic events, such as car accidents and sexual assault, were not "outside the range of (normal) human experience" (APA, 1987) but could still evoke the full range of PTSD reactions. For example, PTSD symptoms have been experienced by individuals following events considered to be normal human experiences, such as childbirth (e.g., Olde et al., 2006); marital affairs, disruption, and divorce (e.g., Burstein, 1995; Dattilio, 2004); unsuccessful adoption arrangements (e.g., Burstein, 1995); money problems and employment stressors (e.g., Scott & Stradling, 1994; Solomon & Canino, 1990); bereavement (Zisook et al., 1998); and losing a close relationship (Solomon, & Canino, 1990). Such findings led researchers, such as Breslau and Davis (1987), to question the validity of explicitly linking "a distinct symptomatic configuration with a distinct class of stressors" (p.255).

The argument was further supported by research demonstrating that the prevalence of traumatic events and PTSD was greater than previously thought. For example, a number of studies showed that up to three quarters of the population in the United States have been exposed to a traumatic event in their lifetime that could meet the DSM-III-R (APA, 1987) PTSD Stressor Criterion (Green, 1994). Vrana and Lauterbach (1994) reported that 84% of a sample of undergraduate students reported experiencing at least one event of sufficient intensity to potentially warrant a PTSD diagnosis, and Kilpatrick and Resnick (1993) found that 75% of a community sample of women reported at least one crime victimisation, with 24-53% reporting a sexual assault. Sexual assault or abuse emerged as one of the most prevalent traumatic events. For example, Feldhaus et al. (2000) reported that 39% of women in an emergency department population had experienced at least one sexual assault/abuse incident in their lifetime, and in Koss et al.'s (1987) study of over 3800 American college women, over 54% nationwide acknowledged experiencing some form of sexual victimisation. Furthermore, Finkelhor et al. (1990) established the prevalence of childhood sexual abuse as 16% of men and 27% of women in a US national phone survey. Taken together, these findings demonstrate that events that can precipitate distress and PTSD symptomatology are quite common and not outside normal human experience.

Such findings led the authors of the DSM-III-R (APA, 1987) to broaden the types of events that could satisfy the Stressor Criterion. It was only in the development of DSM-IV (APA, 1994), however, that an attempt was made to address the issue of how Criterion A1 should be defined during the PTSD field trial. The field trial explored the frequency and symptom severity of PTSD symptoms following from Criterion A1-qualifying traumatic events and non-qualifying events among 400 treatment-seeking and 128 community adults and adolescents. Participants were asked to complete measures of exposure to both Criterion A1 and non-Criterion A1 events using checklists of both types of events (Kilpatrick et al., 1998). Individuals who reported experiencing at least one Criterion A1 event were included in the Criterion A1 group. Most of the A1 group (72%) had also experienced non-A1 events with only 13% (n=66) of the sample identifying only non-A1 events. Results revealed that the lifetime prevalence rate of PTSD among those reporting at least one A1 event was 51% and the current prevalence rate was 36%. In contrast, the lifetime prevalence rate for PTSD for those reporting only non-A1 events was 12% and the current prevalence rate was 9%. Although these results indicate that Criterion A1 events are more likely to be associated with PTSD symptoms than non-A1 events, there are methodological issues. Specifically, A1 and non-A1 events were not assessed separately for the majority of the sample; PTSD symptoms were assessed in reference to multiple events within a person's history. Therefore, PTSD symptoms could relate to either A1 or non-A1 events.

Since the publication of the PTSD field trial in 1998, many researchers have also explored the relation of Criterion A1 and PTSD prevalence rates to symptom levels. These investigations have yielded mixed results. For example, a recent study by Kilpatrick et al. (2009) hypothesized that A1 events may prompt greater PTSD symptoms than non-A1 events. Their results supported this premise with a probability of 6% among adolescents that have experienced an A1 event compared to a probability of 1% among adolescents who had only experienced non-A1 events. In another study, Boals and Schuettler (2009) argued that events that satisfied A1 and A2 were more likely to cause probable PTSD and result in more PTSD symptoms than events that failed to meet the two 'A' criteria. Although their results were supportive of this premise, once variables such as time since the event, depression and perceived stress, were controlled for, A1 events were no longer associated with PTSD symptoms. Other studies have demonstrated that individuals who have experienced qualifying events do not report any more PTSD symptoms than those who experienced non-A1 events (e.g., Green et al., 2000; Spitzer et al., 2000), whereas other researchers have shown non-traumatic events to be associated with greater levels of PTSD symptoms than qualifying events (e.g., Gold et al., 2005; Long et al., 2008). A similar study using a large community sample in the Netherlands also reported greater prevalence of PTSD symptoms among those experiencing non-A1 events (Mol et al., 2005). However, their results were dependent on the amount of time that had elapsed since the event.

2.3 Current status of Criterion A1

The mixed findings can be taken as evidence that there is very little difference in PTSD symptom severity or prevalence rates between A1 and non-A1 events. Many researchers believe that such findings are evidence that Criterion-A1 is flawed (e.g., Gold et al., 2005; Long & Elhai, 2009). This has led some experts to argue that Criterion A1 should be modified to include a wider range of events (e.g., Lev-Wiesel et al., 2006; Olde et al., 2006; Palmieri & Fitzgerald, 2005). Others argue that the data suggest the Stressor Criterion is unnecessary and should be removed entirely from the diagnostic criteria (e.g., Gold et al., 2005; Mol et al., 2005). Some also argue that the inconsistent findings are evidence that the event does not contribute to the presentation of symptoms (e.g., Boals & Schuettler, 2009; Cameron et al., 2010). Instead, they suggest that the individual's emotional and behavioural responses may more accurately predict the risk for PTSD symptomatology. For example, Boals and Schuettler (2009) posit that it is not the event that is related to PTSD symptoms but the individual's emotional response to the event. They argue that if an event elicits intense fear, then fear conditioning may result in the development and maintenance of PTSD symptoms. This premise is in line with many PTSD theories stating that classical conditioning, particularly fear conditioning, underlie PTSD symptoms (e.g., Pitman, 1989; Rothbaum & Davis, 2003). However, different traumas have been found to result in different emotional profiles (Amstadter & Vernon, 2008), implying that the event does play an integral role in the development of PTSD symptoms, even if only to explain the individual's emotional response.

Similarly, Cameron et al. (2010) argued that it is the individual's cognitive and behavioural response to the event, rather than the event itself, that is a significant risk factor for psychological distress. Their study exploring the prevalence and severity of PTSD symptoms among individuals who had experienced criterion-A1 and non-criterion-A1 events, found that those who developed PTSD symptoms, regardless of the event, reported significantly higher tendencies to suppress unwanted thoughts. This is in line with previous studies demonstrating that thought suppression is associated with greater PTSD symptoms (Amstatder & Vernon. 2008), the maintenance of PTSD symptoms (Shipherd & Beck, 2005), and the frequency of negative autobiographical memories (Neufiend et al., 2009). However, Chatard et al. (2011)found that individuals with high levels of PTSD symptoms who were exposed to the possibility of dying, did not suppress death-related thoughts. Instead, mortality salience increased death-related thought accessibility for these individuals. Although Cameron et al. suggests that consideration of the event is unnecessary, some traumas carry a greater chance of dying than other traumas (i.e., assault or war compared to divorce). Therefore, future research may reveal that differences exist in the extent of the thought suppression conducted (i.e., thoughts only related to the event or un-associated information) across different traumatic events.

2.4 How else could these results be interpreted?

Although the inconsistent findings have been interpreted as evidence that the Stressor Criterion is obsolete, the mixed results could also be indicating that a dichotomous categorisation of traumatic versus non-traumatic events based on how "extreme" the stressor is, does not adequately capture the impact that certain events may have on people, or consider the individual differences in people's perceptions, resilience or coping strategies (Weathers & Keane, 2007). Research suggests that such variables affect the individual's response to trauma as well as the course and severity of PTSD symptoms. It is well established that some people do not develop PTSD after a qualifying event (Rubonis & Bickman, 1991); different types of traumatic events are associated with distinct probabilities of developing PTSD (Kessler et al., 1995) and certain types of traumatic events are associated with specific clinical presentations (e.g., Elklit & Christiansen, 2010). The DSM-IV-TR (APA, 2000) text also acknowledges that different types of events can affect the course of PTSD by stating that the "disorder may be especially severe or long lasting when the stressor is of human design (e.g., torture, rape)" (p. 464). The text also describes a specific constellation of symptoms that are commonly seen following an interpersonal stressor such as sexual or physical abuse, or domestic battering (p. 465); this cohort presents with more dissociative symptoms than victims of other trauma types (e.g., Dancu et al., 1996). This suggests that the course and severity of PTSD symptoms vary depending on the type of traumatic event experienced and emphasise the importance of considering the event as part of the causal pathway to PTSD. Thus, to suggest that the inconsistent findings are evidence that the event should be removed from diagnosis seems short sighted.

These findings may in fact reflect our lack of understanding or consideration of the quintessential links shared by traumatic events that can cause PTSD symptoms. The mixed findings may also reflect individual differences in how people respond, interpret, or cope with such events. Many agree that an event is considered traumatic because of the individual's perception and response to that situation (e.g., Hendricks & Byers, 2006; Janoff-

Bulman, 1992). If this is the case, it is possible to conclude from the evidence that the event plays an integral role in the course and symptom profile of the disorder and that the current criteria do not effectively capture those aspects of the event which cause such distress. Many authors agree that the classification of traumatic events is underdeveloped (e.g., Luz et al., 2011) and acknowledge the need for a standardised description (e.g., Braga et al., 2008; Long & Elhai, 2009). Therefore, although the Stressor Criterion may require revision, the etiological connection between the event and the resulting symptoms warrants being retained as the event is likely to hold the key to the best course of treatment, and thus adjustment and recovery.

2.5 Criterion A2 - the emotional response to the stressor

The second part of the Stressor Criterion, CriterionA2, specifies the type and magnitude of the emotional response required to warrant a diagnosis of PTSD. This criterion requires that an individual responds to a traumatic event with "intense fear, helplessness, or horror" (APA, 2000, p. 463). This assumes that all people who develop PTSD symptoms will always respond with these three intense emotions. In support of this premise, a number of studies have demonstrated that individuals who develop PTSD report significantly higher levels of fear, helplessness, and horror than those who did not develop PTSD symptoms (e.g., Brewin et al., 2000; Kilpatrick et al., 1997; O'Donnell et al., 2010) and most individuals who develop PTSD experience these emotions peri- and posttrauma (Bedard-Gilligan & Zoellner, 2008).

Despite such supporting evidence for the current definition of A2, this criterion has also been criticised on a number of grounds. A2 has been said to add very little to the predictive ability of PTSD except with regard to the actual experience of a traumatic event (Bedard-Gilligan & Zoellner, 2008); PTSD prevalence rates remain constant, regardless of the inclusion or exclusion of A2 in diagnosis (Breslau & Kessler, 2001; Kilpatrick et al., 1997; Schnurr et al., 2002); and only a small proportion of those who experience fear, helplessness or horror after a traumatic event subsequently develop PTSD (e.g., Bedard-Gilligan & Zoellner, 2008; O'Donnell et al., 2010).

It also appears that individuals who develop PTSD without experiencing fear, helplessness, or horror, instead experience other intense negative emotions. For example, O'Donnell et al. (2010) found that all of the individuals who developed PTSD in their study reported more intense and comprehensive emotional experiences peri-trauma than those outlined in Criterion A2, compared to those who did not develop PTSD. These included emotions such as sadness, guilt, shame, and frustration. Brewin et al.'s (2000) study using victims of violent crimes also found that guilt and shame were associated with the development of PTSD (B-F Criteria) and Adler et al. (2008) reported that soldiers returning from Iraq who did not meet A2, but developed PTSD, experienced extreme anger at the time of their traumatic event. Similarly, Amstadter and Vernon (2008) found anger to be a stronger emotional response than fear peri- and posttrauma for individuals who had been physically assaulted.

In sum, the evidence indicates that the emotions prescribed by Criterion A2 are not always the most powerful emotions associated with PTSD symptom development (O'Donnell et al., 2010). Individuals who develop PTSD experience a wider range of emotions than currently outlined in the DSM-IV-TR (APA, 2000). This could be interpreted as evidence that Criterion A2 is not necessary for the diagnosis of PTSD and could be removed from PTSD diagnosis.

Many of the these studies, however, have methodological limitations as they require traumatised individuals, with and without PTSD, to retrospectively report on their emotional response at the time of the event (e.g., Bedard-Gilligan & Zoellner, 2008; Breslau & Kessler, 2001). That methodological design is flawed as much research indicates a bias or distortion in declarative memories after trauma (e.g., Amir et al., 2010). Additionally, some trauma victims, especially those involved in motor vehicle accidents, often have no memory of the event or the emotions they experienced (O'Donnell et al., 2010). Indeed, Criterion A2 may, in fact, be preventing individuals with a poor memory of their traumatic event, or those who display different emotional profiles, from receiving a diagnosis and potentially denying them access to healthcare services. There is also the possibility that different traumas result in different emotional responses and that the intensity of emotion may be the essential element of this criterion. If this is the case, this criterion could be expanded to include a wider range of emotional responses. In support of this premise, Amstadter and Vernon (2008) explored different emotional responses peri- and posttrauma to four different types of traumatic events (sexual assault, physical assault, transportation accidents, and illness) and found each type of trauma produced its own emotional profile with different levels of intensity at different time points. Once more, these findings indicate that the event plays an integral role in the course, severity and symptom profile of PTSD.

2.6 Implications of removing the Stressor Criterion

Although we believe that the Stressor Criterion should be retained as it clearly distinguishes PTSD from other disorders and may provide the key to adjustment, some (e.g., Maier, 2007) continue to argue that both parts of Criterion A are redundant and PTSD diagnoses should be based on Criteria B-F. It is argued that without the Stressor Criterion, a greater diversity of posttraumatic experiences will emerge, potentially leading to a better understanding of the impact of trauma. Conversely, it could hinder the discovery of an accurate symptom pattern (McNally, 2003; Simms et al., 2002; Watson, 2005). Removal of Criterion A could also result in professionals mistakenly attributing PTSD symptoms to a mood, psychotic or other anxiety disorder, thus increasing the rate of misdiagnosis. For example, an individual who seeks treatment for hallucinations or other perceptual disturbances that may be present during PTSD "flashbacks", these flashbacks could be misinterpreted as indicators of a psychotic disorder, such as schizophrenia, or dissociative disorders. Similarly, individuals displaying a loss of interest and avoidance of activities that used to be enjoyed, could be misdiagnosed with a mood disorder. This could then lead the person to receive inappropriate medical and psychological treatment, could cause the individual further distress, and could disrupt the recovery process.

Bodkin et al.'s (2007) study provides support for this premise. They found that PTSD Criteria B-F symptoms (symptom clusters B–D, duration of at least 1 month, and impairment of functioning) were commonly reported in a psychiatric outpatient population seeking treatment for depression, regardless of whether or not they had experienced a traumatic event. Furthermore, they found that the prevalence of PTSD was just as high for individuals who had experienced a severe trauma as those who had had no such experience. Spitzer et al. (2007) suggested that these results may have occurred because some of the PTSD symptoms (e.g., difficulty concentrating, difficulty sleeping, diminished interest in activities) are not only commonly found in psychiatric outpatient presentations of depression, but are also included in the criteria of other mental disorders, such as Major Depressive Disorder and Generalised Anxiety Disorder. This suggests that the Stressor Criterion may be the only aspect of this diagnosis, as currently outlined in the DSM-IV-TR (APA, 2000), that clearly distinguishes PTSD from other disorders.

Spitzer et al. (2007), and McHugh and Treisman (2007) have suggested that, instead of discarding the Stressor Criterion, Criteria B, C, and D (re-experiencing, avoidance, and arousal, respectively) should be evaluated for their specificity and ability to differentiate PTSD from other mood and anxiety disorders. On the basis of this, they recommend only to retain symptoms that are directly related to trauma exposure. Spitzer et al. argue that these criteria (B-F) include too many general symptoms of negative effect, and are so broadly interpretable that they could be construed to encompass normal responses. Indeed, this may explain the vast literature reporting PTSD symptoms precipitating from non-traumatic events (e.g., Gold et al., 2005; Mol et al., 2005). Furthermore, Wakefield (in Spitzer et al., 2007) suggests that the symptom descriptions should be more restrictive to ensure that the descriptors are distinct to PTSD and indicative of pathology rather than normal responses to negative life events. In support of this proposal, the authors point out how insufficiently the current criteria separates normal from disordered responses (See Spitzer et al., 2007).

The DSM-V's Posttraumatic Stress Disorder and Dissociative Disorders Sub-Work Group have recently drafted new criteria which broadly support the claims made by Spitzer et al. (2007), McHugh and Treisman (2007), and others. The proposed criteria retain Criterion A1 (Criterion A2 has been removed from Criterion A, expanded to include a wide variety of negative emotional states, and now exists as a new criterion, Criterion D4) and have revised Criteria B-F to represent symptoms directly related to trauma exposure (APA, 2010). The wording of Criterion-A1 has also been revised to distinguish between traumatic events and events that are distressing but do not exceed the traumatic threshold. The list of different types of trauma in the newly drafted criterion A seems to corroborate researchers' beliefs that a better description of the criteria for traumatic events is necessary. Luz et al. (2011) suggest that the list of qualifying events in the new criterion A may contribute to a better definition of this criterion. In turn, this could enable identification of more homogenous groups of traumatised individuals; the recognition of similarities and differences in people's psychological responses; and possibly uncover distinct clinical profiles that are dependent on the type of event that triggered the PTSD symptomatology (Luz et al., 2011).

This line of research is integral to our understanding of the relationship between trauma and PTSD. Although the debate has been ongoing for decades, the discussions have prompted research and highlighted the need for further exploration into the interaction between the type of event and the behavioural, cognitive, and emotional responses that precipitate PTSD. This may provide greater insight into how to predict the risk of subsequent PTSD symptomatology. It is clear that a traumatic event increases the risk of developing PTSD symptoms. However, the role that the characteristics of the event plays, as well as the person's perceptions and responses to the event, to the development of PTSD remains unclear. Thus, until we further understand how traumatic events result in such symptoms, and the variations in symptoms across individuals, the etiological link between the event and the resulting symptoms should be retained as the event distinguishes PTSD from other disorders and may hold the key to the best course of treatment, and thus adjustment and recovery.

3. What kind of changes to the self can occur in the aftermath of trauma?

Trauma research has traditionally focused on the negative symptoms resulting from trauma with much of the literature detailing the severity and chronicity of symptoms and the development of psychological disorders (e.g., Joseph et al., 1993). Although this research has greatly increased our understanding of the negative impact of trauma, the hermeneutic dimensions of experience, and thus the impact on the individual's identity and sense of self, have been largely overlooked. Yet, the negative symptoms of PTSD provide clear indicators of the impact that trauma has on the person's sense of self.

3.1 Negative changes in the self resulting from trauma

The symptoms of PTSD have been said to simply reflect the individual's level of pain and distress (Wilson et al., 2001). However, the experiences of hyperarousal, avoidance and re-experiencing outlined in the PTSD criterion go beyond distress and reflect the disruption of the system and the internal struggles of the person to come to terms with and integrate the event into their self narrative. Such disruptions are often experienced as a fracture in the person's sense of wholeness. Trauma impacts the psychic core, the very soul of the person and thus their identity (Wilson et al., 2001). The alteration to formative processes often lead to a decentring of the self, a loss of relatedness to others, and a loss of sameness and consistency (Lifton, 1976, 1979, 1993; Putnam, 1997). Changes in psychosocial function also occur and include altered ego states and a shift in life-course developmental trajectories (Wilson et al., 2001). Fracturing of ego identity has consequences for psychological stability, well-being, and psychic integration, believed to be a cause of dissociation (van der Kolk et al., 1997). Krystal (1968) and Lifton (1979) also noted that such a fracturing of a person's sense of self and identity may be a precursor to mood disorders and, in extreme cases, suicidality and death. However, it is this shattering of one's core beliefs, and thus the self, that is believed to generate a search for meaning as to why the event occurred as well as drive the person to question, reformulate and reconstruct their very basic core beliefs in an attempt to adjust or recover from the event (Janoff-Bulman, 1992).

Core beliefs are the essence of how we see ourselves, other people, the world, and the future (Janoff-Bulman, 1992). They develop overtime, usually from childhood and through the experience of significant life events. Core beliefs are strongly-held, rigid, and inflexible assumptions about the world that are maintained by the tendency to focus on information that supports the belief and ignore evidence that contradicts it. Once these assumptions are broken, however, people are thrown into disarray, unable to conceive recent events; understand or recognise current experiences and one's own reactions and responses to such events; or consider a possible future, as life now is riddled with inconsistency and unpredictability. Individual variation in the degree of disruption to core beliefs, self-efficacy in coping, and resources may explain the range in the severity of symptoms reported.

Interestingly, the shattering of assumptions has also been found to lead to the experience of many positive changes. In parallel to the exploration of negative symptoms resulting from trauma, researchers and clinicians have documented that many traumatised individuals also report positive changes to the self in the aftermath of trauma. Some survivors mostly experience positive changes and do not develop disorders, such as PTSD (Rubonis & Bickman, 1991). In fact, far more individuals report positive changes following trauma than those reporting psychiatric disorders (Calhoun & Tedeschi, 2004; Salminen et al., 2002). Currently, the most widely used term for positive changes following trauma is Posttraumatic Growth (Tedeschi & Calhoun, 1996).

3.2 Posttraumatic growth and the positive changes in the self resulting from trauma

Posttraumatic Growth (PTG) is the experience of substantial positive psychological change resulting from the struggle to overcome highly challenging life circumstances (Calhoun et al., 2000; Calhoun & Tedeschi, 1999, 2001; Tedeschi & Calhoun, 2004). The term describes the experience of individuals whose development, at least in some areas, has surpassed what was present before the crises occurred. Tedeschi and Kilmer (2005) posited that PTG is different from constructs like resilience, arguing that resilience can be considered as effective coping and adaptation in the face of major life stress, whereas PTG goes beyond resilience and transforms the person. Not only has the person survived, but they have experienced changes that are viewed as important, and exceeding their previous level of adaptation, functioning, or life awareness (Zoellner & Maercker, 2006).

These positive changes are believed to be activated by an event so traumatic that it significantly threatens or shatters the fundamental schemas of the individual (Calhoun &Tedeschi, 2004). This premise is in line with Janoff-Bulman's (1992) theory that traumatic events shatter one's assumptions of the world. Tedeschi and Calhoun's (1996) PTG model compares trauma to an earthquake, claiming that trauma must be "seismic" in nature to significantly threaten or shatter the fundamental schemas of the individual (Calhoun &Tedeschi, 2004). It is through this destruction of schemas that the individual is able to question previous assumptions of the world and start rebuilding or restructuring their lives. In support of this premise, research indicates that the degree of challenge to core beliefs about the world is correlated with the amount of PTG reported (Cann et al., 2010).

Tedeschi and Calhoun (2004) posit that people can experience positive change across three areas of life: relating to others, sense of self, and life philosophy. For example, in regard to changes in how the person relates to others, people often report feeling an increase in closeness and intimacy with their loved ones (Tedeschi & Calhoun, 2004). Constructive changes are also found in relation to the self and a changed philosophy. In relation to the self, individuals exposed to trauma often report feeling a new sense of vulnerability while feeling stronger and more self-efficacious concurrently (Tedeschi & Calhoun, 2006). This may come from learning from the trauma that they are not impervious to harm which in turn reduces the desire to enter into unnecessary risk-taking behaviours. At the same time, the struggle to overcome the trauma can create an improved sense of personal strength and a belief that they can handle adversity in the future.

In respect to changes in philosophy, people report an increased sense of appreciation of life. Through the process of reconstructing the self, people are forced to reassess their lives and their priorities. This leads some to work harder towards areas of their life that they deem important, such as education or families. It can also increase the pleasure obtained from everyday activities; activities that may have previously been taken for granted.

3.3 Research on posttraumatic growth

Since Tedeschi and Calhoun (1996) reintroduced the idea of positive change following adversity into the research community, this phenomenon has been systematically theorised and empirically investigated (e.g., Affleck & Tennen, 1996; Tedeschi & Calhoun, 1996; Tedeschi et al., 2007). Early PTG research focused on the prevalence and occurrence of growth. PTG has been found to emanate from many different types of traumatic events, including sexual assault (e.g., Grubaugh & Resick, 2007), physical assault (e.g., Amstadter & Vernon, 2008), combat (e.g., Maguen et al., 2006), natural disasters (e.g., Cryder et al., 2006), cancer (e.g., Cordova et al., 2001, 2007; Weiss, 2004), terrorism (e.g., Hobfall et al., 2007), and HIV/AIDS (e.g., Milam, 2004).

Prevalence rates for PTG vary widely across studies and trauma types with So-kum (2007) reporting 30% of natural disaster victims demonstrating growth and Pietrzak et al. (2010) reporting rates as high as 72% for war veterans. Although Tedeschi and Calhoun (2006) cite studies reporting PTG prevalence rates ranging from 3% to 100%, they noted that the rates commonly reported in the literature usually span from 30% to 80%.

Recently, the focus of research has shifted from prevalence and occurrence of growth to the cognitive processes involved in producing growth (e.g., Cann et al., 2011); the individual differences and variations in the experience of growth (Lindstrom at al., 2011); and the relationship between PTG and distress (Kunst et al., 2010). This shift was prompted by research suggesting that PTG involves a variety of constructs. Some of these constructs represent a positive outcome, some are related to coping processes, and others involve illusory self-enhancement strategies that enable traumatised individuals to alleviate some of the distress experienced (e.g., Helgeson et al., 2006; Zoellner & Maercker, 2006). Furthermore, although PTG is common, as outlined above, not all trauma survivors experience PTG. In an attempt to understand the differences between those who report growth and those who do not, researchers have explored the relationship between PTSD symptoms and PTG.

3.4 The relationship between PTSD and PTG

As PTSD symptoms are a negative outcome of trauma, and PTG refers to the positive outcomes, it seems logical to view these outcomes as opposite ends of a continuum. Yet, theories of PTG suggest otherwise. In fact, numerous studies show that PTSD symptoms and PTG often coexist in traumatised individuals (e.g., Taku et al., 2008). For example, several researchers have reported that individuals who report severe PTSD symptoms also report more PTG than those experiencing a lower level of PTSD symptoms (McMillen et al., 1997; Park et al., 2008; Park et al., 1996; Snape, 1997). However, other researchers have found the opposite where individuals who experience more severe PTSD symptoms report less growth (e.g., Aldwin et al., 1994; Frazier et al., 2001; Ickovics et al., 2006) and in some studies no relationship is evident between PTG and PTSD symptoms (e.g., Cordova et al., 2001; Powell et al., 2003). Such mixed findings have prompted some researchers to suggest that the relationship between PTSD symptoms and PTG is best explained as a curvilinear relationship where distress is required to start the growth process, but high levels of distress prevent the growth process from occurring (e.g., Butler., 2007; Kleim & Ehlers, 2009; Lechner et al., 2006). However, recent meta-analyses have not found a consistent relationship between PTG, PTSD symptoms and distress (Linley & Joseph, 2004; Stanton et al., 2006; Zoellner & Maercker, 2006). Linley and Joseph (2004) reported mixed results with PTSD symptoms negatively associated with positive life changes following sexual assault, but positively related to stress-related growth in Oklahoma residents following the 1995 bombing. Stanton et al. (2006) found from their meta-analysis that the majority of studies examined did not show a significant relationship between PTG and distress, and Zoellner and Maercker reported weak correlations between PTG and PTSD measures ranging from $r = -.2$ to $r = .2$ among a variety of cohorts.

3.5 Research on the positive and negative changes following trauma

The positive and negative changes to the self that can result from trauma have predominantly been researched independently of each other. Some have argued that focusing solely on the possible positive changes is problematic as this may increase the likelihood of a positive response bias from a desire to appear well adjusted (Tomich & Helgeson, 2004; Park & Lechner, 2006). This biased response style can also inadvertently lead to overly positive self-reports and inflated PTG prevalence ratings. Furthermore, Park and Lechner (2006) claimed that exploring traumatic changes without consideration of the negative consequences of trauma has limited the research and our understanding of the nuances of posttraumatic changes.

Only a few studies have attempted to simultaneously examine the positive and negative consequences (e.g., Joseph et al., 1993; Park et al., 2008). However, these studies examined self-reported positive and negative changes across different domains. For example, Joseph et al. examined positive and negative changes resulting from trauma and their impact on mental health after a shipwreck, whereas Park et al. explored positive and negative changes in health behaviour, such as sleep, diet, and exercise, in cancer survivors. A common finding of these studies was a non-significant relationship between positive and negative changes, suggesting that these experiences of change are independent. These studies concluded that there was a need for a scale that could measure a variety of responses which are believed to be experienced by individuals after a traumatic event. Many other authors have made similar claims, suggesting that a scale that can measure positive and negative changes simultaneously is required (e.g., Dansky et al., 1990; Harvey et al., 2006; Tomich & Helgeson, 2004).

3.6 Simultaneous measurement of the positive and negative effects of trauma

To date, a few scales have been designed to measure the positive and negative changes resulting from trauma simultaneously (e.g., Joseph et al., 1993, 2005; McMillen & Fisher, 1998). However, these scales do not measure the positive and negative effects in the same domains, suggesting that the positive items are still subject to the same response biases as scales that only measure positive changes (Baker et al., 2008).

Recently, Baker et al., (2008) designed an expanded version of the Posttraumatic Growth Inventory (PTGI; Tedeschi & Calhoun, 1996), the Paired Format Posttraumatic Growth Inventory (PTGI-42), which measures posttraumatic growth (PTG) and posttraumatic depreciation (PTD). This scale enables individuals to report both positive and negative changes within the same personal domains. This measure is intended to provide a more detailed understanding of the positive and negative changes experienced by many trauma victims. For example, an individual may report growth in some aspects of social support, such as improved relationships with family members, while concurrently demonstrate reductions in social functioning, such as one's inability to converse with strangers or to trust others. As this scale enables respondents to consider both the positive and negative aspects of their experience, it is thought to reduce the likelihood of positive response biases and overly positive self-reports.

To date, only two studies have examined PTG and PTD simultaneously (Baker et al., 2008; Cann et al., 2010). Interestingly, in both studies PTG and PTD were uncorrelated. This supports previous studies demonstrating that positive and negative changes are independent (e.g., Joseph et al., 1993; Park et al., 2008). This finding also raises the possibility that these two outcomes of a highly stressful life experience, PTG and PTD, might be differently associated with variables assumed to predict growth, and might differentially predict outcome variables assumed to be associated with growth (Cann et al., 2010). For example, it is possible that PTD impacts the type of rumination conducted after trauma. Cann et al.'s study provides some evidence for this premise as they found that PTD was positively related to recent intrusive thoughts and recent intrusive thoughts were negatively correlated with PTG. These findings, however, contradict many studies that have found that intrusive thoughts are negatively related to PTSD (e.g., Shalev, 1992; Snape, 1997) and positively related to PTG and well-being (e.g., Park & Fenster, 2004; Snape, 1997).

Cann et al. (2010) claimed that it was the continuation of intrusive thoughts about the stressful event that appeared to be associated with psychological losses (i.e., depreciation) and posttraumatic symptomatology. Therefore, as PTSD symptoms are thought to be indicative of incomplete emotional processing (Garnefski et al., 2001; Joseph & Linley, 2005); and the distressing elements of the event continue to produce intrusive thoughts until the information is cognitively processed (e.g., Creamer et al., 1992), the amount of cognitive processing conducted after the event may influence or predict whether the potential changes are perceived as positive or negative. Further investigation into the positive and negative changes resulting from trauma and the cognitive processes involved warrant further investigation.

4. What cognitive processes determine whether the changes are positive or negative?

Many post-trauma processing theories claim that trauma-related information must be integrated into a coherent model of the self to enable recovery (e.g., Creamer et al., 1992; Foa & Kozak, 1986). These theories suggest that integration is achieved though an active process of thinking about the traumatic event, as well as the associated feelings and the subsequent implications or consequences, and attempting to make sense of them. This process is thought to enable the individual to regain balance or consistency between the inner and outer worlds (Linley & Joseph, 2004) and has been positively correlated with PTG (Manne et al., 2004).

From this perspective, PTSD can be considered to result from insufficient or incomplete cognitive processing. Many researchers support this premise (e.g., Joseph & Linley, 2005; Park et al., 1996). Joseph and Linley (2005) point out that factors that impede the processing of traumatic information - avoidance of the disturbing situation, refusal or inability to talk, and absence of perceived control - are hallmark symptoms of posttraumatic stress disorder (PTSD) and suggest that PTSD can be conceptualised as indicative of incomplete processing. As the amount of cognitive processing appears to affect the levels of PTSD symptoms and

PTG experienced, it seems possible that cognitive processing may play a moderating role in the relationship between these constructs.

Research into indicators of cognitive processing after trauma have mostly focused on intrusive thoughts (Greenberg, 1995; Horowitz, 1986) and attempts to find the causes or meaning of the trauma (e.g., Taylor, 1983). Intrusions about the trauma have been reported to negatively relate to PTSD (e.g., Patterson et al., 1990; Shalev, 1992; Snape, 1997) and positively to PTG and well-being (e.g., Park & Fenster, 2004; Snape, 1997). Attempts to find the causes or meaning of the trauma also show a positive relation to PTG (e.g., Calhoun et al., 2000; Lepore et al., 2000). Nevertheless, the research on how cognitive processing affects trauma recovery has yielded inconsistent findings. For example, although intrusions are positively related to PTG, a reduction in intrusions can also be associated with better post-trauma adjustment (Lepore, et al., 2000). Furthermore, intrusions lead to avoidance (e.g., Creamer et al., 1992). As high levels of intrusions and avoidance are core elements of PTSD, intrusions can therefore increase PTSD symptoms (e.g., Baum, 1990; Joseph et al., 1996; McFarland et al., 2007).

These findings demonstrate that to date, research has been unable to find meaningful differences in the types of processing that prompt growth and those that do not. This may be due to a focus on inappropriate and problematic indicators of cognitive processing. For example, as intrusions are a core feature of PTSD symptoms, it would be surprising to find that intrusions related more consistently with PTG than PTSD. Additionally, the inconsistent findings may reflect the lack of appropriately sensitive measures. It is difficult to differentiate between "healthy" or "unhealthy" levels of intrusions or "adaptive" or "maladaptive" attempts to find meanings with current scales. Therefore, although the role of cognitive processing in the development of PTG seems to be worthy of exploration, the current focus on intrusions and attempts to find meaning may not be adequate. In response, some researchers have begun to explore whether cognitive processing after trauma might occur through repetitive thought or rumination (e.g., Lindstrom et al., 2011).

4.1 The role of rumination in PTSD and PTG

Rumination, a type of repetitive thought, is commonly defined as a self-focused, negative thinking style about past negative experiences and/or mood that is intrusive, repetitive, cyclical, and uncontrollable (e.g., Nolen-Hoeksema, 1991; Papageorgiou & Wells, 2003; Teasdale, 1999). When defined in this way, research has shown that rumination is a maladaptive type of repetitive thought, and has been linked to significant psychiatric difficulties, such as PTSD, depression and Social Anxiety Disorder (e.g., Kessler et al., 1995; Maercker et al., 2004; Brewin et al., 2010). Rumination is also related to a range of other negative outcomes, such as immune deficiencies, physiological issues, a lowered sense of well-being, and ongoing distress (e.g., Nolen-Hoeksema & Morrow, 1993; Tedeschi & Calhoun, 2004; Watkins, 2008). Rumination is reported to be one of the principal sources of PTSD symptomatology and severity (e.g., Clohessy & Ehlers, 1999; Ehlers & Clark, 2000; Ehlers et al., 2003; Murray et al., 2002; Steil & Ehlers, 2000). However, very little is understood about the mechanisms by which rumination maintains PTSD symptoms (Michael et al., 2007).

Rumination may serve as a cognitive avoidance strategy that inhibits an individual's ability to deploy adaptive coping resources (Fresco et al., 2002). It has been established that those who ruminate about a trauma experience higher levels of PTSD symptoms following naturalistic and experimental trauma (Baum et al., 1993; Nolen-Hoeksema & Morrow, 1991; Sergestorm & Alden, 2000). Furthermore, individuals who are encouraged to ruminate about their traumatic event experience more negative thinking and dysphoric mood, and have difficulty problem solving (Lyubomirsky et al., 1999; Watkins & Baracaia, 2002).

Although the term 'rumination' has traditionally been used to describe a negative repetitive thinking style, rumination has recently been redefined as also being a thoughtfully reflective style of repetitive thought (Nolen-Hoeksema & Davis, 2004), that enables a deliberate, and purposeful re-examination of the traumatic event and related issues (Calhoun et al., 2000). Rumination can include reminiscing and reflecting on events in an attempt to try and understand the event, as well as find possible solutions to life problems (Lindstrom et al., 2011). It can involve consideration of the possible positive repercussions of the event, as well as a conscious and deliberate effort to remind oneself of possible benefits that may have resulted from being challenged with such an event (Affleck & Tennen, 1996; Folkman, 2008; Lindstrom et al., 2011). Although most trauma survivors experience intrusive, negative rumination, many also engage in deliberate rumination whereby they consciously and explicitly decide to think about the event. This deliberate type of rumination is viewed as constructive, adaptive, and related to Posttraumatic Growth (PTG; Affleck & Tennen, 1996; Calhoun et al., 2000). As extensive research demonstrates that rumination can result in both positive and negative outcomes, these findings raise questions about how these opposing outcomes stem from one cognitive process. In an attempt to address this question, Trapnell and Campbell (1999) suggested that the self-focusing process (i.e., the tendency to focus on the inner aspects of the self) is not unidimensional and argued that different forms of self-focused private attention may lead to different outcomes. They posit that two distinct self-focusing processes may exist, namely inquisitive reflection and neurotic rumination, that explain how rumination can lead to both positive and negative outcomes after trauma. In their definition, rumination is focused in the past; is motivated by anxiety; involves chronic negative thinking about losses, threats, and injustices to the self; and is associated with distress and maladjustment. Reflection however, is motivated by curiosity and self-interest; is future oriented; involves new or alternative perceptions of the self; and is associated with increased self-knowledge and accurate self-perceptions (Trapnell & Campbell, 1999).

In a similar model of rumination, Treynor et al. (2003) made a distinction between two types of rumination which they termed “brooding” and “reflective pondering”. Reflective rumination involves a deliberate effort focused on dealing with the situation, and was associated with lower levels of depression over time, whereas brooding rumination is a relatively passive consideration of current conditions and is associated with depression (Nolen-Hoeksema & Davis, 2004). Joormann et al. (2006) investigated the validity of these two factors of rumination and provided supporting evidence that reflective pondering is adaptive and brooding is maladaptive. Many other researchers also provide support for this distinction (e.g., Fresco et al., 2002; Trapnell & Campbell, 1999; Treynor et al., 2003; Siegle et al., 2004; Watkins & Baracaia, 2002; Watkins, 2004).

4.2 Types of rumination and their relationship with PTSD and PTG

As rumination is considered to promote both positive and negative outcomes, Taku et al. (2008) examined how two types of ruminative thought, deliberate and intrusive rumination, related to distress and posttraumatic growth in bereaved Japanese university students. They found that deliberate rumination led to PTG, whereas intrusive rumination led to distress. In a subsequent study by Taku et al. (2009), intrusive rumination soon after the event was shown to be positively associated with PTG, whereas recent deliberate rumination most strongly predicted current levels of PTG. Similarly, Stockton et al. (2011) reported from a cross-sectional study that deliberate, but not intrusive, rumination was significantly related to PTG. Other studies support these findings (e.g., Chan et al., 2011; Morris & Shakespeare-Finch, 2011).

Recently, Stockton et al. (2011) conducted two cross-sectional studies exploring different types of rumination: brooding and reflection, and deliberate and intrusive rumination. Intrusive rumination and brooding showed no association with PTG but related to distress. In contrast, deliberate rumination and reflection were positively associated with PTG, as long as brooding was low. These findings suggest that reflection may enable the individual to approach both positive (i.e., PTG) and negative (i.e., PTSD) outcomes of their traumatic event from a problem-solving perspective as reflection is focused on dealing with the problem. Thus, reflection may activate PTG and strengthen the relationship between PTG and PTSD symptoms. Conversely, brooding may encourage the individual to dwell on the negative consequences of the trauma and prevent them from thinking constructively. Thus, brooding increases PTSD symptoms, hinders the growth process, and weakens the relationship between PTSD and PTG. So far, these results suggest that PTSD symptoms and PTG are dependent on the type of rumination conducted. This raises the question of how these types of rumination are selected or evoked by an individual after a traumatic event. It also raises questions about whether there could be other forms of rumination operating simultaneously and what impact they have on posttraumatic outcomes. Trapnell and Campbell (1999) suggested that cognitive and affective processes may affect the type of rumination conducted which could explain how brooding rumination can lead to distress and maladjustment while reflective rumination results in growth. The possible impact of these factors on rumination, the PTG process, and PTSD symptomatology will be briefly discussed.

4.2.1 Emotion

Traumatic events produce a range of emotions that play an integral role in the eventual outcome (Taku et al., 2009). For example, the DSM-IV-TR's (APA, 2000) PTSD criteria highlight the impact of negative emotions in psychopathology by requiring that individuals respond with "intense fear, helplessness, or horror" (p. 463). Such negative emotions have also been reported to explain a significant amount of the variance in PTSD symptom severity over time (Michael et al., 2007). In contrast, individuals who focus on positive emotions (e.g., interest, love, gratitude) after 9/11 experienced less distress (Fredrickson et al., 2003).

Affective processes also influence the type of rumination or reflective thought undertaken. For example, Boyraz and Efstathiou's (2011) study exploring PTG in bereaved women found that positive affect mediated the relationship between self-focusing tendencies (i.e., rumination) and PTG. Garnefski et al.'s (2001) model of rumination offered further support by arguing that rumination is a strategy to regulate emotions that arise in response to trauma. Furthermore, Joseph and Linley (2005), drawing on Rachman's (1980) concept of emotional processing, suggest that factors that impede the processing of emotions after trauma - avoidance of the disturbing situation, refusal or inability to talk, and absence of perceived control - are hallmark symptoms of posttraumatic stress disorder (PTSD). They suggest that PTSD can be conceptualised as indicative of incomplete emotional processing. In support, many researchers have found that affective and cognitive suppression commonly occurs in individuals after a trauma and this can be adaptive at the time of the trauma (e.g., Bryant & Harvey, 1995 ; Solomon et al., 1988; Valentiner et al., 1996). Yet, suppression over an extended period of time is considered to be maladaptive as it interferes with processing the emotions associated with the trauma, and impedes recovery overtime (e.g. Joseph et al., 1997; Pennebaker et al., 1989).

Research also indicates that different types of trauma result in different emotional responses. For example, Amstadter and Vernon (2008) performed a study exploring the peri- and post-trauma emotional responses of individuals after different types of trauma. They found that different types of traumatic events (sexual assault, physical assault, transportation accidents, and illness) produced distinct emotional profiles with differing levels of intensity. Individuals who were sexually assaulted demonstrated greater emotional responses post-trauma compared to individuals who had been traumatised by physical assault, illness or transportation accidents. They also reported that assault victims, whether physical or sexual, experienced increased PTSD symptom severity compared to those whose trauma resulted from transportation accidents or illness.

If different types of trauma result in different emotional responses, and rumination is a regulatory response to such emotions (Garnefski et al., 2001), it seems plausible that different types of trauma may induce different types of rumination. In support of this premise, research suggests that stress-reactive rumination is a predictor of later depression (Robinson & Alloy, 2003) and later ruminative thinking has been linked to more stressful interpersonal interactions (e.g., Abbot & Rapee, 2004; Harvey et al., 2005; Lundh & Sperling, 2002; Mellings & Alden, 2000). Furthermore, Nolen-Hoeksema and colleagues (Lyubomirsky & Nolen-Hoeksema, 1993, 1995; Nolen-Hoeksema & Morrow, 1993) suggested that negative mood is a necessary component for ruminative thought processes, although they did not define the type of rumination that was explored.

Although negative mood is necessary to evoke ruminative processes, Kross et al. (2005), explored whether individuals can process these negative emotions without becoming overwhelmed by them, and how this is connected to the different types of rumination. The authors explored these questions using Metcalfe and Mischel's (1999) hot/cool systems model of self-regulation. In this model, negative emotional experiences are either mentally represented as concrete and emotionally arousing (i.e., "hot" features) or abstract and informational (i.e., "cool" features). These are then thought to be connected to two different regulatory systems. Concrete and emotionally arousing representations elicit reflexive processing that is predominantly controlled by the negative emotional experience. This is an automatic process that leads to defensive behaviours (e.g., avoidance, blame, intellectualisation) and is thought to increase the intensity of the emotions felt. Conversely, abstract and informational representations enable cognitively directed, reflective processing that is more effortful but effective in inhibiting automatic responses activated by concrete, or "hot", representations. Mentally representing negative emotional experiences in this way is thought to allow the individual to contemplate the event without activating intense levels of affect and negative, or brooding, rumination.

Using Metcalfe and Mischel's (1999) model, Kross et al. (2005) examined the impact of the event the type of self-perspective (the vantage point taken when focusing on emotions, i.e., self-immersed vs. self-distanced) and type of emotional focus (the content of thoughts, i.e., what vs. why) on the recovery process. Their results showed that reflective processing of emotions was facilitated when the individual distanced themselves from the emotion, and focused on the reasons underlying the emotions rather than focus on *what* they had experienced. This enabled individuals to think about their trauma and the emotions elicited in a way that they could make sense of without reactivating and reliving the emotions that resulted from the trauma. Furthermore, they claimed that asking oneself *why* they had experienced the event while self-immersed in the emotional experience may have a detrimental effect by enhancing distress and PTSD symptoms. Overall, these results demonstrate that emotions impact on the cognitive processing of trauma.

4.2.2 Cognition

The literature on social comparison processes demonstrates that interpersonal comparisons are a ubiquitous part of life. Individuals' beliefs about how they compare with other people are influential in determining their self-conceptions, affective states, and expectancies for the future (Suls & Miller, 1977; Suls & Wills, 1991; Wood, 1989). Taylor's (1983) cognitive adaptation model suggests that a traumatic event threatens a person's sense of control and self-esteem (e.g., Abramson et al., 1989; Janoff-Bulman, 1989). His model suggests that to cope with the negative feelings engendered by such events, people may construct a variety of cognitive distortions or illusions that enable them to view the experience and themselves in a more positive light (Taylor & Armor, 1996; Taylor & Brown, 1988). This implies that part of the growth in response to a threatening event may represent exaggerations or illusions of positive temporal change designed to help them cope with the distress experienced.

Similarly, McFarland & Alvaro (2000) suggested that those who have experienced a traumatic event have an acute need for favourable self-evaluations in order to overcome their trauma. They posit that this need for positive self-evaluations can prompt the individual to construct temporal comparisons that reflect positively on the self. A temporal comparison is defined as the consideration of how one's current standing on an attribute relates to one's past standing on the attribute (Albert, 1977; Levine & Moreland, 1987; Suls, Marco, & Tobin, 1991).

Albert (1977) believed that temporal comparison was a corollary to social comparison theory (Festinger, 1954). Whereas social comparisons are interpersonal and ostensibly a-historical, temporal comparisons are intrapersonal and are explicit appraisals of the self over time (Keyes & Ryff, 2000). When an individual makes social comparisons, they are presumed to make temporal comparisons as well in order to understand themselves more clearly or to assess and anticipate their own capabilities.

There is considerable research on the cognitive determinants of temporal comparisons. For example, many researchers have attempted to explore how schema-guided processing may affect perceptions of temporal change (e.g., Suls & Mullen, 1984; Suls, Marco & Tobin, 1991). While some research implies that the person's past qualities are affected by their current beliefs (e.g., Heckhausen et al., 1989; McFarland et al., 1992; Ryff, 1982), other research highlights how people's current qualities are affected by their recollections of their past qualities (e.g., Strack et al., 1985). For example, people assess whether their abilities are improving, whether their memory is deteriorating, and whether they are as happy as they used to be. These "temporal" or "intrapersonal" comparisons may be just as influential as social comparisons in determining our self-evaluations, moods, and expectancies (e.g., Levine & Moreland, 1987; Masters & Keil, 1987; Suls & Mullen, 1982, 1984; Veroff, 1969).

Although the motivational underpinnings of social comparison processes are well documented, the manner in which people's motivations (i.e., needs and desires) affect temporal comparison processes is not yet fully understood. McFarland and Alvaro (2000) explored the affects of motivation on temporal comparisons of traumatised individuals. Their results showed that threatening self-relevant feelings played a causal role in prompting self-enhancing temporal comparisons, and that an individual's perceptions of personal improvement are, in part, motivated illusions designed to help them cope with trauma. Shedler et al.'s (1993) research on the "illusion of mental health" supports McFarland and Alvaro's claim. However, they further suggest that for some individuals, these positive appraisals of improvement may represent defensive denial that is related to maladaptive outcomes. Dohrenwend et al. (2004) suggest that these cognitive distortions may be maladaptive for some but adaptive for others because positive temporal appraisals can represent two different processes: a reformulation of the meaning of the traumatic experience into a positive light which is related to adaptive outcomes; and a defensive denial of the negative features of the traumatic event which is a pathological manoeuvre and related to maladaptive outcomes.

As adaptive appraisals involve a reformulation of the meaning of the event, whereas maladaptive appraisals involve denial, this implies that the manner in which people process information (reflective or ruminative) affects whether their temporal comparisons are adaptive or maladaptive. McFarland et al. (2007) explored the impact of ruminative thought on temporal comparisons and found that people are more likely to view themselves positively when they adopt a reflective orientation to their negative feelings than when they adopt a ruminative orientation. Although this provides partial support for Trapnell and Campbell's (1999) premise that rumination style impacts on cognitive processes involving temporal comparisons, future research into whether temporal comparisons influence the individual's ruminative orientation would provide further information about the relationship between these constructs. Such research may also reveal how adaptive and maladaptive positive appraisals influence whether the changes perceived are temporary or long lasting.

5. Are posttraumatic changes long lasting?

Searching for positive meanings or benefits arising from adversity is believed to reduce PTSD symptoms and to be related to positive outcomes. In support of this premise, cross-sectional studies have associated benefit finding with more positive affect (Tomich & Helgeson, 2002); less negative affect (Revenson et al., 1983); better psychological adjustment (Taylor, 1983; Taylor et al., 1984); better coping (Thompson, 1985); and fewer physical symptoms (van Oyen Witvliet et al., 2010). Although Tedeschi and Calhoun (2004) view growth as a lengthy process, it has been reported soon after the event, even as early as two weeks (Frazier et al., 2001).

McMillen et al. (1997) examined the perceived benefits of individuals after three different types of traumatic events: a tornado, a plane crash, and a mass killing. They found that individuals who perceived benefits 4-6 weeks after the event were less likely to experience PTSD symptoms three years later. Perceived benefits also moderated the impact of the severity of the event on changes to mental health over time. Additionally, the severity of the event was associated with better recovery overtime for those who perceived benefits, whereas the severity of the trauma was associated with worse recovery for those who perceived fewer benefits.

Benefit finding has also been associated with better quality of life (Davis et al., 1998). Davis et al. showed that individuals who perceived some aspect of their experience as positive after 6 months reported lower levels of distress 13 months after the loss of a loved one due to illness. Similarly, in a study by Morrill et al. (2008) on women with early stage breast cancer, benefit finding moderated the relationship between PTSD symptoms, depression and quality of life. Combined, these findings indicate that benefit finding is related to positive outcomes, such as better recovery from trauma and improved quality of life.

Not all studies have shown positive outcomes as a consequence of benefit finding. For example, cross-sectional studies have found that benefit finding does not relate to quality of life, well-being or adjustment in samples of adult bone marrow transplant survivors (Fromm et al., 1996); breast cancer survivors (Cordova et al., 2001); or bereaved individuals (Lehman et al., 1993). In fact, Tomich and Helgeson (2004) found in their study of women with stage II breast cancer, that benefit finding was associated with greater negative affect and reduced mental functioning for individuals with more severe disease. Park et al. (1996, study 3) also found that benefit finding was related to more intrusive and avoidant thoughts in a study of undergraduates who reported negative-stressful events during the past 6 months.

Studies exploring the relationship between posttraumatic growth (PTG) and posttraumatic stress disorder (PTSD) have also yielded mixed results. Some studies have reported a positive relationship (e.g., Wild & Paivio, 2003), whereas others have found a negative relationship (e.g., Hall et al., 2008), some a curvilinear relationship (e.g., Kleim & Ehlers, 2009), and others no relationship at all (e.g., Cordova et al., 2007; Salsman et al., 2009). Contradictory results of the impact of benefit finding on posttraumatic outcomes have been attributed to problems of measurement. For example, Boals et al. (2010) attributed the inconsistent findings to the use of different measures of the construct. In support of Boals et al.'s claim, Helgeson et al.'s (2006) meta-analysis of PTG measures found that the scale administered moderated the relations between benefit finding and anxiety, depression, and distress. This suggests that the current scales may be measuring different aspects of growth. However, these scales have been reported as highly related. For example, Maercker and Langner (2001) reported a correlation of r=.82 between the Posttraumatic Growth Inventory (PTGI, Tedeschi & Calhoun, 1996) and the Stress-Related Growth Scale (SRGS, Park et al., 1996); the two most widely used scales to measure growth. Such a high correlation indicates that these two scales are measuring the same construct.

The inconsistent findings have also raised questions as to whether posttraumatic growth is real or simply an illusion whereby the person construes benefits as a way to relieve distress (e.g., Bonnano, 2005). It has been suggested that self-reported changes resulting from trauma may reflect self-protective and self-enhancing processes that signal a derogation of past selves rather than actual change (e.g., McFarland & Alvaro, 2000). The founders of posttraumatic growth research, Tedeschi and Calhoun (1995) even considered "whether the construal of benefits and the self-perception of growth simply represent another cognitive bias", rather than reflect actual change (p.119).

Gunty et al. (2011) suggested that the relationship between perceived and actual PTG, would best be assessed by longitudinal studies of changes pre- to post-trauma. However, the lack of data on pre-trauma functioning makes it difficult for self-report changes to be verified, leading some researchers to suggest that third-party reports may provide a reliable indicator of PTG (e.g., Park et al., 1996; Weiss, 2002). Measuring third-party responses rather than the individual's subjective perception of change is said to provide stronger evidence of PTG as third-party accounts are not subject to the same memory biases or self-enhancing response distortions as self-reported measures. However, Park et al. (1996) found that the responses of the traumatised and third-party participants correlated between r=.21 and r=.31 suggesting a very weak relationship between their perceptions of change. These results are in accord with other studies showing that traumatised individuals are more likely to report greater improvement in their personal attributes after a traumatic event than their acquaintances (e.g., McFarland & Alvaro, 2000). This evidence suggests that third-party responses may not be the most valid or reliable source of information regarding positive change.

There have also been attempts to verify whether growth is actual or perceived by comparing responses across two time points. Ransom et al. (2008) explored increases in the relative importance of intrinsic versus extrinsic goals and positive attributes of cancer patients before and after radiotherapy. PTG was found to be significantly related with actual, but not perceived, increases in the importance of intrinsic goals, and with perceived, but not actual, increases in positive attributes. Gunty et al. (2011) performed a similar study using the same methodology and produced similar results: perceived growth was more strongly related to actual growth for individuals who reported less distress and more life satisfaction post-trauma.

Although Ransom et al. (2008) and Gunty et al.'s (2011) studies provide important information regarding the extent of actual growth involved in PTG, the research has methodological limitations. These studies asked respondents to complete self-report measures of their current attributes and goal orientations (Ransom, Sheldon, & Jacobsen, 2008), and levels of distress and life satisfaction (Gunty et al., 2011) at two time points. At time 2, the participants were also asked to recall their answers on these measures from time 1. To measure actual change, the authors conducted planned comparisons examining the difference between patients' ratings at the two time points. Perceived change was then measured by exploring the difference between patients' ratings at time 2 and their recalled time 1 ratings.

One problem is that these studies rely on the quality of the participant's memory which is widely reported to be biased or flawed after trauma (e.g., Diener et al., 2010; El-Hage et al., 2006). Additionally, the use of self-report measures to assess people's perceptions of themselves, by definition, provide subjective rather than actual information on growth. Although self-report measures are generally considered an appropriate, if not a superior method for gathering subjective information regarding attitudes and values compared to other approaches (e.g., Howard, 1994; Spector, 1994), the validity of using self-report measures in PTG research has been criticised because such scales are subject to response distortions, such as acquiescence and social desirability (e.g., Andrews, 1998; Linley & Joseph, 2004; Gunty et al., 2011). However, many researchers agree that a traumatic event is characterised not so much by any particular situation as by the individual's perception and response to that situation (Carkhuff & Berenson, 1977; Hendricks & Byers, 2006; Parad, 1971). Therefore, if an event is considered a crisis or not depends on an individual's perception, it seems logical to assess the individual's perception of the event and the possible coinciding growth using self-report measures rather than to use other sources of information.

5.1 Is growth an outcome or a process?

Up until now, growth has been discussed as an outcome of trauma. However, the question has been raised as to whether growth actually reflects a self-enhancing process that assists with the recovery of trauma. For example, Maercker and Zoellner (2004) posit that self-reported posttraumatic growth may partly represent a process of distortion as an attempt to reduce or distance oneself from the event and subsequent emotions experienced after trauma. In support, Park (1999) posited that the inability to find a negative correlation between growth and distress suggests that some people report growth because they are denying the negative impact of the traumatic event, while others are not. Park's argument is plausible as it is generally accepted that reactions to trauma often include denial, avoidance, wishful thinking, and distortions of meaning (Brewin, 1997). Such results raise the possibility that growth is only illusory.

5.2 Is growth only an illusion?

Taylor and colleagues (Taylor, 1983; Taylor and Armor, 1996; Taylor et al., 2000) have explored the illusionary, self-deceptive aspects of growth under the title Positive Illusion (Taylor, 1983). They reported three illusions that commonly characterise people's beliefs after traumatic events or information. These include, mildly distorted positive perceptions of themselves, an exaggerated sense of personal control, and unrealistic optimism. Taylor and colleagues suggest that such illusions or distortions are cognitive attempts to adapt to the situation to regain consistency as well as an understanding of the self and the environment. Such illusions are common in individuals who experience health-related traumas, such as cancer patients. These people often develop a perception of themselves as coping better than other patients (Maercker & Zoellner, 2004) which may explain the high rate of reported positive changes in the self as a result of their illness (Taylor & Armor, 1996).

Although such positive illusions may be used to deny, avoid, hope, or distort the meaning of the event, Taylor and Armor (1996) suggested that positive illusions are indicative of people's beliefs about their personal qualities and degree of perceived control, whereas denial and hope represent a desire for events to be different to how they are. If benefit finding signals denial, benefit finding may then become maladaptive over time as it may interfere with effective coping strategies (Lazarus, 1983) and cognitive processing of the traumatic event.

5.3 The janus face model of posttraumatic growth

The contradictory findings for the potential benefits following trauma led Maercker and Zoellner (2004) to propose a two-factor model of posttraumatic growth, The Janus Face Model. In this model, growth is thought to have a positive, constructive and self-transcending side as described by Tedeschi and Calhoun (1996), as well as a self-deceptive, illusionary side. The authors suggested that the constructive side may develop alongside adjustment and cognitive restructuring of traumatic information, whereas the illusionary side may be related to denial, avoidance, wishful thinking, self-consolidation, or palliation. However, these adaptive and maladaptive outcomes of growth are believed to depend on the timing of the growth, the level of continued distress, and the use of habitual coping styles such as optimism, and openness to experience.

Maercker and Zoellner (2004) also posit that growth can be a coping strategy as well as an outcome. In the immediate aftermath of a trauma, benefit finding can reflect a coping process rather than an outcome that has emerged from the stressful event. They argued that the illusory aspects of growth experienced shortly after the event may represent a coping effort that provides a palliative function. This illusory component illustrates the use of self-enhancement cognitions in an attempt to alleviate acute stress after a threatening event and provide the person with temporary relief, or distance from the distress experienced, to facilitate deliberate and constructive rumination of the traumatic information. During the earlier stages of the trauma, it is expected, therefore, that more illusory aspects of growth will be present. If constructive processing occurs, the illusory side is expected to reduce and more constructive, longer lasting benefits to arise as the trauma becomes more distal. Conversely, if the person does not deliberately reflect or ruminate on the trauma, this illusory component represents an attempt to cope with the situation by denying or repressing the traumatic information, rather than adjusting to or recovering from the experience. As the trauma is not effectively processed, illusory growth is likely to have a deteriorating effect on adjustment, hinder recovery, and the person is expected to experience ongoing distress. Thus, the illusory component of growth can also represent a cognitive avoidant strategy that, over time, has a negative effect on adjustment.

5.4 Evidence for the janus face model of posttraumatic growth

Although the Janus Face model provides a plausible explanation for the inconsistent findings of PTG research, very few studies has tested this model. McFarland and Alvaro's (2000) study exploring the effects of motivation on temporal comparisons of traumatised individuals, provide indirect support for the Janus Face model. They found that threatening self-relevant feelings played a causal role in prompting self-enhancing temporal comparisons, and that individual's perceptions of personal improvement are, in part, motivated illusions designed to help them cope with trauma. Shedler et al.'s (1993) research on the "illusion of mental health" also supports this claim and further suggests that for some individuals, these positive appraisals of improvement may represent defensive denial that is related to maladaptive outcomes. Dohrenwend et al. (2004) posit that these cognitive distortions may be maladaptive for some but adaptive for others because positive appraisals can represent two different processes: a reformulation of the meaning of the traumatic experience into a positive light which is related to adaptive outcomes; and a defensive denial of the negative features of the traumatic event which is a pathological manoeuvre and related to maladaptive outcomes.

Additional support for this model comes from Helgeson et al.'s (2006) meta-analysis of literature pertaining to the relationship between benefit finding and psychological and physical health. They found that the relationship between posttraumatic growth and these outcomes was affected by the amount of time that had passed since the onset of the stressor. Growth or benefit finding was more strongly related to greater positive affect and less depression when the time since the traumatic event was greater than two years, whereas benefit finding was associated with more global distress when the time since the trauma was two years or less. Similarly, Frazier et al., (2001) suggested that encouraging growth too early in the adjustment process may be detrimental to the survivor, based on evidence that early onset growth decreases along with an increase in distress (Wortman, 2004).

Only one study has attempted to directly test the Janus Face Model. Zoellner et al. (2008) explored posttraumatic growth among survivors of motor vehicle accidents in Germany. They operationalised the illusory component of PTG as optimism and the constructive side as openness to experience and intense feelings. Although the relationships between PTG and optimism or openness were non-significant, their results provide some evidence for the Janus Face Model as optimism and openness were found to predict PTSD symptomatology. Individuals with higher levels of PTSD symptoms also had higher levels of optimism and PTG. Conversely, individuals with lower levels of PTSD symptoms also had higher levels of openness and PTG. Further, a relationship was apparent between the severity of trauma and PTG, where more severe trauma was associated with higher levels of PTG. As this is the only study to directly test this model, further research is required to ascertain whether this model is the most appropriate way to explain the inconsistent findings of posttraumatic growth research.

6. Conclusion

This chapter has discussed some of the contemporary views of trauma, outlining the relationship between the disruptive and destructive processes, as well as the constructive processes that can be experienced in the aftermath of a traumatic event. Although research into the impact of trauma has traditionally explored the precipitating negative symptoms of PTSD, the recent advent of the posttraumatic growth research has identified, and started to quantify, the beneficial as well as the detrimental outcomes on a person's sense of self and identity. Despite extensive research, many aspects of the impact of trauma remain poorly understood. Furthermore, the themes discussed here, namely posttraumatic growth and depreciation, rumination, and actual versus perceived growth, have largely been examined independently of each other. Further research is needed to clarify the ways in which the different elements of traumatic response relate to each other and to clarify the nature of several key constructs.

This chapter has examined inconsistencies in the literature in relation to the prevalence and severity of PTSD following qualifying and non-qualifying traumatic events; and whether growth or benefit finding lead to positive change and long lasting improvements. The contradictory findings demonstrate the need for further research on the consequences of trauma. One possible explanation for the inconsistencies is that studies have grouped together distinct types of events and overlooked the nuances of different traumas. Exploration of the differences between traumatic events may reveal that different types of trauma produce specific profiles that could be used to predict the course and severity of symptoms that may ensue. Such research could also enable a more accurate way of categorising traumatic events and the reactions to trauma.

Research on different types of traumas may also reveal that the type of event contributes to the style of cognitive processing conducted. As previously discussed, ruminative thought has been found to prompt growth while also promoting and maintaining PTSD symptoms. Although the literature has distinguished between intrusive and deliberate rumination, and brooding and reflective rumination, a review of the rumination and repetitive thought literature by Watkins (2008) discusses many types of ruminative thought that could potentially impact the processing of a traumatic event (refer to Watkins, 2008 for a review of terms). When you consider the multitude of the different types of repetitive thought identified, as well as the disruption to the individual's cognitions and emotions in the aftermath of trauma, it is difficult to believe that traumatised individuals would only conduct one type of repetitive thought after trauma. Further research on the impact of these different repetitive thinking styles on the outcomes of trauma is therefore warranted. Exploration of how these types of rumination are selected or evoked by an individual may also provide information regarding how adaptive and maladaptive outcomes are formed.

Finally, exploring whether emotional responses after trauma is an externalised or internalised response (i.e., is the emotional response directed at the event, or at the self and one's response to the event) may also contribute to our understanding of the course and severity of symptoms. For example, anger is a strong emotion commonly experienced in the aftermath of trauma (e.g., Adler et al., 2008; Amstadter & Vernon, 2008; Berntsen & Rubin, 2007). Research exploring where the emotion is directed may reveal that anger aimed at the event is processed differently to anger aimed at the self. Anger at the event may become more manageable as the event becomes more distal but anger at how one responded or coped with the event may be more difficult to overcome, be longer lasting and have a greater impact on the reconstruction of the self. Different combinations of emotions may also change the way that the emotions are processed, and the type of ruminative thought conducted, and thus affect the course of PTSD symptoms and/or posttraumatic growth and depreciation. Such data may explain why interpersonal traumas tend to result in specific symptom constellations as well as more severe and longer lasting PTSD symptoms compared to traumas related to natural disasters or illness (APA, 2000). Therefore, research into the emotional profiles of different trauma types is likely to make a major contribution to our understanding of trauma.

7. References

Abbott, M. J., & Rapee, R. M. (2004). Post-event rumination and negative self-appraisal in social phobia before and after treatment. *Journal of Abnormal Psychology*, Vol. 113, No. 1, pp. (136–144), 1939-1846.

Abramson, L. Y., Metalsky, G. I. , & Alloy, L. B. (1989). Hopelessness depression: A theory-based subtype of depression. *Psychological Review*, Vol. 96, No. 2, pp. (358-372), 1939-1471.

Adler, A. B., Wright, K. M., Bliese, P. D., Eckford, R., & Hoge, C. W. (2008). A2 diagnostic criterion for combat-related posttraumatic stress disorder. *Journal of Traumatic Stress*, Vol. 21, No. 3, pp. (301–308), 15736598.

Affleck, G., & Tennen, H. (1996). Construing benefits from adversity: Adaptational significance and dispositional underpinning. *Journal of Personality,* Vol. 64, No. 4, pp. (899-922), 00223506.

Albert, S. (1977). Temporal comparison theory. *Psychological Review,* Vol. 84, No. 6, pp. (485–503), 1939-1471.

Aldwin, C. M., Levenson, M. R., & Spiro, A. (1994). Vulnerability and resilience to combat exposure: Can stress have lifelong effects? *Psychology and Aging,* Vol. 9, No. 1, pp. (34–44), 1939-1498.

American Psychiatric Association. (1952). *Diagnostic and Statistical Manual of Mental Disorders,* Author, Washington, DC.

American Psychiatric Association. (1968). *Diagnostic and Statistical Manual of Mental Disorders,* (2nd ed.), Author, Washington, DC.

American Psychiatric Association. (1980). *Diagnostic and Statistical Manual of Mental Disorders,* (3rd ed.), Author, Washington, DC.

American Psychiatric Association. (1987). *Diagnostic and Statistical Manual of Mental Disorders,* (3rd ed. Revised), Author, Washington, DC.

American Psychiatric Association. (1994). *Diagnostic and Statistical Manual of Mental Disorders,* (4th ed.). Author, Washington, DC.

American Psychiatric Association. (2000). *Diagnostic and statistical manual of mental disorders* (4th ed. Text Revised), Author, Washington, DC.

American Psychiatric Association. (2010). *Diagnostic and statistical manual of mental disorders,* (5th ed., draft). Retrieved from <www.dsm5.org>

Amir, N., Leiner, A., & Bomyea, J. (2010). Implicit memory and posttraumatic stress symptoms. *Cognitive Therapy and Research,* Vol. 34, No. 1, pp. (49-58), 01475916.

Amstadter, A.B., & Vernon, L.L. (2008). Emotional reactions during and after trauma: A comparison of trauma types. *Journal of Aggression, Maltreatment & Trauma,* Vol. 16, No. 3, pp. (391-408), 1545083X

Anders, S.L., Frazier, P.A., & Frankfurt, S.B. (2011). Variations in criterion A and PTSD rates in a community sample of women. *Journal of Anxiety Disorders,* Vol. 25, No. 2, pp. (176-184), 08876185.

Andreasen, N. C. (2004). Acute and delayed posttraumatic stress disorders: A history and some issues. *American Journal of Psychiatry,* Vol. 161, No., 8, pp. (1321–1323), 15357228.

Andrews, B. (1998). Methodological and definitional issues in shame research. In: *Shame: Interpersonal Behavior, Psychopathology, and Culture* P. Gilbert, & B. Andrews, pp. (39–54), Oxford University Press, New York.

Avina, C., & O'Donohue, W. (2002). Sexual harassment and PTSD: Is sexual harassment diagnosable trauma? *Journal of Traumatic Stress,* Vol. 15, pp. (69-75).

Baker, J. M., Kelly, C., Calhoun, L. G., Cann, A., & Tedeschi, R. G. (2008). An examination of posttraumatic growth and posttraumatic depreciation. *Journal of Loss & Trauma,* Vol. 13, No. 5, pp.(450–465), 15325032.

Baum, A. (1990). Stress, intrusive imagery, and chronic stress. *Health Psychology,* Vol. 1, No. 6, pp. (217-236), 1930-7810.

Baum, A., Cohen, L., & Hall, M. (1993). Control and intrusive memories as determinants of chronic stress. *Psychosomatic Medicine,* Vol. 55, No. 3, pp. (274-286), 1534-7796.

Bedard-Gilligan, M.,&Zoellner, L. A. (2008). The utility of the A1 and A2 criteria in the diagnosis of PTSD. *Behaviour Research and Therapy*, Vol. 46, No. 9, pp. (1062-1069), 00057967.

Berntsen, D., & Rubin, D.C. (2006). When a trauma becomes a key to identity: Enhanced integration of trauma memories predicts posttraumatic stress disorder symptoms. *Applied Cognitive Psychology*, Vol. 21, No. 4, pp. (417-431).

Boals, A., & Schuettler, D. (2009). PTSD symptoms in response to traumatic and nontraumatic events: the role of respondent perception and A2 criterion. *Journal of Anxiety Disorders*, Vol. 23, No. 4, pp. (458–462), 08876185

Boals, A., Steward, J.M., & Schuettler, D. (2010). Advancing our understanding of posttraumatic growth by considering event centrality. *Journal of Loss and Trauma*, Vol. 15, No. 6, pp. (518-533), 1532-5032.

Bodkin, A., Pope, H. G., Detke, M. J., & Hudson, J. I. (2007). Is PTSD caused by traumatic stress? *Journal of Anxiety Disorders*, Vol. 21, No. 2, pp. (176–182), 0887-6185.

Bonnano, G.A. (2005). Resilience in the face of potential trauma. *Current Directions in Psychological Science*, Vol. 14, No. 3, pp. (135-138), 0963-7214.

Boyraz, G., & Efstathiou, N. (2011). Self-focused attention, meaning, and posttraumatic growth: The mediating role of positive and negative affect for bereaved women. *Journal of Loss and Trauma*, Vol. 16, No. 3, pp. (13-32).

Braga, L.L., Fiks, J.P., Mari, J.J., Mello, M.F. (2008). The importance of the concepts of disaster, catastrophe, violence, trauma and barbarism in defining posttraumatic stress disorder in clinical practice. *BMC Psychiatry*, Vol. 8, No. 68, pp. (1-8).

Breslau, N., & Davis, G. C. (1987). Posttraumatic stress disorder: The Stressor Criterion. *Journal of Nervous & Mental Disease*, Vol. 175, No. 5, pp. (255–264).

Breslau, N., & Kessler, R. C. (2001). The Stressor Criterion in DSM-IV posttraumatic stress disorder: An empirical investigation. *Biological Psychiatry*, Vol. 50, No. 9, pp. (699–704), 0006-3223.

Brewin, C.R., (1997). Psychological defenses and the distortion of meaning. In: *The Transformation of Meaning in Psychological Therapies*, M. Power & C.R. Brewin, pp. (107-123), Wiley, New York.

Brewin, C. R., Andrews, B., & Valentine, J. D. (2000). Meta-analysis of risk factors for posttraumatic stress disorder in trauma-exposed adults. *Journal of Consulting and Clinical Psychology*, Vol. 68, No. 5, pp. (748−766), 0022-006X.

Brewin, C.R., Lanius, R.A., Novac, A., Schnyder, U., & Galea, S. (2009). Reformulating PTSD for DSM-V: Life after criterion A. *Journal of Traumatic Stress*, Vol. 22, No. 5, pp. (366-373).

Brewin, C.R., Gregory, J.D., Lipton, M., & Burgess, N. (2010). Intrusive images in psychological disorders: characteristics, neural mechanisms, and treatment implications. *Psychological Review*, Vol. 117, No. 1, pp. (210–32), 0033-295X.

Brunner, J. (2002). Identifications, suspicions, and the history of traumatic disorders. *Harvard Review of Psychiatry*, Vol. 10, No. 3, pp. (179–184), 1067-3229.

Bryant, R.A., & Harvey, A.G. (1995). Avoidant coping style and post-traumatic stress following motor vehicle accidents. *Behaviour Research and Therapy*, Vol. 33, No. 6, pp. (631-635).

Burstein, A. (1985). Posttraumatic Stress Disorder. *Journal of Clinical Psychiatry*, Vol. 46, pp. (300−301).

Butler, L.D. (2007). Growing pains: Commentary on the field of posttraumatic growth and Hobfoll and colleagues' recent contributions to it. *Applied Psychology: An International Review*, Vol. 56, pp. (367-378).

Calhoun, L. G., Cann, A., Tedeschi, R. G., & McMillan, J. (2000). A correlational test of the relationship between posttraumatic growth, religion, and cognitive processing. *Journal of Traumatic Stress*, Vol. 13, No. 3, pp. (521–527), 0894-9867.

Calhoun, L.G., & Tedeschi, R.G. (1999). *Facilitating Posttraumatic Growth: A Clinician's Guide*, Lawrence Erlbaum Associates, Inc., Mahah, NJ

Calhoun, L.G., & Tedeschi, R.G. (2001). Posttraumatic growth: The positive lessons of loss. In: *Meaning Reconstruction and the Experience of Loss*, R.A. Neimeyer, pp. (157-172), American Psychological Association, Washington, DC.

Calhoun, R. G., & Tedeschi, L. G. (2004). The foundations of posttraumatic growth: New considerations. *Psychological Inquiry*, Vol. 15, No. 1, pp. (93–102), 1047-840X.

Cameron, A., Palm, K., & Follette, V. (2010). Reactions to stressful life events: What predicts symptom severity? *Journal of Anxiety Disorders*, Vol. 24, No. 6, pp. (645-649), 0887-6185.

Cann, A., Calhoun, L.G., Tedeschi, R.G., & Solomon, D.T. (2010). Posttraumatic growth and depreciation as independent experiences and predictors of well-being. *Journal of Loss and Trauma*, Vol. 15, No. 3, pp. (151-166), 1081-1443.

Cann, A., Calhoun, L.G., Tedeschi, R.G., Triplett, K.N., Vishnevsky, T., & Lindstrom, C.M. (2011). Assessing posttraumatic cognitive processes: The event related rumination inventory. *Anxiety, Stress, & Coping*, Vol. 24, No. 2, pp. (137-156), 1061-5806

Carkhuff, R.R., & Berenson, B.G. (1977). *Beyond Counseling and Therapy* (2nd ed.), Holt, Rinehart and Winston, 0030898129, New York, NY.

Chan, M.W.C., Ho, S.M.Y., Tedeschi, R.G., & Leung, C.W.L. (2011). The valence of attentional bias and cancer-related rumination in posttraumatic stress and posttraumatic growth among women with breast cancer. *Psycho-Oncology*, Vol. 20, No. 65, pp. (544-552), 1057-9249.

Chatard, A., Pyszczunski, T., Arndt, J., Selimbegovic, L., N'Dri Konan, P., & Van der Linden, M. (2011). Extent of Trauma Exposure and PTSD Symptom Severity as Predictors of Anxiety-Buffer Functioning. *Psychological Trauma: Theory, Research, Practice, and Policy*, Advance online publication.

Clohessy, S., & Ehlers, A. (1999). PTSD symptoms, response to intrusive memories and coping in ambulance service workers. *British Journal of Clinical Psychology*, Vol. 38, No. 3, pp. (251-265).

Cordova, M.J., Cunningham, L.L.C., Carlson, C.R., & Andrykowski, M.A. (2001). Posttraumatic growth following breast cancer: A controlled comparison study. *Health Psychology*, Vol. 20, No. 3, pp. (176-185), 0278-6133.

Cordova, M. J., Giese-Davis, J., Gronen, M., Kronenwetter, C., Chang, V., & Spiegel, D. (2007). Breast cancer as trauma: Posttraumatic stress and posttraumatic growth. *Journal of Clinical Psychology in Medical Settings*, Vol. 14, No. 4, pp. (308–319), 1068-9583.

Creamer, M., Burgess, P., & Patterson, P. (1992). Reaction to trauma: A cognitive processing model. *Journal of Abnormal Psychology*, Vol. 101, No. 3, pp. (452-459), 0021-843X.

Cryder, C. H., Kilmer, R. P., Tedeschi, R. G., & Calhoun, L. G. (2006). An exploratory study of posttraumatic growth in children following a natural disaster. *American Journal of Orthopsychiatry*, Vol. 76, No. 1, pp. (65–69), 0002-9432.

Dancu, C. V., Riggs, D. S., Hearst-Ikeda, D., Shoyer, B. G., & Foa, E. B. (1996). Dissociative experiences and posttraumatic stress disorder among female victims of criminal assault and rape. *Journal of Traumatic Stress*, Vol. 9, No. 2, pp. (253–267), 0894-9867.

Dansky, B.S., Roth, S., & Kronenberger, W.G. (1990). The trauma constellation identification scale: A measure of the psychological impact of a stressful life event. *Journal of Traumatic Stress*, Vol. 3, No. 4, pp. (557-572), 0894-9867.

Dattilio, F.M. (2004). Extramarital affairs: The much-overlooked PTSD. *The Behaviour Therapist*, Vol. 27, No. 4, pp. (76-78).

Davis, C.G., Nolen-Hoeksema, S. & Larson, J. (1998). Making sense of loss and benefiting from the experience: Two construals of meaning. *Journal of Personality and Social Psychology*, Vol. 75, No. 2, pp. (561-574), 0022-3514.

De Vries, G., & Olff, M. (2009). The lifetime prevalence of traumatic events and posttraumatic stress disorder in the Netherlands. *Journal of Traumatic Stress*, Vol. 22, No. 4, pp. (259-267).

Diener, S.J., Flor, H., & Wessa, M. (2010). Learning and consolidation of verbal declarative memory in patients with posttraumatic stress disorder. *Journal of psychology*, Vol. 218, No. 2, pp. (135-140), 0044-3409.

Dohrenwend, B.P., Neria, Y., Turner, J.B., Turse, N., Marshall, R., Lewis-Fernandez, R., & Koenen, K.C. (2004). Positive tertiary appraisals and posttraumatic stress disorder in U.S. male veterans of war in Vietnam: The roles of positive affirmation, positive reformulation, and defensive denial. *Journal of Consulting and Clinical Psychology*, Vol. 72, No. 3, pp. (417-433), 0022-006X.

Ehlers, A., & Clark, D. (2000). A cognitive model of posttraumatic stress disorder. *Behaviour Research and Therapy*, Vol. 38, No. 4, pp. (319–345), 0005-7967.

Ehlers, A., Mayou, R.A., & Bryant, B. (2003). Cognitive predictors of posttraumatic stress disorder in children: Results of a prospective longitudinal study. *Behaviour Research and Therapy*, Vol. 41, No. 1, pp. (1-10), 0005-7967.

El-Hage, W., Gaillard, P., Isingrini, M., & Belzung, C. (2006). Trauma-related deficits in working memory. *Cognitive Neuropsychiatry*, Vol. *11*, 33-46

Elklit, A., & Christiansen, D. M. (2010). ASD and PTSD in rape victims. *Journal of Interpersonal Violence*, Vol. 25, No. 8, pp. (1470-1488).

Feldhaus, K,M., Houry, D., & Kaminsky, R. (2000). Lifetime sexual assault prevalence rates and reporting practices in an emergency department population. *Annals of Emergency Medicine*, Vol. 36, No. 1, pp. (23-27), 0196-0644.

Festinger, L. (1954). A theory of social comparison processes, *Human Relations*, Vol. 7, pp. (117-140).

Finkelhor, D., Hotaling, G., Lewis, I.A., & Smith, C. (1990). Sexual abuse in a national survey of adult men and women: Prevalence, characteristics, and risk factors. *Child Abuse & Neglect*, Vol. 14, No. 1, pp. (19-28).

First, M. B., Frances, A., & Pincus, H. A. (2002). *DSM-IV-TR Guidebook*, American Psychiatric Publishing Inc., Washington, DC.

Foa, E., & Kozak, M.J. (1986). Emotional processing of fear: Exposure to corrective information. *Psychological Bulletin*, Vol. 99, No. 1, pp. (20–35), 0033-2909

Folkman, S. (2008). The case for positive emotions in the stress process. *Anxiety, Stress, & Coping,* Vol. 21, No. 1, pp. (3-14), 1061-5806.

Frazier, P., Conlon, A., & Glaser, T. (2001). Positive and negative life changes following sexual assault. *Journal of Consulting and Clinical Psychology,* Vol. 69, No. 6, pp. (1048–1055), 0022-006X.

Fredrickson, B.L., Tugade, M.M., Waugh, C.E., & Larkin, G.R. (2003). What good are positive emotions in crisis? A prospective study of resilience and emotions following the terrorist attacks on the United States on September 11th, 2001. *Journal of Personality and Social Psychology,* Vol. 84, No. 2, pp. (365-376).

Fresco, D.M, Frankel, A.N, Mennin, D.S, Turk, C.L, Heimberg, R.G. (2002). Distinct and overlapping features of rumination and worry: The relationship of cognitive production to negative affective states. *Cognitive Therapy and Research,* Vol. 26, No. 2, pp. (179–188), 0147-5916.

Fromm, K., Andrykowski, M. A., & Hunt, J. (1996). Positive and negative psychosocial sequelae of bone marrow transplantation: Implications for quality of life assessment. *Journal of Behavioral Medicine,* Vol. 19, No. 3, pp. (221–240).

Garnefski, N., Kraaij, V., & Spinhoven, P. (2001). Negative life events, cognitive emotion regulation and emotional problems. *Personality and Individual Differences,* Vol. 30, No. 8, pp. (1311−1327), 0191-8869.

Gold, S. D., Marx, B. P., Soler-Baillo, J. M., & Sloan, D. M. (2005). Is life stress more traumatic than traumatic stress? *Journal of Anxiety Disorders,* Vol. 19, No. 6, pp. (687–698), 0887-6185.

Gould, K.R., Ponsford, J.L., Johnston, L., & Schonberger, M. (2011). The nature, frequency and course of psychiatric disorders in the first year after traumatic brain injury: A prospective study. *Psychological Medicine,* Vol. 41, pp. (2099-2109), 2099-2109.

Green, B.L. (1994). Psychosocial research in traumatic stress: An update. *Journal of Traumatic Stress,* Vol. 7, No. 3, pp. (341-362).

Green, B.L., Goodman, L.A., Krupnick, J.L., Corcoran, C.B., Petty, R.M., Stockton, P., & Stern, N.M. (2000). Outcomes of single versus multiple trauma exposure in a screening sample. *Journal of Traumatic Stress,* Vol. 13, No. 2, pp. (271-286).

Greenberg, M.A. (1995). Cognitive processing of traumas: The role of intrusive thoughts and reappraisals. *Journal of Applied Social Psychology,* Vol. 25, No. 14, pp. (1262-1296).

Grubaugh, A. L., & Resick, P. R. (2007). Posttraumatic growth in treatment-seeking female assault victims. *Psychiatric Quarterly,* Vol. 78, No. 2, pp. (145–155).

Gunty, A., Frazier, P.A., Tennen, H., Tomich, P., Tashiro, T., & Park, C. (2011). Moderators of the relation between perceived and actual posttraumatic growth. *Psychological Trauma: Theory, Research, Practice, and Policy,* Vol. 3, No. 1, pp. (61-66), 1942-9861.

Hall, B.J., Hobfoll, S.E., Palmieri, P.A., Canetti-Nisim, D., Shapira, O., Johnson, R.J., & Galea, S. (2008). The psychological impact of impending forced settler disengagement in Gaza: Trauma and posttraumatic growth. *Journal of Traumatic Stress,* Vol. 21, No. 1, pp. (22-29), 0894-9867.

Harvey, J., Barnett, K., & Rupe, S. (2006). Posttraumatic growth and other outcomes of major loss in the context of complex family lives. In: *Handbook of Posttraumatic Growth: Research and Practice,* L.G. Calhoun & R.G. Tedeschi, pp. (100-120), Lawrence Erlbaum Associates Inc., 0-8058-5196-8, Mahwah, NJ.

Harvey, A. G., Ehlers, A., & Clark, D. M. (2005). Learning history in social phobia. Behavioural and Cognitive Psychotherapy, 33, 257–271.

Heckhausen, J., Dixon, R. A., & Baltes, T. B. (1989). Gains and losses in development throughout adulthood as perceived by different adult age groups. *Developmental Psychology*, Vol. 25, No. 1, pp. (109-121), 0012-1649.

Helgeson, V.S., Reynolds, K.A., & Tomich, P. L. (2006). A meta-analytic review of benefit finding and growth. *Journal of Consulting and Clinical Psychology*, Vol. *74*, No. *5*, pp. (797-816).

Hendricks, J.E., & Byers, B.D. (2006). Historical and theoretical overview, In: *Crisis Intervention in Criminal Justice/Social Service*, J.E. Hendricks & B.D. Byers, pp. (3-36), Charles C Thomas Publisher, Ltd, Retrieved from <http://books.google.com.au>

Hobfoll, S.E., Hall, B.J., Canetti-Nism, D., Galea, S., Johnson, R.J., & Palmieri, P.A. (2007). Refining our understanding of traumatic growth in the face of terrorism: Moving from meaning cognitions to doing what is meaningful. *Applied Psychology: An International Review*, Vol. *56* No. *3*, pp. (345-366).

Horowitz, M. J. (1986). Stress-response syndromes: A review of posttraumatic and adjustment disorders. *Hospital and Community Psychiatry*, Vol. 37, pp. (241–249).

Howard, G.S. (1994). Why do people say nasty things about self-reports? *Journal of Organizational Behavior*, Vol. 15, No. 5, pp. (399-404).

Hunt, N.C. (2010). *Memory, War and Trauma*. Cambridge University Press, New York, NY.+

Ickovics, J. R., Meade, C.S., Kershaw, T.S., Milan, S., Lewis, J.B., & Ethier, K.A. (2006) Urban teens: Trauma, posttraumatic growth, and emotional distress among female adolescents. *Journal of Consulting and Clinical Psychology*, Vol. *74* No. *5*, pp. (841-850).

Janoff-Bulman, R. (1989). Assumptive worlds and the stress of traumatic events: Applications of the schema construct. *Social Cognition*, Vol. 7, No. 2, pp. (113–136), 0278-016X.

Janoff-Bulman, R. (1992). *Shattered Assumptions: Towards a New Psychology of Trauma*. The Free Press, New York, NY

Joorman, J., Dkane, M., & Gotlib, I.H. (2006). Adaptive and maladaptive components of rumination? Diagnostic specificity and relation to depressive biases. *Behaviour Therapy*, Vol. 37, No. 3, pp. (269-280), 0005-7894.

Joseph, S., & Linley, P.A. (2005). Positive adjustment to threatening events: An organismic valuing theory of growth through adversity. *Review of General Psychology*, Vol. 9, No. 3, pp. (262-280), 1089-2680.

Joseph, S., Williams, R., & Yule, W. (1993). Changes in outlook following disaster: The preliminary development of a measure to assess positive and negative responses. *Journal of Traumatic Stress*, Vol. 6, No. 2, pp. (271-279).

Joseph, S., Dalgleish, T., Thrasher, S., Yule, W., Williams, R., & Hodgkinson, P. (1996). Chronic emotional processing in survivors of the Herald of Free Enterprise disaster: The relationship of intrusion and avoidance at 3 years to distress at 5 years. *Behaviour Research and Therapy*, Vol. 34, No. 4, pp.(357-360).

Joseph, S., Dalgleish, T., Williams, R., Yule, W., Thrasher, S. & Hodgkinson, P. (1997). Attitudes towards emotional expression and post-traumatic stress in survivors of the Herald of Free Enterprise disaster. *British Journal of Clinical Psychology*, Vol. 36, No. 1, pp. (133-138), 0144-6657.

Kessler, R. C., Sonnega, A., Bromet, E., Hughes, M., & Nelson, C. B. (1995). Posttraumatic stress disorder in the National Comorbidity Survey. *Archives of General Psychiatry*, Vol. 52, No. 12, pp. (1048–1060), 0003-990X.

Keyes, C.L., & Ryff, C.D. (2000). Subjective change and mental health: A self-concept theory. *Social Psychology Quarterly*, Vol. 63, No. 3, pp. (264-279).

Kilpatrick, D. G., & Resnick, H. S. (1993). PTSD associated with exposure to criminal victimization in clinical and community populations. In *PTSD in Review: Recent Research and Future Directions*, J. R. T. Davidson & E. B. Foa, (pp. 113-143), American Psychiatric Press, Washington, DC.

Kilpatrick, D. G., Acierno, R., Resnick, H. S., Saunders, B. E. & Best, C. L. (1997). A 2-year longitudinal analysis of the relationships between violent assault and substance use in women. *Journal of Consulting and Clinical Psychology*, Vol. 65, No. 5, pp. (834-847), 0022-006X.

Kilpatrick, D. G., Resnick, H. S., & Acierno, R. E. (2009). Should PTSD Criterion A be retained? *Journal of Traumatic Stress*, Vol. 22, No. 5, pp. (374–383), 0894-9867.

Kilpatrick, D. G., Resnick, H. S., Freedy, J. R., Pelcovitz, D., Resick, P., Roth, S., et al. (1998). Posttraumatic stress disorder field trial: Evaluation of the PTSD construct—Criteria A through E. In: DSM-IV sourcebook, T. A. Widiger, A. J. Frances, H. A. Pincus, R. Ross, M. B. First, W. Davis & M. Kline, Vol. 4, pp. (804–844), American Psychiatric Press, Washington, DC.

Kliem, B. & Ehlers, A. (2009). Evidence for a curvilinear relationship between posttraumatic growth and posttrauma depression and PTSD in assault survivors. *Journal of Traumatic Stress*, Vol. 22, No. 1, pp. (45-52).

Koss, M.P., Gidycz, C.A., & Wisniewski, N. (1987). The scope of rape: Incidence and prevalence of sexual aggression and victimization in a national sample of higher education students. *Journal of Consulting and Clinical Psychology*, Vol. 55, No. 2, pp. (162-170), 0022-006X.

Kross, E., Ayduk, O., & Mischel, W. (2005). When asking "why" does not hurt distinguishing rumination from reflective processing of negative emotions. *Psychological Science*, Vol. 16, No. 9, pp.(709-715)

Krystal, E. (1968). *Massive Psychic Trauma*, International Universities Press, New York, NY.

Kunst, M., Winkel, F.W., & Bogaerts, S. (2010). Prevalence and predictors of posttraumatic stress disorder among victims of violence applying for state compensation. *Journal of Interpersonal Violence*, Vol. 25, No. 9, pp.(1631-1654)

Lasiuk, G. C., & Hegadoren, K. M. (2006). Posttraumatic stress disorder part II: Development of the construct within the North American psychiatric taxonomy. *Perspectives in Psychiatric Care*, Vol. 42, No. 2, pp. (72–81), 0031-5990.

Lazarus, R.S. (1983). Psychological stress and coping in aging. *American Psychologist*, Vol. 38, No. 3, pp.(245-254).

Lechner, S.C., Carver, C.S., Antoni, M.H., Weaver, K.E., & Phillips, K.M. (2006). Curvilinear associations between benefit finding and psychosocial adjustment to breast cancer. *Journal of Consulting and Clinical Psychology*, Vol. 74, No. 5, pp. (828–840), 0022-006X.

Lehman, D.R., Davis, C.G., Delongis, A., Wortman, C.B., Bluck, S., Mandel, D.R., et al. (1993). Positive and negative life changes following bereavement and their relations to adjustment. *Journal of Social and Clinical Psychology*, Vol. 12, No. 1, pp. (90-112), 0736-7236.

Lepore, S. J., Ragan, J. D., & Jones, S. (2000). Talking facilitates cognitive-emotional processes of adaptation to an acute stressor. *Journal of Personality and Social Psychology,* Vol. 78, No. 3, pp. (499-508), 0022-3514.

Levine, J. M., & Moreland, R. L. (1987). Social comparison and outcome evaluation in group contexts. In *Social Comparison, Social Justice, and Relative Deprivation: Theoretical, Empirical, and Policy Perspectives,* J. C. Masters & W. P. Smith, pp. (105-127), Erlbaum, Hillsdale. NJ.

Lev-Wiesel, R., Nuttman-Schwartz, O., & Sternberg, R. (2006). Peer rejection during adolescence: Psychological long-term effects: A brief report. *Journal of Loss and Trauma,* Vol. 11, No. 2, pp. (131–142), 1081-1443.

Lifton, R.J. (1976). The human meaning of total disaster. *Psychiatry,* Vol. 39, No. 1, pp.(1-18).

Lifton, R.J. (1979). *The Broken Connection: On Death and the Continuity of Life.* Simon and Schuster, New York, NY.

Lifton, R.J. (1993). *The Protean Self: Human Resilience in an Age of Fragmentation,*Basic Books, New York, NY.

Lindstrom, C.M., Cann, A., Calhoun, L.G., & Tedeschi, R.G. (2011). The relationship of core belief challenge, rumination, disclosure, and sociocultural elements to posttraumatic growth. *Psychological Trauma: Theory, Research, Practice, and Policy,* Advance online publication.

Linley, P. A., & Joseph, S. (2004). Positive change following trauma and adversity: A review. *Journal of Traumatic Stress,* Vol. 17, No. 1, pp. (11–21), 0894-9867.

Long, M.E., & Elhai, J.D. (2009). Posttraumatic stress disorder's traumatic Stressor Criterion: History, controversy, and clinical and legal implications. *Psychological Injury and Law,* Vol. 2, No. 2, pp. (167-178).

Long, M.E., Elhai, J.D., Schweinle, A., Gray, M.J., Grunbaugh, A.L., & Frueh, N.C. (2008). Differences in posttraumatic stress disorder diagnostic rates and symptom severity between criterion A1 and non-criterion A1 stressors. *Journal of Anxiety Disorders,* Vol. 22, No. 7, pp. (1255-1263), 0887-6185.

Lundh, L. G., & Sperling, M. (2002). Social anxiety and the post-event processing of socially distressing events. *Cognitive Behaviour Therapy,* Vol. 31, pp. (129−134).

Luz, M.P., Medlowicz, M., Marques-Portella, C., Gleiser, S., Berger, W., Neylan, T.C., Coutinho, E.S.F., & Figueira, I. (2011). PTSD criterion A1 events: A literature-based categorisation. *Journal of Traumatic Stress,* Vol. 24, No. 3, pp. (243-251).

Lyubomirsky, S., & Nolen-Hoeksema, S. (1993). Self-perpetuating properties of dysphoric rumination. *Journal of Personality and Social Psychology,* Vol. 65, No. 2, pp. (339–349), 0022-3514.

Lyubomirsky, S., & Nolen-Hoeksema, S. (1995). Effects of self-focused rumination on negative thinking and interpersonal problem-solving. *Journal of Personality and Social Psychology,* Vol. 69, No. 1, pp. (176–190).

Lyubomirsky, S., Tucker, K.L., Caldwell, N.D., & Berg, K. (1999). Why ruminators are poor problem solvers: Clues from the phenomenology of dysphoric rumination. *Journal of Personality and Social Psychology,* Vol. 77, No. 5, pp. (1041-1060).

Maercker, A., & Langner, R. (2001). Personliche reifung durch belastungen und traumata: Ein vergleich zweier fragebogen zur erfassung selbstwahr-genommener reifun nach traumatischen erlebnisse [Stress-related personal growth: A comparison of two German questionnaires for self-assessment of personal growth after traumatic events], *Diagnostica*, Vol. 47, pp.(153-162).

Maercker, A., & Zoellner, T. (2004). The Janus face of self-perceived growth: Towards a two-component model of posttraumatic growth. *Psychological Inquiry*, Vol. 15, No. 1, pp. (41-48), 2044-7200.

Maercker, A., Michael, T., Fehm, L., Becker, E. S., & Margraf, J. (2004). Age of traumatisation as a predictor of post-traumatic stress disorder or major depression in young women. *British Journal of Psychiatry*, Vol. 184, No. 6, pp. (482–487), 0007-1250.

Maguen, S., King, L. A., King, D. W., & Litz, B. T. (2006). Posttraumatic growth among Gulf War I veterans: The predictive role of deployment related experiences and background characteristics. *Journal of Loss & Trauma*, Vol. 11, No. 5, pp. (373–388), 1532-5024.

Maier, T. (2007). Weathers' and Keane's, "The criterion A problem revisited: Controversies and challenges in defining and measuring psychological trauma" [Commentary]. *Journal of Traumatic Stress*, Vol. 20, pp. (925–926).

Manne, S., Ostroff, J., & Winkel, G. (2004). Posttraumatic growth after breast cancer: patient, partner, and couple perspectives. *Psychosomatic Medicine*, Vol. 66, No. 3, pp. (442-454), 0033-3174.

Masters, J. C, & Keil, L. J. (1987). Generic comparison processes in human judgment and behaviour. In: *Social Comparison, Social Justice, and Relative Deprivation: Theoretical, Empirical, and Policy Perspectives*, J. C. Masters & W. P. Smith, pp. (11-54), Lawrence Erlbaum Associates Inc., Hillsdale, NJ.

McFarland, C., & Alvaro, C. (2000). The impact of motivation on temporal comparisons: Coping with traumatic events by perceiving personal growth. *Journal of Personality and Social Psychology*, Vol. 79, No. 3, pp. (327-343).

McFarland, C, Ross, M., & Giltrow, M. (1992). Biased recollections in older adults: The role of implicit theories of aging. *Journal of Personality and Social Psychology*, Vol. 62, No. 5, pp. (837-850), 0022-3514.

McFarland, C., Buehler, R., von Ruti, R., Nguyen, L., & Alvaro, C. (2007). The impact of negative moods on self-enhancing cognitions: The role of reflective versus ruminative mood orientations. *Journal of Personality and Social Psychology*, Vol. 93, No. 5, pp. (728-750).

McHugh, P. R., & Treisman, G. (2007). PTSD: A problematic diagnostic construct. *Journal of Anxiety Disorders*, Vol. 21, No. 2, pp. (211–222), 0887-6185.

McMillen, J. C., & Fisher, R. H. (1998). The Perceived Benefit Scales: Measuring perceived positive life changes after negative events. *Social Work Research*, Vol. 22, No. 3, pp. (173–186), 1070-5309.

McMillen, J. C., Smith, E. M., & Fisher, R. H. (1997). Perceived benefit and mental health after three types of disaster. *Journal of Consulting and Clinical Psychology*, Vol. 65, No. 5, pp. (733–739), 0022-006X.

McNally, R. J. (2003). Progress and controversy in the study of posttraumatic stress disorder. *Annual Review of Psychology*, Vol. 54, No. 1, pp. (229–252), 0066-4308.

Mellings, T. M. B., & Alden, L. E. (2000). Cognitive processes in social anxiety: The effects of self-focus, rumination and anticipatory processing. *Behaviour Research and Therapy*, Vol. 38, No. 3, pp. (243–257), 0005-7967.

Metcalfe, J., & Mischel, W. (1999). A hot/cool-system analysis of delay of gratification: Dynamics of willpower. *Psychological Review*, Vol. 106, No. 1, pp.(3-19).

Michael, T., Halligan, S.L., Clark, D.M., & Ehlers, A. (2007). Rumination in posttraumatic stress disorder. *Depression and Anxiety*, Vol. 24, pp. (307-317)

Milam, J. (2004). Posttraumatic growth among HIV/AIDS patients. *Journal of Applied Social Psychology*, Vol. 34, No. 11, pp. (2353–2376), 00219029.

Mol, S. S. L., Arntz, A., Metsemakers, J. F. M., Dinant, G.-J., Bilters-Van Montfort, P. A. P., & Knottnerus, J. A. (2005). Symptoms of post-traumatic stress disorder after non-traumatic events: Evidence from an open population study. *British Journal of Psychiatry*, Vol. 186, No. 6, pp. (494–499), 1472-1465.

Morrill, E.F., Brewer, N.T., O'Neill, S.C., Lillie, S.E., Dees, E.C., Carey, L.A., & Rimer, B.K. (2008). The interaction of post-traumatic growth and post-traumatic stress symptoms in predicting depressive symptoms and quality of life. *Psycho-Oncology*, Vol. 17, No. 9, pp.(948-953).

Morris, B.A., & Shakespeare-Finch, J. (2011). Rumination, post-traumatic growth, and distress: Structural equation modelling with cancer survivors. *Psycho-Oncology*, Vol. 20, No. 11, 1057-9249, pp. (1176-1183).

Murray, J., Ehlers, A., & Mayou, R.A. 2002. Dissociation and posttraumatic stress disorder: Two prospective studies of motor vehicle accident survivors. *British Journal of Psychiatry*, Vol. 180, No. 4, pp. (363–368), 007-1250.

Neufiend, J., Dritschel, B., Astell, A., & MacLeod, M.D. (2009). The effects of thought suppression on autobiographical memory recall. *Behaviour Research and Therapy*, Vol. 47, No. 4, pp. (275-284).

Nolen-Hoeksema, S. (1991). Responses to depression and their effects on the duration of depressive episodes. *Journal of Abnormal Psychology*, Vol. 100, No. 4, pp. (569–582), 0021-843X.

Nolen-Hoeksema, S., & Davis, C. G. (2004). Theoretical and methodological issues in the assessment and interpretation of posttraumatic growth. *Psychological Inquiry*, Vol. 15, No. 1, pp. (60–64), 1047-840X.

Nolen-Hoeksema, S., & Morrow, J. (1991). A prospective study of depression and distress following a natural disaster: The 1989 Loma Prieta earthquake. *Journal of Personality and Social Psychology*, Vol. 61, No. 1, pp. (115-121).

Nolen-Hoeksema, S., & Morrow, J. (1993). Effects of rumination and distraction on naturally-occurring depressed mood. *Cognition & Emotion*, Vol. 7, No. 6, pp. (561–570).

O'Brien, L. S. (1998). *Traumatic Events and Mental Health*, Cambridge University Press, New York, NY.

O'Donnell, M.L., Creamer, M., McFarlane, A.C., Silove, D., & Bryant, R.A. (2010). Should A2 be a diagnostic requirement for posttraumatic stress disorder in DSM-V? *Psychiatry Research*, Vol. 176, No. 2-3, pp.(257-260).

Oakley Brown, M.A., Wells, J.E., Scott, & K.M., McGee, M.A. (2006). Lifetime prevalence and projected lifetime risk of DSM0IV disorder in Te Rau Hinengaro: The New Zealand Mental Health Survey. *Australian and New Zealand Journal of Psychiatry*, Vol. 40, pp. (865-874).

Olde, E., van der Hart, O., Kleber, R., & van Son, M. (2006). Posttraumatic stress following childbirth: A review. *Clinical Psychology Review*, Vol. 26, No. 1, pp. (1–16), 0272-7358.

Palmieri, P. A., & Fitzgerald, L. F. (2005). Confirmatory factor analysis of posttraumatic stress symptoms in sexually harassed women. *Journal of Traumatic Stress*, Vol. 18, No. 6, pp. (657–666), 0894-9867.

Papageorgiou, C., & Wells, A. (2003). An empirical test of a clinical metacognitive model of rumination and depression. *Cognitive Therapy and Research*, Vol. 27, No. 3, pp. (261–273), 0147-5916.

Parad, L.G. (1971). Short-term treatment: An overview of historical trends, issues, and potentials. *Smith College Studies in Social Work*, Vol. 41, No. 2, pp. (119-146), 0037-7317.

Park, C.L. (1999). The roles of meaning and growth in the recovery from posttraumatic stress disorder. In: *Posttraumatic Stress Disorder: A Lifespan Developmental Perspective*, A. Maercker, M. Schutzwohl, & Z. Solomon, pp. (249-264), Hegrefe & Huber, Seattle, WA.

Park, C. L., & Fenster, J. R. (2004). Stress-related growth: Predictors of occurrence and correlates with psychological adjustment. *Journal of Social and Clinical Psychology*, Vol. 23, No. 2, pp. (195–215), 0736-7236.

Park, C. L., & Lechner, S. (2006). Measurement issues in assessing growth following stressful life experiences. In: *Handbook of Posttraumatic Growth: Research and Practice*, L. G. Calhoun & R. G. Tedeschi, pp. (47–67), Lawrence Erlbaum Associates Inc., 0-8058-5196-8, Mahwah, NJ.

Park, C.L., Cohen, L., & Murch, R. (1996). Assessment and prediction of stress-related growth. *Journal of Personality*, Vol. 64, No. 3, pp. (71-105), 0002-9432.

Park, C. L., Aldwin, C. M., Fenster, J. R., & Snyder, L. B. (2008). Pathways to posttraumatic growth versus posttraumatic stress: Coping and emotional reactions following the September 11, 2001, terrorist attacks. *American Journal of Orthopsychiatry*, Vol. 78, No. 3, pp. (300–312), 0002-9432.

Patterson, D. R., Carrigan, L., Robinson, R., & Questad, K. A. (1990). Posttraumatic stress disorder in hospitalized patients with burn injuries. *Journal of Burn Care and Rehabilitation*, Vol. 11, No. 3, pp. (181-184).

Pennebaker, J.W., Barger, S.D., & Tiebout, J. (1989). Disclosure of traumas and health among Holocaust survivors. *Psychosomatic Medicine*, Vol. 51, No. 5, pp. (577-589), 0033-3174.

Pietrzak, R.H., Goldstein, M.B., Malley, J.C., Rivers, A.J., Johnson, D.C., Morgan, C.A.,& Southwick, S.M. (2010). Posttraumatic growth in veterans of operations Enduring Freedom and Iraqi Freedom. *Journal of Affective Disorders*, Vol. 126, No. 1-2, pp. (230-235), 0165-0327.

Pitman, R.K. (1989). Post-traumatic stress disorder, hormones, and memory. *Biological Psychiatry*, Vol. 26, No. 3, pp. (221-223).

Powell, S., Rosner, R., Butollo, W., Tedeschi, R., & Calhoun, L.G. (2003). Posttraumatic growth after war: A study with former refugees and displaced people in Sarajevo. *Journal of Clinical Psychology*, Vol. 59, No. 1, pp. (71-83).

Putnam, F.W. (1997). *Dissociation in Children and Adolescents: A Developmental Perspective*, The Guilford Press, 1572302194, New York.

Rachman, S. (1980). Emotional processing. *Behaviour Research and Therapy*, Vol. 18, No. 1, pp. (51–60).

Ransom, S., Sheldon, K.M., & Jacobsen, P.B. (2008). Actual change and inaccurate recall contribute to posttraumatic growth following radiotherapy. *Journal of Consulting and Clinical Psychology*, Vol. 76, No. 5, pp. (811-819).

Revenson, T.A., Wollman, C.A., & Felton, B.J. (1983). Social supports as stress buffers for adult cancer patients. *Psychosomatic Medicine*, Vol. 45, No. 4, pp.(321-331).

Robinson, M. S., & Alloy, L. B. (2003). Negative cognitive styles and stress-reactive rumination interact to predict depression: A prospective study. *Cognitive Therapy and Research* Negative cognitive styles and stress-reactive rumination interact to predict depression: A prospective study, Vo. 27, No. 3, pp. (275–291), 0147-5916.

Rothbaum, B.O., & Davis, M. (2006). Applying learning principles to the treatment of post-trauma reactions. *Annals of the New York Academy of Sciences*, Vol. 1008, No., 1, pp. (112-121).

Rubonis, A.V., & Bickman, L. (1991). Psychological impairment in the wake of disaster: The disaster-psychopathology relationship. *Psychological Bulletin*, Vol. 109, No. 3, pp. (384-399), 0033-2909.

Ryff, C. (1982). Self-perceived personality change in adulthood and aging. *Journal of Personality and Social Psychology*, Vol. 42, No. 1, pp. (108-115), 0022-3514.

Salminen, E., Heikkila, S., Poussa, T., Lagstrom, H., Saario, R., & Salminen, S. (2002). Female patients tend to alter their diet following the diagnosis of rheumatoid arthritis and breast cancer. *Preventative Medicine*, Vol. 34, No. 5, pp. (529–535), 0091-7435.

Salsman, J.M., Segerstrom, S.C., Brechting, E.H., Carlson, C.R., & Andrykowski, M.A. (2009). Posttraumatic growth and PTSD symptomatology among colorectal cancer survivors: A 3-month longitudinal examination of cognitive processing. *Psycho-Oncology*, Vol. 18, No. 1, pp.(30-41).

Schnurr, P. P., Spiro, A., Vielhauer, M. J., Findler, M. N., & Hamblen, J. L. (2002). Trauma in the lives of older men: Findings from the Normative Aging Study. *Journal of Clinical Geropsychology*, Vol. 8, No. 3, pp. (175–187).

Scott, M. J., & Stradling, S. G. (1994). Posttraumatic stress disorder without the trauma. *British Journal of Clinical Psychology*, Vol. 33, pp. (71–74).

Sergestorm, S., & Alden, L. (2000). Worry and rumination: Repetitive thought as a concomitant and predictor of negative mood. *Cognitive Therapy and Research*, Vol. 24, No. 6, pp. (671-688), 0147-5916.

Shalev, A. Y. (1992). Posttraumatic stress disorder among injured survivors of a terrorist attack. *The Journal of Nervous and Mental Disease*, Vol. 180, No. 8, pp. (505-509), 0022-3018.

Shedler, J., Mayman, M., & Manis, M. (1993). The illusion of mental health. *American Psychologist*, Vol. 48, No. 1, pp. (1117–1131), 0003-066X.

Shipherd, J.C., & Beck, J.G. (2005). The role of thought suppression in posttraumatic stress disorder. *Behavior Therapy*, Vol. 36, No. 3, pp. (277-287).

Siegle, G.J., Moore, P.M., & Thase, M.E. (2004). Rumination: One construct, many features in healthy individuals, depressed individuals, and individuals with lupus. *Cognitive Therapy and Research*, Vol. 28, No. 5, pp. (645-668).

Simms, L. J., Watson, D., & Doebbeling, B. N. (2002). Confirmatory factor analysis of posttraumatic stress symptoms in deployed and nondeployed veterans of the Gulf War. *Journal of Abnormal Psychology*, Vol. 111, No. 4, pp. (637-647), 0021-843X.

Snape, M.C. (1997) Reactions to a traumatic event: The good, the bad and the ugly? *Psychology, Health and Medicine*, Vol. 2, No. 3, pp. (237-242), 1354-8506.

So-kum Tang, C. (2007). Posttraumatic growth of southeast Asian survivors with physical injuries: Six months after the 2004 outheast Asian earthquake-tsunami. *The Australasian Journal of Disaster and Trauma Studies*, Vol. 1, Retrieved from <http://www.massey.ac.nz/~trauma/issues/2007-1/tang.htm>

Solomon, S. D., & Canino, G. J. (1990). Appropriateness of DSM-III-R criteria for posttraumatic stress disorder. *Comprehensive Psychiatry*, Vol. 31, No. 3, pp. (227-237).

Solomon, Z., Mikulincer, M., & Avitzur, E. (1988). Coping, locus of control, social support and combat-related posttraumatic stress disorder: A prospective study. *Journal of Personlaity and Social Psychology*, Vol. 55, No. 2, pp. (279-285), 0022-3514.

Spector, P.E. (1994). Using self-report questionnaires in OB research: A comment on the use of a controversial method. *Journal of Organizational Behavior*, Vol. 15, No. 5, pp. (385-392).

Spitzer, R.L., First, M.B., & Wakefield, J.C. (2007). Saving PTSD from itself in DSM-V. *Journal of Anxiety Disorders*, Vol. 21, No. 2, pp. (233-241), 0887-6185.

Spitzer, C., Abraham, G., Reschke, F.M., Siebel, U., & Freyberger, H.J. (2000). Posttraumatic stress disorder following high- and low-magnitude stressors in psychotherapeutic inpatients. *Clinical Psychology and Psychotherapy*, Vol. 7, No. 5, pp. (379–384), 1063-3995.

Stanton, A.L., Bower, J.E., & Low, C.A. (2006). (2006). Posttraumatic growth after cancer. In: *Handbook of posttraumatic growth: Research and practice*, L. G. Calhoun & R.G. Tedeschi, pp. (138-175), Lawrence Erlbaum Associates Inc., 0-8058-5196-8, Mahwah, NJ.

Steil, R., & Ehlers, A. (2000). Dysfunctional meaning of posttraumatic intrusions in chronic PTSD. *Behaviour Research and Therapy*, Vol. 38, No. 6, pp. (537-558).

Stockton, H., Hunt, N., & Joseph, S. (2011). Cognitive processing, rumination, and posttraumatic growth. *Journal of Traumatic Stress*, Vol. 24, No. 1, pp. (85-92).

Strack, F., Schwarz, N., & Gschneidinger, E. (1985). Happiness and reminiscing: The role of time perspective, affect, and mode of thinking. *Journal of Personality and Social Psychology*, Vol. 49, No. 6, pp. (1460-1469), 0022-3514.

Suls, J., & Miller, R. L. (Eds.). (1977). *Social Comparison Processes: Theoretical and Empirical Perspectives.* Hemisphere, 0898-3038, Washington, DC.

Suls, J., & Mullen, B. (1982). From the cradle to the grave: Comparison of self-evaluation across the life span. In: *Psychological Perspectives on the Self*, Vol. 2, J.M. Suls & A. G. Greenwald, pp. (97-125), Erlbaum, Hillsdale, NJ.

Suls, J., & Mullen, B. (1984). Social and temporal bases of self-evaluation in the elderly: Theory and evidence. *International Journal of Aging and Human Development*, Vol. 18, No. 2, pp. (111-120).

Suls, J., & Wills, T. A. (1991). *Social Comparison: Contemporary Theory and Research*, Erlbaum, Hillsdale, NJ.

Suls, J., Marco, C. A., & Tobin, S. (1991). The role of temporal comparison, social comparison, and direct appraisal in the elderly's self evaluations of health. *Journal of Applied Social Psychology*, Vol. 21, No. 14, pp. (1125- 1144).

Taku, K., Calhoun, L.G., Cann, A., & Tedeschi, R.G. (2008). The role of rumination in the coexistence of distress and posttraumatic growth among bereaved Japanese university students. *Death Studies*, Vol. 32, No. 5, pp. (428-444).

Taku, K., Cann, A., Tedeschi, R.G., & Calhoun, L.G. (2009). Intrusive versus deliberate rumination in posttraumatic growth across US and Japanese samples. *Anxiety, Stress, & Coping*, Vol. 22, No. 2, pp. (129-136), 1061-5806.

Taylor, S.E. (1983). Adjustment to threatening events: A theory of cognitive adaptation. *American Psychologist*, Vol. 38, No. 11, pp. (1161-1173), 0003-006X.

Taylor, S. E., & Armor, D. A. (1996). Positive illusions and coping with adversity. *Journal of Personality*, Vol. 64, No. 4, pp. (873−898), 0022-3506.

Taylor, S.E., & Brown, J.D. (1988). Illusion and well-being: A social psychological perspective on mental health. *Psychological Bulletin*, Vol. 103, No. 2, pp. (193-210), 0033-2909.

Taylor, S.E., Lichtman, R.R., &Wood, J.V. (1984). Attributions, beliefs about control, and adjustment to breast cancer. *Journal of Personality and Social Psychology*, Vol. 46, No. 3, pp. (489-502).

Taylor, S.E., Kemeny, M.E., Reed, G.M., Bower, J.E., & Gruenewald, T.L. (2000). Psychological resources, positive illusions, and health. *American Psychologist*, Vol. 55, No. 1, pp. (99-109).

Teasdale, J.D. (1999). Emotional processing, three modes of mind and the prevention of relapse in depression. *Behaviour, Research and Therapy*, Vol. 37, pp. (53–77).

Tedeschi, R.G., & Calhoun, L.G. (1995). *Trauma and Transformation: Growing in the Aftermath of Suffering*, Sage, Thousand Oaks, CA.

Tedeschi, R.G., & Calhoun, L.G. (1996). The posttraumatic growth inventory: Measuring the positive legacy of trauma. *Journal of Traumatic Stress*, Vol. 9, No. 3, pp. (455-471), 089-9867.

Tedeschi, R. G., & Calhoun, L. G. (2004). Posttraumatic growth: Conceptual foundations and empirical evidence. *Psychological Inquiry*, Vol. 15, No. 1, pp.(1–18), 1047-840X.

Tedeschi, R.G., & Calhoun, L.G. (2006). Time of change? The spiritual challenges of bereavement and loss. *Journal of Death and Dying*, Vol. 53, No. 1-2, pp. (105-116).

Tedeschi, R.G. & Kilmer, R.P. (2005). Assessing strengths, resilience, and growth to guide clinical interventions. *Professional Psychology: Research and Practice*, Vol. 36, No. 3, pp. (230-237).

Tedeschi, R.G., Calhoun, L.G. & Cann, A. (2007). Evaluating resource gain: Understanding and misunderstanding posttraumatic growth. *Applied Psychology*, Vol. 56, No. 3, pp. (396-406), 0259-994X.

Thompson, S. C. (1985). Finding positive meaning in a stressful event and coping. *Basic and Applied Social Psychology*, Vol. 6, No. 4, pp. (279–295), 0197-3533.

Tomich, P.L., & Helgeson, V.S. (2002). Five years later: A cross-sectional comparison of breast cancer survivors with healthy women. *Psycho-Oncology*, Vol. 11, No. 2, pp. (154-169).

Tomich, P. L., & Helgeson, V. S. (2004). Is finding something good in the bad always good? Benefit finding among women with breast cancer. *Health Psychology*, Vol. 23, No. 1, pp. (16–23), 0278-6133.

Trapnell, P. D., & Campbell, J. D. (1999). Private self-consciousness and the five-factor model of personality: Distinguishing rumination from reflection. *Journal of Personality and Social Psychology*, Vol. 76, No. 2, pp. (284–304), 0022-3514.

Treynor, W., Gonzalez, R., & Nolen-Hoeksema, S. (2003). Rumination reconsidered: A psychometric Analysis. *Cognitive Therapy and Research*, Vol. 27, No. 3, pp. (247-259), 0147-5916.

Valentiner, D.P., Foa, E.B., Riggs, D.S., & Gershuny, B.S. (1996). Coping strategies and posttraumatic stress disorder in female victims of sexual and nonsexual assault. *Journal of Abnormal Psychology*, Vol. 105, No. 3, pp. (455-458).

Van der Kolk, B. A. (1996). History of trauma in psychiatry. In: *Traumatic Stress: The Effects of Overwhelming Experience on Mind, Body, and Society*, B. A.Van der Kolk, A. C. McFarlane & L. Weisæth, pp. (47–74), Guilford, New York, NY.

Van der Kolk, B., McFarlane, A.C., & Weisaeth, L. (1996). *Traumatic Stress*. Guilford Publications, New York, NY.

Van Oyen Witvliet, C., Knoll, R.W., Hinman, N.G., & DeYoung, P.A. (2010). Compassion-focused reappraisal, benefit-focused reappraisal, and rumination after an interpersonal offense: Emotion-regulation implications for subjective emotion, linguistic responses, and physiology. *The Journal of Positive Psychology*, Vol. 5, No. 3, pp. (226-242).

Veroff, J. (1969). Social comparison and the development of achievement motivation. In: *Achievement-Related Motives in Children*, C. P. Smith, pp. (46-101), Sage, . New York, NY.

Vrana, S., & Lauterbach, D. (2001). The relationship among personality variables, exposure to traumatic events, and severity of posttraumatic stress symptoms. *Journal of Traumatic Stress*, Vol. 14, No. 1, pp. (29–45), 0894-9867.

Watkins, E. (2004). Adaptive and maladaptive ruminative self-focus during emotional processing. *Behaviour Research and Therapy*, Vol. 42, No. 9, pp. (1037–1052), 0005-7967.

Watkins, E.R. (2008). Constructive and unconstructive repetitive thought. *Psychological Bulletin*, Vol. 134, No. 2, pp. (163-206).

Watkins, E.R. & Baracaia, S. (2002). Rumination and social problem-solving in depression. *Behaviour Research and Therapy*, Vol. 40, No. 10, pp. (1179–1189), 0005-7967.

Watson, D. (2005). Rethinking the mood and anxiety disorders: A quantitative hierarchical model for DSM-V. *Journal of Abnormal Psychology*, Vol. 114, No. 4, pp. (522–536), 0021-843X.

Weathers, F.W., & Keane, T.M. (2007). The criterion A problem revisited: Controversies and challenges in defining and measuring psychological trauma. *Journal of Traumatic Stress*, Vol. 20, No. 2, pp. (107-121).

Weiss, D. S. (2004). The impact of event scale—revised. In: *Assessing Psychological Trauma and PTSD Second Edition*, J. P. Wilson & T. M. Keane, pp. (168–189), Guilford Press, New York, NY.

Weiss, T. (2002). Posttraumatic growth in women with breast cancer and their husbands: An intersubjective validation study. *Journal of Psychosocial Oncology*, Vol. 20, No. 2, pp. (65-80), 0734-7332.

Wild, N.D. & Paivio, S.C. (2003). Psychological adjustment, coping, and emotion regulation as predictors of posttraumatic growth. *Journal of Aggression, Maltreatment, & Trauma*, Vol. 8, No. 4, pp. (97-122).

Wilson, J.P., Friedman, M.J., & Lindy, J.D. (2001). *Treating Psychological Trauma and PTSD*. The Guilford Press, New York, NY.

Wood, J. V. (1989). Theory and research concerning social comparisons of personal attributes. *Psychological Bulletin*, Vol. 106, No. 2, pp. (231-248), 0033-2909.

World Health Organization. (1992). *The ICD-10 Classification of Mental and Behavioural Disorders*, Author, Geneva, Switzerland.

Wortman, C. B. (2004). Posttraumatic growth: Progress and problems. *Psychological Inquiry*, Vol. 15, No. 1, pp. (81−90).

Zisook, S., Chentsova-Dutton, Y., & Shuchter, S. R. (1998). PTSD following bereavement. *Annals of Clinical Psychiatry*, Vol. 10, No. 4, pp. (157−163), 1040-1237.

Zoellner, T., & Maercker, A. (2006). Posttraumatic growth in clinical psychology: A critical review and introduction of a two component model. *Clinical Psychology Review*, Vol. 26, No. 5, pp. (626–653), 0272-7358.

Zoellner, T., Rabe, S., Karl, A. & Maercker, A. (2008). Posttraumatic growth in accident survivors: Openness and optimism as predictors of its constructive or illusory sides. *Journal of Clinical Psychology*, Vol. 64, No. 3, pp. (245-263).

9

Depression in Women Experiencing Intimate Partner Violence

J.Y.H. Wong, D.Y.T. Fong and A. Tiwari
School of Nursing, Li Ka Shing Faculty of Medicine
The University of Hong Kong
Hong Kong S.A.R.,
China

1. Introduction

Intimate partner violence (IPV) is a well recognized public health issue. According to the U.S. Centers for Disease Control and Prevention, IPV is defined as:

"physical and/or sexual violence, or threats of such violence, or psychological/ emotional abuse including coercive tactics; between persons who are current or former spouses, marital or non-marital partners, same or opposite sex partners and boyfriend/girlfriends or dating partners. They may be co-habiting, but need not be." (Saltzman, 1999)

In the past two decades, there has been a rapid increase in the awareness of IPV and the incidents of IPV reported in different countries. In 2002, the issue was raised at the international level by the World Health Organization (WHO) in its first report on health and violence against women (Krug, 2002). According to the report, the lifetime prevalence of physical assaults by intimate partners against women was between 10 and 69 percent among 48 population-based surveys worldwide (Krug, 2002).

IPV is known to be strongly associated with depression (Golding, 1999), which is often found in abused women staying with abusive partners. Also, depression has persistently been found in abused women after they have separated from abusive partners (Anderson, Saunders, Yoshihama, Bybee, & Sullivan, 2003; Amy E. Bonomi et al., 2009; J. C. Campbell, 2002; J. C. Campbell, Kub, & Rose, 1996; Dienemann et al., 2000; Hegarty, Gunn, Chondros, & Small, 2004; O'Campo et al., 2006). In a meta-analysis of 18 studies, the pooled prevalence of depression among abused women was 47.6 percent, which is much higher than the lifetime rate of 18.6 percent in the general population (Golding, 1999). Also, as shown in a 2009 study, the relative risk of depression in abused women is three times higher than that of non-abused women (Amy E. Bonomi, et al., 2009).

Depression has been predicted to be the leading cause of disability and the second leading contributor to the global burden of disease by the year of 2020 (Pollock, Manaseki-Holland, & Patel, 2006). Also, numerous studies have revealed that depression is associated with higher rates of physical and mental illness, such as headaches, back pain, sexually transmitted diseases, appetite loss, digestive problems, and gynaecological problems (Amy E. Bonomi, et al., 2009; J. Campbell et al., 2002), chronic pain (Humphreys, Cooper, &

Miaskowski, 2010; Wuest et al., 2008), loss of consciousness, diminished cognitive abilities, memorization and concentration problems (Valera & Berenbaum, 2003), greater functional disability and higher healthcare resource utilization (D. S. Brown, Finkelstein, & Mercy, 2008; Jones et al., 2006; Ulrich et al., 2003). There is, therefore, an urgent need to address this common and persistent adverse consequence of IPV.

2. Organization

In this chapter, we aim to enhance the understanding of depression in abused women. It includes the following sections:

a. An examination of the definition of depression and how it is different from depressive symptoms.
b. An introduction to the different ways of measuring depression and depressive symptoms according to current knowledge.
c. An illustration of the possible etiology of depression in women, in particular, related to IPV given that there are a variety of causes of depression.
d. Finally, an identification of the risk factors that have contributed to depressive symptoms in women experiencing IPV based on empirical evidence from literature. Both consistent and inconsistent findings are discussed.

3. Depression versus depressive symptoms

Most, if not all, individuals occasionally feel emotionally sad or blue. These symptoms may develop into a medical illness or disorder, termed as depression in psychopathology. According to the *Diagnostic and Statistical Manual IV* (DSM IV) (Association, 2000), depression consists of a major depressive episode that must include at least five out of nine symptoms for two weeks or more. The nine depressive symptoms are:

a. depressed mood
b. significant reduced level of interest in most activities
c. loss or gain weight
d. insomnia
e. agitated or slowed down behaviour
f. guilt
g. inability to concentrate
h. feeling fatigue
i. thoughts of death

The symptoms should be intense, prolonged and interfere with the person's daily functioning. This distinct definition can clearly differentiate depression from unhappiness and sadness. An individual may possess depressive symptoms but may not necessarily have depression if there are fewer than five depressive symptoms or the symptoms are not intense, prolonged or interfere with daily functioning.

Unfortunately, many abused women suffer from depression without being diagnosed or receiving any treatment. They simply are not willing or are not aware of the need to seek medical advice (WHO, 1990).

4. Diagnosis and assessment of depression

The medical diagnosis of depression is conventionally conducted using the Structural Clinical Interview (SCID), which is a clinical assessment administered by a licensed clinician or clinical psychologist. In order to allow researchers and clinicians to assess for mental disorders, WHO (1990) developed the first Composite International Diagnostic Interview (CIDI), which is a structured interview designed to assess for mental disorders according to the International Classification of Disease (ICD) and DSM-IV that can be administered by trained lay interviewers. The CIDI is now widely used in research and clinical practice to diagnose depression.

Although SCID and CIDI are gold standard tools used to diagnose depression, their administration requires professional or trained personnel which can be costly and time consuming. Therefore, self-report questionnaires have been developed to assess depressive symptoms without the need for trained personnel. A valid and reliable depression questionnaire can facilitate the self-assessment of depression. This allows not only individuals to assess their level of depression on their own but also clinicians to identify individuals with potential depression problems in a busy clinical setting. It also facilitates assessment of depression in research studies, especially in large-scale epidemiologic studies where self-report measurement tools are very functional.

Self-report assessment tools for depression require rigorous evaluation of their psychometric performance before they are used in practice. An evaluation often includes the checking of reliability, validity, sensitivity and responsiveness (Fong, in press). There are depression assessment tools with evidence supporting satisfactory psychometric performance in measuring depression for clinical settings (Maercker, Michael, Fehm, Becker, & Margraf, 2004; Pokorski & Siwiec, 2006; Rohde et al., 2008). The common tools are described in the next section.

5. Common self-report measurements of depression

Beck Depression Inventory

The Beck Depression Inventory (BDI) was developed in 1961 by A.T. Beck, a remarkable scholar in the study of depression (Maraste, Brandt, Olsson, & Ryde-Brandt, 1992). He defined depression as the self-conception of worthless, outer world meaninglessness, and future hopelessness (Beck, 1971). These self-concepts are what can be observed in a person experiencing depression because of an irreversible loss or disappointment which is very significant in their life (Beck, 1971; G. W. Brown, & Harris, T.O., 1978). In 1996, the BDI was revised as BDI-II to reflect changes in the DSM-IV. The BDI-II is a 21-item questionnaire addressing the severity of depressive symptoms in the past week. The symptoms include:

a. sadness
b. pessimism
c. past failure
d. loss of pleasure
e. guilt feelings
f. punishment feelings
g. self-dislike

h. self-criticalness
i. suicidal thoughts
j. crying
k. agitation
l. loss of interest
m. indecisiveness
n. worthlessness
o. loss of energy
p. changes in sleeping patterns
q. irritability
r. changes in appetites
s. difficulty in concentrating
t. tiredness
u. loss of interest in sex

Each item scores in the range 0 (symptom not presents) to 3 (symptom strongly presents), giving a total score from 0 to 63. The higher the total score, the more severe the depression is. It can be further categorized to define the level of depression. An individual is considered to be at a minimal depression level when their total score is between 0 and 13, mildly depressed with a score between 14 and 19, moderately depressed with a total score between 20 and 28, and severely depressed with a total score between 29 and 63.

Center for Epidemiologic Studies of Depression Scale

The Center for Epidemiologic Studies of Depression Scale (CES-D) is a questionnaire that comprises 20 items covering the most common depressive symptoms in the general population (Newcomb & Carmona, 2004). The items were selected based on previously validated depression scales. It includes the components of

a. depressed mood
b. feelings of worthlessness
c. feelings of helplessness and hopelessness
d. loss of appetite
e. sleep disturbance

Similar to the BDI, the recall period is also one week. However, CES-D does not include some of the items the BDI does, including feelings of guilt, psychomotor retardation and suicidal thoughts. Each CES-D item is rated on a 4-point Likert scale, ranging from 0 (rarely or none of the time) to 3 (most all of the time). The plausible range of score is 0 to 60, with higher scores indicating higher depression severity. A CES-D score ≥ 16 indicates the presence of depression but no further categorization by severity is available. The CES-D has been widely used in all age groups and in both health care and community settings. It has been developed and translated into many different languages and is free for non-profit use.

Patient Health Questionnaire

The Patient Health Questionnaire (PHQ-9) is a multi-purpose questionnaire for both diagnosing and measuring the severity of depression. It incorporates the DSM-IV depression diagnostic criteria (Rohde, et al., 2008). It consists of 9 items, covering nine depressive symptoms. They are:

a. depressed mood
b. significant reduced level of interest in most activities
c. loss of appetite
d. insomnia
e. agitated or slowed down behaviour
f. guilt
g. poor concentration
h. feeling fatigue
i. thoughts of death

For each item, both the frequency of the symptoms experienced, and how difficult the problem makes the person's life are rated on a 4-point Likert scale ranging from 0 (not at all) to 3 (nearly every day) . The scoring system allows the classification of depression severity where 1 - 4 = minimal depression, 5 - 9 = mild depression, 10 - 14 = moderate depression, 15 - 19 = moderately severe depression and 20 - 27 = severe depression.

Although the PHQ-9 is a short questionnaire, there is a briefer version, named PHQ-2 (Eisenman et al., 2009), which consists of only two case-finding questions:

1. "During the past month, have you often been bothered by feeling down, depressed, or hopeless?"
2. "During the past month, have you often been bothered by little interest or pleasure in doing things?"

The PHQ-2 is a very useful and feasible measure for screening depression in community and primary care settings.

6. Etiology of depression in abused women

Lenore Walker (1984) was among the first to explore the etiology of depression in IPV victims. She developed what she termed a Cycle of Abuse to describe the behavioural pattern of abusers and the responses of abused women to the violence (A. E. Bonomi, Anderson, Cannon, Slesnick, & Rodriguez, 2009). Figure 1 shows the three phases in Walker's Cycle of Abuse:

a. Tension building phase: In this phase interpersonal tension builds up between the abuser and the abused woman. The abuser may become increasingly jealous and short tempered. The abuser's anger is always irrational. However, the abused woman usually uses placating coping strategies to avoid triggering the abuser's outburst.
b. Acting out phase: This phase is characterized by violent incidents. The abused woman is in a very dangerous situation as she may be injured or even killed by the abuser. In this phase, the abused woman is often too frightened to seek help.
c. Honeymoon phase: Following a violent incident, the abuser becomes apologetic. He promises that it will not happen again and becomes loving, caring and affectionate. As the abuser's behaviours are usually convincing, the abused woman is often very eager to forgive him and believes that the abuser will change. This phase is often short lived and the interpersonal tension starts to build again and even involves mildly violent behaviours. The cycle continues.

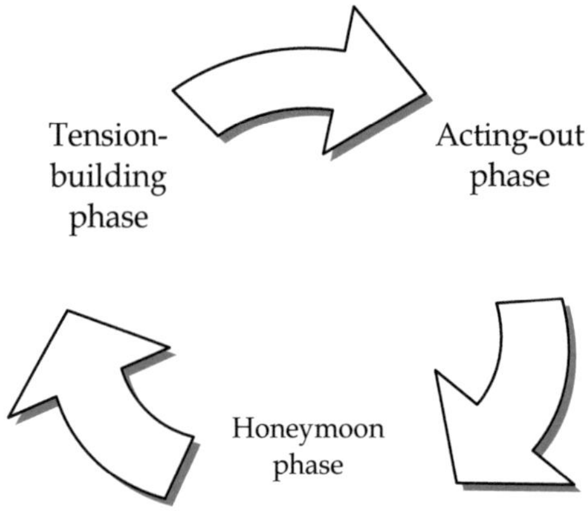

Fig. 1. *Cycle of Abuse.*

Under the Cycle of Abuse, woman may develop Battered Women Syndrome, a term also introduced by Lenore Walker (Walker, 1979). Battered Women Syndrome explains why abused women are often reluctant to leave abusive relationships where they experience physical and psychological suffering. Battered Women Syndrome is a subcategory of posttraumatic stress disorder (PTSD), which comprises symptoms of:

a. re-experiencing the battering even though it is not re-occurring,
b. avoiding the psychological impact of abuse by avoiding personal emotions, family and friends, and social activities,
c. hyperarousal or hypervigilance,
d. disrupted interpersonal relationships,
e. body image distortion or other somatic problems, and
f. sexuality and intimacy issues.

All these symptoms may become manifest after a traumatic experience. They can be very distressing and lead to depression. In the book, Social Origin of Depression, a strong causal link between stressful life events and depression was found, especially when a stressful event was severe or threatening events were of remarkably long duration (G. W. Brown, & Harris, T.O., 1978); an example of which would be IPV.

Battered Women Syndrome was developed after Martin Seligmen's (1975) classical Learned Helplessness Theory, which describes the phenomenon where a person has learned to behave helplessly even though there is an opportunity to escape from an unpleasant situation. However, this does not imply abused women are helpless at all. Rather, abused women may choose to stay in abusive relationships but give up the belief that they are able to escape from their abusers because of chronic suffering. As a result, they develop sophisticated coping strategies to minimize their physical and psychological suffering. Unfortunately, the more pessimistic they become, the less likely they will be able to escape from the relationship; and even worse, the more likely it is they will develop a sense of guilt and self-blame leading to depression. Depression can pull abused women down, and normally, they will try to get rid of the painful feelings. However, as long as the cyclical pattern of abuse persists, abused women will feel increasingly discouraged and may eventually feel there is nothing that they can do.

There is no unique cause of depression in abused women. In fact, the causes may vary largely across different women. Public health approaches, instead of understanding the causes of depression in individuals, may understand what factors tend to affect some groups of individuals more than others. Risk group identification is essential for addressing public health problems because actions can be taken to alleviate IPV and ameliorate its adverse impact on women's mental health. Risk factors associated with depression in abused women are discussed in the next section and are listed in Table 1.

7. Risk factors associated with depression in abused women

a. **Young age**. Studies have demonstrated that younger abused women are more likely to report depression (Hazen, Connelly, Soriano, & Landsverk, 2008; Wrangle, Fisher, & Paranjape, 2008). This is consistent with other epidemiology studies conducted in women with no history of abuse (Scarinci et al., 2002). However, in most of the studies conducted on abused women, the mean age of participants was between 30 and 50 years. In some other studies that investigated the relationship between depression and age in participants covering full adulthood, a U-shaped relationship was found (Kasen, Cohen, Chen, & Castille, 2003; Mirowsky & Ross, 1992). In other words, levels of depression decreased with age among young and middle-aged adults but increased among older adults.

b. **Low socioeconomic status**. Socioeconomic status is associated with depression. Economic deprivation due to low income or unemployment has been shown to be one of the most significant risk factors for depression in abused women (J. C. Campbell, Kub, Belknap, & Templin, 1997; Deyessa et al., 2009; Hazen, et al., 2008; Mburia-Mwalili, Clements-Nolle, Lee, Shadley, & Yang, 2010) because it limits abused women's access to community resources and medical care, thus making them much more vulnerable and economically dependent on their abusers. Economic dependency amongst women of low socio-economic status reduces their ability to leave their abusers, which may cause feelings of hopelessness resulting in the development of depression.

   Education attainment is another socioeconomic factor associated with depression. Numerous studies have reported that lower education is a risk factor for depression in abused women (Carlson, McNutt, Choi, & Rose, 2002; Mburia-Mwalili, et al., 2010; Newcomb & Carmona, 2004; Wong, Tiwari, Fong, Humphreys, & Bullock, 2011; Wrangle, et al., 2008). Women with lower educational attainment may have fewer chances of employment or acquiring sufficient resources to free themselves from economic deprivation and/or abusive relationships. It also appears that poorly educated women may have less knowledge about IPV and have less information about ways to protect themselves from it. These result in abused women perceiving that they are unable to control abusive situations and may result in depression.

c. **History of child abuse**. A number of studies have found that child abuse underpins adult depression in abused women (J. C. Campbell, et al., 1997; Koopman et al., 2007; Rohde, et al., 2008; Shan A, 1995; Widom, DuMont, & Czaja, 2007). In particular, severe forms of child sexual abuse with penetration or attempted penetration is strongly association with adult depression (Cheasty, Clare, & Collins, 1998). Child abuse and neglect acts are traumatic past experiences that may make abused women much more sensitized to the stress response from current abuse and lead them down the path of depression. In addition, fear, increased arousal and low self-esteem developed over the years since the trauma may also contribute to depression in adulthood. At the same time, the child abuse experience may be linked to PTSD which follows the women into adulthood (Pederson et al., 2004), leading again to depression. Recently, there has been emerging evidence of an interaction in the genome of abused child that relates to adult depression (Bradley et al., 2008; Nikulina, Widom, & Brzustowicz, 2011). This new finding improves our understanding of why some children with a history of abuse develop depression in adulthood while others do not.

d. **Abuse experience**. Although there is a strong link between depression and IPV, evidence on the relative influence of the different types of IPV as risk factors for depression has been inconclusive. Some studies suggest that physical or sexual abuse is a stronger predictor of depression (Ali, Israr, Ali, & Janjua, 2009; J. C. Campbell, et al., 1997), while others suggest that psychological abuse is a stronger predictor of depression in abused women (Follingstad, 2007; Pico-Alfonso et al., 2006; Wong, et al., 2011). Hazen and her colleagues (2008) also examined the impact of different types of psychological abuse on the mental health of abused women. They found that dominance-isolation was significantly associated with depression in abused women but emotional-verbal abuse was not.

   Nevertheless, caution should be taken when examining the findings of these studies in terms of their methods of assessing the frequency and severity of IPV. In our previous study (Wong, et al., 2011), we found that different types of abuse made no significant difference to depression in abused women. However, once the frequency of abuse was considered, the findings revealed that psychological abuse was significantly associated with depression but not physical or sexual abuse. A consistent finding of other studies has been that the longer abuse endures in an abusive relationship the more it is significantly associated with depression (Lindhorst & Beadnell, 2011; Rodriguez et al., 2008).

e. **Little or no social support**. There is much evidence that abused women are particularly vulnerable to depression if they lack social support (J. C. Campbell, et al., 1997; Mburia-Mwalili, et al., 2010; Rodriguez, et al., 2008; Wong, et al., 2011). Social support includes various forms of support including tangible resources, a support network and perceived support, which are extremely important as they act as buffers, especially after a person has experienced a stressful life event (Cohen & Hoberman, 1983). In some cases, perceived support is much more important than tangible support for abused women. When a woman suffers an abusive experience, she may consider that the threat and fear begin with her perceived ability to cope with the abuse; therefore, perceived availability of support will have an important buffering effect for women coping with abuse. Hence, social support always serves as a protective factor against depression in abused women. Moreover, some abusers use social isolation to control and assault women, which makes it more difficult for abused women to reach out for help from others. Without social support, abused women will be psychologically entrapped in abusive relationships and thus prone to developing depression.

f. **Coping styles.** Coping has a direct influence on psychological adaptation to stress in women who experience abuse. Thus, coping is also strongly associated with depression. There have been no conclusions reached in the current literature as to which coping styles are most prominently associated with the development of depression in abused women. From a historical perspective, active coping styles are always adaptive and problem-focused while passive coping styles are always maladaptive and avoiding. A study conducted to investigate the relationship among IPV, depression and coping styles (Haden & Scarpa, 2008) found that an avoidant coping style is a risk factor for depression in abused women. However, an inconsistent result was found in a study conducted in Japan (Yoshihama, 2002) where passive coping styles were perceived as more effective and resulted in less psychological distress for abused Japanese women. Conversely, more active coping strategies adopted by Japanese abused women, resulted in less reduction is their psychological distress. Therefore, evidence shows that effective coping styles may be culture dependent. In other words, strategies adopted by abused women may be culturally consistent and may not necessary lead to maladaptive coping.

Risk Factors for depression in abused women:
• Young age • Low socioeconomic status (low education, low income and unemployment) • History of child abuse • Abuse experience (type, frequency and severity) • Lack of social support • Coping styles

Table 1. Risk factors for depression in abused women.

8. Conclusion

No woman expects that she will be hurt by a loved one. Depression, being one of the most prevalent mental health problems, is strongly associated with IPV. Some abused women have been found to be more vulnerable to developing depression than others; therefore, it is important to understand the risk factors associated with depression in abused women. It is expected that these findings may encourage health professionals to identify groups of women at high risk of developing depression, and devise appropriate and effective measures or behavioural interventions to help abused women reduce their depression.

9. References

Ali, F. A., Israr, S. M., Ali, B. S., & Janjua, N. Z. (2009). Association of various reproductive rights, domestic violence and marital rape with depression among Pakistani women. *BMC Psychiatry, 9*, 77.

Anderson, D. K., Saunders, D. G., Yoshihama, M., Bybee, D. I., & Sullivan, C. M. (2003). Long-term Trends in Depression among Women Separated from Abusive Partners. *Violence Against Women, 9*(7), 807-838.

Association, A. P. (2000). *Diagnostic and statistical manual of mental disorders : DSM-IV-TR* (4th ed., text revision. ed.). Washington, D.C.: American Psychiatric Association.

Beck, A. T. (1971). Cognition, affect and psychopathology. *Archives of General Psychiatry, 1*, 495-500.

Bonomi, A. E., Anderson, M. L., Cannon, E. A., Slesnick, N., & Rodriguez, M. A. (2009). Intimate partner violence in Latina and non-Latina women. *Am J Prev Med, 36*(1), 43-48.

Bonomi, A. E., Anderson, M. L., Reid, R. J., Rivara, F. P., Carrell, D., & Thompson, R. S. (2009). Medical and Psychosocial Diagnoses in Women With a History of Intimate Partner Violence. *Arch Intern Med, 169*(18), 1692-1697.

Bradley, R. G., Binder, E. B., Epstein, M. P., Tang, Y., Nair, H. P., Liu, W., . . . Ressler, K. J. (2008). Influence of child abuse on adult depression: moderation by the corticotropin-releasing hormone receptor gene. *Arch Gen Psychiatry, 65*(2), 190-200.

Brown, D. S., Finkelstein, E. A., & Mercy, J. A. (2008). Methods for estimating medical expenditures attributable to intimate partner violence. *J Interpers Violence, 23*(12), 1747-1766.

Brown, G. W., & Harris, T.O. (1978). *Social Origins of Depression: A Study of Psychiatric Disorder in Women*. London: Tavistock Publications.

Campbell, J., Jones, A., Dienemann, J., Kub, J., Schollenberger, J., O' Campo, P., . . . Wynne, C. (2002). Intimate partner violence and physical health consequences. *Arch Intern Med, 162*, 1157-1163.

Campbell, J. C. (2002). Health consequences of intimate partner violence. *Lancet, 359*(9314), 1331-1336.

Campbell, J. C., Kub, J., Belknap, R. A., & Templin, T. N. (1997). Predictors of Depression in Battered Women. *Violence Against Women, 3*(3), 271-293.

Campbell, J. C., Kub, J. E., & Rose, L. (1996). Depression in battered women. *J Am Med Womens Assoc, 51*(3), 106-110.

Carlson, B. E., McNutt, L.-A., Choi, D. Y., & Rose, I. M. (2002). Intimate Partner Abuse and Mental Health: The Role of Social Support and Other Protective Factors. *Violence Against Women, 8*(6), 720.

Cheasty, M., Clare, A. W., & Collins, C. (1998). Relation between sexual abuse in childhood and adult depression: case-control study. *BMJ, 316*(7126), 198-201.

Cohen, S., & Hoberman, H. M. (1983). Positive Events and Social Supports as Buffers of Life Change Stress. *Journal of Applied Social Psychology, 13*(2), 99-125.

Deyessa, N., Berhane, Y., Alem, A., Ellsberg, M., Emmelin, M., Hogberg, U., & Kullgren, G. (2009). Intimate partner violence and depression among women in rural Ethiopia: a cross-sectional study. *Clin Pract Epidemol Ment Health, 5*, 8.

Dienemann, J., Boyle, E., Baker, D., Resnick, W., Wiederhorn, N., & Campbell, J. (2000). Intimate partner abuse among women diagnosed with depression. *Issues Ment Health Nurs, 21*(5), 499-513.

Eisenman, D. P., Richardson, E., Sumner, L. A., Ahmed, S. R., Liu, H., Valentine, J., & Rodriguez, M. (2009). Intimate partner violence and community service needs among pregnant and postpartum Latina women. *Violence Vict, 24*(1), 111-121.

Follingstad, D. R. (2007). Rethinking current approaches to psychological abuse: Conceptual and methodological issues. *Aggression and Violent Behavior, 12*(4), 439-458.

Fong, D. Y. T. (Ed.). (in press). Research Instruments for Domestic Violence Studies in Hong Kong. Hong Kong: HKU Press.

Golding, J. M. (1999). Intimate Partner Violence as a Risk Factor for Mental Disorders: A Meta-Analysis. *Journal of Family Violence, 14*(2), 99-132.

Haden, S. C., & Scarpa, A. (2008). Community violence victimization and depressed mood: the moderating effects of coping and social support. *J Interpers Violence, 23*(9), 1213-1234.

Hazen, A. L., Connelly, C. D., Soriano, F. I., & Landsverk, J. A. (2008). Intimate partner violence and psychological functioning in Latina women. *Health Care Women Int, 29*(3), 282-299.

Hegarty, K., Gunn, J., Chondros, P., & Small, R. (2004). Association between depression and abuse by partners of women attending general practice: descriptive, cross sectional survey. *BMJ, 328*(7440), 621-624.

Humphreys, J., Cooper, B. A., & Miaskowski, C. (2010). Differences in depression, posttraumatic stress disorder, and lifetime trauma exposure in formerly abused women with mild versus moderate to severe chronic pain. *J Interpers Violence, 25*(12), 2316-2338.

Jones, A. S., Dienemann, J., Schollenberger, J., Kub, J., O'Campo, P., Gielen, A. C., & Campbell, J. C. (2006). Long-term costs of intimate partner violence in a sample of female HMO enrollees. *Womens Health Issues, 16*(5), 252-261.

Kasen, S., Cohen, P., Chen, H., & Castille, D. (2003). Depression in adult women: age changes and cohort effects. *Am J Public Health, 93*(12), 2061-2066.

Koopman, C., Ismailji, T., Palesh, O., Gore-Felton, C., Narayanan, A., Saltzman, K. M., . . . McGarvey, E. L. (2007). Relationships of depression to child and adult abuse and bodily pain among women who have experienced intimate partner violence. *J Interpers Violence, 22*(4), 438-455.

Krug, E., Dahlberg, I., Mercy, J., Zwi, A., & Rafael, L. (2002). World Report on Violence and Health (W. H. Organization, Trans.). Geneva.

Lindhorst, T., & Beadnell, B. (2011). The long arc of recovery: characterizing intimate partner violence and its psychosocial effects across 17 years. *Violence Against Women, 17*(4), 480-499.

Maercker, A., Michael, T., Fehm, L., Becker, E. S., & Margraf, J. (2004). Age of traumatisation as a predictor of post-traumatic stress disorder or major depression in young women. *Br J Psychiatry, 184*, 482-487.

Maraste, R., Brandt, L., Olsson, H., & Ryde-Brandt, B. (1992). Anxiety and depression in breast cancer patients at start of adjuvant radiotherapy. Relations to age and type of surgery. *Acta Oncol, 31*(6), 641-643.

Mburia-Mwalili, A., Clements-Nolle, K., Lee, W., Shadley, M., & Yang, W. (2010). Intimate Partner Violence and Depression in a Population-Based Sample of Women: Can Social Support Help? *J Interpers Violence, 25*(12), 2258-2278.

Mirowsky, J., & Ross, C. E. (1992). Age and depression. *J Health Soc Behav, 33*(3), 187-205.

Newcomb, M. D., & Carmona, J. V. (2004). Adult trauma and HIV status among Latinas: effects upon psychological adjustment and substance use. *AIDS Behav, 8*(4), 417-428.

Nikulina, V., Widom, C. S., & Brzustowicz, L. M. (2011). Child Abuse and Neglect, MAOA, and Mental Health Outcomes: A Prospective Examination. *Biol Psychiatry*, article in press.

O'Campo, P., Kub, J., Woods, A., Garza, M., Jones, S., Gielen, A. C., . . . Campbell, J. (2006). Depression, PTSD, and Comorbidity Related to Intimate Partner Violence in Civilian and Military Women. *Brief Treatment and Crisis Intervention, 6*(2), 99-110.

Pederson, C. L., Maurer, S. H., Kaminski, P. L., Zander, K. A., Peters, C. M., Stokes-Crowe, L. A., & Osborn, R. E. (2004). Hippocampal volume and memory performance in a community-based sample of women with posttraumatic stress disorder secondary to child abuse. *Journal of Traumatic Stress, 17*(1), 37-40.

Pico-Alfonso, M. A., Garcia-Linares, M. I., Celda-Navarro, N., Blasco-Ros, C., Echeburua, E., & Martinez, M. (2006). The impact of physical, psychological, and sexual intimate male partner violence on women's mental health: depressive symptoms, posttraumatic stress disorder, state anxiety, and suicide. *J Womens Health (Larchmt), 15*(5), 599-611.

Pokorski, M., & Siwiec, P. (2006). Memory, depression, and progressing old age in women. *J Physiol Pharmacol, 57 Suppl 4*, 297-304.

Pollock, J. I., Manaseki-Holland, S., & Patel, V. (2006). Detection of depression in women of child-bearing age in non-Western cultures: a comparison of the Edinburgh Postnatal Depression Scale and the Self-Reporting Questionnaire-20 in Mongolia. *J Affect Disord, 92*(2-3), 267-271.

Rodriguez, M. A., Heilemann, M. V., Fielder, E., Ang, A., Nevarez, F., & Mangione, C. M. (2008). Intimate partner violence, depression, and PTSD among pregnant Latina women. *Ann Fam Med, 6*(1), 44-52.

Rohde, P., Ichikawa, L., Simon, G. E., Ludman, E. J., Linde, J. A., Jeffery, R. W., & Operskalski, B. H. (2008). Associations of child sexual and physical abuse with obesity and depression in middle-aged women. *Child Abuse Negl, 32*(9), 878-887.

Saltzman, L. E., Franslow, J. L., McMahon, P. M., & Shelley, G. A. (1999). Intimate partner violence surveillance: uniform definitions and recommended data elements, version 1.0 *National Center for Injury Prevention and Control, Centers for Disease Control and Prevention*. Atlanta, GA.

Scarinci, I. C., Beech, B. M., Naumann, W., Kovach, K. W., Pugh, L., & Fapohunda, B. (2002). Depression, socioeconomic status, age, and marital status in black women: a national study. *Ethn Dis, 12*(3), 421-428.

Shan A, J. (1995). A meta-analysis of the relationship of child sexual abuse to adult psychological adjustment. *Child Abuse & Neglect, 19*(6), 715-728.

Ulrich, Y. C., Cain, K. C., Sugg, N. K., Rivara, F. P., Rubanowice, D. M., & Thompson, R. S. (2003). Medical care utilization patterns in women with diagnosed domestic violence. *American Journal Of Preventive Medicine, 24*(1), 9-15.

Valera, E. M., & Berenbaum, H. (2003). Brain injury in battered women. *J Consult Clin Psychol, 71*(4), 797-804.

Walker, L. E. (1979). *The battered woman*. New York: Harper and Row

Walker, L. E. (1984). Battered women, psychology, and public policy. *Am Psychol, 39*(10), 1178-1182.

WHO. (1990). *Composite International Diagnostic Interview*. Geneva, Switzerland: World Health Organization.

Widom, C. S., DuMont, K., & Czaja, S. J. (2007). A prospective investigation of major depressive disorder and comorbidity in abused and neglected children grown up. *Arch Gen Psychiatry, 64*(1), 49-56.

Wong, J. Y. H., Tiwari, A., Fong, D. Y. T., Humphreys, J., & Bullock, L. (2011). Depression Among Women Experiencing Intimate Partner Violence in a Chinese Community. *Nursing Research, 60*(1), 58-65

Wrangle, J., Fisher, J. W., & Paranjape, A. (2008). Ha sentido sola? Culturally competent screening for intimate partner violence in Latina women. *J Womens Health (Larchmt), 17*(2), 261-268.

Wuest, J., Merritt-Gray, M., Ford-Gilboe, M., Lent, B., Varcoe, C., & Campbell, J. C. (2008). Chronic pain in women survivors of intimate partner violence. *J Pain, 9*(11), 1049-1057.

Yoshihama, M. (2002). Battered Women's Coping Strategies and Psychological Distress: Differences by Immigration Status. *American Journal of Community Psychology, 30*(3), 429-452.

10

Adolescent Cigarette Use in the Americas: The Link with Depression

Cristina B. Bares[1], Jorge Delva[2], Marya Hynes[3] and Ninive Sanchez[2]
[1]*School of Social Work, Virginia Commonwealth University, Richmond, VA*
[2]*School of Social Work, University of Michigan, Ann Arbor, MI*
[3]*Inter-American Drug Abuse Control Commission (CICAD), Secretariat for Multidimensional Security, Organization of American States, Washington, D.C.*
USA

1. Introduction

While society's understanding of the burden of disease associated with substance use and mental health disorders continues to grow, serious gaps remain in our ability to help all individuals with these disorders. It has been estimated that the use of tobacco and alcohol each represent 8.7% and 3.8% of all deaths worldwide. In addition, the Disability-Adjusted Life Years (DALYs) caused by alcohol, tobacco and illicit drug use are estimated to be 4.4%, 3.7% and 0.9%, respectively (WHO, 2009). Unfortunately, these gaps are likely to be substantially larger among racial and ethnic minorities and culturally diverse populations.

The purpose of this chapter is to describe the extent of comorbidity between depressive symptoms and tobacco use among adolescents in North, Central and South America. We accomplish this purpose via a thorough literature review of the subject and by empirically exploring the association between depressive symptoms and cigarette use among adolescents using data from several studies conducted in the Americas. These studies are (1) the National Survey of Drug Use and Health (NSDUH), a national household representative study of drug use and mental health in the United States; (2) the National Longitudinal Survey of Youth (NLSY), a longitudinal study of youth and their families also conducted in the United States; (3), data from several national studies of drug use conducted by various Latin American countries carried out in collaboration with the Organization of American States - Inter-American Drug Abuse Control Commission; and (4) the Santiago Longitudinal study (SLS), a longitudinal study of substance use among adolescents and their families underway in Santiago, Chile. We conclude the Chapter with a discussion of implications for prevention and treatment by reviewing the corresponding literature.

1.1 Depressive disorders and symptoms in the Americas

Data from the United States suggest that about 11% of the adolescent population experiences a depressive disorder in their lifetime (Merikangas et al., 2010). The lifetime prevalence of depression among adolescents in Canada is estimated to be around 7% (Cheung & Dewa, 2006). In Mexico City, the prevalence rate of major depression among 12-

to 17-year-old adolescents has been estimated to be approximately 7.6% (Benjet et al., 2009). Because we were not able to identify studies of mental health disorders in Latin American countries that used nationally representative samples to obtain country-wide estimates, we provide a brief review of findings from studies using adult populations. Overall, studies with adult populations in Latin America have found that depressive disorders account for approximately 7% of the disease burden in the region (WHO, 2003). Studies have estimated the prevalence rate of Major Depressive Disorder to be around 30% among the adult population seeking health care services in Emergency Departments in various countries in Latin America (Castilla-Puentes et al., 2008). Using the World Mental Health Composite International Diagnostic Interview in various countries in the Americas, the 12-month prevalence rate of mood disorders among adults, including major depression, ranges from 4.8% in Mexico, to 10% in Colombia, and 18.2% in the United States (WHO, 2004).

Data on depressive symptoms among adolescent populations are available for a few Latin American geographic areas and cities. For example, using a representative sample of adolescents residing in the Brazilian San Gonzalo municipal area, the second most populous area of the state of Rio de Janeiro, Avanci and colleagues (Avanci, Assis, & Oliveira, 2008) assessed depressive symptoms using the Self-Rating Questionnaire for Depression (SRQ-20) scale (Harding et al., 1980). The results suggested that 10% of this group exhibited depressive symptoms (Avanci, Assis, & Oliveira, 2008). In another study of Brazilian youth, one of children and adolescents attending public schools in the municipality of Ribeirão Preto, and using the Child Depression Inventory, it was found that 6.4% of the 5,000 6- to 18-year-olds exhibited depressive symptoms (Golfeto, D'Oliveira, Baptista, & Bisson, 2011). In addition, Camacho and colleagues (2009) carried out a school-based survey in the Colombian providence of Santander and found that the prevalence of major depressive disorder using the Spanish translation of the Center for Epidemiological Studies Depression Scale (CES-D) among adolescents was 11.5% (Camacho et al., 2009). Furthermore, the prevalence of depressive episodes among 12- to 17-year-old adolescents representing three urban cities in Peru was estimated to be 5.7% (Vargas et al., 2010) using the Mini International Neuropsychiatric Interview (Sheehan et al., 1998). Finally, among a representative sample of Chilean adolescents residing in the capital, Santiago, the prevalence rate of depressive symptoms was estimated to be 6.9% (Florenzano et al., 2009).

The results of the aforementioned studies provide varying rates of depressive symptoms among adolescents in Latin America. However, none of these studies used samples that allow for generalizations to the general population of adolescents in their respective countries, let alone the entire region. In fact, these studies have used samples representative of specific geographical regions or cities within individual countries. Further, each of the studies mentioned above have used different assessment tools when measuring depressive symptoms and depressive disorders. Thus, the varying estimates of depressive symptoms might be partly due to differences in how the assessment tools assess depression, rather than reflect true country-based differences in depressive symptoms. Our literature review indicates that there are currently no national representative studies of depressive symptoms or depressive disorders among adolescents in Latin America.

1.2 Cigarette use among adolescents in the Americas

Data from the Monitoring the Future study, an ongoing yearly survey of drug use among school-attending adolescents in the United States, suggests that in 2010 7.1% of 8th-graders,

13.6% of 10th-graders, and 19.2% of 12th-graders in the United States had used cigarettes in the past 30 days (Johnston, O'Malley, Bachman, & Schulenberg, 2011). To further illustrate the extent of cigarette use among adolescents in the United States, we used publicly available data from the 2004-2009 NSDUH to obtain estimates of past-month cigarette use among adolescent males and females (see Table 1). The NSDUH, conducted by the U.S. Substance Abuse and Mental Health Services Administration, samples the civilian, noninstitutionalized population of the United States (including civilians living on military bases) 12 years of age or older (SAMHSA, 2009). The NSDUH is an annual nationwide survey that interviews about 70,000 randomly selected individuals aged 12 to 64 years. Only participants 12 to 17 years old were selected for the analyses conducted for the purpose of this Chapter. The survey has been carried out annually since 1991 but for the purpose of this Chapter we used data from 2004-2009. We restricted the data to these years because later in the Chapter we present data on depression among adolescents 12-17 years old using the NSDUH. The NSDUH included questions on adolescent depression only for the 2004-2009 years (see Table 3 later in the Chapter).

As shown in Table 1, the percent of adolescent males and females who have smoked a cigarette in the past month has shown a slight decrease since 2004. Perhaps more interesting, the percents of male and female recent smokers are fairly similar. This could suggest that the male risk factor for cigarette use is no longer applicable (Brook et al., 2008), or, that adolescent females are taking similar risks and engaging in similar risky behaviors as adolescent males. In fact, the same risk factors (such as lower parental education, living in a one parent family) for being a daily smoker have been identified to have an effect on both female and male adolescents (Voorhees, Schreiber, Schumann, Biro, & Crawford, 2002). Despite the sharing of risk factors, certain risk factors appear to more specifically influence adolescent females. Higher drive for thinness and higher stress levels during the transition to puberty are two such factors (Voorhees et al., 2002).

Gender	2004	2005	2006	2007	2008	2009
Total adolescent sample	18,294	18,678	18,314	17,727	17,842	17,705
Males	11.2	10.5	10.1	10.2	8.7	9.2
Females	12.5	11.1	11.1	9.7	9.0	8.6

Table 1. Percent of adolescents 12-17 years old who consumed cigarettes in the past month, by gender and year, in the United States: National Survey of Drug Use and Health (NSDUH) 2004-2009.

In Latin America, trend data are more limited but, as shown in Table 2, we find that there is considerable variety in the proportion of 12- to 17-year-olds in the region who have smoked cigarettes in the previous 30 days. Using data from the Organization of American States Inter-American Drug Abuse Control Commission indicate that Chile, Uruguay, and Argentina show the highest prevalence of past-month cigarette use across a range of years. In the most recent year for which data are available for Chile (2009), 35.6% of adolescent females and 30.6% of adolescent males smoked cigarettes in the past month. In Uruguay, data from the same year indicate that 21.1% of adolescent females and 15.5% of adolescent males have used cigarettes the past month. Data from 2007 for Argentina indicate that 22%

of adolescent females and 21.6% of adolescent males have smoked cigarettes in the previous 30 days. The countries that exhibit the lowest rates of previous 30 day smoking by adolescents are the Bahamas, Panama and Venezuela.

Country	2004		2005		2006		2007		2008		2009	
	M	F	M	F	M	F	M	F	M	F	M	F
Argentina			21.0	21.3			21.6	22.1				
Antigua			2.7	1.1			20.2	19.4				
Bahamas									1.6	1.6		
Barbados					3.6	3.2						
Bolivia	22.7	11.0							18.9	8.4		
Chile			38.4	44.3			32.7	37.9			30.6	35.6
Colombia	27.7	18.6										
Costa Rica					10.0	7.2					9.5	7.7
Ecuador			29.6	13.8								
El Salvador									13.2	5.9		
Honduras			12.89	5.91								
Panama									6.0	3.8		
Paraguay			17.7	12.3								
Peru			21.5	12.4			13.6	7.4				
Uruguay			21.1	29.5			19.9	24.3			15.5	21.1
Venezuela			5.2	2.8							2.8	6.6

Table 2. Percent of adolescents 12-17 years old who consumed cigarettes in the past month by year in Latin American countries.

1.3 Comorbidity of depression and cigarettes use: Etiological considerations

A variety of studies have suggested a relationship between cigarette smoking and depressive disorders and depressive symptoms. Although the exact mechanisms responsible for this relationship remain uncovered (Audrain-McGovern, Rodriguez, Cuevas, & Rodgers, 2009), the association between cigarette smoking and depressive disorders can be explained in several ways. First, depressive disorders may lead to cigarette use (Nezami et al., 2005; Wu & Anthony, 1999). Using data from the National Longitudinal Study of Adolescent Health, Munafò and colleagues (2008) found that among individuals who had never smoked at baseline, increases in depressive symptoms lead to smoking initiation but not to becoming regular smokers (Munafò, Hitsman, Rende, Metcalfe, & Niaura, 2008). Some have suggested that mood disorders may lead individuals to smoke due to their need to alleviate distressing symptoms they may be experiencing (Khantzian, 1997). The self-medication hypothesis, proposed by Khantzian (1985), states that individuals choose to use certain substances because they offer the individual alleviation from painful emotional states. The proposed pathway through which the self-medication hypothesis is thought to work involves individuals having low self-efficacy in the control of their own emotional states, which in turn, create a vulnerability for depressive symptoms that then is controlled through the use of tobacco (Minnix, Blalock, Marani, Prokhorov, & Cinciripini, 2011). Another suspected pathway, one that may particularly apply to females, suggests that adolescent females' expectations that smoking will reduce their negative affect may help explain the relationship between depression and cigarette use (Morrell, Cohen, & McChargue, 2010). Furthermore, others have suggested that depression increases adolescents' risk of smoking by increasing their susceptibility to peer pressure from peers who smoke (Patton et al., 1998).

Second, cigarette smoking might lead to depressive disorders. Empirical investigations in the United States have shown that higher levels of depression are observed among adolescents who are current smokers, compared to levels of depression among adolescents who have never smoked and those who are former smokers (Martini, Wagner, & Anthony, 2002), but the exact mechanisms for this association have yet to be uncovered. For example, using longitudinal data from the United States National Longitudinal Study of Adolescent Health, Steuber and Danner (2006) found that current smokers were more likely to experience depressive symptoms, even after controlling for prior level of depression (Munafò et al., 2008; Steuber & Danner, 2006). For the past two decades, a considerable amount of empirical attention has been devoted to understanding the genetic factors associated with cigarette smoking. The result of such attention has been the uncovering of specific genes that may predispose individuals to experiencing a reward upon consuming nicotine (Barrueco, Alonso, & Gonzalez-Sarmiento, 2005; Gerra et al., 2005; Lerman et al., 1999). Nicotine itself has been found to have an influence on the neurotransmitter systems that are involved in the development of depression (Morisano, Bacher, Audrain-McGovern, & George, 2009). It has been hypothesized that neurochemical changes in the brain caused by depression, specifically in the cholinergic system (Dagyte, Den Boer, & Trentani, 2011), may create a vulnerability to seek the rewarding effects of smoking (Lerman et al., 1998). Of particular importance to this chapter is the research on genetic predisposition to smoking among adolescents who experience depression (Audrain-McGovern, Lerman, Wileyto, Rodriguez, & Shields, 2004). This research suggests that 11-th grade adolescent smokers with an DRD2 A1 allele are particularly susceptible to depressive symptoms. The interactions between depressive symptoms and the genetic predisposition may lead to a progression towards smoking.

A third explanation suggests that shared risk factors are involved in the etiology of both problems. Several studies from various countries have provided evidence that depressive disorders and cigarette use share similar, if not the same, environmental and genetic precursors (Fergusson, Boden, & Horwood, 2011; Hu, Davies, & Kandel, 2006; Kendler et al., 1993; Mykletun, Overland, Aaro, Liabo, & Stewart, 2008; Rohde, Lewinsohn, Brown, Gau, & Kahler, 2003). Using longitudinal data from New Zealand, Boden and colleagues (2003) found that even after controlling for environmental (e.g., experienced stressful life events, unemployment, and affiliation with deviant peers, among others) and genetic risk factors associated with cigarette use (e.g., nicotinic achetylcholine receptors CHRNA5, CHRNA3 and CHRNB4 (Chen et al., 2009)) and depressive symptoms (SLC6A15 (Kohli et al., 2011)) there remained a significant association between these two variables (Boden, Fergusson, & Horwood, 2010; Fergusson, Goodwin, & Horwood, 2003). Certainly more research is needed to understand the mechanisms responsible for the association between cigarette use and depressive symptoms (Munafò & Araya, 2010).

Regardless of the initiating factor, it has also been hypothesized that a reciprocal relationship exists between cigarette use and depressive symptoms whereby a feedback loop is likely to occur once smoking or depression symptoms manifest themselves (Breslau, Peterson, Schultz, Chilcoat, & Andreski, 1998). For instance, it has been found that individuals who use nicotine are at an increased risk for developing depression because of the effect that nicotine has on the acetylcholine and catecholamine systems (Pomerleau & Pomerleau, 1984), which themselves have been implicated in the onset of depression (Carmody, Vieten, & Astin, 2007).

1.3.1 Studies of cigarette use and depression with North and Latin American populations

1.3.1.1 North America

Studies using national representative samples of adolescents in the United States have found that those who report greater depression symptoms are at greater risk for smoking initiation (Moon, Mo, & Basham, 2010). Similarly, data from adolescents in California suggest that those who report greater depression during 6th grade are at greater risk for smoking initiation two years later (Weiss, Mouttapa, Cen, Johnson, & Unger, 2011). Further, higher levels of depressive symptoms at age 14 have been associated with a steeper rate of smoking progression (Audrain-McGovern, Rodriguez, & Kassel, 2009). Depressive symptoms also have been found to be particularly associated with increases in cigarette use among adolescent females (Whitbeck, Yu, McChargue, & Crawford, 2009). On the other hand, adolescent females who smoke cigarettes have been found to be at greater risk for depressive symptomatology (Groth & Morrison-Beedy, 2011).

We again used publicly available data from the U.S. NSDUH 2004-2009 to report the prevalence of a depression symptom and of lifetime and past-year major depressive episodes (MDE) (see Table 3). We then used data from the 2009 NSDUH to examine the bivariate correlation between these measures of depression and past-month cigarettes use among adolescent 12-17 years old (see Table 4).

As shown in Table 3, in 2009 approximately 38% of adolescent males and 53% adolescent females reported ever having had a period of time lasting several days or longer when most of the day they felt sad, empty, or depressed. This corresponds to approximately 4.7 and 6.3 million boys and girls, respectively. In the same year, 8.4% and 17.8% of boys and girls, respectively, were estimated to have a MDE in their lifetime which corresponds to an estimated one million boys and 2.1 million girls. Finally, approximately 4.9% and 11.3% of boys and girls were estimated to have a MDE in the past year or an estimated 606 thousand and 1.3 million boys and girls, respectively. The NSDUH classified adolescents as having a MDE using the diagnostic criteria set forth in the 4th edition of the *Diagnostic and Statistical Manual of Mental Disorders* (DSM-IV) (APA, 2000) which specifies a period of 2 weeks or longer during which there is either (1) depressed mood or (2) loss of interest or pleasure and at least four other symptoms (out of 9) that reflect a change in functioning, such as problems with sleep, eating, energy, concentration, and self-image.

As shown in Table 4, a significantly higher percent of adolescent males who indicated they had "Ever felt sad, empty, or depressed most of the day lasting several days or longer" had smoked cigarettes in the past month (10.8%) than those who did not endorse this depression question (8.3%). Similarly, a considerably greater percent of adolescent females who indicated having felt sad, empty or depressed, reported smoking cigarettes in the past month (11.7%) compared to those who did not indicate feeling that way (5.0%). Once again, similar differences are observed in the percent of past-month smoking among adolescent males and females who met criteria for lifetime and past-year MDE compared to those who did not meet this criteria (see Table 4).

Depression Measure and Gender	2004	2005	2006	2007	2008	2009
Total adolescent sample	18,161	18,527	18,144	17,566	17,670	17,531
Ever felt sad, empty, or depressed most of the day lasting several days or longer						
Males	41.3***	41.2***	39.4***	37.8***	38.3***	38.0***
Females	56.3	55.9	54.6	51.8	52.4	53.0
Lifetime Major Depressive Episode						
Males	8.5***	7.9***	7.4***	7.5***	7.3***	8.4***
Females	19.6	19.8	18.4	18.0	18.8	17.8
Past-year Major Depressive Episode						
Males	5.0***	4.5***	4.2***	4.6***	4.3***	4.9***
Females	12.8	13.1	11.9	12.1	12.6	11.3

*$p < 0.05$, **$p < 0.01$, ***$p<0.001$.

Table 3. Percent of male and female adolescents who had ever in their lives had a period of time lasting several days or longer when most of the day they felt sad, empty, or depressed, and by whether they met criteria for lifetime and past-year Major Depressive Episode: NSDUH 2004-2009.

Depression measure	% of adolescents who smoked cigarettes in the past month	
	Male	Female
Ever felt sad, empty, or depressed most of the day lasting several days or longer		
Yes	10.8**	11.7***
No	8.3	5.0
Lifetime Major Depressive Episode		
Yes	14.2***	16.2***
No	8.7	6.9
Past-year Major Depressive Episode		
Yes	16.0***	17.9***
No	8.8	7.3

*$p < 0.05$, **$p < 0.01$, ***$p<0.001$.

Table 4. Percent of male and female adolescents who smoked cigarettes in the past month by whether they had ever in their lives had a period of time lasting several days or longer when most of the day they felt sad, empty, or depressed, and by whether they met criteria for lifetime and past-year Major Depressive Episode: NSDUH 2009.

Table 4 also shows that a slightly higher percent of females than males who reported depression symptoms and who were estimated to have a lifetime and past-year MDE reported smoking in the past month. However, these differences are not large (17.9% of girls vs. 16.0% of boys with past-year MDEs smoked in the past month).

To further examine the association between depression symptoms and cigarette use, we used data from the National Longitudinal Survey of Youth cohort that was first followed in 1997. The NLSY97 dataset consists of a nationally representative sample of U.S. residents who were born between 1980 and 1984 (OSU, 2007). Adolescents were first sampled and interviewed in 1997 and then were assessed yearly until 2008. The survey assesses adolescents' development in several areas; educational, labor market experiences, mental health, and drug use. The questions about mental health that relate to depressive symptoms were included in Waves 4, 6, and 8, that is, in years 2000, 2002, and 2004. Thus, the analyses we present below were based on these three waves of data. A total of 8,162 adolescents (Mean age at wave 4 = 17.9, SD=1.44, 49% female) were included in the analyses.

At each wave, the NLSY survey asked participants to report on the frequency with which they (a) felt down, (b) depressed, and (c) nervous in the past month. Response options for each of these questions ranged from "All of the time=4" to "None of the time=1". These responses were added to create a composite score of depression symptoms that could range from 3 to 12, with higher scores representing more depression symptoms. Two dependent variables measuring cigarette use were created. One measure consisted of a dichotomous Yes-No answer to a question about past-year cigarette use. The second measure was the total number of cigarettes smoked in the past 30 days, a variable created by multiplying the answers to the questions about the number of days youth indicated they had smoked cigarettes and the number of cigarettes they indicated they would usually smoke each day, in the past month. These variables were also created at each wave.

These data were used to examine if changes in depression symptoms over two successive waves, two years apart, were associated with changes in smoking status (no changes, initiated smoking, or quit smoking) over the prior year and, among smokers, with the total number of cigarettes smoked in the past month. Data were analyzed using multinomial logit regression and with ordinary least square regression, respectively.

Table 5 indicates that change in depression symptoms over two successive periods is a strong predictor of changes in smoking status over the same period, with or without controlling for age, age squared, and parental education ($p<0.01$). In other words, adolescents experiencing more depression symptoms over time were considerably more likely to have initiated smoking over the prior year, and, they also were less likely to quit smoking if they were smokers the year prior. Males were more likely to have smoked in the past year ($p<0.01$). However, the interaction of the variables, changes in depression symptoms with gender, was not significant suggesting that the association between changes in depression symptoms and smoking status over time is similar between adolescent males and females.

As shown in Table 6, adolescents who experience higher level of depressive symptoms over time have a greater risk of increasing the total number of cigarettes they smoke in the past 30 days, even after controlling for age, age squared, and parental education. And although adolescent males smoke more cigarettes, the interaction of changes in depression with

Variables	Quitter (1)	Initiated (2)	Quitter (3)	Initiated (4)	Quitter (5)	Initiated (6)
ΔDepression	**-0.06*** **	**0.11*** **	**-0.06*** **	**0.10*** **	**-0.06** **	**0.09*** **
	(0.02)	(0.02)	(0.02)	(0.02)	(0.02)	(0.03)
Male=1			**0.05**	**0.35*** **	**0.05**	**0.34*** **
			(0.06)	(0.06)	(0.06)	(0.06)
(ΔDepression)*male					0.01	0.02
					(0.04)	(0.03)
Age			0.36	-1.19***	0.36	-1.18***
			(0.35)	(0.31)	(0.35)	(0.31)
Age squared			-0.01	0.03***	-0.01	0.03***
			(0.01)	(0.01)	(0.01)	(0.01)
Parental education			-0.00	0.01	-0.00	0.01
			(0.01)	(0.01)	(0.01)	(0.01)
Constant	-2.28***	-2.10***	-5.32	10.15***	-5.34	10.12***
	(0.03)	(0.03)	(3.34)	(2.93)	(3.34)	(2.93)
Observations	14,557	14,557	13,486	13,486	13,486	13,486

Note: Δ=Changes in. Robust standard errors in parentheses. Observations are pooled samples.
* p<0.1, ** p<0.05, *** p<0.01.

Table 5. Results of multinomial logit analysis to examine if changes in depression symptoms over two waves would be associated with adolescents being more likely to initiate or quit smoking (if they were smokers) two years later when compared to adolescents whose smoking status did not change between waves: NLSY97 Waves 4 (2000), 6 (2002), and 8 (2004).

gender was not significant. This suggests that the link between changes in depression symptoms and total number of cigarettes smoked in the past 30 days is similar among adolescent males and females.

The findings shown in Tables 4, 5 and 6 are interesting because if indeed depression symptoms are such important predictors of smoking, one would expect a much higher proportion of females becoming smokers. That this is not the case is an important indication of the complex etiology of smoking behaviors and the more likely scenario that any behavior such as smoking is influenced by genetic and environmental factors, including cultural, familial and societal that are inter-related.

To our knowledge, no studies in Latin America have examined the association between mental disorders and rates of cigarette use among adolescents with the exception of Mexico. It has been posited that in Latin America depressive symptoms are the most common risk factors that predispose adolescents to begin using cigarettes, second only to having a parent who has used substances (Baptista et al., 2006). Researchers in Mexico have examined baseline data from an ongoing cohort study of a representative sample of adolescents for different factors that might be associated with being experimenters (having tried a cigarette one or two times) compared to being a regular smoker (having smoked in the past 30 days).

Variables	Bivariate	Includes controls	Controls and Interaction
ΔDepression	**7.79*** **	**6.60** **	**10.75*** **
	(2.68)	(2.81)	(3.78)
Male=1		**21.36** **	**20.17** **
		(9.44)	(9.43)
(ΔDepression) * male			-7.92
			(5.62)
Age		-126.52**	-129.63**
		(56.56)	(56.82)
Age squared		2.98**	3.06**
		(1.47)	(1.48)
Parental education		-1.50	-1.44
		(1.70)	(1.70)
Constant	31.70***	1,363.55**	1,394.15**
	(4.57)	(539.80)	(542.29)
Observations	3,790	3,511	3,511

Note: Δ=Changes in. Robust standard errors in parentheses. Observations are pooled samples.
* $p<0.1$, ** $p<0.05$, *** $p<0.01$.

Table 6. Results of multiple regression analysis predicting if changes in adolescents depression symptoms over two waves predict changes in the total number of cigarettes smoked in the past 30 days between the waves: NLSY97 Waves 4 (2000), 6 (2002), and 8 (2004).

The results of this cross-sectional study of Mexican adolescents found that depression, as measured by the Zung scale, was associated with smoking, but only for adolescents who were regular smokers, not with experimenting with tobacco use (Arillo-Santillan et al., 2005). Among the adult, urban population in Mexico, current tobacco users have been found to have twice the odds of reporting elevated depressive symptoms than individuals who have never used tobacco (Benjet, Wagner, Borges, & Medina-Mora, 2004).

1.3.1.2 Central America and the Caribbean

Depressive symptoms have been found to be associated with increased odds of tobacco use among a convenience sample of about 5,000 Costa Rican adolescents that included students in private and public schools, adolescents in treatment for substance use, as well street youth (Obando, Kliewer, Murrelle, & Svikis, 2004). Similarly, a study of six Central American countries (Costa Rica, El Salvador, Guatemala, Honduras, Nicaragua, and Panama) including the Dominican Republic using national representative samples found that tobacco use was 2.9 times more likely to occur among adolescents with moderate behavioral problems (Vittetoe, Lopez, Delva, Wagner, & Anthony, 2002).

1.3.1.3 South America

The relationship between depressive symptoms and cigarette use in South America has been primarily examined among adults. Among a Brazilian adult sample, individuals with moderate and severe scores of depression, measured by the Beck Depression Inventory, were more likely to smoke (Bortoluzzi, Kehrig, Loguercio, & Traebert, 2011). One of the few studies examining this association among adolescents was conducted in Colombia. The study sampled about 500 adolescents attending four high schools in a large city in Colombia. They found that adolescents with clinically relevant depressive symptoms had odds of using cigarettes that were 1.91 times higher than those without clinically relevant depressive symptoms (Campo-Arias et al., 2007).

To further examine the potential association between depression symptoms and cigarette smoking among Latin American adolescents, we used data from a longitudinal study of substance use presently underway in Santiago, Chile. The study, called the Santiago Longitudinal study (Bares, Andrade, Delva, & Grogan-Kaylor, 2011; Bares, Andrade, Delva, Grogan-Kaylor, & Kamata, 2011; 2011), is a collaborative project between U.S. and Chilean institutions with funding from the U.S. National Institute on Drug Abuse (NIDA). The sample for the present analyses consisted of 660 adolescents with data on the variables of interest in both Waves 1 and 2, assessed about 1.5-2 years apart. Youth at Wave 1 were approximately 14 years old, 48% female, and of mid-to-low socioeconomic status. The average number of years of parental education was 9.9 years and the average monthly family income was 315,000 pesos (500 Chilean pesos is approximately $1.00 US dollar). About 68% of the youth lived with both their father and mother. Participants for this study were recruited from a sample of approximately 1,700 families that participated in a study of nutrition when the youth were in infancy and 1,200 when the youth were 10 years old (Lozoff, et al., 2003). Between 2007 and 2010, over 1000 youth were successfully recruited. In 2007-2010, youth completed Wave 1 assessments consisting of a 2-hr interviewer-administered questionnaire with comprehensive questions on demographics, mental health, peer, family, and school characteristics. Wave 2 assessments have begun and will be completed in 2012. For the purpose of this Chapter we examined if depression symptoms at Wave 1 were associated at Wave 2 (1.5-2 years later) with (1) smoking initiation, quitting among those who had reported smoking in Wave 1, or no changes in smoking or non-smoking status and (2) if the total number of cigarettes smoked in the past month changed between waves.

Depressive symptoms were assessedby the ASEBA School-Age Form Youth Self Report (YSR) that measures levels of depression-anxiety and withdrawn-depression symptoms (Achenbach & Rescorla, 2001). The stem question for the thirteen items that make up these two scales is "Below is a list of items that describe kids. For each item that describes you now or within the past 6 months, please tell me if the item is *(3) very true or often true, (2) somewhat or sometimes true, or (1)* is *not true (0).*

We conducted two types of analyses. First, we used multinomial logit regression to examine if depression scores at Wave 1 for both variables (withdrawn-depression and anxious-depression) were associated with changes in lifetime smoking status 1.5-2 years later (Wave 2). The dependent variable, Smoking Changes, consisted of three categories: quitter, initiator, and no changer (the reference group). Then we used multiple regression analysis to examine if, among adolescents who had smoked at Wave 1, their withdrawn-depression and anxious-depression, symptoms were associated with changes in the total number of cigarettes smoked in the past month between the two waves.

Table 7 presents the results of the multinomial logit regression that examined if adolescents withdrawn-depression symptoms at Wave 1 were associated with changes in smoking status at Wave 2 (initiated smoking, quit smoking, or status did not change between waves).

Variables	Quitter (1)	Initiated (2)	Quitter (3)	Initiated (4)	Quitter (5)	Initiated (6)
Withdrawn-Depression	-0.00	0.03	-0.03	0.05	-0.01	0.02
	(0.08)	(0.03)	(0.08)	(0.03)	(0.11)	(0.05)
Male=1			0.09	0.12	0.25	-0.19
			(0.44)	(0.19)	(0.79)	(0.35)
Withdrawn-depression * male					-0.04	0.07
					(0.16)	(0.07)
Age			0.23	8.63***	0.21	8.47***
			(6.11)	(2.95)	(6.13)	(2.95)
Age squared			0.01	-0.32***	0.01	-0.32***
			(0.22)	(0.11)	(0.22)	(0.11)
SES			-0.14*	0.06*	-0.14*	0.05
			(0.08)	(0.03)	(0.08)	(0.03)
Constant	-3.03***	-1.23**	-7.67	-58.78***	-7.63	-57.53***
	(0.39)	(0.17)	(42.13)	(19.96)	(42.22)	(19.97)
Observations	663	663	660	660	660	660

Note: Robust standard errors in parentheses.
* p<0.1; ** p<0.05, *** p<0.01.

Table 7. Results of multinomial logit analysis to examine if adolescents with higher withdrawn-depression symptoms at Wave 1 would be more likely to initiate or quit smoking (if they were smokers) one-and-a-half to two years later (Wave 2) when compared to adolescents whose smoking status did not change between waves (never smoked at Wave 1 and neither at Wave 2 or smoked at Wave 1 and remained a smoker at Wave 2).

The first two columns in Table 7 present the bivariate analysis of the depression-cigarette status changes while columns (3)-(4) adds age, age squared, and SES as controls. Finally, columns (5)-(6) adds the controls and an interaction term representing the depression variable with gender (male) interaction. There was no significant association between adolescents' withdrawn-depressive symptoms at Wave 1 and changes in smoking behavior between Waves 1 and 2 (about 1.5-2 years apart). Age was positively associated with smoking initiation and higher SES was inversely associated with quitting, that is youth with higher SES are less likely to quit smoking.

Table 8 below presents the results of the multinomial logit regression that examined if adolescents anxious-depression symptoms at Wave 1 were associated with changes in smoking status at Wave 2 (initiated smoking, quit smoking, or status did not change between waves).

Variables	Quitter (1)	Initiated (2)	Quitter (3)	Initiated (4)	Quitter (5)	Initiated (6)
Anxious-Depression	0.08	0.01	0.08	0.02	0.02	-0.02
	(0.05)	(0.02)	(0.05)	(0.03)	(0.07)	(0.03)
Male=1			0.29	0.13	-0.50	-0.51
			(0.45)	(0.19)	(0.87)	(0.36)
Anxious-Depression*male					0.12	**0.11****
					(0.11)	(0.05)
Age			1.00	8.51***	1.48	8.47***
			(6.21)	(2.95)	(6.23)	(2.95)
Age squared			-0.02	-0.32***	-0.04	-0.32***
			(0.22)	(0.11)	(0.23)	(0.11)
SES			-0.12	0.05	-0.13	0.05
			(0.08)	(0.03)	(0.08)	(0.03)
Constant	-3.55***	-1.18***	-13.34	-58.02***	-16.29	-57.52***
	(0.42)	(0.17)	(42.79)	(19.92)	(42.96)	(19.94)
Observations	663	663	660	660	660	660

Note: Robust standard errors in parentheses.
* p<0.1; ** p<0.05, *** p<0.01.

Table 8. Results of multinomial logit analysis to examine if adolescents with higher anxious-depression symptoms at Wave 1 would be more likely to initiate or quit smoking (if they were smokers) one-and-a-half to two years later (Wave 2) when compared to adolescents whose smoking status did not change between waves (never smoked at Wave 1 and neither at Wave 2 or smoked at Wave 1 and remained a smoker at Wave 2).

As was the case with the earlier analysis, the first two columns present the bivariate analysis of the depression-cigarette status changes while columns (3)-(4) adds age, age squared, and SES as controls. Also, columns (5)-(6) adds the controls and an interaction term representing the depression variable with gender (male) interaction. As shown in Table 8, males with higher anxious-depression symptoms at Wave 1 were more likely to have started smoking at Wave 2. Age was positively associated with smoking onset but in this case, when controlling for anxious-depression symptoms, SES was not associated with quitting as had been the case earlier.

Then, we examined if, among smokers at Wave 1, there were changes in the total number of cigarettes smoked in the past 30 days between Waves 1 and 2 as a function of the adolescents' depression symptoms. The total number of cigarettes was created by multiplying two variables – the average number of cigarettes adolescents reported smoking on a given day in the past 30 days by the number of days they reported smoking in the past 30 days. Table 9 presents the results of the multiple regression analysis predicting if withdrawn-depression symptoms at Wave 1 predicted changes in the total number of cigarettes smoked between waves. There were no significant findings. Similarly, Table 10 presents the results of the multiple regression analysis predicting if anxious-depression symptoms at Wave 1 predicted changes in the total number of cigarettes smoked between waves. There were also no significant findings.

Variables	**Bivariate**	**Includes controls**	**Controls and Interaction**
Withdrawn-Depressed	1.17	0.98	2.09
	(3.49)	(3.26)	(5.07)
Male=1		3.04	15.62
		(10.80)	(23.66)
Withdrawn-Depressed * male			-2.97
			(5.70)
Age		53.78	60.77
		(159.01)	(159.64)
Age squared		-1.83	-2.07
		(5.87)	(5.88)
SES		-3.08	-2.89
		(2.22)	(2.14)
Constant	32.50**	-361.79	-417.42
	(12.85)	(1,072.43)	(1,078.68)
Observations	154	153	153

Note: Robust standard errors in parentheses.
* p<0.1; ** p<0.05, *** p<0.01.

Table 9. Results of multiple regression analysis predicting if adolescents' withdrawn-depression symptoms at Wave 1, among smokers at Wave 1, predicted changes in the total number of cigarettes smoked in the past 30 days between Waves 1 and 2.

Variables	**Bivariate**	**Includes controls**	**Controls and Interaction**
Anxious-Depressed	-0.95	-1.06	-1.01
	(1.92)	(1.94)	(2.82)
Male=1		0.17	1.00
		(11.25)	(22.73)
Anxious-Depressed * male			-0.14
			(3.62)
Age		53.33	53.09
		(160.26)	(161.71)
Age squared		-1.80	-1.79
		(5.93)	(5.99)
SES		-3.30	-3.31
		(2.33)	(2.36)
Constant	43.86***	-348.82	-347.56
	(11.46)	(1,081.20)	(1,089.32)
Observations	154	153	153

Note: Robust standard errors in parentheses.
* p<0.1; ** p<0.05, *** p<0.01.

Table 10. Results of multiple regression analysis predicting if adolescents' anxious-depression symptoms at Wave 1, among smokers at Wave 1, predicted changes in the total number of cigarettes smoked in the past 30 days between Waves 1 and 2.

These findings suggest that anxious-depression is not associated with changes in the number of cigarettes smoked in the past 30 days. Although the results in Table 9 suggest that anxious-depression is associated with being a current smoker, changes in symptoms of anxious-depression among this adolescent population does not change the number of cigarettes smoked.

2. Discussion

Data for the United States suggest that about 10% of 12- to 17-year-old adolescents have used cigarettes in the previous 30 days. The prevalence of past 30-days cigarette use among 12- to 17-year-old adolescents in Latin America vary greatly from a low of 1.6% in the Bahamas to a high of 35.6% in Chile. Data from the United States indicate that about 11% of adolescents experience a depressive disorder in their lifetime while data from Mexico suggest that the rate there is about 7.6% of adolescents. The rate of depression symptoms for adolescents in two municipal areas in Brazil were 6.4% and 10%. After a thorough search, we were not able to identify any studies of depression symptoms among adolescents in Latin American countries.

High rates of co-occurrence have been reported for cigarette use and depressive symptoms (McKenzie, Olsson, Jorm, Romaniuk, & Patton, 2010; Weiss et al., 2011). The available evidence suggests that adolescents with a substance use disorder and a mental disorder are more psychologically distressed (Essau, 2011; Oesterle, 2008). Although a great deal of literature supports the link between cigarette use and depression symptoms during adolescence much of this work comes from the United States. In fact, our analysis using a nationally representative sample of adolescents in the United States indicate that adolescent males and females experiencing more depression symptoms over time were considerably more likely to have initiated smoking and were less likely to have quit smoking if they were smokers the year prior. Among the Chilean adolescent sample, males with higher anxious-depression symptoms over time, but not withdrawn-depression symptoms, were more likely to smoke than males who experience less changes in these symptoms. These findings suggest the way(s) by which we understand the link between depressive symptoms and cigarette use among adolescents might be specific to the stressors experienced by youth in their respective countries.

Given the large variations in smoking among adolescents in the Americas, examining the association between smoking and depression symptoms in each country warrants further attention. Doing so might elucidate some of the unique risk and protective factors in place throughout the region.

The analyses we conducted to further examine the potential associations between the two variables, smoking and depressive symptoms, showed that changes in depressive symptoms are strong predictors of adolescent initiating cigarette use and with smoking greater number of cigarettes. The results of the analyses conducted to examine the relationship between depressive symptoms and cigarette use among adolescents Santiago, Chile, indicate that the positive association between anxious-depression symptoms and ever smoking 1.5 to 2 years later was found to only occur among adolescent males and not females. This suggests that anxious-depression might be creating a special vulnerability among adolescent males to seek the effects of nicotine to dampen their distress while adolescent females might have a different way of coping with distressing depressive symptoms. Future work devoted to understanding the mental health of adolescents in Latin America is needed to better understand the differential relationship between gender, depression symptoms, and smoking.,

Because adolescents with a substance use disorder and a mental disorder are more psychologically distressed (Essau, 2011; Oesterle, 2008), some have suggested that they also exhibit a greater need for health care services. In fact, Georgiades and colleagues have found that among those who use tobacco during adolescence, 26.5% go on to develop major depressive disorder in adulthood (2007). In addition, individuals with clinical scores of depression at a baseline measurement have been found to be more susceptible to initiate smoking 18 months later (Minnix et al., 2011) further stressing the need to help youth prevent smoking and help smokers quit as well as find better ways to treat youth who suffer from depression. Interventions for adolescent smokers who experience depressive symptoms might target modifiable factors, rather than those that may not be modifiable at this point in time (Green & Kreuter, 2005). Modifiable risk factors could include adolescents' self-efficacy (Stevens, Colwell, Smith, Robinson, & McMillan, 2005) and perceptions of body image (Rodríguez-Esquivel, Cooper, Blow, & Resor, 2009), which have been found to be associated with both cigarette use and depressive symptoms (Kulbok et al., 2008). Because many countries in Latin America are involved in the production of tobacco products, it may be necessary to implement social-influence interventions for these high risk populations (Noland et al., 1998). At this point, interventions to reduce genetic susceptibility to depressive symptoms and progression of cigarette smoking might not be feasible.

Interventions and treatment programs for adolescent tobacco use and tobacco prevention need to be sensitive to the adolescents' gender, developmental stage and cultural backgrounds, among other identities. Some preventive interventions for cigarette use are currently available for minority youth in the United States (Prokhorov et al., 2010) but the existence of tobacco prevention and research on the effectiveness of such interventions among adolescents in Latin America are lacking. Because interventions that are effective with one group of adolescents may not be effective with other groups of adolescents (Foraker, Patten, Lopez, Croghan, & Thomas, 2005), there is a critical need for the development and evaluation of interventions targeting cigarette use but also comorbid cigarette use and depressive symptoms among adolescents in Latin America.

3. References

APA, A. P. A. (2000). *Diagnostic and statistical manual of mental disorders*: DSM-IV-TR. Washington, DC.

Arillo-Santillan, E., Lazcano-Ponce, E., Hernandez-Avila, M., Fernández, E., Allen, B., Valdes, R., & Samet, J. (2005). Associations between individual and contextual factors and smoking in 13,293 Mexican students. *American Journal of Preventive Medicine, 28*(1), 41-51. doi: 10.1016/j.amepre.2004.09.002

Audrain-McGovern, J., Rodriguez, D., Cuevas, J., & Rodgers, K. (2009). The Role of Depression in Adolescent Smoking Trajectories. *Journal of Dual Diagnosis, 5*(2), 179-190. doi: 10.1080/15504260902870145

Audrain-McGovern, J., Rodriguez, D., & Kassel, J. D. (2009). Adolescent smoking and depression: evidence for self-medication and peer smoking mediation. *Addiction, 104*(10), 1743-1756. doi: 10.1111/j.1360-0443.2009.02617.x

Avanci, J. Q., Assis, S. G., & Oliveira, R. V. C. (2008). Sintomas depressivos na adolescência: estudo sobre fatores psicossociais em amostra de escolares de um município do Rio de Janeiro, Brasil. *Cadernos de Saúde Pública, 24*, 2334-2346.

Baptista, F., Cabrera, J., Montilla, M., Ortiz, R., Salomon, A., Testa, M., . . . Morales, A. (2006). Prevalencia del consumo de alcohol, patron de consumo y factores de riesgo asociados en adolescentes del sector las delicias de la comunidad de Tamaca. *Boletin Medico de Postgrado, 12*(3).

Bares, C., Andrade, F., Delva, J., & Grogan-Kaylor, A. (2011). Examining the factor structure of anxiety and depression symptom items among adolescents in Santiago, Chile. *Journal of the Society for Social Work Research, 2*(1).

Bares, C., Andrade, F., Delva, J., Grogan-Kaylor, A., & Kamata, A. (2011). Differential item functioning due to gender between depression and anxiety items among Chilean adolescents. *International Journal of Social Psychiatry*. doi: 10.1177/0020764011400999

Barrueco, M., Alonso, A., & Gonzalez-Sarmiento, R. (2005). Genetic basis of tobacco dependence. *Medicina Clinica, 124*(6), 223-228. doi: 10.1157/13071764

Benjet, C., Borges, G., Medina-Mora, M. E., Méndez, E., Fleiz, C., Rojas, E., & Cruz, C. (2009). Diferencias de sexo en la prevalencia y severidad de trastornos psiquiátricos en adolescentes de la Ciudad de México. (Spanish). *Sex differences in the prevalence and severity of psychiatric disorders in Mexico City adolescents. (English), 32*(2), 155-163.

Benjet, C., Wagner, F. A., Borges, G. G., & Medina-Mora, M. E. (2004). The relationship of tobacco smoking with depressive symptomatology in the Third Mexican National Addictions Survey. *Psychological Medicine, 34*(5), 881-888. doi: 10.1017/s0033291703001600

Boden, J. M., Fergusson, D. M., & Horwood, L. J. (2010). Cigarette smoking and depression: tests of causal linkages using a longitudinal birth cohort. *The British Journal Of Psychiatry: The Journal Of Mental Science, 196*(6), 440-446.

Bortoluzzi, M. C., Kehrig, R. T., Loguercio, A. D., & Traebert, J. L. (2011). Prevalência e perfil dos usuários de tabaco de população adulta em cidade do Sul do Brasil (Joaçaba, SC). *Ciência & Saúde Coletiva, 16*, 1953-1959.

Breslau, N., Peterson, E. L., Schultz, L. R., Chilcoat, H. D., & Andreski, P. (1998). Major Depression and Stages of Smoking: A Longitudinal Investigation. *Arch Gen Psychiatry, 55*(2), 161-166. doi: 10.1001/archpsyc.55.2.161

Brook, D. W., Brook, J. S., Chenshu, Z., Whiteman, M., Cohen, P., & Finch, S. J. (2008). Developmental trajectories of cigarette smoking from adolescence to the early thirties: Personality and behavioral risk factors. *Nicotine & Tobacco Research, 10*(8), 1283-1291. doi: 10.1080/14622200802238993

Camacho, P. A., Rueda-Jaimes, G. E., Latorre, J. F., Navarro-Mancilla, Á. A., Escobar, M., & Franco, J. A. (2009). Validez y confiabilidad de la escala del Center for Epidemiologic Studies-Depression en estudiantes adolescentes de Colombia. *Biomédica, 29*, 260-269.

Campo-Arias, A., Dallos Bareño, C. M., González Rueda, S. J., Rodríguez Rodríguez, D. C., Sánchez Herrera, Z. M., & Díaz Martínez, L. A. (2007). Consumo de cigarrillo y síntomas depresivos en estudiantes de Bucaramanga, Colombia. *Archivos argentinos de pediatría, 105*, 12-16.

Carmody, T. P., Vieten, C., & Astin, J. A. (2007). Negative affect, emotional acceptance, and smoking cessation. *Journal Of Psychoactive Drugs, 39*(4), 499-508.

Castilla-Puentes, R. C., Secin, R., Grau, A., Galeno, R., Feijo de Mello, M., Pena, N., & Sanchez-Russi, C. A. (2008). A multicenter study of major depressive disorder among emergency department patients in Latin-American countries. *Depression And Anxiety, 25*(12), E199-E204.

Chen, X. N., Chen, J. C., Williamson, V. S., An, S. S., Hettema, J. M., Aggen, S. H., . . . Kendler, K. S. (2009). Variants in Nicotinic Acetylcholine Receptors alpha 5 and alpha 3 Increase Risks to Nicotine Dependence. *American Journal of Medical Genetics Part B-Neuropsychiatric Genetics, 150B*(7), 926-933. doi: 10.1002/ajmg.b.30919

Cheung, A. H., & Dewa, C. S. (2006). Canadian community health survey: major depressive disorder and suicidality in adolescents. *Healthcare Policy = Politiques De Santé, 2*(2), 76-89.

Dagyte, G., Den Boer, J. A., & Trentani, A. (2011). The cholinergic system and depression. *Behavioural Brain Research, 221*(2), 574-582. doi: 10.1016/j.bbr.2010.02.023

Essau, C. A. (2011). Comorbidity of substance use disorders among community-based and high-risk adolescents. *Psychiatry research, 185*(1-2), 176-184.

Fergusson, D. M., Boden, J. M., & Horwood, L. J. (2011). Structural models of the comorbidity of internalizing disorders and substance use disorders in a longitudinal birth cohort. *Social Psychiatry and Psychiatric Epidemiology, 46*(10), 933-942. doi: 10.1007/s00127-010-0268-1

Fergusson, D. M., Goodwin, R. D., & Horwood, L. J. (2003). Major depression and cigarette smoking: results of a 21-year longitudinal study. *Psychological Medicine, 33*(8), 1357-1367.

Florenzano, R., Cáceres, E., Valdés, M., Calderón, S., Santander, S., & Casassus, M. (2009). Conductas de riesgo, síntomas depresivos, auto y heteroagresión en una muestra de adolescentes escolarizados en la Región Metropolitana de Santiago de Chile, 2007. *Revista chilena de neuro-psiquiatría, 47*, 24-33.

Foraker, R. E., Patten, C. A., Lopez, K. N., Croghan, I. T., & Thomas, J. L. (2005). Beliefs and attitudes regarding smoking among young adult Latinos: A pilot study. *Preventive Medicine, 41*(1), 126-133. doi: 10.1016/j.ypmed.2004.10.018

Georgiades, K., & Boyle, M. H. (2007). Adolescent tobacco and cannabis use: young adult outcomes from the Ontario Child Health Study. *Journal of Child Psychology and Psychiatry, 48*(7), 724-731. doi: 10.1111/j.1469-7610.2007.01740.x

Gerra, G., Garofano, L., Zaimovic, A., Moi, G., Branchi, B., Bussandri, M., . . . Donnini, C. (2005). Association of the serotonin transporter promoter polymorphism with smoking behavior among adolescents. *American Journal of Medical Genetics Part B-Neuropsychiatric Genetics, 135B*(1), 73-78. doi: 10.1002/ajmg.b.30173

Golfeto, J. H., D'Oliveira, A. B., Baptista, C., & Bisson, F. (2011). Prevalencia da sintomatologia depressiva nas cidades de Ribeirao Preto e regiao/Prevalence of depressive symptoms in Ribeirao Preto and neighboring cities. *Pediatria Moderna, 47*(1).

Green, L. W., & Kreuter, M. W. (2005). *Health Program Planning: An Educatinal and Ecological Approach* (4th ed.). New York: McGraw-Hill.

Groth, S., & Morrison-Beedy, D. (2011). Smoking, Substance Use, and Mental Health Correlates in Urban Adolescent Girls. *Journal of Community Health, 36*(4), 552-558. doi: 10.1007/s10900-010-9340-8

Harding, T. W., de Arango, M. V., Baltazar, J., Climent, C. E., Ibrahim, H. H., Ladrido-Ignacio, L., Wig, N. N. (1980). Mental disorders in primary health care: a study of their frequency and diagnosis in four developing countries. *Psychological Medicine, 10*(2), 231-241.

Hu, M. C., Davies, M., & Kandel, D. B. (2006). Epidemiology and correlates of daily smoking and nicotine dependence among young adults in the United States. *American Journal of Public Health, 96*(2), 299-308. doi: 10.2104/ajph.2004.057232

Johnston, L., O'Malley, P., Bachman, J., & Schulenberg, J. (2011). Monitoring the Future national survey results on drug use, 1975-2010. *Institute for Social Research, The University of Michigan*. Ann Arbor, MI.

Kendler, K. S., Neale, M. C., MacLean, C. J., Heath, A. C., Eaves, L. J., & Kessler, R. C. (1993). Smoking and major depression. A causal analysis. *Archives Of General Psychiatry, 50*(1), 36-43.

Khantzian, E. J. (1985). The self-medication hypothesis of addictive disorders: focus on heroin and cocaine dependence. *Am J Psychiatry, 142*(11), 1259-1264.

Khantzian, E. J. (1997). The self-medication hypothesis of substance use disorders: A reconsideration and recent applications. *Harvard Review of Psychiatry, 4*(5), 231-244. doi: 10.3109/10673229709030550

Kohli, M. A., Lucae, S., Saemann, P. G., Schmidt, M. V., Demirkan, A., Hek, K., . . . Binder, E. B. (2011). The Neuronal Transporter Gene SLC6A15 Confers Risk to Major Depression. *Neuron, 70*(2), 252-265. doi: 10.1016/j.neuron.2011.04.005

Kulbok, P. A., Rhee, H., Botchwey, N., Hinton, I., Bovbjerg, V., & Anderson, N. L. R. (2008). Factors Influencing Adolescents' Decision Not to Smoke. *Public Health Nursing, 25*(6), 505-515. doi: 10.1111/j.1525-1446.2008.00737.x

Lerman, C., Caporaso, N., Main, D., Audrain, J., Boyd, N. R., Bowman, E. D., & Shields, P. G. (1998). Depression and self-medication with nicotine: The modifying influence of the dopamine D4 receptor gene. *Health Psychology, 17*(1), 56-62. doi: 10.1037/0278-6133.17.1.56

Lerman, C., Caporaso, N. E., Audrain, J., Main, D., Bowman, E. D., Lockshin, B., . . . Shields, P. G. (1999). Evidence suggesting the role of specific genetic factors in cigarette smoking. *Health Psychology, 18*(1), 14-20. doi: 10.1037/0278-6133.18.1.14

Martini, S., Wagner, F. A., & Anthony, J. C. (2002). The association of tobacco smoking and depression in adolescence: Evidence from the United States. *Substance Use & Misuse, 37*(14), 1853.

McKenzie, M., Olsson, C. A., Jorm, A. F., Romaniuk, H., & Patton, G. C. (2010). Association of adolescent symptoms of depression and anxiety with daily smoking and nicotine dependence in young adulthood: findings from a 10-year longitudinal study. *Addiction, 105*(9), 1652-1659. doi: 10.1111/j.1360-0443.2010.03002.x

Merikangas, K. R., He, J. P., Burstein, M., Swanson, S. A., Avenevoli, S., Cui, L., . . . Swendsen, J. (2010). Lifetime Prevalence of Mental Disorders in U.S. Adolescents:

Results from the National Comorbidity Survey Replication-Adolescent Supplement (NCS-A). *Journal of the American Academy of Child & Adolescent Psychiatry, 49*(10), 980-989. doi: 10.1016/j.jaac.2010.05.017

Minnix, J. A., Blalock, J. A., Marani, S., Prokhorov, A. V., & Cinciripini, P. M. (2011). Self-efficacy mediates the effect of depression on smoking susceptibility in adolescents. *Nicotine & Tobacco Research: Official Journal Of The Society For Research On Nicotine And Tobacco, 13*(8), 699-705.

Moon, S., Mo, B., & Basham, R. (2010). Adolescent Depression and Future Smoking Behavior: A Prospective Study. *Child & Adolescent Social Work Journal, 27*(6), 405-422. doi: 10.1007/s10560-010-0212-y

Morisano, D., Bacher, I., Audrain-McGovern, J., & George, T. P. (2009). Mechanisms Underlying the Comorbidity of Tobacco Use in Mental Health and Addictive Disorders. *Canadian Journal of Psychiatry-Revue Canadienne De Psychiatrie, 54*(6), 356-367.

Morrell, H. E. R., Cohen, L. M., & McChargue, D. E. (2010). Depression vulnerability predicts cigarette smoking among college students: Gender and negative reinforcement expectancies as contributing factors. *Addictive Behaviors, 35*(6), 607-611. doi: 10.1016/j.addbeh.2010.02.011

Munafò, M. R., & Araya, R. (2010). Cigarette smoking and depression: a question of causation. *The British Journal of Psychiatry, 196*(6), 425-426. doi: 10.1192/bjp.bp.109.074880

Munafò, M. R., Hitsman, B., Rende, R., Metcalfe, C., & Niaura, R. (2008). Effects of progression to cigarette smoking on depressed mood in adolescents: evidence from the National Longitudinal Study of Adolescent Health. *Addiction, 103*(1), 162-171.

Mykletun, A., Overland, S., Aaro, L. E., Liabo, H. M., & Stewart, R. (2008). Smoking in relation to anxiety and depression: Evidence from a large population survey: The HUNT study. *European Psychiatry, 23*(2), 77-84. doi: 10.1016/j.eurpsy.2007.10.005

Nezami, E., Unger, J., Tan, S., Mahaffey, C., Ritt-Olson, A., Sussman, S., . . . Johnson, C. A. (2005). The influence of depressive symptoms on experimental smoking and intention to smoke in a diverse youth sample. *Nicotine & Tobacco Research: Official Journal Of The Society For Research On Nicotine And Tobacco, 7*(2), 243-248.

Noland, M. P., Kryscio, R. J., Riggs, R. S., Linville, L. H., Ford, V. Y., & Tucker, T. C. (1998). The Effectiveness of a Tobacco Prevention Program With Adolescents Living in a Tobacco-Producing Region. *American Journal of Public Health, 88*(12), 1862-1865.

Obando, P., Kliewer, W., Murrelle, L., & Svikis, D. S. (2004). The comorbidity of substance abuse and depressive symptoms in Costa Rican adolescents. *Drug And Alcohol Dependence, 76*(1), 37-44.

Oesterle, S. (2008). Positive functioning and alcohol-use disorders from adolescence to young adulthood. *Journal of Studies on Alcohol and Drugs, 69*(1), 100-111.

OSU, O. S. U. (2007). National Longitudinal Study of Youth 1997. In C. f. H. R. Research (Ed.). Ann Arbor, MI: Inter-university Consortium for Political and Social Research.

Patton, G. C., Carlin, J. B., Coffey, C., Wolfe, R., Hibbert, M., & Bowes, G. (1998). Depression, anxiety, and smoking initiation: A prospective study over 3 years. *American Journal of Public Health, 88*(10), 1518-1522. doi: 10.2105/ajph.88.10.1518

Pomerleau, O. F., & Pomerleau, C. S. (1984). Neuroregulators and the reinforcement of smoking: towards a biobehavioral explanation. *Neuroscience And Biobehavioral Reviews, 8*(4), 503-513.

Prokhorov, A. V., Kelder, S. H., Shegog, R., Conroy, J. L., Murray, N., Peters, R., . . . Ford, K. H. (2010). Project ASPIRE: An Interactive, Multimedia Smoking Prevention and Cessation Curriculum for Culturally Diverse High School Students. *Substance Use & Misuse, 45*(6), 983-1006. doi: 10.3109/10826080903038050

Rodríguez-Esquivel, D., Cooper, T. V., Blow, J., & Resor, M. R. (2009). Characteristics associated with smoking in a Hispanic sample. *Addictive Behaviors, 34*(6/7), 593-598. doi: 10.1016/j.addbeh.2009.03.030

Rohde, P., Lewinsohn, P. M., Brown, R. A., Gau, J. M., & Kahler, C. W. (2003). Psychiatric disorders, familial factors and cigarette smoking: I. Associations with smoking initiation. *Nicotine & Tobacco Research, 5*(1), 85-98. doi: 10.1080/1462220031000070507

SAMHSA, S. A. a. M. H. S. A. (2009). National Survey on Drug Use and Health. Rockville, MD: Office of Applies Studies.

Sheehan, D. V., Lecrubier, Y., Sheehan, K. H., Amorim, P., Janavs, J., Weiller, E., . . . Dunbar, G. C. (1998). The Mini-International Neuropsychiatric Interview (M.I.N.I.): the development and validation of a structured diagnostic psychiatric interview for DSM-IV and ICD-10. *The Journal Of Clinical Psychiatry, 59 Suppl 20*, 22-33.

Steuber, T. L., & Danner, F. (2006). Adolescent smoking and depression: Which comes first? *Addictive Behaviors, 31*(1), 133-136. doi: 10.1016/j.addbeh.2005.04.010

Stevens, S. L., Colwell, B., Smith, D. W., Robinson, J., & McMillan, C. (2005). An exploration of self-reported negative affect by adolescents as a reason for smoking: implications for tobacco prevention and intervention programs. *Preventive Medicine, 41*(2), 589-596. doi: 10.1016/j.ypmed.2004.11.028

Study, S. L. (2011). Welcome, from www.umich.edu/~slsgroup/Santiago_Longitudinal_Study/Welcome.html

Vittetoe, K., Lopez, M. F., Delva, J., Wagner, F., & Anthony, J. C. (2002). Behavioral problems and tobacco use among adolescents in Central America and the Dominican Republic. *Revista Panamericana De Salud Pública = Pan American Journal Of Public Health, 11*(2), 76-82.

Voorhees, C. C., Schreiber, G. B., Schumann, B. C., Biro, F., & Crawford, P. B. (2002). Early Predictors of Daily Smoking in Young Women: The National Heart, Lung, and Blood Institute Growth and Health Study. *Preventive Medicine, 34*(6), 616-624. doi: 10.1006/pmed.2002.1026

Weiss, J. W., Mouttapa, M., Cen, S., Johnson, C. A., & Unger, J. (2011). Longitudinal Effects of Hostility, Depression, and Bullying on Adolescent Smoking Initiation. *Journal of Adolescent Health, 48*(6), 591-596. doi: 10.1016/j.jadohealth.2010.09.012

Whitbeck, L. B., Yu, M., McChargue, D. E., & Crawford, D. M. (2009). Depressive symptoms, gender, and growth in cigarette smoking among indigenous adolescents. *Addictive Behaviors, 34*(5), 421-426.

WHO. (2004). Prevalence, Severity, and Unmet Need for Treatment of Mental Disorders in the World Health Organization World Mental Health Surveys. *JAMA: The Journal of the American Medical Association, 291*(21), 2581-2590. doi: 10.1001/jama.291.21.2581

WHO. (2009). Global health risks: Mortality and burden of disease attributable to selected major risks. Geneva, Switzerland: World Health Organization.

Wu, L. T., & Anthony, J. C. (1999). Tobacco smoking and depressed mood in late childhood and early adolescence. *Am J Public Health, 89*(12), 1837-1840. doi: 10.2105/ajph.89.12.1837

11

Violence in the Nursing Homes: Understandings, Management, Documentation and Impact of Resident to Resident Aggression

Stephen Soreff
President, Education Initiatives
USA

1. Introduction

There has been a growing recognition of resident-to-resident aggression (RRA) in long term care facilities. This article reviews these concerns for this and looks at the events themselves. It explores the reasons for its current attention, delineates the types of RRA and examines dynamics of both the resident aggressor and the resident victim. It discusses ways to prevent RRA and interventions during these incidents. It outlines ways to review the RRA event after it has occurred. It highlights required documentation and evaluates the impact of such aggression on the quality of life for all nursing facility residents and staff.

2. RRA Scenario

Bob "Bull" Jones, age 79 strolls into the dining area and is about to sit in his usual seat. However, Dan Walker age 85 with moderate dementia of the Alzheimer Type is already at the table in Bob's chair. Dan yells "I was here first". Bob shoves him hard and says, "It's my chair". Staff quickly separates the two and each will have his meal in his room. Most of the other residents in the dinning are upset; some leave; others eat less than they would have had the incident not occurred; and still seem obvious to the event. Staff will have a mountain of reports to file and many family members to contact.

3. Background

3.1 Reports of RRA incidents

The statistics of resident-to resident violence are striking and the incidents are growing. "RRA is a ubiquitous phenomenon in nursing home settings with important consequences for affected individuals and facilities." (Rosen et al 2008, pp 1398) "Resident to resident injuries are on the rise in health care facilities. In fact, a nursing home resident has a 1-in-400 chance of being injured by another resident. " (Prevention, 2011) For example, one study over a two week period in a long-term care facility, noted that 2.4% of the residents said that they had been victims of physical aggression by another resident and 7.3% reported being victims of verbal aggression. (Cornell University, 2011) Another investigation looked at occurrence RRA for one eight hour shift. Here, twelve nurses acting as observers witnessed

30 RRA events of which 17 were physical. (Cornell University, 2011) The world wide press has drawn attention to RRA. In 2000, Manhattan woman was suffocated by her 90-year-old roommate in a New York City Long term care facility. (Zambito, 2000) " Residents of New York City nursing homes have been killed, sexually assaulted and beaten by unlikely assailants in the past few years, their fellow residents" (Zambito, 2000) And in 2009 "Fear in nursing Homes: Assault claims soar" as Packham reported in an Australian newspaper "Violence and sexual assaults against the elderly are increasing, according to new figures. More than 1400 assault allegations were made by nursing-home residents in the past fiscal year -- a record, and a 52 per cent rise on the previous year's figures." (Packham, 2009 page 22)

There has been a history of reports in both the nursing facilities' literature and the press about this phenomenon. (Cohen-Mansfield et al, 1990, Packham, 2009, Zambito, 2000) In 1990, Cohen-Mansfield noted that of all the victims of resident physical aggression, 62% were other Residents, 37%, staff and 1% , visitors. (Cohen-Mansfield et al , 1990). However, it was the article by Shinoda –Tagawa in the JAMA *"Resident-to-Resident Violent Incidents in Nursing Homes"* that galvanized attention to RRA. (Shinoda-Tagawa et al 2004). These authors looked at an 1132 initial reports from nursing facilities in 2000 in Massachusetts of resident- to- resident violence. They refined this number ultimately 294 cases in which the resident victim had demonstrated physical evidence of the attack. The injuries included 39 fractures, 6 dislocations, 105 bruises,113 lacerations and 31 redden region. Still more recently, the works of Rosen and his colleagues that have drawn attention to RRA. (Rosen et al, 2010 and 2008)

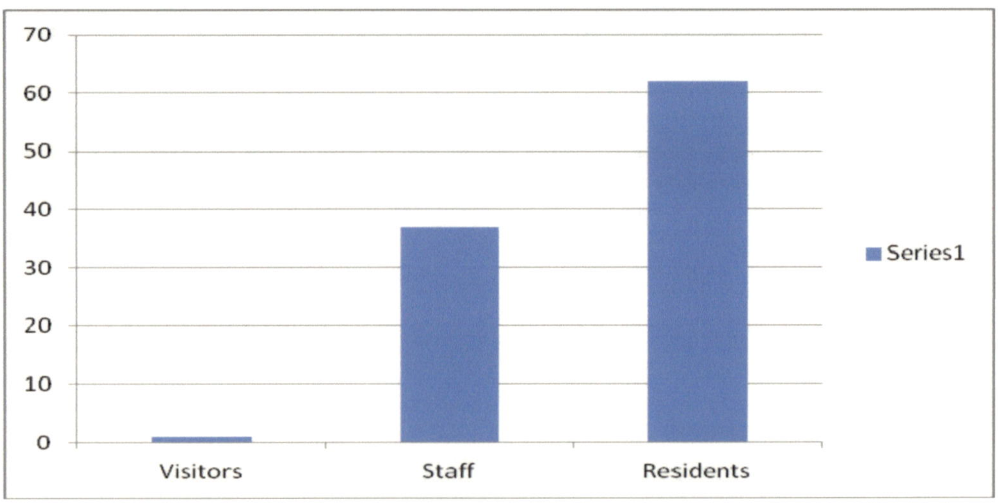

Fig. 1. Who are the victims of Resident Aggression (Cohen-Mansfield et al , 1990).

This author having consulted to long-term care facilities for over a decade has found that staff were much more attentive and more concerned about resident aggression toward staff than RRA. In discussions and training sessions with line staff in over one hundred nursing homes, when asked who is the greatest victim of resident aggression, their answer was staff. When this author cited the work of Cohen-Mansfield, nurses aids, nurses and hospital administrators expressed surprise about the number of RRA incidents. (Cohen-Mansfield et al , 1990) The statistics made them look more for carefully at resident to resident aggressive interactions.

One way to verify that number of RRA in a long term care facility is to have a hidden camera in the day room. (Sifford KS, Bharucha A, 2010) Without the presence of staff, many RRA events were recorded. These were incidents of verbal and physical aggression. Those videoed observations showed pushing, bullying and uninvited touching.

3.2 Reasons for the growing attention to RRA

There is an emerging concern about RRA and there are a number of reasons for this attention. The growing reports of RRA incidents have generated more awareness and the need for focus on them. The series of cited studies in the background have provided key statistical information as to the number of incidents. These incidents in turn have brought attention to the phenomenon. Perhaps, nursing facilities are dealing better with resident -to-staff aggression which allows them to look more on these events. Maybe staff is simply becoming aware of these disruptions. Certainly, more patients with psychiatric histories are becoming residents of nursing homes rather than being in state hospitals. Then, there is the aging Viet Nam veteran population who are starting to enter nursing facilities. Many of them have a Post Traumatic Stress Disorder (PTSD) which can be accompanied by aggressive behavior. The number of residents with dementia especially of the Alzheimer's type are increasing in nursing homes. (Isaksson U, 2011) In fact, that person with dementia living in the community may have become aggressive due to the cognitive deficiency. That aggressive episode led to that person's admission to a nursing home. Finally, residents' unmet needs can result in RRA. (Sifford, 2010)

Accrediting and government surveying agencies are paying more attention to RRA. For example, Massachusetts Department of Public Health using Complaint and Incident Reporting System had been accumulating data for years. It was through the analysis by Shinoda-Tagawa that that data on RRA caught clinical and public attention. (Shinoda-Tagawa et al 2004). Legal concerns and litigation websites have also contributed to RRA awareness. (A-nursing-home-abuse, 2011) Finally, a number well publicized of homicides as a result of RRA have caught the public's attention. (Zambito, 2000)

4. Types of RRA

The nature of the resident to resident aggression takes three forms: verbal, physical assaults and sexual advances. Rosen and colleagues have delineated 35 types of violence. (Rosen et al , 2008) Furthermore, physical and sexual violence are not necessarily mutually exclusive. There are a wide variety of types of physical attacks ranging from a shove to homicidal attack, from slap to a protracted punching episode and from pushing someone out of the way to pushing someone down a stair way. Similarly sexual violations range from a brief fondling to rape. (Rosen et al, 2010) This paper focuses on physical encounters. It should be remembered that the actual aggression spectrum ranges from yelling, verbal assaults, offensive gestures, pinching, throwing objects, hitting, punching, assaults to homicide . (Soreff & Siddle, 2003)

5. Understanding RRA: The residents- assaulters, their victims, the staff and the environment

There are four key aspects in looking at resident-to-resident aggression: resident who assaulted another resident, the assaulted resident, the staff and the unit's environment.

5.1 The assaulter

What are the defining features of an assaulting resident? There are a number of cognitive issues, personality characteristics, family dynamics, background events, medical illnesses, mental health histories, and nursing home situations which provide clues and explanations for the assaults. Although I will discuss each of these qualities, individuals often have more than one. And commonly, the two or more may interact synergistically. For example, a resident with dementia of the Alzheimer's type may also have a history of being impulsive and was a pugilist (boxer). That combination can result in an individual who is at risk to strike out at other residents.

5.1.1 Cognitive deficiencies

Rosen and colleagues noted that between 80% to 90 %residents in nursing homes have an incidence of cognitive impairment and that disorder leads to behavioral disruptions and aggression. (Rosen, 2008) The question now becomes how do cognitive deficiencies result in RRA. Let us first, review so of the features of cognitive difficulties. These include memories problems, orientation issues and loss of judgment. Cognitive impairment often takes the form of dementia. The most commonly encountered dementia in nursing facilities' population are those of the Alzheimer's type.

5.1.1.1 Memory difficulties

Memory difficulties would be evidenced by not recalling events. Often, residents early in their dementia history would exhibit an inability to recall recent events; e.g. what they had had for breakfast later in the day. Meanwhile, they would have preserved their long term memory. As a result, these persons might keep repeating stories of their youth without appreciating how annoying these adventures are to others hearing them for the thousandth time. As the dementia progressed they would lose distant collections. Recent memory loss becomes distressful to those experiencing it. They in turn may become agitated and then aggressive. For example, one resident 86 year old Bill M has loss of recent memory. He was bothered by this and slightly depressed. He kept asking others what he had for breakfast. They became infuriated with him; he became inpatient with them. One afternoon he shoved another resident who refused to answer Bill 's one thousandth inquiry about his breakfast.

Recent recollection loss can result in RRA incident in other way. In this scenario example, Mary W age 79 years old has middle stage Alzheimer's. She places her eye glasses in her dresser top draw in the morning after breakfast. Later that day when she cannot remember where her glasses are, she accuses her roommate Betty K age 86 of stealing them. Betty protests. Mary insists that thief has occurred and she has been robbed. Before staff can intervene she pushes Betty into a chair. In this dynamic, the resident compensates for the memory loss by blaming others and making accusations. In turn, this led to an RRA situation.

5.1.1.2 Orientation issues

Residents with dementia have orientation problems. Orientation can be evaluated in three dimensions: time, place and person. As the dementia progresses the first to go is sense of time: time of day, day of the week, month, and year. The next area to have problems with is the sense of place. The residents do not where they are. Questions like what is your room number , the facility's address, and your state's name will reveal problems here. Finally in severe dementia, the residents lose their sense of who they are. Some will not recall their names.

Orientation loss leads to RRA in several ways. In one scenario the residents wanders into other residents' room believing it is their and altercations ensue. In another instance, for example, Sam H age 78 years old wakes from a nightmares in which he believes he is in jail. He does not recognize his room or roommate. He becomes combative as he demands his freedom.

5.1.1.3 Loss of judgment

Dementia erodes judgment. Residents with dementia at an earlier point in their lives, knew that waiting in line is part of life. Historically, they would patiently stand in line for medications or in a much earlier time they were used to grocery store check-out lines. So with dementia they now become pushing and striking out, when waiting in lines at the nursing home.

5.1.1.4 Problems with executive functions

Dementia robs residents of their executive functions. Remember the old slogan: engage mind before putting mouth in gear. Before dementia they used to know there was a time and place for things. For example, Walter K age 74 years old had evidence of middle stage of Alzheimer's. He had led a privileged life with a nanny and his family had other live-in help. However, as an owner of local Southern five and dime store he had learned to keep his prejudices to himself and his close friends. As he aged and his executive functions slipped, he began to tell everyone exactly what he thought of them. In called several of the African-American nursing aids *slaves.* He did not limit his opinions to just staff. He regularly insulted other residents. He called one woman out for being too fat. He then questioned her birth and heritage. His insults resulted in many heated discussions at that nursing home and one RRA event.

5.1.2 Personality elements and gender issues

Many authors have attributed RRA to the initiator's personality. (Cohen-Mansfield et al , 1990; Enmarker et al, 2011; Soreff & Siddle, 2003,) Enmarker et al in the landmark article, *Management of person with dementia with aggressive and violent behaviour: a systematic literature review* wrote "The results could be summarized in two themes: 'origins that may trigger violence' and 'activities that decrease the amount of violent behaviour'. Together, the themes showed that violence was a phenomenon that could be described as being connected to a premorbid personality ..."(Enmarker et al, 2011, pp. 153) A study of nursing assistants stated "Findings gained from semi-structured interviews revealed that CNAs perceive initiators of RRA to be 'more with it' and to have 'strong personalities', a 'short fuse' and 'life history' that make them prone to inflict harm on other residents." (Sifford-Snellgrove,

2011, pp 1) And although the majority of residents in many nursing homes are women, often it is males who are most of the RRA instigators.

What are the personalities related to RRA? They include the following characteristics: impulsiveness, a controlling posture, angry, aggressiveness, inflexibility, quarrelsomeness, jealousy, demanding, bullying, and impatience. It is easy to envision these qualities resulting a resident who might engage in RRA. Joe M age 72 years liked to describe himself at a demanding S.O.B. who always got things done quickly. His theme song was Frank Sinatra's *"I did my way"*. He regularly fought with other residents in the day room over which television show was to be watched. On more than one occasion he pushed others out of the way so he could see his baseball game.

One particular personality pattern associated with residents becoming aggressive is paranoia. The residents see or feel that others are arrayed against them. They view others are plotting against them and wanting to take things from them. They look at their environment as harmful and threatening. They are always on guard. They believe others getting more attention or privileges than they have. In turn, their persecutory view of the view may indeed provoke others to be distant and distrustful of them. For example, Jerry G age 77 years old believed others get better care and food than he did. He saw unit rules as deliberating designed to make him miserable. Finally, he dumped all his food on his table mate's lap, proclaiming that his portions were smaller than all the other residents.

5.1.3 Intrapersonal dynamics

In understanding RRA there are two interconnected senses and one defense mechanism which can be responsible for a resident striking out. The two inter-related attitudes are the sense of loss and the feeling of dependency. The defense mechanism is displacement.

5.1.3.1 Sense of loss

Let us first look at residents' sense of loss as a possible trigger for RRA. Long term care facilities serve a vital component in the continuum of geriatric care. Yet, to enter such an institution, regardless of the needs it serves and the importance of the care it provides, many residents feel a sense of loss. Imagine condensing your life's possessions into one room. And that resident may be sharing that room with a person who is initially a stranger. Furthermore, this is for people who up until their nursing home admission, had been living on their own, making all their daily decisions and arranging their own affairs. Often, the residents have a sense of loss which can result in the feelings depression or anger or both. Some people react aggressively in response to this sense of loss when they are first admitted. Sarah H age 79 years old resented her family placing her in a nursing home. She stroke out at anyone who attempted to placate her.

5.1.3.2 Loss of independence

Not only do residents give up their homes upon entering a long-term care facility, they also must accept a level of dependency. In the United States, independence is a valued quality and highly prized. The American state of New Hampshire has as its motto, "Live free or Die". Iconoclastic figures; such as John Wayne in the movies displays a national pride in being and maintaining autonomy. Nursing homes by their very nature require a degree of dependency. And as with the sense of loss, residents may rebel against curtailment of freedoms with belligerent behavior toward staff and other residents.

5.1.3.3 Displacement

Displacement is the classic psychological mechanism where one person (person A) is frustrated or angry at one individual (person B). But instead of telling B one's feelings, that individual transfers them to a third person (person C). The common example involves you being annoyed and irritated at your boss. However, you are not secure in your employment status; you dare not voice disapproval. Instead, you go home and yell at the family dog. The displacement means taking it from one object and putting on another. This displacement frequently happens when the object of anger is someone in authority ; .e.g. a police officer, physician or a teacher. Let us connect this to nursing homes . Staff do have authority over residents. And yes, on occasion staff can mistreat residents. (Natan, 2010). However, the resident is still dependent on that staff. For example, Sally K age 85 years old has just been refused a p.r.n.(as needed and asked for) medication for her headache by a nurse. She is very annoyed at the staff nurse but also likes her and does not want to be seen as a complainer. On the way back from the nursing station, after the nurse has been again told Her that she cannot have that medication, she kicks Heather T's wheelchair. This is a classic example of displacement resulting in a RRA incident.

5.1.4 Interpersonal interplays

Of all the thus far discussed causes, interpersonal relationships leading to a physical altercation is the easiest to comprehend and perhaps prevent. Nursing homes represent in the words of Goffman a total institution. (Goffman, 1961) That means residents sleep, play and work in the same place. Residents live there. Living together can promote great friendships and also create protracted conflicts. Their daily interactions can lead to antagonist relationships. Little idiosyncrasies over days and weeks can be wearing on others. For example, William T age 77 years old liked to command attention at meals and enjoyed 'guiding' the table conservations. Over time he became very annoyed with Victor L's age 81 years old cracking his knuckles at the table. At lunch one day William slapped Victor's hand. Staff quickly separated the two.

The same interpersonal bond or antagonism can develop between roommates. In this situation the interaction is much more intensified. Because of this roommate dynamic, their interaction is much more heightened and prolonged. It is not just sporadic or at meal times; it is all day and night. Again that type of sustained, seemingly relentless interaction can magnify differences and disputes. Most acts of RRA are either in the victim's room or in the hallway. (Shinoda-Tagawa et al 2004) The roommate interpersonal conflict may account for that observation of the resident's room as the site of RRA.

5.1.5 Biographical contributions

Residents' past life can finish clues as to their present behavior and potential for RRA. Although it may occur in many ways, let us focus on two particular life experiences: family dynamics and prior profession.

5.1.5.1 Family dynamics

5.1.5.1.1 Birth order

One's place in the family can often be viewed as determent of certain life-long characteristics. (birth order, 2011) The only child may be self-centered and have difficulty sharing. The oldest child may become bossy and demanding. The middle child get lost in the family and the youngest is 'the baby' and feels inferior. Although these are stereotypes and there are many exceptions, others have found some validity to this concept. So certain residents may carry this birth order baggage into their new surroundings. For example, Paula P age 77 years old was the oldest of seven children. Since both her parents worked she was the 'family boss". She was in charge when the parents were not around. She carried this mantle into her marriage and into all of her activities. In the nursing home she often told other residents what to do. One day pulled too hard on her roommates blouse when her roomie refused to pick up some paper from the floor.

5.1.5.1.2 Nuclear family position

The nuclear family usually consists of the mother, the father and the children. If there is an extended family there can be also be grandparents and therefore grand children too. In some families these positions can carry certain roles and responsibilities. In the great musical *Fiddler on the Roof*, there is one song featuring ideas: "*I'm the papa*" and "*I'm the mama*". Some residents carry these roles in their long-term care environment. So as the father or the mother they excrete their roles on other residents and perhaps initiating an RRA incident.

5.1.5.2 Previous career

The potential for RRA can be found in the assaulter professional background. Certain jobs carry with them authority, power and prestige. It is often hard for those individuals to relinquish the controls built-in to their prior occupations. Although not limited to this list some of the jobs that come to mind include the following: physicians, people of the cloth, those in law enforcement, teachers, judges, top executives , military officers and lawyers. They were used to commanding immediate attention and people following their orders. In the setting of a nursing home those commands often go unheeded. One resident, a retired army general. George P age 77 years old even into his 'golden years' wanted everyone to call him the "the General" and if he could, he would love to have people salute him. One day another resident wanders into his path; he pushed him aside and announced "the General" coming through.

5.1.6 Medical problems

Medical problems especially those unrecognized by the resident and the staff can play a big part of RRA. Here is where the convergence of a cognitive deficient and a physical problem meet. Often, if the residents were unaware of the condition, they therefore cannot alert staff to the issue. An acute medical disorder such as a urinary tract infection (UTI) or even constipation can move that person to aggression. One resident with Alzheimer's developed pneumonia. Her response to lung insult was to hit another resident. Once her infection was treated with an antibiotic, she was no longer violent.

5.1.7 Pain

There is a close connection between the medical condition called pain and RRA. (Leone, 2 009) As Leone and associates noted, "Many SNF [Skilled Nursing Facility} and NH [Nursing

Home] have not adopted a uniform plan to assess and treat pain for their residents despite published literature that demonstrates that the implementation of scales improves detection and treatment of pain." (Leone, 2009, pp 67) The source of the pain could come after either an acute or chronic medical illness. Again, if the residents had full cognition often they would complain staff and hopefully get relief. Instead, aggression becomes the manifestation of that discomfort. Grammy Nancy J age 69 years old used to love to knit. As arthritis of her hands not only curtailed her knitting but also became a huge source of her pain. She liked to see herself as a bit of a stoic but when her pain flared so did her temper and she shoved her friend aside. Attention and proper treatment of residents' pains can forestall aggression results. (Leone et al 2009)

5.1.8 Mental disorders

Many residents in nursing homes have mental illnesses and in some cases that disorder can contribute to RRA. There has been a general increase of residents with both mental illnesses and dementia in the last decade and especially those with depression. (Fullerton et al 2009)As in the area of a medical condition, treating the mental illness may decrease the RRA. These residents with mental illnesses can experience their symptoms heightened if they also have cognitive difficulties. For example, a resident with both an anxiety disorder such General Anxiety Disorder (GAD) and Alzheimer's' may experiences more episodes of uncontrollable fear , apprehension and terror than if that person only had dementia. Bagchi and associates have noted "The NNHS [National Nursing Home Survey], produced the most valid national-level estimates of residents with a mental illness--nearly 102,000 with a primary diagnosis in 2004 (6.8% of residents), of which about 23,000 were under age 65 and 79,000 were aged 65 and older."(Bagchi et al, 2009 pp. 958)

Rather than review of all mental illnesses that residents may have, let us look at several serious and persistent mental disorders and show how each might contribute to RRA. These are Bipolar Disorder, Major Depression, Schizophrenia, Posttraumatic Stress Disorder (PTSD) and Generalized Anxiety Disorder (GAD).

5.1.8.1 Bipolar disorder

Bipolar Disorder also known as Manic-Depressive Disorder has as its dominant feature extreme mood swings over time from periods of severe, debilitating, profound depression and then times of super-energy, high productivity, distractibility, and not sleeping called mania. (DSM IV, 2000) The section on Major Depression will address the RRA aspects of the depressed phase; here the focus is on mania. It can be very destructive in terms of the resident's behavior. The grandiosity of mania can involve delusions of elevated self worth and self-power. Some persons in manic phase have thoughts that they have great power and proclaimed to themselves to be a deities, presidents or kings or queens.. It is accompanied by agitated, sleeplessness and irritability. John H age 67 years old had a life-long history of Bipolar Disorder. When he stopped taking his mood stabilizing medication, in this case Lithium he would become high. As he mood increased so did he sense of his power and this was accompanied by demands of people literally bow down for him. When another resident refused this gesture, John struck him. Later after a brief psychiatric hospitalization, he returned to the nursing home on the proper dose of medication and apologized to the other resident.

5.1.8.2 Major depression

The **5.1.3 Intrapersonal dynamics** section looked at the sense of loss and loss of dependence as mental situations which cause the resident to feel sad. Here the focus is on a clinical depression. Depression is commonly encountered within the nursing home residents. (Fullerton et al 2009) Furthermore, the incidence of depression within the nursing home population has been increasing. (Lemke SP, Schaefer JA, 2010) A Major Depression is often similar in features to the depressed phase of the Bipolar Disorder. Both are characterized by loss of appetite, weight loss, sleep difficulty, thoughts of death, inability to function, suicidal ideation and loss of concentration. In the feelings of despair and futility they may strike at others residents. Again, the treatment of the depression with antidepressants can decisive.

5.1.8.3 Schizophrenia

Like Bipolar Disorder, schizophrenia represents a life-long illness. It is marked by hallucinations and delusions. The hallucinations can include hearing voices. In certain cases the hallucinations can take the form of commands telling the resident to hurt themselves or others. Delusions are false beliefs often of the persecutory type such as that FBI or the KGB are after them. Hallucinations and delusions can lead to RRA. For example, Beatrice K age 77 years of age had a life-long history of schizophrenia and many psychiatric hospitalizations . When she was off her medications delusions others plotting to harm her or take sexual advance of her emerged. One night she thought her roommate was going to attack her so she slapped her and ran from the room. As a result of her attack, she was committed to local psychiatric unit. Once her anti-psychotic medication regime was re-instated , her delusions decreased.

5.1.8.4 Posttraumatic Stress Disorder (PTSD)

In PTSD the resident carries within one's self often for a lifetime the residue of a traumatic event. The incident could be a violent attack, a sexual assault as a child or as an adult, combat, the Holocaust, 9-11, an earthquake or a bad accident. The traumatic event could have been short lived or prolonged. The residents would have had experiences in which their lives were endangered. There are three major categories of symptoms: re-experiencing, avoidance and hyperarousal. (DSMIV 2009) Any one of these three types of reactions can result in RRA. In the first the resident relives often seeming in real time the dreadful episode. This vivid recollection is a flashback. Suddenly, they are re-experiencing it in the present moment. A loud noise might lead one to believe he is combat again. Nightmares reflect a method of re-experiencing the traumatic event and can be very disturbing. In avoidance some residents will isolate themselves. With hyper vigilance the resident is always on heightened alert ; they are perceiving danger at any time. For many veterans of Vet Nam the war still rages in the minds and when in a nursing home it can continue to play out there. For example, Al G age 65 years of old, a combat veteran of Southeast Asia, kept having flashbacks and nightmares. In one flashback triggered by a flash of lightning, he suddenly threw three other residents out of the way as he ran for cover.

5.1.8.5 Generalized Anxiety Disorder (GAD)

What is the difference between fear and anxiety? In fear you know the danger and have the sensations and emotions of arousal. In anxiety you are on edge and anxious without any identifiable source. This is very distressing. Residents with prolonged, protracted anxiety find themselves literately grabbing on to other residents and clinging on to them. This might perceived as the other resident as an assault.

5.1.9 Substance abuse

Substance abuse either in current usage or in the past occurs within the nursing home population and can result in RRA in several ways. According to an investigation of 368 residents in France long- term facilities, the researchers found "The study confirms that the prevalence of chronic at risk consumption is high in nursing homes" (Leurs et al, 2010,pp 280). The first way involves a long history alcohol use resulting in dementia. In turn, that dementia as outlived in the 5.1.1 Cognitive deficiencies can lead to RRA. A second mechanism usually occurs with newly admitted residents with unrecognized alcohol or other substance problems. In these instances the resident undergoes withdrawal. For some withdrawal can usher in combative behavior.

The third situation happens when the resident becomes acutely intoxicated with alcohol. On face value this seems unlikely. But it does occur. In one scenario the family may take the resident out for a celebration usually for a birthday. While away, the resident drinks too much and returns intoxicated. Another example happened with Bill W age 55 years of age. He had a history of drinking before entering the facility and had been admitted because of several severe medical problems. His room was on the first floor and the nursing home was located in moderate sized city. Not infrequently Bill would slip out of his room's window and go to a nearby pub. On one of his forays into town he consumed more whiskey than his usual amount. He returned late at night drunk and belligerent. When his roommate attempted to comfort him, Bill pushed him over.

Each resident is unique; each nursing home is unique. However, the above review of causes of RRA provides a beginning to understanding the assaulter. It also offers clues as to prevention and intervention.

5.2 The three types of resident victims

5.2.1 The un-intentional victim

Often another resident unwittingly may become the object of an assault. This most frequently occurs when that other resident has dementia. (Shinoda-Tagawa et al 2004) Out of this cognitive deficient, that resident may unintentionally provoke another resident. This could happen if one resident wandered into another's room. The assault may see that action as an invasion of one's space and privacy and retaliate physically. Or that resident forgets one's seat in the dining area and innocently antagonize another resident by taking the other's chair as in the article's initial scenario. The victim may simply wanders into the path of an angry resident. It is not uncommon that two residents with dementia through mutual misunderstandings may precipitate a physical altercation.

5.2.2 The provoking victim

Then there are residents who deliberately antagonize others. Living together over a protracted time can lead to close and supportive relationships between residents or as in this case result in bitter feuds. Imagine two frustrated, annoyed, and disgusted residents arguing about some small item leading a physical fight.

5.2.3 The bystander victim

Finally, some residents are simply innocent by-standers. Sadly, this could be called 'being in the wrong place at the wrong time'. A belligerent resident strikes out at any one whom he happens to pass in the hallway that day. Kevin J age 75 years of age was enraged at being 'there' in the nursing home. He hated the food and wanted to just go out and have beer. He charged down the too narrow corridor knocking over any staff and residents in his path.

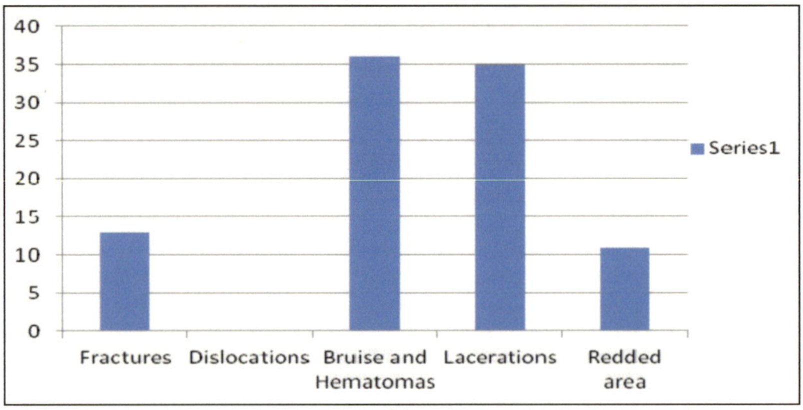

(a)

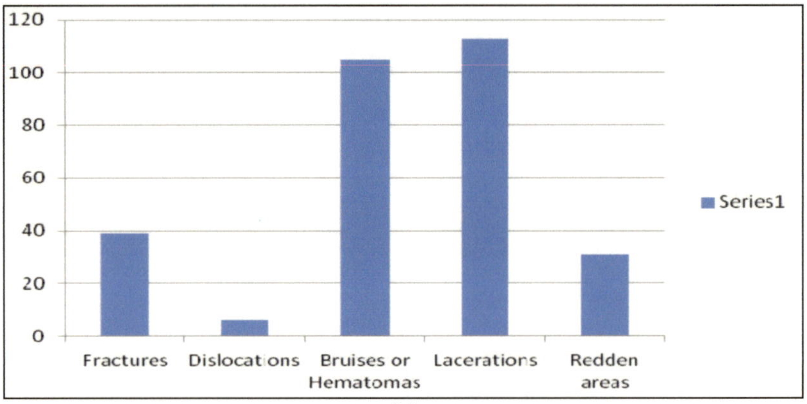

(b)

Results During the first incident, 294 residents sustained fractures (n = 39), dislocations (n = 6), bruises or hematomas (n = 105), lacerations (n = 113), and reddened areas (n = 31).
Graphs from data provided by Shinoda-Tagawa, T., Leonard, R., Pontikas, J., McDonough, JE., Allen, A., Dreyer, PI, *Resident-to-Resident Violent Incidents in Nursing Homes JAMA* 291:591-598. Feb. 2004.

Fig. 2. Resident-to-resident violent incidents in nursing homes: injuries to the victim: (a) by percentages, (b) by number of types of injuries to the resident victim.

5.3 The staff

Although not the focus of this chapter, staff can contribute to RRA in a number of ways. Insufficient numbers of clinical staff, in general and specifically nursing aides can result in residents' needs not being fully attended to. As a consequence, a resident feels neglected.

(Sifford, 2011) In turn, the annoyed resident can displace one's frustration on another resident as outlined in 5.1.3. 3 Displacement. In some facilities, many of the staff have as their first language one that is different than the residents. This results in communication problems and agitation leading to RRA. For example, Sara B age 79 years old was in a long-term facility where many of the aides spoke primarily Spanish. She had cognitive impairment and her language was English. She told her family that she was in a Mexican hospital. Out of her miss perception and frustrations, she struck out at her roommate.

5.4 Environmental contributions

Lastly, the environment itself can contribute to the aggressive episode in several ways.

5.4.1 Too stimulating

The milieu may be too stimulating, confusing, and hectic. Crowdedness especially in certain areas such as the nursing station, dining room or day room can produce a noisy, disrupting and discomforting situation. These circumstances challenge residents especially if they have cognitive deficient. Certain television programs which are too loud and violent can be instigators as well as radio stations featuring music which appeals to a younger generation. The time of day can be a factor with early morning with the transition from sleep to activity being a particularly aggressive period in many facilities.

5.4.2 Architectural contribution

Aspects of the architecture have been implicated. Too narrow hallways, too little area around the nurses' station and too constrained access to the elevator can contribute to RRA. In one unit had many residents who needed wheel chairs. This resulted combative behavior at the bottleneck of all of them trying to get into one small elevator. Location can play a role in that many assaults occur either in the resident victim's room or in the hallway. Shinoda-Tagawa et al 2004) Therefore, rooms where staff cannot watch what is occurring can contribute to RRA.

In one long-term care facility housed a large number of veterans in wheel chairs. The building was old and had just one slow elevator. Most of the residents lived on the first floor; the majority of their daily activities e.g. meals, recreation, crafts rooms and day room were on the second floor. As a result of this architecture residents fought for their place on the elevator. Daily they would ram others in wheel chairs striving to gain access to the elevator. Both staff and residents were aware of the situation, but solutions to that problem eluded them. Finally, low lighting can be a factor. Decreased lighting such as in the winter months coupled with visual difficulty can lead to *sun-downing*, agitation because of decreased sun light.

6. Prevention

The best way to manage RRA is to prevent it. The key to prevention is to understand the causes of RRA and then address them. That is the reason for the detailed review of possible etiologies.

First, let us review some of specific causes and methods to approach then. This will be followed by some general ideas to decrease RRA.

6.1 Specific indications

6.1.1 For the assaulter

6.1.1.1 Cognitive deficiencies

Residents with cognitive deficiencies not only are clinically challenging but also require approaches geared to their issues. They need more supervision and monitoring than other residents. Staff should have training focused on their problems. Care plans should incorporate interventions tailored to that resident's uniqueness as well as dementia care issues in general.

6.1.1.2 Sense of loss

As the sense of loss can be underlying RRA, so then methods to provide a sense of gain should be initiated. If going to the nursing home represents a loss, then being there can offer an opportunity to have a sense of place and achievement. Individualizing the residents' rooms and tailing activities can help. Provide residents with individualized activities and events such as a birthday party. Many residents overtime develop a sense of pride in their room and unit. Grammy Gail B age 87 years old welcomed visitors to her room. She had decorated it with pictures of her family and friends. She had her own sitting and entertaining area within it which she loved. Although protesting her family's decision to 'institutionalize' her, eventually she has come to see that facility and especially her room as her 'home'.

6.1.1.3 Loss of independence

Many residents see themselves as trapped and 'jailed' in a nursing home. They feel robbed of their autonomy. Perhaps, as they see it there is some reality to that perception. However, the more choices residents have the more they can feel in command of their lives. Whenever possible, the more decisions they can make, the better they may feel about their lives. Areas where they can make determinations include in their meals, daily schedule, activities, entertainment and visitors.

6.1.1.4 Address medical problems

A medical problem can be behind a RRA. Here early detection and treatment represent the keys to solving those issues. Regular medical, dental and podiatrist evaluations help. Charting of vital signs can offer clues in changes in their physical status. Once identified, medical issues must be addressed. Medical problems which cause discomfort and pain are the subject of the next prevention section.

6.1.1.5 Recognize and manage pain

Pain constitutes one of the cardinal determinants of RRA. Many authors have commented on this. "It was found that if the origin of violent actions was the residents' pain, it was possible to minimize it through nursing activities." (Enmarker et al, 2011, pp. 153) Using a system of charting pain can be very useful. Asking and then recording the residents' pain levels not only focuses staff attention to pain but also allows one to see it direction overtime. Many nursing homes use pain charts with illustrations or a series faces smiling ☺ to frowning ☹ for residents to identify their pain level. This is especially effective if the resident has cognitive deficits. By staff taking the initiative and asking residents about their pain level, the residents with dementia can have their discomfort recognized and treated.

6.1.1.6 Treat mental illness

Mental illness must be detected and treated. One of the great achievements of modern psychiatry has been its ability to provide treatment to patients with mental disorders. Psychiatry has ushered in an era of psychopharmacology. Historically, patients with mental illness were placed in large institutions with little hope of relief of their symptoms. Now there are specific medications for specific diagnoses. For residents with Major Depression, antidepressants are effective. Those residents with Bipolar Disorder, mood stabilizers such as Lithium have proved quite useful. For residents with schizophrenia a number of anti-psychotic medications that has proven valuable. Mental illnesses such a Bipolar Disorder and Schizophrenia are severe and persistent illnesses. (Soreff, 1996) They are life-long and therefore, they go with the resident into the nursing home . But they can and should be treated throughout the persons' life including in the long-term care facilities.

6.2 The victims

There are a number of ways to prevent other residents from being victims of an aggressive resident depending on the type of victim: un-intentional, provoking and bystander. In the first instance, the un-intended victim, the resident with cognitive deficits may wanders into the path of aggressive resident. The key here is to prevent that resident from being in the area of the assaulter. With the provoking resident, separation of the two antagonists remains the best way to avoid an altercation leading to RRA event. In the bystander situation, good practice involves keeping other residents away from an assaulting resident.

6.3 The staff

Staff and staffing remains the key ingredient in prevention. This means insuring an adjacent number of trained staff for the number of residents. Furthermore, administrators must develop and deploy nurse education programs on how to deal with residents with dementia. (Narevic et al 2011; Williams et al 2005) The formula is simple: the more the combative your resident population, the more personnel you need. But it not just numbers alone. Those doing direct care must be trained in understanding and dealing with resident aggression. (Soreff & Siddle, 2003)

6.4 Environment

Two facets of the environment prove key to decreasing RRA. The first is creating a comforting and safe milieu. The second encompasses architectural elements.

6.4.1 The milieu

The goal remains to create and maintain a not too stimulating, comforting and safe milieu. This can be accomplished in a number of ways. As noted deploy staff in appropriate numbers who have training to work with residents with dementia and deal with aggressive residents. Then control the noise in the building, the corridors and the day room. Make sure there is a system to monitor the television programming and the TV's volume. As will be discussed under general aspects, have ample recreational activities.

6.4.2 Architecture

Building design and unit arrangements can decrease RRA. As Shinoda-Tagawa and his colleagues have pointed out the resident victim's room was the site of the assault. Therefore, the residents' rooms if possible should be visible from the nursing station. (Shinoda-Tagawa et al 2004) Ideally, there would be a central nurse station from which all residents' rooms could be observed. Rooms farthest from that station stand at higher risk for incidents to occur. Additionally, attention must be paid to the roommate selection process.

The more lighting means less aggression. Dark areas and 'sunning downing' can promote aggression. One nursing home each day as evening comes on, simultaneously increase the hallway and day room lights. Eliminate congested areas at the nursing station and the elevator entrances. This can be done by limiting the number of residents served per station; e.g. 24 residents for each station can decrease the number of residents seeking help at that station. Since many of the assaulting residents have impulse control problems, having two elevators per unit minimizes the residents' waiting time. The two elevators were particularly effective when there were many residents in wheel chairs. Wide corridors promote easy passage through the unit and can decrease residents bumping into each other.

6.5 Documentation for prevention

As will be discussed in 10.0 Documentation, using the unit records of RRA can actually be used to decrease violence. By tracking aggressive episodes the facility can have a better idea of times and areas where the assaults occur. For example, if there are many incidents on weekends or on a certain unit, then they can deploy more staff then and there.

6.6 General approaches

Two general approaches to nursing home care can serve to decrease RRA and increase residents' satisfaction, improve their quality of life, promote their autonomy and challenge their sense of loss. The first are individualized treatment plans. The second is activity therapy.

6.6.1 Individualized therapy

"The optimal management of aggressive and violent actions from residents with dementia living in nursing homes was a person-centered approach to the resident." (Enmarker et al, 2011, pp. 153) Each resident must have a detailed and specific treatment plan. Each resident is unique and that plan must reflect that person's individual characteristics. This is where information about the resident's family, birth order, profession, interests, hobbies and fears can be complied. The more the care is tailored to the individual resident, the better the care and the less the RRA.

6.6.2 Activity therapy

"Activities that decrease the amount of violent behavior'." (Enmarker et al, 2011, pp. 153)Certain programs can help prevent aggressive episodes. Having residents engaged in unit activities and physical activities not only benefits the participants but also can remove the residents from a situation which an assault might have occurred. Through these activities the residents can regain their sense of independence and become creative. In one facility the activities were based in part on the residents' interests and hobbies. Life-long hobbies could finally be achieved.

Here is an example of a creative activity which decreased RRA. One unit developed an activity group for those residents who had gastronomy tubes and therefore they could not eat in the conventional way. For them, not being able to eat and having to mix with eating residents during meal times was stressful. Certain of these residents had been known to be disruptive when they saw other residents enjoying breakfast, lunch or supper. By those with gastronomies having their own group activity away from the dining area at meal times, the members felt less stressed and more satisfied and their number of RRA episodes decreased.

7. Interventions

The focus of these interventions is those conducted by staff within the facility. In some incidences police are involved. (Lachs et al, 2007) The intervention is two phased based upon whether the resident-to-resident violence is about occur or if it is actually in progress. The former is an extension of the prevention process while the latter involves halting the assault.

7.1 RRA is imminent

There are a number of de-escalation techniques which can often avert a pending resident-to-resident attack. These include redirection and fib-lets. A comprehensive knowledge of the residents proves invaluable. Here is another example of a prevention when RRA is imminent. In the situation of the provoking victim, if staff recognizes that two particularly antagonistic residents are about to be alone in the day room, they can act to separate them before there is an altercations.

7.1.1 Redirection

One key approach involves the redirection of the threatening resident. This technique can be especially effective if the resident has dementia. Molly S age 77 years old was getting herself very distraught over the way others with were behaving in the day room. She demanded that they all watch one particular television show. The other residents preferred a different program already in progress. A nurse's aide observing this build up of Molly emotions quietly went to her side and asked if she would like a cup of tea. Molly agreed and they went off together and the crisis was averted. Molly S through re-direction of her attention was diverted from the television show.

7.1.2 Fib-lets

Another method is the use of fib-lets or little white lies. This is designed for residents with dementia. By staff acknowledging the reality of the resident's perception, they can often calm one of them down. (Soreff 2003) In one nursing home, many of the residents used to work in a local mill. Their lives revolved around that factory's schedule. One resident Betsy

G age 87 year old had moderate cognitive impairment. She insisted every day at 4 PM she had to get the bus home to take care of her children. When staff had pointed out to her that she was not a worker anymore and that her children were adults, Betsy would hear none of it. She insisted that she must get the bus at 4 PM. Ultimately, they staff came up with an idea, they contact a local bus company and obtained a Bus Stop sign. They placed it next to a bench in the corridor. At 4 PM when Betsy clamored that she must get to the bus, a nurse's aide walked her over to the 'bus stop'. Within a few minutes Betsy had forgotten about getting home and moved on to another activity.

7.2 During RRA episode

Once a violent episode erupts swift, focused, decisive and firm intervention is required. This means immediately separating the two residents and moving all other residents from the area. Securing physical distance between the two residents is the top priority. Yet at the same time all other residents must be removed for the combat zone. The intervention must be a well orchestrated and coordinated team effort. Having many staff available and working in a directed, coordinated fashion can bring the combative behavior to a prompt conclusion. The assaulting resident must be removed from the area but also not be left alone.

The initial scenario illustrates many of these points. Bob "Bull" Jones, age 79 strolls into the dining area and is about to sit in his usual seat. However, Dan Walker age 85 with moderate dementia of the Alzheimer Type is already at the table in Bob's chair. Dan yells "I was here first". Bob shoves him hard and says, "It's my chair". Staff quickly separates the two and each will have his meal in his room. Most of the other residents in the dinning are upset; some leave; others eat less than they would have had the incident not occurred; and still seem obvious to the event. Staff will have a mountain of reports to file and many family members to contact.

That scenario highlights many of the major aspects of intervention: swiftness and decisiveness. For the intervention, there must be staff training, preparation drills, and team work. During the eruption there were many tasks which had to be done: separation of two residents, moving other residents out of the way, and protecting visitors.

Immediately after the RRA has been handled, staff must physically assess both the victim and the assaulter and treat any medical problems. .

8. After the intervention

After a RRA event things hopefully return to normal in the facility. However, it has been the author's experience that several meetings should be held afterwards. One should be with the assaulting resident; one with the victim; one for all the other residents; one with the assaulter's family; one with the victim's family and finally one for the staff.

8.1 The assaulter

This meeting with the resident initiating the violence is most effective if the assaulter is cognitively competent. If the resident has dementia, this may not be too productive. It does give that resident an opportunity to talk about the event and in some cases actually leads to an apology. Minnie L age 90 years old has severe and painful arthritis. One afternoon when her joint pain was particularly severe she weakly slapped her roommate Mary M. The staff immediately separated the two. When Minnie met with the social worker, she was mortified by her own behavior and then apologized to the staff member and her roommate.

8.2 The victim

After the RRA event, staff should meet with the victim. Again this is best when the resident is cognitively aware. This gives the resident an opportunity express one's feelings about the attack.

8.3 The family of the attacker

It is important that staff notify and meet with the initiating resident's family. In some cases where transfer is appropriate, the family will want to know the reason. The family or guardian of the resident will then hear about the event from the staff rather than from other sources. In some cases the meeting may prompt that family to provide useful care information which could help prevent another of the episode. Neil G age 86 years old became agitated while watching a documentary on World War II and shoved his nursing home friend. Later when staff met with his family, his son mentioned his father's south Pacific combat experiences. This information helped staff to better care for Neil and to pay attention to the television programs he might watch.

8.4 The victim's family

Again it is important that staff inform the family before they hear it from other sources. All too often a family member coming on a regular visit could be shocked to hear for the first time that the loved one had been attacked. This also gives staff an opportunity to tell the family steps taken to insure their loved one's safety.

8.5 Meeting with other residents

Residents having witnessed the attack may feel threatened and not safe. Again this type of meeting is particularly relevant when most of the resident are cognitively aware. The meeting allows to residents to voice their concerns and gives staff an opportunity to assure them of their safety.

8.6 Staff meeting

Finally, there should be a staff meeting to review the entire episode which will serve many purposes. The tone of the meeting should be assuring, educational, healing rather than punitive and fault finding. It gives staff a chance to express their feelings about attack. Furthermore, staff often can be discouraged by working a stressful combative environment. They had sought employment to help people not to be 'policemen'. It offers an opportunity to learn from the RRA episode. What did they do right? And in what areas could they improve their response? It also provides the nursing home leadership an opportunity to be supportive of their staff.

9. Documentation

Documentation plays an important role in RRA as both a record of the intervention and as for prevention. In both cases those documents become critical in risk management and for accreditation.

9.1 Recording the intervention

Each RRA event must be documented. It should recorded in the assaulter's and the victim's charts. Those charts are one of the key places to best document care issues. However, in those charts, only identify the resident whose chart you are writing in. Therefore, in the victim's chart, do not identify by name or medical record number the assaulter. And in the attacker's chart, do not identify the victim. Document the event without specifically identifying of the other party. This fulfills the HIPAA, the United States' Health Information Privacy requirement. *"Minimum Necessary. A central aspect of the Privacy Rule is the principle of "minimum necessary" use and disclosure. A covered entity must make reasonable efforts to use, disclose, and request only the minimum amount of protected health information needed to accomplish the intended purpose of the use, disclosure, or request"*. (Health Information Privacy, 2011) However, in the incident report, record both parties and the events completely. The incident report if done thoroughly and competently can be very effective as a risk management document.

9.2 Prevention

Documentation can be used in RRA prevention in several ways.

Documentation prevention involves the use of a Preadmission Behavioral Review. This form consists of a list of the behavioral concerns for a new admission. It offers staff insights into residents who are about to be joining their unit. This is particularly useful since the entrance for the new resident to any unit can be both stressful to the unit and the resident. One specific interesting aspect of this form has been the place for staff to initial that they have read it. Staff by initialing the form , helps to assure effective transmission resident care information. This form provides an excellent place to put in information about the resident's life such as birth order and profession.

A companion piece to the Preadmission Behavioral Review is the Individual Treatment Plan. This form not only outlines specific behavior concerns but also should contain information about emergency management techniques if the resident becomes aggressive. Here again the Treatment Plan offers an excellent place for information about the resident's life such as birth order and profession.

There is one other useful way to record RRA events. This is one master list of all RRA incidents in the facility by time and place. By documenting each RRA event, clinical staff and administration have an important method to track and see patterns of resident aggression. If they identify certain times and units of high RRA events, they use that information to deploy staff to forestall violence episodes.

10. Conclusion the impact of RRA

The impact of resident-to-resident violence is both profound and pervasive. It affects both the actual residents involved, their families, the witnessing residents, the clinical staff and the administration. RRA plays a significant role in the quality of life in the nursing home. Incidents of RRA can lead to residents feeling unsafe and anxious. It can result increased staff turn-over.

There are a number of identifiable causes of RRA. An appreciation of the roots of residents' aggression can lead to ways of preventing RRA. RRA must be dealt with swiftly and decisively. And after the RRA episode, it must be reviewed . Finally, each RRA event must be thoroughly documented.

11. Acknowledgements

David Siddle, Ph.D. has contributed much to my appreciation and understanding RRA. For several years he and I worked together in the Commonwealth of Massachusetts in a training program sponsored its Department of Industrial Accidents, Office of Safety in a day long workshop entitled *A Nurse Safety Program dealing with Resident Aggression in Long-term Care Facilities to Reduce Injuries and Lost Work Days: A Comprehensive Approach.* We trained over a thousand nursing home staff member in over one hundred facilities. He also co-authored *A Caregiver's Guide to Working with Combative Resident.* Thanks also to Elaine Bunker of Daniel Webster College for helping in formatting this chapter.

12. References

A nursing home abuse lawyer, accessed 8/22/11, <www.a-nursing-home-abuse-lawyer.com>

American Psychiatric Association. 2000. *Diagnostic and Statistical Manual of Mental Disorders, Fourth Edition, Text Revision, DSM-IV-TR.* Washington, DC

Bagchi AD, Verdier JM, Simon SE., How many nursing home residents live with a mental illness? *Psychiatr Serv.*;60(7):958-64. Jul 2009 Birth order, accessed 9/5/11 http://www.childdevelopmentinfo.com/development/birth_order.shtml>.

Cohen-Mansfield, J., Billig, N., Lipson, S., Rosenthal, A.S., Pawlson, L.G., Medical correlates of agitation in nursing home residents, *Gerontology* 36:3, 150-158, 1990.

Cornell University (2008, June 4). Aggression Between Nursing-home Residents More Common Than Widely Believed, Studies Find. *ScienceDaily.* accessed 8/22/ 2011, from <http://www.sciencedaily.com/releases/2008/06/080602170924.htm>

Enmarker I, Olsen R, Hellzen O., Management of person with dementia with aggressive and violent behavior: a systematic literature review. *Int J Older People Nurs.* ;6(2):153- 62. Jun 2011

Fullerton CA, McGuire TG, Feng Z, Mor V, Grabowski DC, Trends in mental health admissions to nursing homes, 1999-2005. *Psychiatr Serv.*;60(7):965-71. Jul 2009

Goffman, E. Asylums, Garden City, NJ, Anchor, 1961.

Health Information Privacy, accessed 9/19/11, http://www.hhs.gov/ocr/privacy/hipaa/understanding/summary/index.html

Lachs M, Bachman R, Williams CS, O'Leary JR. Resident-to-resident elder mistreatment and police contact in nursing homes: findings from a population-based cohort. *J Am Geriatr Soc.* Jun;55(6):840-5. 2007

Lemke SP, Schaefer JA., Recent changes in the prevalence of psychiatric disorders among VA nursing home residents. *Psychiatr Serv.* 61(4):356-63. Apr;2010

Leone AF, Standoli F, Hirth V., Implementing a pain management program in a long-term c are facility using a quality improvement approach. *J Am Med Dir Assoc.* Jan;10(1):67-73. 2009

Leurs P, Huvent-Grelle D, Lelievre-Leroy S, Roche J, Puisieux F; Comité Scientifique de la Société Septentrionale de Gérontologie Clinique. Alcohol consumption patterns in older people living in nursing homes, *Presse Med.* 39(12):e280-8. Dec; 2010

Narevic E, Giles GM, Rajadhyax R, Managuelod E, Monis F, Diamond F., The effects of enhanced program review and staff training on the management of aggression among clients in a long-term neurobehavioral rehabilitation program. *Aging Ment Health.* Jan;15(1):103-12. 2011

Natan MB, Lowenstein A, Eisikovits Z., Psycho-social factors affecting elders' maltreatment in long-term care facilities. *Int Nurs Rev.* 57(1):113-20. Mar; 2010

Packham, B, Fear in nursing homes Assault claims soar, Herald Sun (Australia) December 14, 2009 Monday 1 - FIRST Edition, page 22

Preventing Resident to Resident Altercations in Nursing Homes. accessed 9/3/2011 <http://www.intergens.com/featurearticle-38.html >

Rosen T, Lachs MS, Pillemer K. Sexual aggression between residents in nursing homes: literature synthesis of an underrecognized problem.*J Am Geriatr Soc.* ;58(10):1970-9. Oct . 2010

Rosen T, Lachs MS, Bharucha AJ, Stevens SM, Teresi JA, Nebres F, Pillemer K. Resident-to-resident aggression in long-term care facilities: insights from focus groups of nursing home residents and staff.*J Am Geriatr Soc.* 56(8):1398-408. Aug;2008

Sifford-Snellgrove KS, Beck C, Green A, McSweeney JC., Victim or Initiator?: Certified Nursing Assistants' Perceptions of Resident Characteristics that Contribute to Resident-To-Resident Violence in Nursing Homes. *Res Gerontol Nurs.* 15:1-9. Jun. 2011

Sifford, Krista Susan, *Caregiver perceptions of unmet needs that lead to resident-to-resident violence involving residents with dementia in nursing homes, dictatorial dissertation* 2010, accessed 8/25/11< http://gradworks.umi.com/34/10/3410295.html >

Sifford KS, Bharucha A., Benefits and challenges of electronic surveillance in nursing home research. *Res Gerontol Nurs.* 3(1):5-10, Jan;2010

Shinoda-Tagawa, T., Leonard, R., Pontikas, J., McDonough, JE., Allen, A., Dreyer, PI, Resident-to-Resident Violent Incidents in Nursing Homes *JAMA.* 291:591-598. Feb. 2004

Soreff, S and Siddle, D, *A Caregiver's Guide to Working with Combative Residents* Needham, MA, Lighthouse CCUNIV Pub. Ltd. 2003 ISBN 0-9719578-4-3- 5200

Soreff, S. Editor, *Handbook for the Treatment of the Seriously Mentally Ill,* Seattle, Washington, Hogrefe & Huber, 1996.ISBN 0-88937-123-7

Williams CL, Hyer K, Kelly A, Leger-Krall S, Tappen RM.Development of nurse competencies to improve dementia care. *Geriatr Nurs.*;26(2):98-105. Mar-Apr 2005

Zambito, T., Violent Patients Loose in Home, The New York Daily News, December 18, 2000, accessed 8/22/11 <http://www.globalaging.org/elderrights/us/violentpatients.htm,>

Zhang Z, Schiamberg LB, Oehmke J, Barboza GE, Griffore RJ, Post LA, Weatherill RP, Mastin T, Neglect of older adults in Michigan nursing homes .*J Elder Abuse Negl.*;23(1):58-74. Jan 2011

Section 3

Effectiveness of Selected Mental Health Therapies and Interventions

12

Effectiveness of Participative Community Singing Intervention Program on Promoting Resilience and Mental Health of Aboriginal and Torres Strait Islander People in Australia

Jing Sun[1,3] and Nicholas Buys[2,3]
[1]*Griffith Health Institute and School of Public Health, Griffith University, Australia*
[2]*Griffith Health Institute and Health Group, Griffith University, Australia*
[3]*Peking University, Beijing, China*

1. Introduction

Aboriginal and Torres Strait Islander people are more likely to have a higher prevalence of mental illness than non-Indigenous people, which may be caused by multiple factors (Australian Bureau of Statistics, 2008; Australian Institute of Health and Welfare, 2008; Pink & Allbon, 2008). These factors have been shown to be closely related to resilience. The concept was introduced by Masten and Coatsworth (1998) and includes key factors that affect recovery from illness and maintenance of health. The key factors of resilience entail (1) an ability of bouncing back, through which a person can recover from stressful event quickly; (2) a sense of family support, through which a person can manage a stressful event process; and (3) a sense of social connectedness, through which a person feels supported and connected to the community and social environment in a stressful event (Masten & Coatsworth, 1998; Weinberger, Schwartz & Davidson, 1979; Werner & Smith, 2001). Previous studies have shown an association with the sense of resilience score and depression. A high resilience score is related to a lower degree of depression (Weinberger et al., 1979), a lower level of anxiety (Weinberger et al., 1979), and a lower mental or physical stress response (Werner & Smith, 2001). These studies suggest the importance of resilience for coping with stress and adverse events and to prevent mental illness. A community participative singing approach (CPSA) is an effective intervention in promoting resilience and mental health in a range of population groups (Cohen et al., 2006, 2007). The CPSA programme is modelled on the work of Clift and colleagues at the Canterbury Christ Church University in England (Clift & Hancox, July 2008; Clift et al., 2007).

The programme is based on the principle of multi-psychosocial functions development, 'divided into environmental and social processes (interpersonal mechanisms) and cognitive and emotional processes (intrapersonal mechanisms). These processes are bi-directional, as the interpersonal mechanisms can trigger intrapersonal responses, and vice versa' (Lob et al., 2011, p. 46). The goal of the CPSA programme is to guide participants through breathing exercises, group singing, and social interaction and collaboration. It aims to maximise their collective experience in a non-judgemental and accepting way, one where individuals feel a sense of belonging and safety, and to build relationships in which individuals socialise with others and are able to work on their social skills in a safe setting. A second aim is to develop individuals' inner psychological state such as competence, purposefulness, managing emotions and wellbeing, and creating a meaningful life. It is effective for mood disturbance and stress symptoms (Lob et al., 2011), for quality of life (Cohen et al., 2006, 2007) and the immune profile (Clift et al., 2008). However, few studies have examined interventions for mental health promotion in the Aboriginal and Torres Strait Islander population. Thus, the present study was performed to investigate the efficacy of community participative singing on the sense of resilience and psychological wellbeing of Aboriginal and Torres Strait Islander people. The study was performed for Aboriginal and Torres Strait Islanders who reside in five Aboriginal and Torres Strait Islander communities in South East Queensland, Australia. These Aboriginal and Torres Strait Islander people may be under particular stress and have a mental illness status since many of them have gone through the colonisation process and had traumatic experiences related to it. The aim of the study was to assess the effectiveness for Aboriginal and Torres Strait Islander people of active engagement in community music activities on measures of resilience, mental health, and quality of life.

It is hypothesised that Aboriginal and Torres Strait Islander people will have increased resilience, mental health and quality of life after they participate in a community singing intervention programme for six months.

2. Methods

The study used the participatory community singing approach and the prospective intervention method for the intervention trial. A multi-method design was used to monitor and evaluate the programme. Participants were invited to participate in the project in June 2010 and completed questionnaires towards the end July 2010, and they were asked to fill in the questionnaire again in January and February 2011. They were also asked over the course of the project to provide qualitative comments on their experiences. The present paper only focuses on changes over a six-month period from July 2010 to the January 2012 based on the quantitative results. The study was granted ethical approval by Research Ethics Committee at Griffith University with GU Ref No: PBH/13/10/HREC

2.1 Participants and data collection procedure

Participants were adults aged 18 and above. They were all able to speak English, provide informed consent and complete questionnaires. Individuals who were unable to provide informed consent or complete questionnaires were excluded from the study.

Researchers, in conjunction with five Community Controlled Health Services (CCHSs) providing the intervention, sought suitable venues across five South East Queensland communities to conduct intervention activities. Advertisements seeking participants were placed in each CCHS and in local newspapers, and leaflets were delivered to homes within the vicinity of the venues. Two 'taster sessions' were held in each venue, which included the provision of information, an invitation for questions and an opportunity for individuals to sample the nature of the proposed intervention programme. A dedicated phone line and email address was set up to deal with responses and queries and a checklist was devised to collate details of those volunteering to participate.

2.2 Participatory community singing intervention approach

The chief investigator met with Queensland Aboriginal and Islander Health Council (QAIHC) representatives to discuss the initial concept. QAIHC representatives met with and discussed the concept with each Chief Executive Officer (CEO) from each Aboriginal and Islander CCHS. A reference committee was established made up of CEOs, health workers, counsellors and music therapists, the majority of which identified as Aboriginal and/or Torres Strait Islander. QAIHC took on an active role in meeting with community elders via each local council.

Each singing group was led by a skilled and experienced singing group leader. Leaders were provided with five days of training and met regularly throughout the project to ensure a broadly consistent approach. The singing programme took place in the five groups over two three-month blocks. Groups came together at the end of each block for a choral performance event. Each session lasted 120 minutes, with a break for socialising. Sessions commenced with 30 minutes of relaxation, posture, breathing and vocal exercises followed by singing. Two performances for five communities were organised after three months and again after six months of intervention. Monthly performances for each community were held after six months.

2.3 Measures

A number of reliable and valid questionnaires was used to assess the effectiveness of the participative community singing programme on improving resilience and quality of life, and reducing depression symptoms of the participants.

Resilience: The Brief Resilience Scale is a five-item scale used to assess resilience and individual strength, defined as the ability to bounce back and recover from stress (Smith et al., 2008).

Depression: The Indigenous Risk Impact Screen (IRIS) scale is a six-item scale used to assess depressive symptoms and it is designed for use with the Aboriginal and Torres Strait population (Schlesinger et al., 2007). Scores range from six to 18, with higher scores reflecting greater levels of depressive symptoms, and a score of 11 is the cut-off point (Schlesinger et al., 2007). Sensitivity and specificity of the measure was checked by using a depression total score against clinical diagnosed depression results.

Singing questionnaire: The singing questionnaire, consisting of eight questions, was modified based on Clift and colleagues (2010) to measure the improvement of quality of life through community participative singing activities. These questions were designed to measure participants' feelings about their emotional, physical health, spiritual, and social aspects of health. An example question is 'Singing has spiritual significance for me personally'. For each question, participants were asked to choose one of the answers from the three options 'never', 'sometimes' or 'all the time'. The more participants that choose the answer 'all the time', the more likely it is that the participative singing programme has impacted on the quality of life of participants.

3. Results

Table 1 shows that there are statistically significant differences between the pre- and post-intervention phases through a decreased depression rate, improved quality of life, and a reduction of depression symptoms, reduced medication use in participants after six months of intervention activities. This indicates that the participative community singing is effective in improving Aboriginal and Torres Strait Islander participants' resilience, quality of life and mental health.

Variables	Pre (%) N=217	Post (%) N=50	difference	χ^2	p
Resilience1: It takes me a long time to get through stressful events (all the time)	52(24.2%)	5(9.6%)	14.6%	6.47	0.04
Resilience2: I tend to take a long time to get over difficult things in my life (all the time)	55 (25.7%)	5(9.6%)	14.1%	7.60	0.02
Depression (yes)	80(37.2%)	14 (28.2%)	9% decrease	6.61	0.03
Singing is something I like to do	58(26.5%)	42(80.8%)	Significant increase		
Singing has spiritual significance to me personally	50(22.9%)	42(80.8%)	Significant increase	75.92	0.001
Singing really helps to improve my general wellbeing	61(27.9%)	41(78.8%)	Significant increase	63.38	0.001
I find singing helps me to relax and deal with the stresses of the week	55(25.1%)	41(78.8%)	Significant increase	69.11	0.001
Singing helps to give me a positive attitude to life	61(27.9%)	44(84.6%)	Significant increase	69.30	0.001
Being in a singing group and singing is a very important part of my life	51(23.3%)	43(82.7%)	Significant increase	73.13	0.001
Singing helps to make me a happier person	61(27.9%)	44(84.6%)	Significant increase	67.93	0.001
Singing is an activity that has made me physically healthier	45(20.5%)	35(67.3%)	Significant increase	73.19	0.001

Table 1. Improved mental health, resilience and quality of life post-intervention time.

Medication use for Chronic disease	Pre	Post	Differences	χ^2	p
Medication use (yes)	44.2%	31.9%	12.3% decrease	6.35	<0.01
Medication reduced the last 6 month	18.3%	27.3%	9% medication reduction	7.91	<0.01

Table 2. Difference in medication use between the pre- and post-intervention phases

4. Discussion

4.1 Changes in resilience

Our findings show a statistically significant improvement in the percentage of participants who are able to recover from stress and difficult events in post-intervention phase. It should be remembered that the sample in the study is people with Aboriginal and Torres Strait Islander background. It includes not only people with current mental health and chronic diseases issues, but also individuals with a history of colonisation, 49% of whom gave depression scores below the clinical cut-off point. The significant change in the resilience scores indicate that the community singing programme helps to build participants' resilience. This result confirmed the findings of a previous study that choir singing enhanced confidence and self-esteem, gave a sense of purpose and of achievement (Tonneijck et al., 2008). In the present study, the community singing programme has resulted in improved sense of ability to recover and bounce back from the stressful and difficult events in life.

4.2 Change in singing-related quality of life

Statistically significant changes are also found for aspects within the singing-related quality of life questionnaire regarding physical health, social and emotional health, stress reduction, spiritual significance, suggesting that group singing helps to create improvements in all these areas equally. The findings of our study are consistent with those of other studies that singing carries benefits to physical, mental and social health. Clift et al. (2010) and Clift et al. (2008) examined the effects of choral singing on wellbeing in participants with relatively low psychological wellbeing, as assessed by the World Health Organization Quality of Life (WHOQOL)-BREF, and high scores on the singing scale, indicating a strong perceived impact of singing on a sense of personal wellbeing. In Clift et al.'s (2010) study, it was found that singing provided support in coping with challenges in four aspects: enduring mental health problems, family and relationship problems, physical health challenges and recent bereavement.

4.3 Change in depression

Our results show a statistically significant reduction in the percentage of participants who had depression in the post-intervention phase. It should be noted that the sample includes not only people with current mental health issues, 37.8% of whom gave depression scores below the clinical cut-off point. There was 9% reduction in the percentage of people who had depression, suggesting that the singing programme helps some people with mental illness to recover from the depression status. This is consistent with a recent study by Clift and Morrison (2011), who also found that singing programmes significantly reduce the depression rate among participants with depression.

The findings of our study indicate that a participative community singing programme is effective in preventing the deterioration of depression, and in improving resilience and quality of life. A CPSA can foster a sense of happiness, positive attitude towards life, and feelings of the significance of life. Singing is considered by participants a means to release stress, and deal with worries and negative emotions. Singing is also regarded as a way to make them physically healthy as indicated in the reduced level of medication use.

A community-based participatory research approach can foster a sense of self-determination, create greater commitment and can ultimately improve self-esteem and increase a sense of belonging.

5. Limitations

There are a number of limitations for the study. The first limitation is lack of control group as a comparison to intervention group in the post intervention phase. The difference between pre intervention and post intervention in resilience, quality of life and depression would not be attributable to the singing activities. The second limitation is that the standard measure of depression, for example, Beck's Depression Scale, and WHO Quality of Life Questionnaire were not used, and this may have limited the generalisation of the study results to other populations. Further study is needed to ensure the control group data are collected to strengthen the methodology and evidence of the present study. In addition, standard measures are needed in the next step of the study so that the results can be compared with previous published literature, and be generalised to wide population groups.

6. Conclusion

The results of the study found that the community singing programme is effective in promoting social and emotional wellbeing, and preventing the deterioration of depression and chronic conditions. The results of the study may inform future studies of preventative and treatment interventions for high-risk populations that integrate community singing into prevention and intervention strategies in the Aboriginal and Torres Strait Islander population in Australia.

7. Acknowledgement

The authors received financial support from Griffith Health Institute and Provost Chancellor Office at Logan Campus at Griffith University, and Queensland Aboriginal and Islander Health Council. The authors also wish to acknowledge the support of the following Aboriginal Community Controlled Health Services: *Brisbane Kambu Medical Service Centre Pty Ltd, Kalwun Health Service, Aboriginal and Torres Strait Islander Community Health Service Brisbane Ltd, Goolburri Health Advancement Corporation, and Warwick Peace Festival Community. The authors also wish to thank all participants' participation from five Aboriginal and Torres Strait Islander communities.* In addition, authors wish to express great thanks to Lindsay Johnson, Dion Tatow, Lennart Dahlen in Queensland Aboriginal and Islander Health Council for their contribution in data collection and intervention coordination work.

8. References

Australian Bureau of Statistics. (2008). The Health and Welfare of Australia's Aboriginal and Torres Strait Islander Peoples, ABS, Canberra.

Australian Institute of Health and Welfare. (2008). Australia's Health, Canberra.

Clift, S. & Hancox, G. (July 2008, in press). The significance of choral singing for sustaining psychological welbeing: Findings from a survey of choristers in England, Germany and Australia. Paper presented at the ISME Commision Seminar on Community Music, Rome.

Clift, S., Hancox, G., Morrison, I., Hess, B., Kreutz, G. & Stewart, D. (2007, November). Choral singing and psychological wellbeing: Findings from English choirs in a cross-national survey using the WHOQoL-BREF. Paper presented at the Proceedings of the International Symposium on Performance Science, Porto.

Clift, S., Hancox, G., Staricoff, R. & Whitmore, C. (2008). A systematic mapping and review of research on singing and health-non-clinical studies. Canterbury: Canterbury Christ Church University College.

Clift, S., Hancox, G., Morrison, I., Hess, B., Kreutz, G., & Stewart, D. (2010). Choral singing and psychological wellbeing: Quantitative and qualitative findings from English choirs in a cross-national survey. Journal of Applied Arts and Health doi: 10.1386/jaah.1.1.19/1: 19-34.

Clift S, Morrison I. (2011). Group singing fosters mental health and wellbeing: findings from the East Kent "singing for health" network project. Mental Health and Social Inclusion. 2011 Vol. 15(No.2):88-97.

Cohen, G. D., Perlstein, S., Chapline, J., Kelly, J., Firth, K. M. & Simmens, S. (2006). The impact of professionally conducted cultural programs on the physical health, mental health, and social functioning of older adults, The Gerontologist Vol. 46(No. 6): 726–734.

Cohen, G. D., Perlstein, S., Chapline, J., Kelly, J., Firth, K. M. & Simmens, S. (2007). The impact of professionally conducted culturally programs on the physical health, mental health and social functioning of older people-2 year results, Journal of Aging, Humanities and the Arts Vol. 1: 5–22.

Lob, G. V., Camic, P. & Clift, S. (2011). The use of singing in a group as a response to adverse life events, International Journal of Mental Health Promotion Vol. 12(No. 3): 45–53.

Masten, A. S. & Coatsworth, J. D. (1998). The development of competence in favorable and unfavorable environments: lessons from research on successful children, American Psychologist Vol. 53: 205–220.

Pink, B. & Allbon, P. (2008). The Health and Welfare of Australia's Aboriginal and Torres Strait Islander Peoples 2008, Australian Bureau of Statistics, and Australian Institute of Health and Welfare, Canberra.

Schlesinger, C. M., Ober, C., McCarthy, M. M., Watson, J. D. & Seinen, A. (2007). The development and validation of the Indigenous Risk Impact Screen (IRIS): A 13-item screening instrument for alcohol and drug and mental health risk, Drug and Alcohol Review Vol. 26: 109–117.

Smith, B. W., Dalen, J., Wiggins, K., Tooley, E., Christopher, P. & Bernard, J. (2008). The Brief Resilience Scale: Assessing the ability to bounce back, International Journal of Behavioral Medicine Vol. 15: 194–200.

Tonneijck, H. I. M., Kinebanian, A. & Josephsson, S. (2008). An exploration of choir singing: Achieving wholeness through challenge, Journal of Occupational Science Vol. 15(No. 3): 173–180.

Weinberger, D. A., Schwartz, G. E. & Davidson, R. J. (1979). Low-anxious, high-anxious, and repressive coping styles: Psychometric patterns and behavioral and physiological responses to stress, Journal of Abnormal Psychology Vol. 88: 369–380.

Werner, E. E. & Smith, R. S. (2001). Journeys from childhood to midlife: Risk, resilience, and recovery. Introduction to the special issue on resilience, Substance Use & Misuse Vol. 39(No. 5): 657–670.

13

Antipsychotics Versus Cholinesterase Inhibitors for the Treatment of Psychosis in Alzheimer's: A Critical Review

Emmanuelle Lévy[1], Howard C Margolese[2] and Serge Gauthier[3]
[1]*Douglas Institute of Mental Health, Department of Psychiatry, McGill University, Montreal,*
[2]*Clinical Psychopharmacology Unit, McGill University Health Centre and Department of Psychiatry, McGill University, Montreal,*
[3]*Professor of Neurology, Neurosurgery and Medicine, McGill University, and Director of the Alzheimer's disease Research Unit, McGill Centre for Studies in Aging, Montreal, Canada*

1. Introduction

In the later stages of dementia, more than 50% of patients will experience behavioral and psychological symptoms of dementia (BPSD) including psychosis (Hemels, 2001). These symptoms reputably cause distress in both patients and care-giving family members. Caregivers typically have reduced quality of life and see increases in the cost of care (Finkel, 1997; Herrmann, 2001), whereas patients tend to increase resource utilization and form a high-risk group for institutionalization (Daniel, 2000). Behavioral disorders being paramount, it is surprising that there is little agreement on the actual description of these symptoms (Stoppe, 1999). This reason among others, contributes to the perception that "*treating secondary symptoms of AD is more of an art than a science*" (Corey-Bloom, 1995).

In seeking pharmacological treatment options for psychotic symptoms in Alzheimer's disease, this review will attempt to address the following four questions: 1) What is the definition and clinical presentation of BPSD? 2) What is the prevalence and impact of psychotic symptoms on the progression of dementia in AD? 3) What are the indications for the use of antipsychotics in the treatment of BPSD? 4) What are the evidence-based treatments for BPSD?

2. Definition and clinical presentation of behavioral and psychological symptoms of dementia (BPSD)

In 1996, the International Psychogeriatric Association consensus group defined behavioral and psychological symptoms of dementia (BPSD) as: "*symptoms of disturbances of perception, thought content, mood or behavior frequently observed in demented patients*".

Many classifications of BPSD have been proposed. When pharmacological treatment is concerned, classifying BPSD by syndromes is most useful. Although it is often difficult to subgroup behavioral symptoms, psychological symptoms can be grouped into three syndromes: psychotic, depressive and delirious. A more descriptive classification summarizes the characteristic symptoms of BPSD in table 1.

Different BPSD appear at different stages of the illness. Affective symptoms tend to appear in the early stages of dementia (Reisberg et al., 1989; Rubin et al., 1988), whereas psychotic symptoms and agitation are more frequent in patients with moderate cognitive dysfunction. In fact, most BPSD are present prior to the later stages of the illness, when they abate possibly because of the physical and neurological deterioration of the patient (Tariot & Blazina, 1994).

3. Prevalence and impact of psychotic symptoms in dementia

In a review of 30 studies of patients with AD, affective and psychotic symptoms were found to occur in 30%-40% of patients (Wragg & Jeste, 1989). However, up to 90% of patients living in institutions may suffer BPSD (Finkel, 1998). In patients with AD, the prevalence of psychotic symptoms alone is quite variable and was found to cluster around 20%-40% (Raskind & Barnes, 2002). In a study following patients longitudinally from the beginning to the later stages of AD, presence of psychotic symptoms was documented in over 50% of patients, and was more common at moderate and severe stages of dementia (42 to 84%) (Drevets & Rubin, 1989). Furthermore, in a one year longitudinal study, recurrence rates of psychotic symptoms in untreated patients have been estimated at 95% (Levy et al., 1996).

The two most common psychotic symptoms that develop in AD are delusions and hallucinations. The median prevalence of delusions is 36%, ranging between 9% and 63% (Ropacki and Jeste, 2005). Among the most frequent types of delusions identified are persecutory (involving theft) in 18-43% of patients followed by delusions of abandonment in 3-18% and delusions of jealousy (involving infidelity) in 1-9% (Tariot & Blazina, 1994). Hallucinations were estimated to vary between 4-41% hallucinations with a median of 18% (Ropacki and Jeste, 2005). Visual hallucinations were reported in up to 30% of moderately demented patients, whereas auditory hallucinations may occur in up to 10% of patients (Swearer, 1994). Other types of hallucinations such as olfactory, tactile, gustatory and haptic are rarely observed (Tariot & Blazina, 1994).

Aggression, one of the major behavioral symptoms in dementia, causes great distress in caregivers and can lead to earlier institutionalization (Chenoweth & Spencer, 1986; Rabins PV et al., 1982; Rabins et al., 1982). Delusions, mainly persecutory, have been identified as a risk factor for physical and verbal aggression in patients with AD (Deutsch et al., 1991). For instance, Deutsch et al. (1991) reported that out 181 AD patients, 43.5% suffered delusions, of which 29.6% were noted to be physically aggressive. Furthermore, delusions preceded and were significantly associated with aggressive behavior (Deutsch et al., 1991). The converse has also been shown in another study where 80% of patients with high levels of aggression (more than one episode/month) also presented with delusions (Gilley et al., 1997). This suggests that the presence of delusions predicts the frequency of physically aggressive behavior.

Increased rates of cognitive deterioration are also associated with psychotic symptoms in AD particularly in patients manifesting psychosis earlier in the course of dementia (Jeste et al., 1992; Lopez et al., 1991; Stern et al., 1987). Interestingly, patients manifesting earlier psychotic symptoms were found to live longer than those without psychosis (Drevets & Rubin, 1989).

4. Use of antipsychotics in the elderly

Though outside of the official FDA indication, in the elderly, atypical antipsychotics are most frequently prescribed for the treatment of behavioral symptoms of dementia. In May 2004, the FDA issued a warning of an increased death risk in elderly patients using atypical antipsychotics (Jeste et al., 2008). This warning was based on a meta-analysis of seventeen randomized double-blind controlled trials revealing a drug-related death risk increasing by 1.6-1.7 times when compared to placebo (Jeste et al., 2008). Most frequent causes of death were cardiovascular (heart failure or sudden death) and infectious (pneumonia). In April 2005, the FDA followed suit with a black box warning cautioning against the use of atypical antipsychotics in the elderly. Later the same year, a meta-analysis of 15 randomized controlled trials (Schneider *et al.*, 2005) examined the mortality risk between placebo and atypical antipsychotics as well as a comparison between various atypical antipsychotics (aripiprazole, olanzapine, quetiapine, risperidone). This study found a small increased mortality risk compared to placebo (OR = 1.54; 95%CI: 1.06-2.23). No difference was found between antipsychotics.

Given that this meta-analysis and the FDA warning did not apply to typical antipsychotics, the remaining assumption was that typical agents could be warranted in the treatment of BPSD. However, a study published in the New England Journal of Medicine compared the use of typical and atypical antipsychotics in the elderly and found that typical antipsychotics were associated with a significantly higher risk of death than atypical antipsychotics (Wang *et al.*, 2005). Hence, typical antipsychotics should not be used to replace atypical agents in the treatment of BPSD.

Currently, the FDA has not approved of any treatment for BPSD. Facing agitation in the elderly and consequent caregiver distress, clinicians are left with unclear choices. In the treatment of BPSD, what are the evidence-based alternatives?

5. Evidence-based treatment-options for BPSD

Non-pharmacological options

In the treatment of BPSD, an initial assessment of the underlying causes of behavioral changes is necessary. Co-morbid medical illnesses and sensory impairment should be corrected prior to medication use. It has even been suggested that non-pharmacological approaches, including music therapy, light therapy, changes in stimulation, and specific behavioral techniques such as positive reinforcement could be attempted before medication (Beck & Shue, 1994; Opie et al., 1999). Although pharmacological treatment of BPSD should not be first line, high rates of psychotropic drug use have been reported, particularly in very old patients living in institutions (Giron, 2001). Between 39% and 51% of elderly institutionalized patients were found to be treated with antipsychotics (Avorn et al., 1989; Lantz et al., 1990). In the pharmacological treatment of BPSD, antipsychotic are the agents that have been most frequently studied (Stoppe, 1999). In mild or moderate BPSD cases, particularly when symptoms are not interfering strongly with functioning, clinicians may opt not to treat BPSD. In such mild to moderate cases, psychosocial interventions (eg music therapy, cognitive therapy, behavioral management techniques, caregiver education) may have modest effectiveness (Cohen-Mansfield, 2001; Livingston et al, 2005).

In severe cases where psychotic symptoms and agitation interfere with functioning and cause significant caregiver distress, lack of treatment may be dangerous. Below we review the pharmacological treatment options for BPSD.

Antipsychotics

A number of well-controlled trials predating the 2005 FDA warnings had examined the effectiveness of atypical antipsychotics in the treatment of BPSD. These studies are summarized and presented in Table 2. In the treatment of BPSD, atypical antipsychotics seem to be of significant though modest effectiveness. However, given the FDA black box warnings, much caution is necessary in using antipsychotics in the elderly.

The large NIMH funded Clinical Antipsychotic Trial of Intervention Effectiveness study for Alzheimer's Disease (CATIE-AD) trial found that olanzapine, quetiapine, and risperidone were no better than placebo in the treatment of psychotic symptoms of dementia. However, in a review of 15 randomized controlled trials (RCTs) of atypical antipsychotics for the treatment of BPSD, only risperidone was found to significantly improve psychosis scores (Schneider et al (2006).

Cholinesterase inhibitors

There is some evidence supporting the relationship between cholinergic neurotransmission and behavioral symptoms of AD (Cummings & Kaufer, 1996). Given that neuropsychiatric changes in AD are associated with cholinergic deficits, one expects neuropsychiatric changes to respond to cholinergic therapy. Supporting this cholinergic hypothesis, Cummings (2000b) linked cholinergic deficits to behavior by identifying the following four dimensions of behavioral symptoms: "1) *induction of AD-like behaviours in normal individuals by administration of anticholinergic drugs;* 2) *the exaggeration of behavioural disturbances in AD patients by anticholinergic agents;* 3) *the correlation of the distribution of cholinergic deficits of AD with regions that are relevant to the observed behaviours, i.e. frontal and temporal regions; and* 4) *improvement of behavioural disturbances in AD patients treated with cholinergic receptor agonists and cholinesterase inhibitors*" (Cummings, 2000b).

Cummings also provides some compelling evidence that cholinesterase inhibitors have positive psychotropic effects in AD (Cummings, 2000a). For instance, patients with anticholinergic delirium (agitation and psychosis) were found to be similar to AD patients with non-cognitive symptoms (hallucinations and agitation). Given that these symptoms responded well to treatment enhancing cholinergic activity (Cummings, 1993), adjusting acetylcholine levels can reduce psychosis.

Displayed in table 3 are open label and double-blind studies on cholinesterase inhhibitors (tacrine, donepezil, metrifonate, galantamine and rivastigmine) that have found reductions of non-cognitive behaviors over placebo.

A systematic review and meta-analysis quantified the efficacy of cholinesterase inhibitors as a group for neuropsychiatric symptoms in patients with mild to moderate AD (Trinh et al., 2003). This study found a modest beneficial impact on neuropsychiatric and functional outcomes. Other studies looking at the effects of galantamine (Hermann et al, 2005), donepezil (Holmes et al., 2004) and metrifonate (Kaufer, 1998) showed a modestly better outcome in behavioral symptoms than placebo-treated subjects. Another study compared memantine and placebo in AD patients treated with donepezil (Cummings et al., 2006 Neurology). Patients treated with donepezil and memantine had better behavioral outcomes that those treated with donepezil and placebo. Finally, a recent pooled analysis from six RCTs found a small but significant benefit from memantine in behavioral outcome scores (Gauthier et al., 2008).

Finally, one pilot open-label study assessed the safety of co-administration of rivastigmine with risperidone in dementia patients with behavioral disturbances (Weiser et al., 2002). The authors' main findings were two-fold: first, both these agents could be co-administered with no significant adverse effects and second, significant improvement in NPI scores were found in the rivastigmine-risperidone group of patients. These findings suggest that combination of these two agents might be more efficacious than either one alone (Weiser et al., 2002).

6. Conclusion

Addressing behavioral and psychological symptoms of dementia is paramount. Psychotic symptoms in AD occur in a majority of patients, and have a very high recurrence rate. Untreated BPSD can result in increased rates of hospitalization, institutionalization, cost of care and diminished quality of life for both patients and caregivers. Pharmacological treatment of BPSD should not be first line. Initial assessments of the underlying causes of BPSD are warranted and co-morbid medical illnesses should be corrected before initiating pharmacological treatment. In mild to moderate cases, non-pharmacological approaches (including music therapy, light therapy, changes in stimulation, and behavioral techniques) could be attempted before medications are used (Beck & Shue, 1994; Opie et al., 1999).

Given the FDA warnings, atypical antipsychotics should only be considered in moderate to severe cases on a case-by-case basis after careful evaluation of the risk-benefit ratio. The preferred antipsychotic seems to be risperidone as it was the only agent found in a meta-analysis of six RCTs to non-significantly increase mortality (Haupt et al., 2006) while another meta-analysis of fifteen trails found it to significantly improve psychosis scores (Schneider et al., (2006).

Facing the paucity of safe and effective medications available, cholinesterase inhibitors may be used as first line pharmacotherapy. Cholinesterase inhibitors have positive psychotropic effects in AD and are modestly effective in the treatment of BPSD. However, many AD patients are taking cholinesterase inhibitors and nevertheless develop BPSD. In such cases, the augmentation with memantine (Cummings et al, 2006) or risperidone (Weiser et al, 2002) may be warranted. More studies examining the combination of cholinesterase inhibitors with other agents are warranted.

Behavioral Symptoms	Psychological Symtpoms
Aggression	Delusions
Wandering	Hallucinations
Agitation	Depressed mood
Yelling	Insomnia
Disinhibition	Anxiety
Pacing	Misidentification

Table 1. Slassification of behavioral and psychological symptoms of dementia (BPSD).

Reference	Study Type / Duration	n	Rx types	Dose (mg/d)	Neuro scales	Outcome
(Frenchman & Prince, 1997)	Retrospective chart review	186	Risperidone (n=60) Haloperidol (n=83) Thioridazine (n=43)	-Mean risperidone= 1 mg/d -Mean haloperidol= 2 mg/d -Mean thioridazine= 33 mg/d		Target behaviors (including paranoia and delusions) improved in more patients on risperidone (94%) than haloperidol (65%), and thioridazine (67%) (p < .001).
(Goldberg & Goldberg, 1997)	Open / 6 months	109	Risperidone	0.5-1 (range)		Delusions improved in 75% of patients and Hallucinations in 73%.
(Irizarry et al., 1999)	Retrospective / 16 months	41	Risperidone	1.8 1.4 (mean sd)	4-point-scale constructed by authors	Psychosis improved partially in 41% with AD, completely in 15%.
(Katz et al., 1999)	Double-blind / 12 wk	625	Risperidone	0.5-2 (range)	BEHAVE-AD	Improvement in total scores and psychosis sub-scale scores of BEHAVE-AD for 1-2mg/d.
(De Deyn et al., 1999)	Double-blind / 12 wk	344	Risperidone Haloperidol	0.5-4 1.1	BEHAVE-AD	Significant difference from baseline in total scores of BEHAVE-AD in risperidone group only.
(Jeste et al., 2000)	Open / 12 month	330	Risperidone	0.5-2 (range)	BEHAVE-AD	Improvement on total and psychosis sub-scale scores of BEHAVE-AD for 0.75-1.5mg/d (p=0.03).
(Street et al., 2000)	Double-blind / 6 wk	206	Olanzapine	Fixed doses of 5-10-15 mg/d or placebo	NPI-NH	Significant improvement at 5mg/d (p<0.001) and 10 mg/d (p=0.006) on core symptoms including hallucinations & delusions.

Table 2. Part I.

(Clark et al., 2001)	Double-blind / 6 wk	206	Olanzapine	Fixed doses of 5-10-15mg/d vs. placebo	NPI-NH	-Significantly greater emergence of delusions and hallucinations for placebo vs olanzapine (p=0.006) in patients without at baseline. -Significantly greater emergence of hallucinations for placebo vs olanzapine (p=0.026) in patients without at baseline.
(Street et al., 2001)	Open / 18 wk	105	Olanzapine	5-15	NPI-NH	Significant improvement in 'Core total items' on NPI-NH (p=0.002) and NPI-NH total scores (p<0.001).
(Satterlee et al., 1995)	Double-blind / 8 wk	238	Olanzapine	1-8	BEHAVE-AD	No statistical significant differences between placebo and olanzapine.
(McManus et al., 1999)	Open / 52 wk	151	Quetiapine	25-800	BPRS (18- item) & CGI-severity of illness	Significant improvement at 12 wks on both BPRS (p<0.0001) and CGI (p<0.01).
(Scharre & Chang, 2002)	Open / 12 wk	10	Quetiapine	50-150	NPI	Significant improvement on total NPI score (p=0.002) and delusion sub-scale score (p=0.02) at wk 12.
(Chengappa et al., 1995)	Retrospective chart review / 30 month	12	Clozapine	25-300	survey	2/12 showed significant and 5/12 moderate improvement in psychosis.
(Oberholzer et al., 1992)	Open / 0.2-22 months	18	Clozapine	12.5-200	NOSIE[1] & SCAG[2]	Improvement in NOSIE score for psychotic symptoms but not significant (p=0.76).
(Salzman et al., 1995)	Retrospective chart review / 2-14 months	20	Clozapine	Average dose=208	NA	Modest reduction in psychotic symptoms.

Part II

1 - NOSIE = Nurses' Observation Scale for Inpatient Evaluation
2 - SCAG = Sandoz Clinical Assessment Geriatric Scale
NPI = Neuropsychiatric Inventory, NPI-NH: Neuropsychiatric Inventory Nursing Home Version
BEHAVE-AD = Behavioural Pathology in Alzheimer's Disease Rating Scale
BPRS = Brief Psychiatric Rating Scale
CGI-S = Clinical Global Impression-Severity of Illness Scale
NA = Not Available

Table 2. Treatment of psychosis in AD: Atypical antipsychotics.

Reference	Study Type / Duration	n	Rx types	Dose (mg/d)	Neuro scales	Outcome
(Kaufer et al., 1996)	Open / 24 wks	28	Tacrine	40-160	NPI	-Mean NPI score was markedly decreased at 120mg/d (p=0.04) and 160mg/d (p=0.01) of tacrine. -Symptoms including hallucinations were most improved.
(Raskind et al., 1997)	Retrospective analysis of Randomized-Placebo-controlled / 30wk	415	Tacrine	160	ADAS-non-cog	Significant improvement or stabilization on ADAS-non-cog scores for scale items including delusions (p<0.05).
(Qizilbash et al., 1998)	Meta-analysis of double-blind trials / 12 wk	2021	Tacrine	20-160	ADAS-non-cog	Small but significant difference in ADAS-non-cog favoring tacrine at 12 wks (p=0.006).
(Knapp et al., 1994)	Double-blind / 30wk	663	Tacrine	40-160	ADAS-non-cog	No significant difference between placebo and doses of 80, 120, 160 mg/d.
(Farlow et al., 1992)	Double-blind / 12wk	468	Tacrine	20-80	ADAS-non-cog	No statistical differences at week 6 & 12 for dose-related improvement.
(Davis et al., 1992)	Double-blind / 6 wk	215	Tacrine	40 or 80	ADAS-non-cog	No statistical differences in mean scores in both groups.
(Feldman et al., 2001)	Double-blind / 24wk	219	Donepezil	5-10	NPI	Significant difference in favor of donepezil at wks 4 (p=0.03) & 24 (p=0.008).
(Gauthier et al., 2002)	Double-blind / 24 wk	207	Donepezil	5-10	NPI	Significant differences with placebo at wk 4 & 24 (p=0.0022).
(Mega et al., 1999)	Open label retrospective study	86	Donepezil	5-10	NPI	-Improvement in 41% of patients; 28% worsened and 31% unchanged. -Responders had worse delusions at baseline (p=0.04). -Significant change from baseline for delusions in responders (p=0.004) and worsening in non-responders (p=0.003).
(Matthews et al., 2000)	Open / 18 months	80	Donepezil	5-10	NPI	37% of patients improved at 3 months; of those patients, improvements were sustained at 18 months.
(Tariot et al., 2001)	Double-blind / 24 wk	208	Donepezil	5-10	NPI-NH	No statistical difference in mean NPI total scores between placebo and donepezil.
(Winblad et al., 2001)	Double-blind / 52 wk	286	Donepezil	5-10	NPI-NH	No statistical differences in total NPI scores.

Table 3. Part I

Part II

(Morris et al., 1998)	Double-blind / 36 wk	408	Metrifonate	30-60	NPI & ADAS-non-cog	-Significant differences for mean total NPI scores (p=0.0161). -No statistical differences favoring metrifonate with ADAS-non-cog.
(Kaufer, 1998)	Double-blind / 26 wk	408	Metrifonate	30-60	NPI	Statistically significant mean change differences in total NPI scores (p=0.07) and in symptoms including hallucinations (p=0.0002).
(Cummings et al., 1998)	Double-blind / 26 wk	1218	Metrifonate	Low dose (LD): 50 fixed or 30-60 or High dose (HD): 60 or 80	NPI	-Both HD (p=0.0392) and LD (p=0.002) significantly improved total NPI scores. -Hallucinations were most responsive to metrifonate in a dose-related manner (p=0.028 for LD; p=0.012 for HD).
(Raskind et al., 1999)	Double-blind / 26 wk	264	Metrifonate	50	NPI & ADAS-non-cog	Improvement in total NPI scores (p=0.013) but not with ADAS-non-cog.
(Tariot et al., 2000)	Double-blind / 5 mo	978	Galantamine	8 or 16 or 24	NPI	16 & 24mg/d groups improved significantly on total NPI scores (p<0.05) but 8mg/d and placebo groups deteriorated on total NPI scores.
(Bullock et al., 2001)	Open / 26wk	113	Rivastigmine	3-12	NPI-NH	-53% of patients with behavioral symptoms showed improvement. -Up to 93% of patients without behavioral symptoms did not develop these symptoms.
(Etemad, 2001)	Open / 26 wk	181	Rivastigmine	12	NPI-NH	Significant behavioral improvement (decrease by 4 points on mean total NPI score).
(Cummings et al., 2000a)	Open / 26 wk	173	Rivastigmine	3-12	NPI-NH	-Significant behavioral improvement (decrease by 3.25 points on mean total NPI score). -Significant improvement in psychosis sub-scale scores.
(Rosler et al., 1998)	Placebo-controlled / 26 wk Open / 104 wk	34	Rivastigmine	6-12	CIBIC-Plus	Statisitcal difference in the groups (p=0.02). Significant behavioral improvement at week 52 for hallucinations.

CIBIC-Plus: Clinician's Interview-Based Impression of Change Plus scale
ADAS-non-cog: Non-Cognitive portion of the Alzheimer's Disease Assessment Scale

Table 3. Cholinesterase inhibitors for psychosis in AD.

7. References

Avorn, J., Dreyer, P., & Connelly, K. (1989). Use of psychoactive medication and the quality of care in rest homes: findings and policy implications of a statewide study. *N Engl J Med, 320,* 227-232.

Barnes, R., Veith, R., Okimoto, J., Raskind, M., & Gumbrecht, G. (1982). Efficacy of antipsychotic medications in behaviorally disturbed dementia patients. *Am J Psychiatry, 139,* 1170-1174.

Beck, C. K. & Shue, V. M. (1994). Interventions for treating disruptive behavior in demented elderly people. *Nurs Clin North Am, 29,* 143-155.

Bullock, R., Moulias, R., & Steinwachs, K. C. (2001). Effects of Rivastigmine on behavioral symptoms in nursing home patients with Alzheimer's disease. *International Psychogeriatrics, 13,* 241.

Bymaster, F. B., Calligro, D. O., & Falcone, J. F. (1996). Radioreceptor binding profile of the atypical antipsychotic olanzapine . *Neuropsychopharmacology, 14,* 87-96.

Chengappa, K. N., Baker, R. W., Kreinbrook, S. B., & Adair, D. (1995). Clozapine use in female geriatric patients with psychoses. *J.Geriatr.Psychiatry Neurol., 8,* 12-15.

Chenoweth, B. & Spencer, B. (1986). Dementia: the experience of family caregivers. *Gerontologist, 26,* 267-272.

Clark, W. S., Street, J. S., Feldman, P. D., & Breier, A. (2001). The effects of olanzapine in reducing the emergence of psychosis among nursing home patients with Alzheimer's disease. *J.Clin.Psychiatry, 62,* 34-40.

Cohen-Mansfield, J. (2001). "Nonpharmacologic interventions for inappropriate behaviors in dementia: a review, summary, and critique." American Journal of Geriatric Psych 9(4): 361.

Corey-Bloom, J. (1995). Adjunctive therapy in patients with Alzheimer's disease. *Drugs & Aging, 7,* 79-87.

Cummings, J. L. (2000a). Cholinesterase inhibitors: A new class of psychotropic compounds. *Am.J.Psychiatry, 157,* 4-15.

Cummings, J. L. (2000b). The role of cholinergic agents in the management of behavioural disturbances in Alzheimer's disease. *Int. J. Neuropsychopharmacol., 3,* 21-29.

Cummings, J. L., Anand, R., & Koumaras, B. (2000a). Rivastigmine provides behavioral benefits to Alzheimer's disease patients residing in a nursing home: findings from a 26-week trial. *Neurology, 54,* A468.

Cummings, J. L., Donohue, J. A., & Brooks, R. L. (2000b). The relationship between donepezil and behavioral disturbances in patients with Alzheimer's disease. *Am.J.Geriatr.Psychiatry, 8,* 134-140.

Cummings, J. L., Cyrus, P. A., Ruzicka, B. B., & Gulanski, B. (1998). The Efficacy of Metrifonate in Improving the Behavioral Disturbances of Alzheimer's Disease Patients. *Neurology, 50,* Suppl.4, A251.

Cummings, J. L. & Kaufer, D. (1996). Neuropsychiatric aspects of Alzheimer's disease: the cholinergic hypothesis revisited. *Neurology, 47,* 876-883.

Cummings, J. L., Mega, M., Gray, K., Rosenberg-Thompson, S., Carusi, D. A. et al. (1994). The Neuropsychiatric Inventory: comprehensive assessment of psychopathology in dementia. *Neurology, 44,* 2308-2314.

Cummings, J. L., Gorman, D. G., & Shapira, J. (1993). Physostigmine ameliorates the delusions of Alzheimer's disease. *Biol.Psychiatry, 33,* 536-541.

Daniel, D. G. (2000). Antipsychotic treatment of psychosis and agitation in the elderly. *Journal of Clinical Psychiatry, 61,* 49-52.

Davis, K. L., Thal, L. J., Gamzu, E. R., Davis, C. S., Woolson, R. F. et al. (1992). A double-blind, placebo-controlled multicenter study of tacrine for Alzheimer's disease. The Tacrine Collaborative Study Group. *N.Engl.J.Med., 327,* 1253-1259.

De Deyn, P. P., Rabheru, K., Rasmussen, A., Bocksberger, J. P., Dautzenberg, P. L. et al. (1999). A randomized trial of risperidone, placebo, and haloperidol for behavioral symptoms of dementia. *Neurology, 53,* 946-955.

Deutsch, L. H., Bylsma, F. W., Rovner, B. W., Steele, C., & Folstein, M. F. (1991). Psychosis and Physical Aggression in Probable Alzheimer's Disease. *Am J Psychiatry, 148,* 1159-1163.

Devanand, D. P., Marder, K., Michaels, K. S., Sackeim, H. A., Bell, K. et al. (1998). A Randomized, Placebo-Controlled Dose-Comparison Trial of Haloperidol for Psychosis and Disruptive Behaviors in Alzheimer's Disease. *Am J Psychiatry, 155,* 1512-1520.

Drevets, W. C. & Rubin, E. H. (1989). Psychotic symptoms and the longitudinal course of senile dementia of the Alzheimer type. *Biological Psychiatry, 25,* 39-48.

Etemad, B. (2001). Behavioral and cognitive effects of rivastigmine in nursing home patients - a 26-week follow up. *International Psychogeriatrics, 13,* A246.

Farlow, M., Gracon, S. I., Hershey, L. A., Lewis, K. W., Sadowsky, C. H. et al. (1992). A controlled trial of tacrine in Alzheimer's disease. The Tacrine Study Group. *JAMA, 268,* 2523-2529.

Feldman, H., Gauthier, S., Hecker, J., Vellas, B., Subbiah, P. et al. (2001). A 24-week, randomized, double-blind study of donepezil in moderate to severe Alzheimer's disease. *Neurology, 57,* 613-620.

Finkel, S. I. (1998). The signs of the behavioral and psychological symptoms of dementia. *Clinician, 16,* 33-42.

Finkel, S. I. (1997). Managing the behavioral and psychological signs and symptoms of dementia. *International Clinical Psychopharmacology, 12,* 25-28.

Frankenburg, F. R. & Kalunian, D. (1994). Clozapine in the elderly. *J.Geriatr.Psychiatry Neurol., 7,* 129-132.

Frenchman, I. B. & Prince, T. (1997). Clinical experience with risperidone, haloperidol, and thioridazine for dementia-associated behavioral disturbances. *Int.Psychogeriatr., 9,* 431-435.

Gauthier, S., Feldman, H., Hecker, J., Vellas, B., Emir, B. et al. (2002). Functional, cognitive and behavioral effects of donepezil in patients with moderate Alzheimer's disease. *Curr.Med.Res.Opin., 18,* 347-354.

Gauthier, S., H. Loft, et al. (2008). "Improvement in behavioural symptoms in patients with moderate to severe Alzheimer's disease by memantine: a pooled data analysis." *International journal of geriatric psychiatry* 23(5): 537-545.

Gilley, D. W., Wilson, R., Beckett, L. A., & Evans, D. A. (1997). Psychotic Symptoms and Physically Aggressive Behavior in Alzheimer's Disease. *J Am Geriatr Soc, 45,* 1074-1079.

Giron, M. S. (2001). Psychotropic drug use in elderly people with and without dementia. *International Journal of Geriatric Psychiatry, 16,* 900-906.

Goldberg, R. J. & Goldberg, J. (1997). Risperidone for dementia-related disturbed behavior in nursing home residents: a clinical experience. *Int.Psychogeriatr., 9,* 65-68.

Gorman, D. G., Read, S., & Cummings, J. L. (1993). Cholinergic therapy of behavioral disturbances in Alzheimer's disease. *Neuropsychiatry Neuropsychol Behav Neurol, 6,* 229-234.

Haupt, M., A. Cruz-Jentoft, et al. (2006). "Mortality in elderly dementia patients treated with risperidone." Journal of Clinical Psychopharmacology 26(6): 566.

Helms, P. M. (1985). Efficacy of antipsychotics in the treatment of the behavioral complications of dementia: a review of the litterature. *J Am Geriatr Soc, 33,* 206-209.

Hemels, M. E. (2001). Clinical and economic factors in the treatment of behavioral and psychological symptoms of dementia. *Drugs & Aging, 18(7),* 527-550.

Herrmann, N., K. Rabheru, et al. (2005). "Galantamine treatment of problematic behavior in Alzheimer disease: post-hoc analysis of pooled data from three large trials." American Journal of Geriatric Psych 13(6): 527.

Herrmann, N. (2001). Recommendations for the management of behavioral and psychological symptoms of dementia. *Canadian Journal of Neurological Sciences, 28-Suppl 1,* 96-107.

Holmes, C., D. Wilkinson, et al. (2004). "The efficacy of donepezil in the treatment of neuropsychiatric symptoms in Alzheimer disease." Neurology 63(2): 214.

Irizarry, M. C., Ghaemi, S. N., Lee-Cherry, E. R., Gomez-Isla, T., Binetti, G. et al. (1999). Risperidone treatment of behavioral disturbances in outpatients with dementia. *J.Neuropsychiatry Clin.Neurosci., 11,* 336-342.

Jeste, D. V., D. Blazer, et al. (2007). "ACNP white paper: update on use of antipsychotic drugs in elderly persons with dementia." Neuropsychopharmacology 33(5): 957-970.

Jeste, D. V., Okamoto, A., Napolitano, J., Kane, J. M., & Martinez, R. A. (2000). Low incidence of persistent tardive dyskinesia in elderly patients with dementia treated with risperidone. *Am.J.Psychiatry, 157,* 1150-1155.

Jeste, D. V., Wragg, R. E., Salmon, D. P., Harris, M. J., & Thal, L. J. (1992). Cognitive deficits of patients with Alzheimer's Disease With and Without Delusions. *Am J Psychiatry, 149,* 184-189.

Katz, I. R., Jeste, D. V., Mintzer, J. E., Clyde, C., Napolitano, J. et al. (1999). Comparison of risperidone and placebo for psychosis and behavioral disturbances associated with dementia: a randomized, double-blind trial. Risperidone Study Group. *J.Clin.Psychiatry, 60,* 107-115.

Kaufer, D. (1998). Beyond the cholinergic hypothesis: the effect of metrifonate and other cholinesterase inhibitors on neuropsychiatric symptoms in Alzheimer's disease. *Dement.Geriatr.Cogn Disord., 9 Suppl 2,* 8-14.

Kaufer, D. I., Catt, K., Pollock, B. G., Lopez, O. L., & DeKosky, S. T. (1998). Donepezil in Alzheimer's disease: relative cognitive and neuropsychiatric responses and impact on caregiver distress. *Neurology, 50(4),* A89.

Kaufer, D. I., Cummings, J. L., & Christine, D. (1996). Effect of tacrine on behavioral symptoms in Alzheimer's disease: an open-label study. *J.Geriatr.Psychiatry Neurol, 9,* 1-6.

Knapp, M. J., Knopman, D. S., Solomon, P. R., Pendlebury, W. W., Davis, C. S. et al. (1994). A 30-week randomized controlled trial of high-dose tacrine in patients with Alzheimer's disease. The Tacrine Study Group. *JAMA, 271,* 985-991.

Lanctot, K. L., Best, T. S., Mittmann, N., Liu, B. A., Oh, P. I. et al. (1998). Efficacy and Safety of Neuroleptics in Behavioral Disorders Associated with Dementia. *J Clin Psychiatry, 59,* 550-561.

Lantz, M. S., Louis, A., & Lowenstein, G. (1990). A Longitudianal study of psychotropic prescriptions in a teaching nursing home. *Am J Psychiatry, 147,* 1637-1639.

Livingston, G., K. Johnston, et al. (2005). "Systematic review of psychological approaches to the management of neuropsychiatric symptoms of dementia." American Journal of Psychiatry 162(11): 1996.

Levy, M. L., Cummings, J. L., Fairbanks, L. A., Bravi, D., Calvani, M. et al. (1996). Longitudinal Assessment of Symptoms of Depression, Agitation, and Psychosis in 181 Patients With Alzheimer's Disease. *Am J Psychiatry, 153,* 1438-1443.

Lopez, O. L., Becker, J. T., & Brenner, R. P. (1991). Alzheimer's disease with delusions and hallucinations: neuropsychological and electroencephalographic correlates. *Neurology, 41,* 906-912.

Maixner, S. M., Mellow, A. M., & Tandon, R. (1999). The efficacy, safety, and tolerability of antipsychotics in the elderly. *J Clin Psychiatry, 60,* 29-41.

Matthews, H. P., Korbey, J., Wilkinson, D. G., & Rowden, J. (2000). Donepezil in Alzheimer's disease: eighteen month results from Southampton Memory Clinic. *Int.J.Geriatr.Psychiatry, 15,* 713-720.

McManus, D. Q., Arvanitis, L. A., & Kowalcyk, B. B. (1999). Quetiapine, a novel antipsychotic: experience in elderly patients with psychotic disorders. Seroquel Trial 48 Study Group. *J.Clin.Psychiatry, 60,* 292-298.

Mega, M. S., Masterman, D. M., O'Connor, S. M., Barclay, T. R., & Cummings, J. L. (1999). The spectrum of behavioral responses to cholinesterase inhibitor therapy in Alzheimer disease. *Arch.Neurol, 56,* 1388-1393.

Molchan, S. E., Vitiello, B., Minichiello, M., & Sunderland, T. (1991). Reciprocal changes in psychosis and mood after physostigmine in a patient with Alzheimer's disease. *Arch.Gen.Psychiatry, 48,* 1113-1114.

Morris, J. C., Cyrus, P. A., Orazem, J., Mas, J., Bieber, F. et al. (1998). Metrifonate benefits cognitive, behavioral, and global function in patients with Alzheimer's disease. *Neurology, 50,* 1222-1230.

Oberholzer, A. F., Hendriksen, C., Monsch, A. U., Heierli, B., & Stahelin, H. B. (1992). Safety and effectiveness of low-dose clozapine in psychogeriatric patients: a preliminary study. *Int.Psychogeriatr., 4,* 187-195.

Opie, J., Rosewarne, R., & O'Connor, D. W. (1999). The efficacy of psychosocial approaches to behavior disorders in dementia: a systematic literature review. *Aust NZ J Psychiatry, 33,* 789-799.

Overall, J. E. & Gorham, D. R. (1962). The Brief Psychiatric Rating Scale. *Psychol Rep, 10,* 799-812.

Petrie, W. M., Ban, T. A., & Berney, S. (1982). Loxapine in psychogeriatrics: a placebo- and a standard-controlled clinical investigation. *J Clin Psychopharmacol, 2,* 122-126.

Pitner, J. K., Mintzer, J. E., Pennypacker, L. C., & Jackson, C. W. (1995). Efficacy and adverse effects of clozapine in four elderly psychotic patients. *J.Clin.Psychiatry, 56,* 180-185.

Qizilbash, N., Whitehead, A., Higgins, J., Wilcock, G., Schneider, L. et al. (1998). Cholinesterase inhibition for Alzheimer disease: a meta-analysis of the tacrine trials. Dementia Trialists' Collaboration. *JAMA, 280,* 1777-1782.

Rabins, P. V., Mace, N. L., & Lucas, M. J. (1982). The impact of dementia on the family. *JAMA, 248,* 333-335.

Raskind, M. A. & Barnes, R. F. (2002). Alzheimer Disease: Treatment of non-cognitive behavioral abnormalities. In K. L. Davis, D. Charney, J. T. Coyle, & C. Nemeroff (Ed.), *Neuropsychopharmacology: The fifth generation of progress* (pp. 1253-1265). American College of Neuropsychopharmacology.

Raskind, M. A., Cyrus, P. A., Ruzicka, B. B., & Gulanski, B. I. (1999). The effects of metrifonate on the cognitive, behavioral, and functional performance of Alzheimer's disease patients. Metrifonate Study Group. *J.Clin.Psychiatry, 60,* 318-325.

Raskind, M. A., Sadowsky, C. H., Sigmund, W. R., Beitler, P. J., & Auster, S. B. (1997). Effect of tacrine on language, praxis, and noncognitive behavioral problems in Alzheimer disease. *Arch.Neurol, 54,* 836-840.

Reisberg, B. M., Franssen, E., & Sclan (1989). Stage specific incidence of potentially remediable behavioral symptoms in aging and Alzheimer's disease: a study of 120 patients using the BEHAVE-AD. *Bull Clin Neurosc, 54,* 95-112.

Reisberg, B., Borenstein, J., Salob, S. P., Ferris, S. H., Franssen, E. et al. (1987). Behavioral Symptoms in Alzheimers-Disease - Phenomenology and Treatment. *Journal of Clinical Psychiatry, 48,* 9-15.

Rosen, W. G., Mohs, R. C., & Davis, K. L. (1984). A new rating scale for Alzheimer's disease. *Am.J.Psychiatry, 141,* 1356-1364.

Rosler, M., Retz, W., Retz-Junginger, P., & Dennler, H. J. (1998). Effects of two-year treatment with the cholinesterase inhibitor rivastigmine on behavioural symptoms in Alzheimer's disease. *Behav Neurol, 11,* 211-216.

Rubin, E., Morris, J. C., & Berg, L. (1988). The progression of personality changes in senile dementia of the Alzheimer's type. *J Am Geriatr Soc, 35,* 721-725.

Salzman, C., Vaccaro, B., Lieff, J., & Weiner, A. (1995). Clozapine in Older Patients with Psychosis and Behavioral Disruption. *American Journal of Geriatric Psychiatry, 3*, 26-33.

Satterlee, W. G., Reams, S. G., Burns, P. R., & . (1995). A clinical update on olanzapine treatment in schizophrenia and Alzheimer's disease patients. *Psychopharmacolgy Bulletin, 31*, 534.

Scharre, D. W. & Chang, S. I. (2002). Cognitive and behavioral effects of quetiapine in Alzheimer disease patients. *Alzheimer Dis.Assoc.Disord., 16*, 128-130.

Schneider LS, Dagerman KS, Insel P (2005). Risk of death with atypical antipsychotic drug treatment for dementia: meta- analysis of randomized placebo-controlled trials. J Am Med Assoc 294: 1934–1943.

Schneider LS, Dagerman K, Insel PS (2006). Efficacy and adverse effects of atypical antipsychotics for dementia: meta-analysis of randomized, placebo-controlled trials. Am J Geriatr Psychiatry 14: 191–210.

Schneider, L. S., Pollock, V. E., & Lyness, S. A. (1990). A metaanalysis of controlled trials of neuroleptic treatment in dementia. *J Am Geriatr Soc, 38*, 553-563.

Small, G. W., Donohue, J. A., & Brooks, R. L. (1998). An economic evaluation of donepezil in the treatment of Alzheimer's disease. *Clin.Ther., 20*, 838-850.

Small, J. G., Milstein, V., Marhenke, J. D., Hall, D. D., & Kellams, J. J. (1987). Treatment outcome with clozapine in tardive dyskinesia, neuroleptic sensitivity, and treatment-resistant psychosis. *J.Clin.Psychiatry, 48*, 263-267.

Stern, Y., Mayeux, R., & Sano, M. (1987). Predictors of disease course in patients with probable Alzheimer's disease. *Neurology, 37*, 1649-1653.

Stoppe, G. (1999). Behavioral problems associated with dementia: the role of newer antipsychotics. *Drugs & Aging, 14*, 41-54.

Street, J. S., Clark, W. S., Kadam, D. L., Mitan, S. J., Juliar, B. E. et al. (2001). Long-term efficacy of olanzapine in the control of psychotic and behavioral symptoms in nursing home patients with Alzheimer's dementia. *Int.J.Geriatr.Psychiatry, 16 Suppl 1*, S62-S70.

Street, J. S., Clark, W. S., Gannon, K. S., Cummings, J. L., Bymaster, F. P. et al. (2000). Olanzapine treatment of psychotic and behavioral symptoms in patients with Alzheimer disease in nursing care facilities: a double-blind, randomized, placebo-controlled trial. The HGEU Study Group. *Arch.Gen.Psychiatry, 57*, 968-976.

Swearer, J. M. (1994). Behavioral disturbances in dementia. In J. C. Morris (Ed.), *Handbook of dementing illnesses* (pp. 499-527). New York: Marcel Dekker Inc.

Tandon, R. (1998). Antipsychotic agents. In F. M. Quintin, D. C. Adams, & C. L. Bowden (Ed.), *Current psychotherapeutic drugs* (pp. 120-154). Philadelphia (PA): Current Medicine Inc.

Tariot, P. N., Cummings, J. L., Katz, I. R., Mintzer, J., Perdomo, C. A. et al. (2001). A randomized, double-blind, placebo-controlled study of the efficacy and safety of donepezil in patients with Alzheimer's disease in the nursing home setting. *J.Am.Geriatr.Soc., 49*, 1590-1599.

Tariot, P. N., Solomon, P. R., Morris, J. C., Kershaw, P., Lilienfeld, S. et al. (2000). A 5-month, randomized, placebo-controlled trial of galantamine in AD. The Galantamine USA-10 Study Group. *Neurology, 54,* 2269-2276.

Tariot, P. N. & Blazina, L. (1994). The psychopathology of dementia. In J. C. Morris (Ed.), *Handbook of dementing illnesses* (pp. 461-474). New York: Marcel Decker Inc.

Trinh NH, Hoblyn J, Mohanty S, Yaffe K (2003). Efficacy of cholinesterase inhibitors in the treatment of neuropsychiatric symptoms and functional impairment in Alzheimer disease: a meta-analysis. J Am Med Assoc 289: 210–216.

Wang, P. S., S. Schneeweiss, et al. (2005). "Risk of death in elderly users of conventional vs. atypical antipsychotic medications." New England Journal of Medicine 353(22): 2335-2341.

Weiser, M., Rotmensch, H. H., Korczyn, A. D., Hartman, R., Cicin-Sain, A. et al. (2002). A pilot, randomized, open-label trial assessing safety and pharmakokinetic parameters of co-administration of rivastigmine with risperidone in dementia patients with behavioral disturbances. *Int.J.Geriatr.Psychiatry, 17,* 343-346.

Winblad, B., Engedal, K., Soininen, H., Verhey, F., Waldemar, G. et al. (2001). A 1-year, randomized, placebo-controlled study of donepezil in patients with mild to moderate AD. *Neurology, 57,* 489-495.

Wragg, R. E. & Jeste, D. V. (1989). Overview of Depression and Psychosis in Alzheimer's disease. *Am J Psychiatry, 146,* 577-587.

14

The Relative Efficacy of Live Graded Exposure, Live Modeling, and Computer-Based Symbolic Modeling in the Treatment of Spider Phobia: A Perspective of Emotion

Ahmed M. Hassan*
Department of Anatomy, School of Medicine, and Department of Psychology, Leeds University, UK

1. Introduction

This chapter describes a research work that investigated whether a computer-based symbolic modeling procedure could be successfully used in the treatment of a maladaptive emotional condition, namely spider phobia. It also examined whether the procedure would prove to be as effective as other conventional treatments for the same clinical condition.

The efficacy of any therapeutic strategy presumably depends considerably on the accuracy with which the systems of the human body, as well as the ways in which they function, are conceived. Accordingly, an accurate model of human emotional functioning is crucial for the construction of a therapeutic framework that expresses an integral set of scientifically established facts about emotion and sets forth relevant objectives and specific principles for clinical application. A major line of investigation in this research was concerned with the diversity of existing concepts of emotion (such as fear and anxiety) and its components, which has led the various therapeutic approaches to emphasize different emotional components as the major target of their therapeutic techniques. The objective in this respect was to investigate whether specific conceptualizations of emotion, fear and anxiety in particular, could be consolidated to form a coherent theoretical basis for the proposed, computer-based, delivery system. In this respect, a specific psychological problem (i.e., specific phobia) was targeted to provide a reference point in exploring the theoretical and clinical dimensions of this investigation. This principal line of research is reviewed in detail in the next section below.

Another line of investigation in this research concerned the usability of computers in delivering treatment for behavioral problems such as anxiety-related disorders including phobias. The objective was to verify the efficacy of a self-administered, computer-based, treatment technique in producing effective therapeutic change, hence providing theoretical and empirical bases for expanding behavioral treatment to meet a substantial proportion of the current demand. This line of research is outlined in section 3 on human-computer interaction.

---

* Current Address: *Department of Mental Health, King Faisal Specialist Hospital & Research Center, Riyadh, Saudi Arabia*

Subsequently, a prototype computer-based symbolic modeling technique for the treatment of spider phobia, which was constructed on the basis of a proposed theoretical concept of emotion, was described in section 4. The effectiveness of the technique was compared with that of two conventional methods for treating spider phobia in order to validate its clinical efficacy. Spider phobia was selected as the clinical problem of investigation mainly because of its clinical specificity. The clinical results, described and discussed in sections 5 and 6, further suggest that the effect induced in either of the cognitive or overt verbal response systems underlying respective fear components is likely to similarly and equally affect the fear component manifested by the other systems. The findings of this work may warrant the development of similar techniques for the treatment of other similar behavioral problems concerned with anxiety and fear.

2. Emotion: review and implications

The literature on emotion shows that the nature of emotion and the mechanisms involved in its experience and expression constitute a field of long-standing controversy (e.g., James, 1890/1950; Cannon, 1927; Papez, 1937; MacLean, 1950; Schachter, 1964; Lazarus, 1984; Zajonc, 1984; Panksepp, 1988, 1990; Gray, 1982, 1990; Hassan and Ward, 1991). The result of this controversy has been a set of concepts of emotion that are neither exclusive nor complementary, and which have projected a range of divergent clinical implications (e.g., Rachman, 1981). In fact, different theories of emotion are found to be emphasizing different response systems as being underlying the mechanisms involved in emotional experience or expression (Leventhal and Tomarken, 1986, 1988). A brief outline of controversies about emotion will follow.

Early theories of emotion (e.g., James, 1950/1890; Lange, 1967/1885; Zajonc, 1980, 1984) point out that the autonomic processes are the prime determinant of emotion, or that emotion is potentially independent of cognition. Further, the primary role of subcortical structures within the brain in mediating emotional functioning is emphasized by yet another set of theories on emotion (e.g., Cannon, 1927; Papez, 1937; McLean, 1950). Each of these theories offers its own concepts of emotion and proposes specific mechanisms for its experiencing and expression. One major implication of such controversy on psychotherapy is that the various therapeutic approaches tend to place a primary emphasis on one response system to the relative neglect of the others (Wilson, 1978). This can be clearly observed by looking to the therapeutic strategies of these approaches in the treatment of an emotion such as fear. For example, behavioral approaches to therapy focus on overt behavior as the subject matter of therapy. They explain emotional responses in terms of learning principles (e.g., Eysenck, 1987). They argue that fear reactions, for instance, are learned as a way of reducing the anxiety elicited by a particular object or situation. Therefore, exposure to the feared stimulus without harmful consequences leads to extinction of the fear; hence, exposure to the un-reinforced conditioned stimulus (i.e., the harmless object of fear) is the conceptual basis of behavior therapy. Wolpe's (1958) counter-conditioning approach emphasizes autonomic responsiveness. Based on his theory of reciprocal inhibition, Wolpe argues that the induction of an autonomic responsiveness of relaxation can reduce or eliminate pre-existing anxiety symptoms since the autonomic states of relaxation and anxiety are incompatible and cannot co-exist. Cognitive approaches, on the other hand, conceptualize emotion as a post-cognition phenomenon (e.g., Beck, 1976; Lazarus, 1982, 1984). Generally speaking, these approaches argue that an individual's emotional reactions are determined by the way he/she interprets events (Greenberg and Safran, 1987). Therefore, these personal meanings of events are the primary targets of change in cognitive therapy; hence they focus on maladaptive thought patterns and related cognitive processes.

These, rather 'skewed', concepts of the emotion of fear, which underlie the therapeutic approaches so far outlined, are probably a contributory factor in the frequently observed discordance between autonomic, somatic motor, and cognitive components of fear in their rate of response to treatment (Rachman, 1978, 1990). However, despite the diverse notions about emotion, there seems to be a consensus on the multi-component nature of emotion (Lang, 1971, 1985; Scherer, 1984; Frijda, 1986; Gray, 1990). Lang's (1968, 1971) three-system model of emotion conceptualizes fear and anxiety in terms of overt behavioral, cognitive, and autonomic components. Further, Rachman (1977) has found that the response systems underlying these three components of fear do not always co-vary and, therefore, a treatment procedure that affects only one or two response systems may result in incomplete treatment in terms of residual fear in other response systems. On the basis of this proposition, an effective treatment of, for example, phobia would be expected to induce a therapeutic change in all response systems. Nevertheless, different theoretical and therapeutic perspectives of emotion tend to emphasize the primacy of one component over the others. Rachman (1981), for example, suggests that behaviorally-based treatments will probably prove more effective than cognitive treatments of emotional disorders. Further, Zajonc (1984) proposes the independence of emotion from cognition (For a critical review of Zajonc's (1984) proposition on the primacy of emotion, see Hassan and Ward, 1991). Accordingly, one may logically argue that if a behaviorally based treatment of an irrational emotional state, such as phobia, would prove effective, then there must be a central mechanism whereby the behaviorally induced therapeutic change also mediates cognitive and autonomic change. This proposition is pursued below after reviewing some major concepts of emotion.

The cognitive-appraisal theories of emotion (e.g., Schachter, 1964; Lazarus, 1982, 1984; Scherer, 1984) argue for the primacy of cognitive processes in determining an emotional state. They hold that an emotional state is the product of an interaction between two components: physiological arousal, and cognition about the cause of that arousal. Therefore, the perception or attribution of a causal connection between the two components is necessary for the generation of an emotional state. According to these theories, cognitions determine the quality of emotions, while arousal determines the intensity of these emotions. Hence, like Cannon's (1927) assertion, it is proposed that arousal in itself is emotionally non-specific. However, the various studies conducted to test the predictions derived from the cognitive-appraisal theory, concerning the mis-attribution of drug-induced arousal to emotional or neutral cues, revealed that the evidence for the theory was generally weak (Leventhal and Tomarken, 1986). Further, some studies (e.g., Rogers and Deckner, 1975; Marshal and Zimbardo, 1979; Maslach, 1979) showed that the unexplained arousal was in fact found to induce heightened negative affect. Similarly, the manipulation of attributions concerning anxiety and other negative emotional states, in clinical settings, have generally failed (e.g., Bootzin, Herman and Nicassio, 1976; Chamblis and Murray, 1979; Cotton, Baron and Borkovec, 1980).

On the other hand, Leventhal (1984) identifies a hierarchical emotional processing mechanism, consisting of a series of temporal stages, in the cognitive system. He argues that the mechanism mediates, in a fast acting and rapidly processed manner, between stimulus situations and response. The first stage involves the reception and coding of information, which results in the construction of a 'representation' of the stimulus situation and an 'emotional representation' (or experience) of the situation. The second, 'coping', stage involves the generation and execution of action to cope with the perceived situation and with the emotional reaction to it. The third, 'appraisal', stage involves setting criteria and evaluating the outcome of coping efforts. Accordingly, the creation of an emotional representation (or experience) is a product of a multi-level system that is usually simultaneously active and congruent in their emotional output, although at times may act differently or become in conflict with each other. The lowest level is a 'sensory-motor' processing, followed by a 'schematic processing' level, with the highest level is the 'conceptual processing'. This model of emotion proposes a reciprocal relationship between emotion and cognition, rather than the primacy of one over another. According to this model, emotion is either elicited by cognition or it generates cognition by activating schematic memory once aroused.

Leventhal's (1984) model provides a basis for explaining some clinical observations, such as the fear reactions of individuals with phobia despite their acknowledgement of the irrationality of their fears. According to the model, although the individual may recognize, at the conceptual processing level, the non-harmfulness of the object of his/her fear, yet he/she displays strong sensory-motor reactions of anxiety when confronted with the same object. The model suggests that emotion is experienced and generated centrally, with the expressive responses (verbal reports; overt motor responses, such as bodily movements; and autonomic reactions, such as sweating) being an outer reflection of an inner emotional state. That is, outer emotional expression and inner emotional experience are linked in sensory-motor processing and in emotional schematic processing. Similarly, outer emotional expression, the theory proposes, can initiate, strengthen, or sustain inner experience by the same two routes of processing. However, outer expression is more frequently preceded by the activation of an emotional state; for example, a stimulus situation may evoke an expressive-motor process.

Leventhal's (1984) model of cognitive processing of emotion reflects an integrative image of emotion and emotional processing. For example, emotional reflexes (activated by sensory-motor processing) are integrated with concrete (schematic processing) and abstract (conceptual processing) memory structures in the presence of fear and anxiety. In addition, the model reflects a concept of emotional processing that proposes a number of interactions among the systems of behavioral machinery. This proposition of systemic interactivity may be extended to assume, for example in the case of phobias, that the influence of environmental factors may affect cognitive responding, or that cognitive events may be sufficient to induce behavioral and autonomic change. The latter proposition has been hypothesized by Lang (1971) in relation to the three-system model of fear and anxiety. The accuracy of Leventhal's (1984) conceptual model of emotion may be examined at a neuro-biological level of analysis.

The neuro-biological perspective of emotion attempts to explain the nature of emotional experience and expression by exploring the different neural systems implicated in emotion. The belief (e.g., Panksepp, 1988) is that the neuro-biological approach has a better chance of generating factual knowledge about brain structures, pathways, and processes implicated in emotionality. This approach represents a molecular level of analysis, and the evidence yielded by which may help guide the search for solid understanding of emotion at the psychological level. All psychological phenomena can not be reduced to intrinsic brain processes (Panksepp, 1988); therefore, the two domains can reciprocate to produce a much more accurate model of human emotional functioning (Hassan and Ward, 1991). Cannon's (1927) theory of emotion proposes that the thalamus is the center that mediates the various processes associated with emotional expression (somatic-motor, autonomic, and subjective/cognitive). The theory argues that, upon the discharge of 'thalamic processes', bodily changes occur almost simultaneously with the emotional experience. The evidence quoted for supporting this proposition included the observation that emotional expressions could be elicited in decorticated and decerebrated animals (Cannon, 1927), but not when thalamic structures were additionally ablated (Bard and Rioch, 1937). This theory was later challenged by Papez (1937) and MacLean (1950), who concluded that the anatomical interconnections among limbic structures in the forebrain were responsible for emotional experience, and that the limbic portion of the brain was the locus of emotion. However, Wall and Pribram (1950) have shown the relationship between the limbic structures and emotion to be non-conclusive. They demonstrated that other cerebral regions, when electrically stimulated, also evoke a visceral response. In addition, they observed that emotional changes were found to accompany lesions in forebrain centers other than the limbic areas. When the limbic structures themselves were stimulated, behavior of a cognitive nature, such as problem-solving and memory deficiencies, was affected in ways which could not be related to emotional changes.

Following the above review on emotion, certain conclusions may be summarized. First, emotion seems to be unexplainable in terms of the processes of a single brain structure. Second, the neuro-biological basis of emotion seems to give the forebrain cortex, rather than peripheral (i.e., visceral) processes, a central role in emotional control and experience. Third, the evidence on central neural interconnections (Dimond, 1980; Brodal, 1981) shows that a convergence of information as sensory impulses of different kinds is evident in many regions of the cerebral cortex. This fact suggests that highly integrative processes occur in the brain, whether in emotional or non-emotional states.

What are the implications of this line of evidence on the propositions that advocate the primacy of one response system over the others?

First, there does not seem to be, at least in the available literature, strong evidence for assuming that overt behavior is the primary indicator of an emotional state. The same probably applies to cognitive responding and autonomic reactions associated with such a state.

Second, the brain seems to sustain a dynamic two-way exchange with external as well as internal environment (Panksepp, 1988). In so doing, the brain is equipped with intrinsic but experientially refined sensory, attentional, perceptual, emotional, and motor systems. The richness of neural interconnections of the CNS adds to the complexity of ways in which these systems interact to mediate different behaviors, including emotional ones, whether normal or abnormal.

Third, intrinsic perceptual and memory properties of the brain suggest that the latter probably never remains empty or still (Panksepp, 1988). Leventhal's (1984) model, and particularly his concept of central schematic and propositional storage, may explain how emotional states are influenced by previous emotional and non-emotional events. This proposition gives a significant importance, but not primacy, to the cognitive system with regard to emotional processing.

With this view of human emotional functioning in mind, one would hypothesize that different effects produced by cognitively directed or behaviorally based techniques are not necessarily the result of targeting a specific, presumably prime, response system. It is rather due to the interactive nature of brain processes. This conclusion seems to favor the view suggested by Lang (1971) that the three response systems (overt behavioral, cognitive, and autonomic) tend to mutually augment, sustain, or attenuate each other. For example, high levels of physiological arousal during an emotional state are likely to affect cognitive performance (Williams, Watts, MacLeod and Mathews, 1988). Williams, et al., (1988) argues that phobic clients are usually highly sensitive to stimuli in their environment that represent their fear; they become more vigilant towards, or preoccupied with ideas related to, these stimuli than others. This attentional bias is demonstrated by Watts, McKenna, Sharrock and Trezise (1986) in a study involving spider-avoidant subjects. Subjects were required to name the color of words in two lists: one containing words such as fear, death, and grief; the other consisted of spider-related words, such as hairy and crawl. They found that the subjects showed little disruption in responding to the first list, but a very large disruption in colour-naming spider words. Following treatment, these subjects showed significant reduction in disruption in comparison to controls.

On the other hand, factors associated with cognitive processing during an emotional state may be the underlying source of the reported dissociation between different response systems in phobias (Rachman and Hodgson, 1974; Rachman, 1977; Hugdahl, 1989). Leventhal's (1988) model offers an explanation for the effects of such factors on other response systems. For example, people with specific phobias may acknowledge the irrationality of their fear reactions at the conceptual level of cognitive processing; yet, they may show fear reactions at the sensory-motor level, in the form of overt avoidance responses and/or autonomic reactions, when faced with the object of their phobia.

The proposition, therefore, is that a cognitively directed treatment of specific phobia is likely to prove effective if it takes into consideration all relevant, cognitive and non-cognitive, components of emotion. For example, in conducting a therapeutic symbolic modeling procedure, the adequacy of modeled behaviors in instigating lasting effects (whether in terms of overt responses or autonomic functioning) on observing clients is likely to depend on clients' previous and subsequent overt behavioral responses, and the autonomic events associated with such behaviors. By means of graded sequence of fear-provoking symbolic stimuli, the level of arousal induced by these stimuli in clients is likely to be reasonably below the threshold that may instigate avoidance. In addition, a coping, rather than mastering, style of the model in performing approach responses to these stimuli is expected to contribute positively and to match the cognitive image of the observing phobic client. The same applies to behaviorally based therapies. This proposition, which reflects the core of the conceptual framework of the symbolic modeling technique, is examined empirically in Section 4.

3. Human-computer interaction

The practical help that computers provide in many domains of today's human life is well recognized (e.g., Zoltan and Chapanis, 1982). The usability of computers by humans has been thoroughly investigated (e.g., Rasmussen, 1986; Woods and Roth, 1988). In this respect, a usable computer system is defined by Landauer (1988) as the one that is "easy and pleasant to learn and operate" (p. 905). This definition involves two factors, knowledge and attitude, which seem to be interrelated. However, several studies (e.g., Zoltan and Chapanis, 1982; Bertino, 1985) concluded that the mere lack of knowledge about, or experience with, computers may not be in itself a sufficient condition for negative attitudes towards computers; having such knowledge or experience is also not likely to be sufficient for producing positive attitudes towards computers. However, the use of computers for treatment or in treatment-related contexts, where a patient is required to interact with a computer rather than a human clinician, raises important issues. Of these, the more salient are: whether the adoption of such procedures is justified; the acceptability of the procedure by patients; and the validity of clinical outcome of these computer-based procedures.

Patients have been required to interact with computers in many different situations, which included medical history taking (Slack, Hicks, Reed and Van Cura, 1966; Slack and Van Cura, 1968; Greist, Gustafson and Stauss, 1973; Lucas, Mullin, Luna and McIlroy, 1977; Fitter and Cruickshank, 1982; Carr, Ghosh and Ancill, 1983), behavioral assessment (Carr and Ghosh, 1983a), and psychiatric assessment (Lewis, Pelosi, Glover, Wilkinson, Stansfeld, Williams and Sheperd, 1988; Wright, 1990). Various justifications have been offered in these previous studies for using computer-based methods to achieve certain clinical objectives, ranging from pressures of short appointment times and differing abilities of individual doctors (Wright, 1990) that may result in failure to detect problems, to shortage of experienced staff and limited availability of treatment to patients in areas away from appropriate treatment centers (Carr and Ghosh, 1983a). All the reported studies so far on computer-based clinical procedures have agreed that the results that emerged from such interactions were as accurate and valid as those obtained by human clinicians. Further, Carr and Ghosh (1983b), in a study on phobia patients, concluded that some of their clients found the computer-based interview more acceptable and found it easier to communicate with the computer than with the clinician.

However, the use of computers in all the previous studies was restricted to history taking and assessment. That is, there has been no attempt to use computers for delivering active behavioral treatment. Nevertheless, there seems to be a broadly held conviction that behavioral and emotional malfunctioning constitutes a problem of a considerable prevalence (e.g., Sines, 1980). Existing therapeutic procedures often require the expertise and the actual involvement of specialist therapists and lengthy durations of management (Carr and Ghosh, 1983b; Carr, Ghosh and Ancill, 1983). This situation effectively has meant the restriction of such expertise to specialist behavioral units, out of reach of many sufferers (Carr and Ghosh, 1983b), as well as long client waiting lists. Given the findings of Carr and Ghosh (1983a) that a computer interview was as acceptable as a conventional interview to clients with phobia, and that computer-derived target behaviors for treatment were accurate, a subsequent question may be whether a computer-based exposure treatment of phobia will be equally accurate and acceptable to such clients. One possible justification for raising such a question is that treatment of phobias, and specific phobias in particular, has frequently involved exposure to the phobic object, whether *in vivo*, imagined or as symbolic representations. In fact, equipment other than computers, such as film projectors (e.g., Bandura, 1965; Bandura, Blanchard and Ritter, 1969) has been utilized in treating specific phobias by symbolic representations of the phobic object. Therefore, it seems reasonable to investigate whether computers can be used in the same context. Since no empirical evidence for answering this question was available at the time of this study, some encouraging indications of relevance to this issue have been derived from the study by Lang, Melamed and Hart (1970) on an automated treatment of snake phobia. Computers were not involved in the study by Lang, et al. (1970), and, instead, an apparatus consisting of audio transmitters to convey imagery instructions and buttons for clients to interact with the equipment were used. Nevertheless, the principle of automated behavioral treatment was applied. The findings were that the automated procedure was found to be effective in inducing the desired behavioral change, and the technique was acceptable to all clients. Along these lines, a computer-based symbolic modeling technique was conceived, constructed, and then applied in order to examine the clinical validity and efficacy of such a computer-based therapeutic approach to behavioral treatment.

In this study, the knowledge of a group of individuals with spider phobia about computers, as well as their attitudes towards a proposition of using computers in behavioral treatment, were investigated using a questionnaire designed and validated for the purpose. The results showed a generally positive attitude towards interacting with a computer for treatment purposes. This positive attitude was independent of the level of computer knowledge acquired by respondents.

4. Method and procedure

Sample

A group of self-identified spider phobic individuals responded to an advertisement in the local media offering treatment for spider phobia. Of the 44 individuals who attended the first pre-treatment session, 42 were found suitable for psychological treatment of their spider phobia, decided on the basis of (a) a clinical interview; and (b) a behavioral approach test (BAT). Consequently, the 42 individuals were identified as having spider phobia on the basis of the BAT results and in accordance with the DSM-III-R (American Psychiatric Association, 1987) criteria for the diagnosis of simple phobia.

Using a matched-group design technique, four client groups matched on the basis of their BAT scores were obtained and each client was then designated, on a random basis, to one of the four treatment conditions: Live Graded Exposure (LGE), Live Modeling (LM), Computer-Based Symbolic Modeling (CBSM), and Waiting List Control (WLC) groups. Of the 42 clients, three failed to attend subsequent sessions; a fourth client decided to withdraw from the study (because she was self-convinced that her anxiety and fear of spiders were "beyond treatment"). The final number of clients included in the study was, therefore, 38 (8 males and 30 females); the mean age was 28.7 (SD = 13.3). The LGE group contained 2 males and 7 females, the LM group contained one male and 10 female, and the CBSM group contained 3 males and 7 females, while the WLC group contained 2 males and 6 females. Clients in the four groups of the study received pre- and post-treatment assessment, whereas clients in the three treatment conditions also received a follow-up assessment at least 45 days after the completion of treatment.

Treatments

1. Live Graded Exposure (LGE)

It involved exposing the client with spider phobia to live spiders in a graded sequence of fear provoking items/tasks, whereas the client made his/her progression through the increasingly fearful steps of the sequence with the help of muscle relaxation exercises. Two sets of pictorial representations of the spiders were used as a baseline exposure. Three live tarantula spiders, of different sizes, and a garden spider were used in the live exposure sessions.

2. Live Modeling (LM)

The client with phobia here first observed the therapist performing a similarly graded sequence of tasks involving live spiders. Next, the client was required to repeat what he/she had observed the therapist performing. The procedure continued, with the help of muscle relaxation exercises in response to client's anxiety or fear, until the client was capable of performing all the tasks in the graded sequence without experiencing anxiety or fear. Two sets of pictorial representations of the spiders were used as a baseline exposure. Three live tarantula spiders and a garden spider, identical to those used with the LGE group, were used in the LM sessions.

3. Computer-Based Symbolic Modeling (CBSM)

This prototype treatment procedure was based on Bandura's (1969) principles of modeling and the findings of studies on human-computer interaction for behavioral treatment purposes (Hassan, 1992, unpublished PhD Thesis). The system used in this technique involved an optical disc that contained the programmed audio-visual therapeutic material. The therapeutic material included real life pictures of spiders, filmed human-spider interactions, as well as a filmed demonstration of muscle relaxation exercises. A laser vision player was used to control the display of the optical disc material on an interconnected TV screen. A computer system (IBM PS/2), consisting of a Guide programme (prepared by the researcher with the help of a computer specialist), was used to control the laser vision player. The client's interaction with the programme was effected using a computer mouse. Communication with the laser vision player and the display of material from the optical disc were achieved using labeled buttons created with Guide programme and displayed on the computer screen.

The procedure, which involved the use of still and motion pictures in a graded sequence of fear provoking pictures or instructions, consisted of an adult female who approached the spiders in a coping, rather than mastering, manner. The contents of the CBSM programme were prepared so that all information necessary for a client's interaction with the equipment were provided by the system directly to the client. The therapist, however, was present in the treatment room during sessions to monitor the smooth running of equipment, and to answer queries related to that matter; otherwise, no help was offered to clients in this group or, in fact, was requested by them.

4. Waiting List Control (WLC)

The clients in this group were left untreated until the treatment sessions of the other three groups were completed, and then the WLC clients were assessed for the second time using the same assessment procedures as used in the pre-treatment assessment protocol. Finally, all clients in the WLC group were provided with treatment of their spider phobia condition.

Measures

1. Behavioral Approach Test (BAT)

The BAT objectively observed and then scored each client's overt behavioral approach responses to the spiders. It involved 11 increasingly fearful tasks. A completed task was scored 2, an attempted but not completed task was scored 1, and a score of 0 was given if the task was not attempted. A video recorder was mounted in the BAT room, so that it monitored the full length of the room, to record each client's performance during the BAT.

2. Fear Scale (FS)

The FS was designed by the researcher to identify, in a self-report form, the fear reactions of clients to various dimensions of spiders - type, size, color, proximity, movement, and various physical contacts with spiders. Clients' responses to each item were made on an 8-point scale, ranging from no fear (0) to extreme fear (7).

3. Spider Phobia Questionnaire (SPQ)

To be answered at a computer screen, the researcher adopted the SPQ (Watts and Sharrock, 1984), which focused on clients' responsiveness relevant to their spider phobia (rather than the dimensions of the phobic object).

4. Anticipatory Fear Arousal (assessed in terms of HR acceleration)

This index of fear was measured in terms of the acceleration in heart rate (HR) in response to anticipatory fear. The measure was represented in terms of the difference between 'baseline HR' and 'the HR during an instruction phase' - involving verbal statements describing to clients the tasks of the BAT that they were required to perform.

Procedure

1. Pre-treatment sessions

The first of the two pre-treatment sessions involved educating each client on the study's objectives, carrying out a semi-structured clinical interview, and then explaining the treatment procedures to the 'suitable' client and obtaining an informed consent from him or her. Also, the client was required to answer the SPQ at the computer screen. Then, the client was given: (a) the written instructions on muscle relaxation training, and was instructed to exercise the steps at least once daily at home and to report any difficulties experienced at the second assessment session; (b) the FS, to complete at home; the clients were also required to rate the 20 items of the FS in terms of fear or anxiety induced by each, starting from the most fearful downward. The rankings were then used to build the standard graded hierarchy of the phobic object.

In the second pre-treatment session, clients' performance in the relaxation exercise was reviewed and difficulties were dealt with accordingly. Then, clients' HR was measured using the Grass polygraph machine and disposable surface electrodes. The procedure consisted of a baseline recording and a subsequent instructional phase recording during which the client listened to the BAT instructions.

2. Treatment sessions

All treatment procedures provided specific and essentially similar factual knowledge about spiders, either verbally by the therapist (as in the LGE and LM conditions) or contained in the audio-visually presented dialogue between two adult females (as in the CBSM condition). The treatment sessions, across the conditions, lasted for 40 minutes each, and were held twice a week for each client. The sessions in the LGE and LM conditions continued until the client was capable of performing all approach tasks, involving live spiders, fearlessly and confidently. In the CBSM condition, the sessions continued until the client was confident that he or she would perform the subsequent BAT fearlessly and confidently. Otherwise, each treatment condition progressed as described above.

3. Post-treatment assessment

It was carried out approximately one weak after the completion of treatment, and consisted of the measurements as those contained in the pre-treatment assessment.

4. Follow-up assessment

It took place at least 45 days from the date of the post-treatment assessment. It followed, in assessing treatment effects, the same procedure as that of the pre-treatment assessment. However, clients were not asked to complete the FS because the SPQ and the FS were found to be showing a high positive correlation.

5. Results

Table 1 shows the distribution of age, sex, and occupation of clients in the four study groups. On the pre-treatment data, an Anova procedure showed no significant difference between the four groups on age, sex, or duration of phobia. As the four groups were matched on the basis of their pre-treatment BAT scores, subsequent analysis of variance for BAT scores confirmed the appropriateness of the matching procedure [$F(3, 37) = .292$; $p>.10$].

Group	N	Sex		Age		Occupation		
		M	F	Mean	SD	Employed	Unemployed	Student
LGE	09	02	07	32.89	14.66	05	02	02
LM	11	01	10	27.27	12.63	07	01	03
CBSM	10	03	07	31.30	11.98	07	01	02
WLC	08	02	06	22.88	14.31	01	01	06
Total	38	08	30	28.74	13.31	20	05	13

Key: LGE = Live Graded Exposure; LM = Live Modeling; CBSM = Computer-based Symbolic Modeling; WLC = Waiting List Control; M = Male; F = Female; SD = Standard Deviation.

Table 1. Distribution of Age, Sex, and Occupation in the Four Study Groups.

5.1 The statistical significance of results

The Statistical Analysis of Treatment Effects (post-treatment)

Table 2 shows the mean scores and the standard deviations (SD) of the three treated groups and the WLC group, before and after treatment, in each of the four measures of fear (BAT, FS, SPQ, and HR acceleration). The table also shows that the four groups differed significantly in terms of the difference between pre-treatment and post-treatment scores on BAT, FS, and SPQt (i.e., SPQ total score). The four groups, however, showed a non-significant difference between their pre-treatment and post-treatment scores on the HR acceleration. It is note worthy that subsequent *Scheffe's test* results showed a significant difference (at the 0.05 level) between the WLC group and each of the three treated groups (LGE, LM, and CBSM) in respect of post-treatment BAT, FS, and SPQt. No other significant differences were obtained among the groups.

GROUPS	BAT				FS				SPQt				HR Acceleration			
	Before		After		Before		After		Before		After		Before		After	
	M	SD	M	SD	M	SD	M	SD	M	SD	M	SD	M	SD	M	SD
LGE	8.2	3.3	22.0	0.0	88.1	17.5	21.2	17.0	36.1	10.9	17.2	7.8	09.4	5.9	6.1	2.8
LM	7.1	4.4	21.6	1.2	92.6	17.1	18.0	14.5	41.4	08.7	18.2	6.5	11.5	6.9	7.3	4.9
CBSM	7.8	4.2	21.8	0.6	81.7	20.0	13.6	11.3	37.8	10.7	18.7	9.9	07.7	7.1	4.6	3.1
WLC	6.6	3.3	09.8	2.8	85.5	12.2	75.1	07.5	42.1	06.0	41.6	5.5	04.9	2.7	2.6	4.3
Treatment Effects (Post-treatment Assessment)	F(3, 33) = 143.8; p<.001				F(3, 32) = 40.3; p<.001				F(3, 26) = 28.4; p<.001				F(3, 32) = 1.797; p>.10			

Groups: LGE = Live Graded Exposure; LM = Live Modeling; CBSM = Computer-Based Symbolic Modeling; WLC = Waiting List Control
Measures: BAT = Behavioral Approach Test; FS = Fear Scale; SPQt = Spider Phobia Questionnaire (total score); HR Acceleration = Heart Rate Acceleration.
Statistics: M = Arithmetic means; SD = Standard Deviations; Before = Before treatment; After = After treatment.

Table 2. Means and Standard Deviations for the Four Study Groups in BAT, FS, SPQt, and HR Acceleration Before and After Treatment, and Treatment Effects at Post-Treatment Assessment.

A combined fear index (*CFI*) was calculated for the analysis of treatment effects. That is, the focus was on the overall pattern of groups' responding to treatment, since no single phobic client will load in only one component of fear but will rather show more or less activation in each of the three systems of responding. The *CFI* was computed by transforming pre- and post-treatment scores in each of the four fear indices into z scores, then adding together each client's resultant z scores in each of the two stages of assessment to form his or her *CFI* for that stage of assessment. Each client's BAT score was adjusted to represent an avoidance (indicating a fearful response), rather than approach, score so as to unify the directionality of all combined scores. The Anova procedure on the post-treatment *CFI* of the four groups, with the pre-treatment *CFI* serving as a covariate, showed a significant group difference [F (3, 37) = 53.63; p<.001], indicating that the four groups differed significantly in terms of their post-treatment *CFI*. The pre-treatment *CFI* emerged as a significant source of variation [F (1, 33) = 11.02; p<.01]. Further, to examine the source of the observed group difference and to determine whether the different treatment conditions produced differential effects, *Scheffe's test* was computed. The result showed that the WLC group (Mean *CFI* = 4.28) differed significantly (at the 0.05 level) from each of the three treatment groups (which had the following *CFI* means: LGE = -1.14; LM = -0.88; CBSM = -1.73), such that the WLC group's combined fear score was significantly higher than that of each of the treatment groups. No other significant differences were obtained among the groups. These results indicate that all treatment groups showed improvement that was significantly greater than what was obtained by the WLC group as a function of time or repeated exposure to the phobic object in pre- and post-treatment assessments. These results also indicate that the three treated groups did not differ significantly from each other in the degree of change produced by treatment in them.

An Anova procedure was performed on post-treatment BAT scores of the four groups, with the pre-treatment BAT scores serving as a covariate, to specifically examine the efficacy of treatment in affecting the overt behavioral component of fear (assessed by the BAT). This is because the overt behavioral component is a necessary criterion in the definition of specific phobia (formerly simple phobia) that the spider phobia is a subtype (American Psychiatric Association, 1987). The Anova results showed a significant group difference [F (3, 33) = 143.81; p<.001], such that the four groups differed significantly in terms of their post-treatment BAT scores. The pre-treatment BAT did not emerge as a significant source of this variation. Subsequent *Scheffe's test* results showed that the WLC group differed significantly (at the 0.05 level) from each of the other three groups. No other significant differences were observed among the groups. This result indicates that the three treated groups showed pre- to post-treatment improvement in the overt behavioral component of fear that was significantly greater than that shown by the WLC group. The result also indicates that the three treatment procedures induced analogous effects in the overt behavioral component of their clients' phobic behavioral responses.

The Statistical Analysis of Treatment Effects (Follow-up)

Each treated client's 45-day follow-up assessment scores on the BAT, HR acceleration, and SPQt (i.e., SPQ total score) were transformed into z scores and added together to obtain that client's combined fear index (*CFI*). Clients' post-treatment *CFI* scores were adjusted accordingly. Hence, the Manova procedure included the post-treatment *CFI*, the follow-up *CFI*, and the three treated groups that represented the three levels of the between-groups factors. Manova results showed that there was no overall significant difference between the three treated groups. The same result of non-significant difference was obtained when the three treated groups were compared in terms of differences between post-treatment and follow-up *CFIs* (i.e., there was no Group X Measure interaction). Finally, the within-group results showed no significant difference between post-treatment and follow-up measures (*CFIs*). These results indicate that the treated groups maintained the improvement over at least 45 days after the completion of treatment.

Manova procedure was also performed on the treated groups' follow-up BAT scores and their post-treatment equivalent. The result showed that there was no overall significant group difference. The results related to within-group effects also showed no significant Measure difference, indicating that the three treated groups' scores in these two BAT measures did not differ significantly. Finally, there was no significant Group X Measure interaction, such that the non-significant difference between the two BAT measures was true across the three treated groups. These results indicate that all the three treated groups had maintained their improvement in terms of overt behavioral approach responses at the follow-up stage.

An Anova procedure was performed on treated clients' pre-treatment and follow-up HR acceleration scores, to examine if treated clients' HR scores in these two stages of treatment differed significantly. The results showed that the pre-treatment to follow-up difference in HR acceleration was significantly different [$F(1, 24) = 13.02$; $p<.01$], such that clients' HR acceleration at the follow-up stage was significantly smaller than that observed in the pre-treatment assessment. The *Scheffe's test* results showed that the three treated groups did not differ significantly (at the 0.05 level) in this respect. These results suggest that clients' HR acceleration scores reflected a delayed response to treatment across the three treatment conditions.

5.2 The clinical significance of results

Introductory

The treatment effects presented in the previous section were inferred on the basis of the conventional method of statistical comparisons between mean changes resulting from the four treatment conditions (LGE, LM, CBSM, and the WLC). However, it has been argued (e.g., Kendall and Norton-Ford, 1982; Jacobson, Follette and Revenstorf, 1984) that such use of statistical significance tests to evaluate treatment efficacy has at least one major limitation: the tests provide no information on the variability of response to treatment in terms of *individual members of the sample*. In addition, the clinical significance of a treatment's effects is seen to refer to the treatment's impact on clients and to its ability to induce a change in their respective pattern of functioning (Jacobson and Truax, 1991). In this respect, Jacobson and Truax (1991) argue that conventional statistical comparisons between groups provide limited information about the efficacy of psychotherapy. Along the line of these arguments, Jacobson, Follette and Revenstorf (1984) proposed that a clinically significant change is the therapeutic change which returns a client to normal functioning. In other words, clients entering therapy are viewed as belonging to a dysfunctional population; whereby those completing the treatment are viewed as no longer belonging to that population. It follows, from this conception of clinically significant change, that a precise method is needed to classify respective clients, upon the completion of treatment, as "changed" or "unchanged" on the basis of the clinical significance conceptualization. For the purpose of this study, the application of a method that may provide information about the treatment impact on individual clients was deemed relevant. Hence, the treatment effects described in the previous sections were also examined on the basis of the clinical significance criterion. Jacobson and Truax (1991) have outlined three alternative methods for putting this process into operational terms. Generally speaking, these methods differ in terms of the information (the mean and standard deviation) from functional and dysfunctional populations that their execution may require. The method used here does not require data from a normative sample; rather, it uses the mean and standard deviation of the dysfunctional sample. This method defines the range of the dysfunctional population as extending, in the direction of functionality, to two standard deviations beyond the mean for that population. Hence, the level of functioning following treatment is expected to fall outside this range. In other words, of the treated clients, the post-treatment scores of those whose treatment was clinically significant would be expected to fall beyond the 'cutoff' point for clinically significant change. The cutoff point is defined by Jacobson and Truax (1991) as "the point that the client has to cross at the time of the post-treatment assessment in order to be classified as changed to clinically significant degree" (p. 13).

The Clinical Significance of Treatment Effects (post-treatment stage)

Accordingly, the method for assessing the clinical significance of change was applied to the three treatment groups (LGE, LM, and CBSM) of this study to examine the clinical significance of changes induced by the treatment in the fear indices on *individual clients* in the three treated groups. The scores of clients in the WLC group were also included to demonstrate that these clients were still within the range of dysfunctional population, and that the change in treated clients' scores was a function of the treatment they had received rather than the effect of time or repeated assessment.

Figure 1, which specifies the cutoff point (denoted 'a') for BAT, shows that all clients in the three treated groups crossed the cutoff point (a). That is, they were able, at the post-treatment assessment, to perform all or most of the tasks specified in BAT. This result indicates that the clients in these groups have changed to a clinically significant degree as far as the overt behavioral index of fear is concerned. On the other hand, all clients in the WLC group remained, at the post-treatment assessment, below the cutoff point; in other words, they were still among the dysfunctional population in terms of the overt behavioral index of fear.

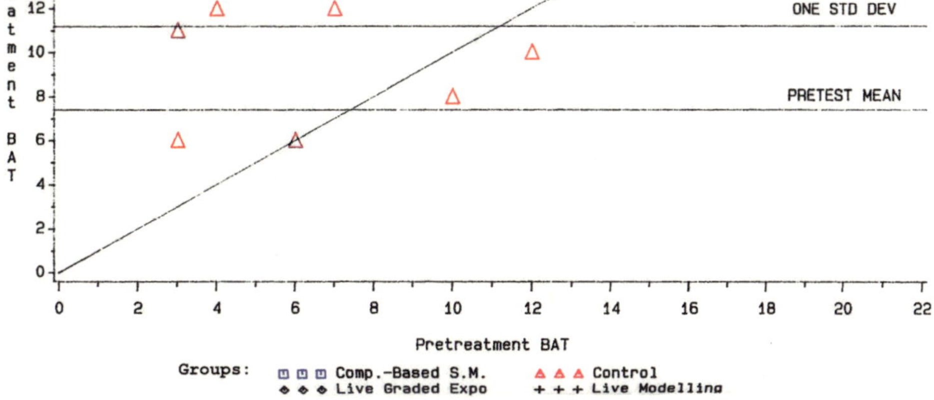

Fig. 1. The clinical significance of change in BAT at post-treatment assessment.

With regard to the cognitive/subjective fear, as assessed by the FS, **Figure 2** shows that all clients in the LGE, LM and CBSM groups crossed the cutoff point, indicating that they were improved to a clinically significant degree. Their post-treatment scores in the FS indicated 'less fear' and, therefore, appeared below the cutoff point and outside the range of dysfunctional population. The figure also shows that all clients in the WLC group remained above the cutoff point and within the range of dysfunctional population, which indicates that the amount of fear expressed by clients in the WLC group at the post-treatment assessment did not differ significantly, in clinical terms, from what they had reported at the pre-treatment assessment.

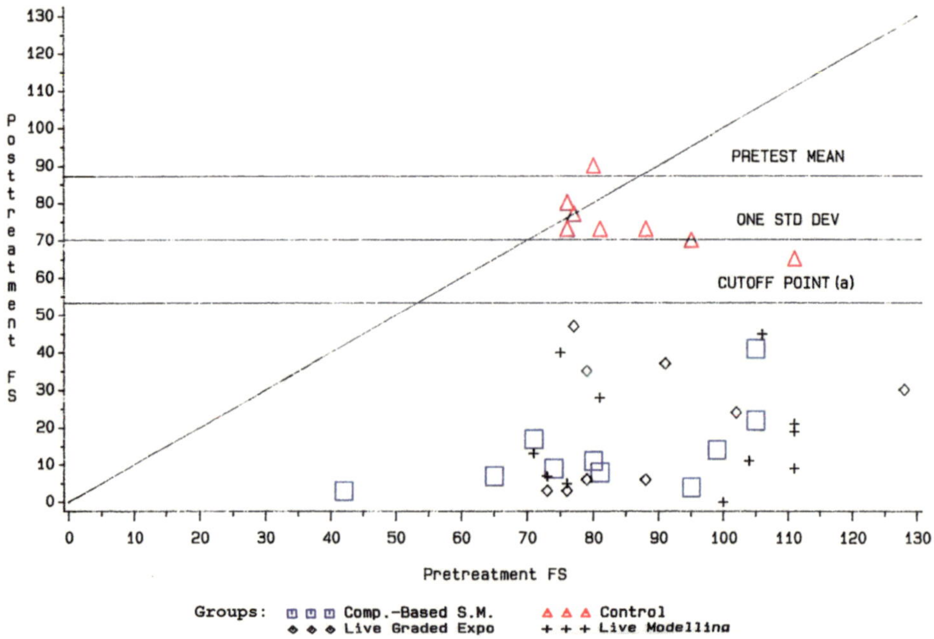

Fig. 2. The clinical significance of change in FS at post-treatment assessment.

Figure 3 shows the clinical significance of change induced by treatment in the treated clients as assessed by the SPQ total score (SPQt). From the figure, it is clear that few clients from the treated groups did not cross the cutoff point (a) into the range of functional population below the cutoff line. In fact, 4 clients from the LM and 2 clients from the LGE group appeared within one standard deviation above the cutoff point and in the range of dysfunctional population; the scores of 2 clients from the CBSM were more than one standard deviation above the cutoff point and in the range of dysfunctional population. The rest of the treated clients crossed the cutoff point into the range of functional population. On the other hand, all the WLC clients remained above the cutoff point and within the range of dysfunctional population. This result indicates that the improvement induced by each of the three treatment methods in its respective clients, as far as the SPQt measure is concerned, was of similar clinical significance. It also indicates that the improvement of clients in each of the treated groups was clinically more significant than that of the clients in the WLC group. One important observation is that the results of the clinical significance of change in clients' fear as assessed by the SPQt were less impressive than those related to the other cognitive measure of fear (i.e., the FS). This might be due to the fact that the SPQt contained an assessment of clients' vigilance, preoccupation, cognitive-behavioral, and avoidance/coping responses associated with fear; whereas the FS assessed only those phobic responses which were of behavioral nature (such as escape and avoidance).

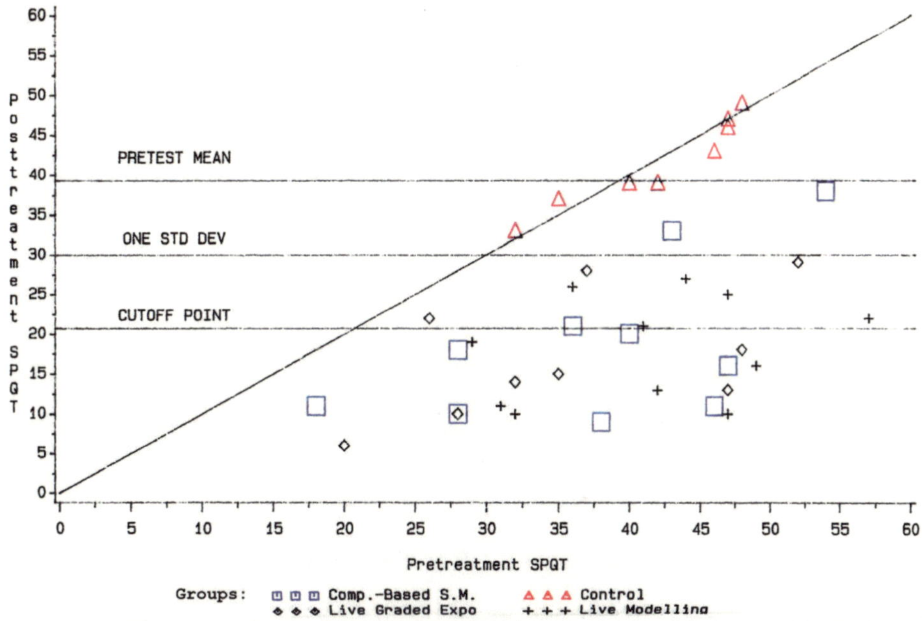

Fig. 3. The clinical significance of change in SPQ (total score) at post-treatment assessment.

Figure 4 shows the clinical significance of change induced by the treatment in HR Acceleration. The scales presented in the figure represent the HR Acceleration in response to fear-provoking instructions before and after the treatment. Hence, for a client's improvement to be classified as clinically significant (as far as the psychophysiological index of fear was concerned), his or her post-treatment heart rate was required to be indicative of no physiological arousal and, hence, sufficiently low; in other words, at least two standard deviations below the pre-treatment mean. An initial observation is that none of the clients in any of the groups crossed the cutoff point (of two standard deviations below the treatment mean) into the range of a functional population. Another equally important observation is that the scores of two clients in the WLC group were more than one standard deviation *below* the pre-treatment mean; the score of a third client from the WLC group was, in fact, on the cutoff point itself. These latter observations suggest that some factors other than the treatment (such as exposure to the phobic object during assessment) had contributed to the improvement of these three untreated clients from the WLC group to levels above those reached by treated clients in other groups. However, none of the treated groups was particularly uniformly *better* than the others with respect to improvement in HR index of fear. Generally speaking, decrement in HR responses to the fear-provoking instructions did not reflect a clinically significant improvement at the post-treatment stage. The latter conclusion was true for all treated groups. It is noteworthy that, of the treated clients, only six scored more than one standard deviation below the pre-treatment mean. Of these clients, three were from the CBSM group, two from the LM group, and one from the LGE group.

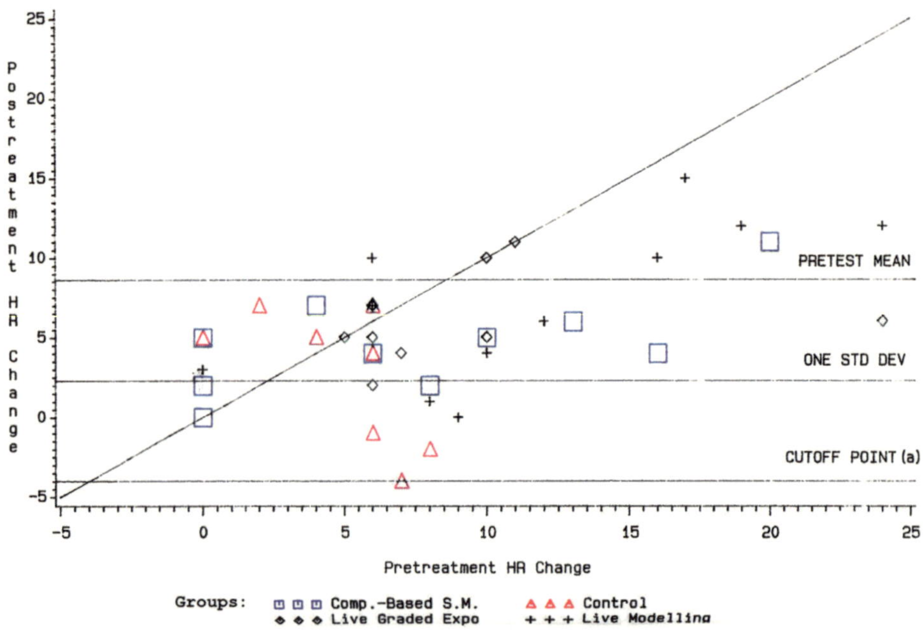

Fig. 4. The clinical significance of change in HR acceleration at post-treatment assessment.

The Clinical Significance of Treatment Effects (Follow-up Stage)

The clinical significance of treatment effects at the follow-up stage was also examined following the concept and procedure outlined above for the post-treatment assessment. Despite the non-significant difference observed, using statistical significance tests, between clients' post-treatment and follow-up scores (hence, proving that the clients did sustain their significant improvement at least 45 days after treatment completion), the clinical significance of treatment effects was examined at the follow-up stage since this procedure, as explained earlier, provides information about treatment impact on 'individual' clients rather than in terms of the overall 'group' performance.

The follow-up assessment involved clients' scores in the BAT, HR and SPQt, and included the Live Graded Exposure (LGE), Live Modeling (LM), and Computer-Based Symbolic Modeling (CBSM) groups.

Figure 5 shows that all clients retained a clinically significant change in their approach behavior (as assessed by BAT). That is, the BAT scores of clients in each of the three treated groups appeared well above the cutoff line (a), two standard deviations away from the pre-treatment (i.e., dysfunctional stage) mean in the direction of functionality. This observation confirms that the impact of each of the three treatment methods on the overt behavioral component of each individual client proved to be clinically significant, as was also proved to be statistically significant, after at least a 45-day follow-up period. From the figure, it is clear that this observation is applicable to all three treatment methods such that the treatment effects on overt behavior were sustained at the follow-up stage by the clients in each of the three treatment conditions.

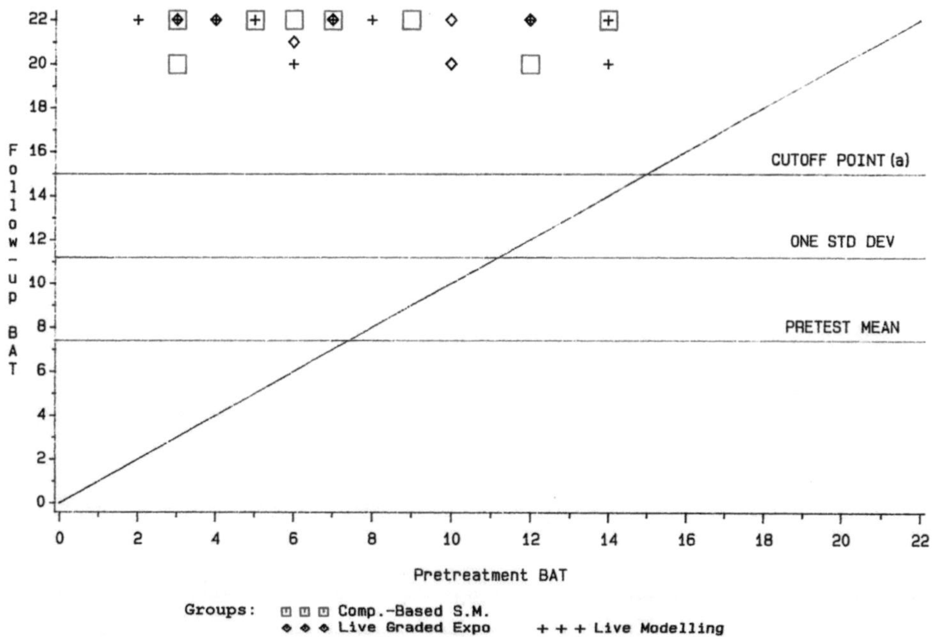

Fig. 5. The clinical significance of change in BAT acceleration at follow-up assessment.

Figure 6 represents the clinical significance of change induced by treatment in the cognitive/subjective component of fear as assessed by the SPQt. The majority of clients either crossed the cutoff point (a) into the range of normal functioning, or they reached it. The scores of additional 3 clients (2 from the LM group, and one from the LGE group) appeared just below the cutoff point and within the range of dysfunctional population. The scores of two clients from the CBSM group, however, remained within the range of dysfunctional population (within one and two standard deviations, respectively, below the pre-treatment mean). From the distribution of individual clients in Figure 6, it can be concluded that the effects of the three treatment procedures on the cognitive/subjective component of fear (as assessed by the SPQt) were similar in terms of their clinical significance on individual clients. When compared with Figure 3, this figure indicates that some clients in the conventional treatment groups (i.e., LGE and LM groups) showed a clear improvement from post-treatment to follow-up assessment with regard to their cognitive/subjective component of fear as assessed by the SPQt. Some improvement, although less dramatic than that shown by the latter groups, was also shown by two clients in the CBSM group.

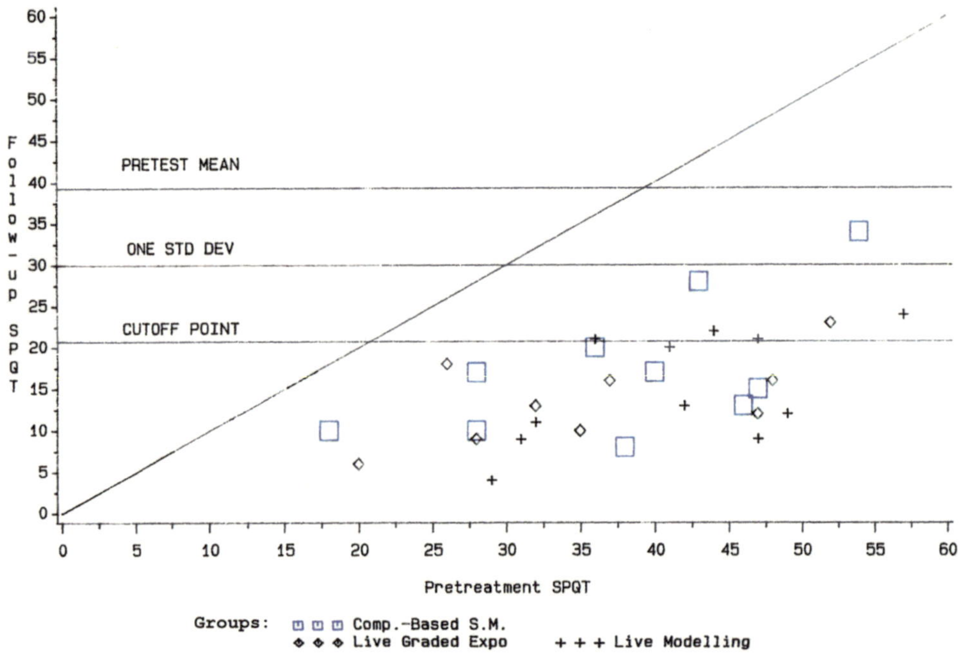

Fig. 6. The clinical significance of change in SPQ (total score) at follow-up assessment.

Figure 7 shows the clinical significance of changes in HR responses to fear-inducing instructions at the follow-up stage. Although none of the clients crossed the cutoff point into the range of a functional population, the figure shows a slight improvement when compared with that for the post-treatment assessment (see Figure 4). In this figure, the scores of only six clients remained above the pre-treatment mean (indicating relatively high HR responses to fear-inducing verbal instructions), compared to eight at the post-treatment stage. Similarly, the scores of seven treated clients were more than one standard deviation below the pre-treatment mean, compared to six at the pre-treatment stage. Of these seven clients, five belonged to the CBSM group, compared to three in the pre-treatment assessment. This observation suggests that the CBSM procedure induced a relatively more effect in the physiological component of fear than the other non-symbolic procedure did (i.e., the LGE and LM). To conclude, the figure showed a consistent trend in the direction of functionality, although no client actually moved into the range of functionality.

To conclude, this method of examining the clinical significance of the therapeutic change induced by the treatment provided additional information to the results obtained by inferential statistics procedures. The method has confirmed the clinical significance of the statistically significant change induced in clients' BAT and indicated the significance of change induced by treatment in the two indices of self-reported fear (i.e., FS and SPQt). The effect of the treatment on the psychophysiological component of fear (in terms of HR Acceleration in response to fear-inducing instructions) was shown not to be clinically significant, at least in the post-treatment assessment. It confirmed that the three treatment methods produced similar improvement which, with the exception of HR fear index, was significantly more than the WLC condition did.

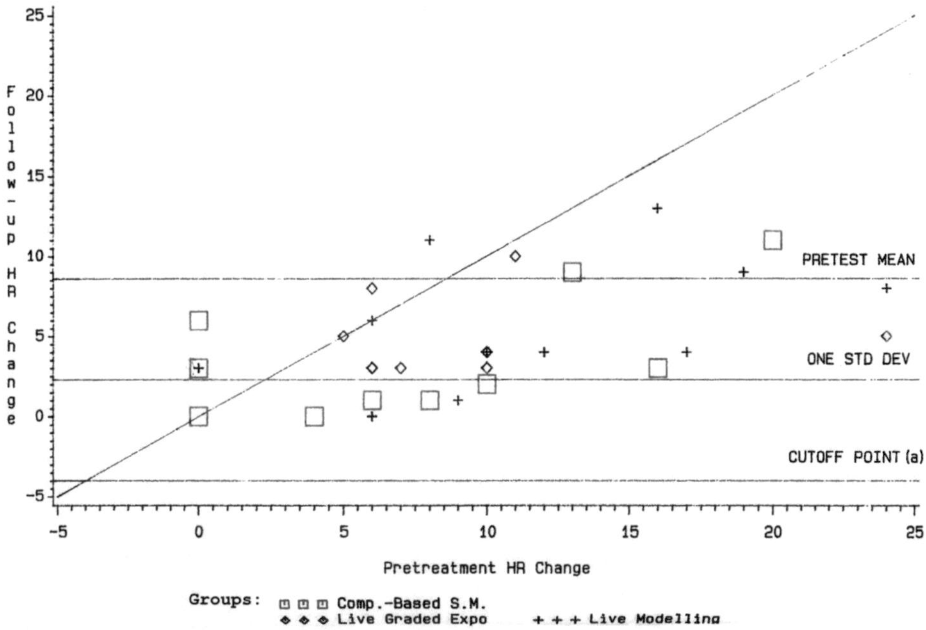

Fig. 7. The clinical significance of change in HR acceleration at follow-up assessment.

6. Discussion

The results described above have revealed that the therapeutic effects induced by the prototype CBSM technique in clients' fear components (including the overt behavioral and cognitive components) were similar to that induced by the conventional live exposure and modeling techniques. All treated groups, however, showed only a delayed *statistically* significant improvement (i.e., at the follow-up stage) over the control group on the measure of autonomic fear component that was assessed in terms of HR acceleration scores. It might be suggested that a direct measure of clients' HR during exposure to the fear object would have reflected the significance of the fear object as a fear-provoking entity and, hence, a clear picture of the treatment effect on the heart rate as a fear index might have been obtained. In this respect, Lang, Melamed and Hart (1970), who observed the heart rate of clients with snake phobia while imagining fear-relevant scenes, have demonstrated a positive correlation of heart rate acceleration and self-reported fear intensity. Sartory, Rachman and Grey (1977), however, showed that the linear relationship between heart rate acceleration and fear intensity was consistent only at relatively intense fear levels. Thus, one may argue that fear-eliciting material in the form of verbal instructions was probably insufficient for provoking levels of fear intensity that were capable of differentiating between groups in terms of change in heart rate acceleration. Such an argument, however, may not hold firmly since the treated groups in this study did show a relatively clear, and statistically significant, therapeutic reduction in the heart rate acceleration to the same fear-eliciting material in the follow-up assessment. A possible reason why the treated groups did not show a similar reduction in their heart rate acceleration scores in the post-treatment assessment is that the clients were not sufficiently relaxed during the recording of their baseline heart rate. This might be because the clients were anticipating an eventual encounter with the phobic object during the subsequent BAT session. That is, as ethical considerations required, all clients were briefed ahead of each session about what that session would involve. Other arguments may include that clients' baseline heart rate measures were contaminated with some anticipatory fear arousal, or they were a reflection of the differential effect of clients' age groups on the change in the heart rate acceleration. At present, the results related to change in clients' heart rate acceleration from pre-treatment to post-treatment and follow-up stages suggest an overall delayed treatment effect on the autonomic fear component across the three treated groups. In looking for the possible causes of such a delay, the issue of interaction between treatment factors and individual characteristics may be raised. That is, some individuals may be high physiological responders while others are medium or low in that respect (e.g., Ost, Johansson and Jerremalm, 1982; for more detail).

The three treated groups did not show a substantial difference in terms of the average number of sessions required for the completion of treatment. Hence, the CBSM treatment did not seem to be more demanding than the two conventional treatments (LGE and LM) in terms of the time required for treatment completion (the three treatments: LGE, LM, and CBSM required 3.34, 3.19, and 4.45 hours, respectively).

With respect to the therapist involvement, the CBSM did not require the active involvement of the therapist in the treatment process since the clients interacted with the computer system directly and at their own rate of progression. The therapist involvement throughout this prototype clinical intervention was restricted to monitoring the treatment sessions and ensuring the smooth running of equipment. However, because the concept of self-help was also emphasized for all clients in the two conventional treatment conditions, the therapist's role was restricted to a large extent in administering the exposure according to the pre-determined sequence and at the discretion of the client.

To conclude, the computer-Based version of treatment was shown to be capable of producing therapeutic results that were as clinically effective as those produced by conventional procedures. It has been observed (Hassan, 1992; unpublished PhD Thesis) that clients' positive opinion about the role that the computer can play in delivering behavioral treatment did not seem to be associated with the degree of improvement that they obtained from the treatment delivered by this technique. In fact, most clients maintained this positive view after the treatment was given, regardless of the level of their improvement. Nevertheless, the difficulty perceived by the majority of clients of interacting with a computer for treatment purposes raises an important implication. That is, further research work and clinical trials may focus on ensuring that the mechanisms of client-computer interaction for therapeutic purposes are made even simpler and easier. Achieving such an end will help making behavioral treatments more widely available for those in need for.

7. References

American Psychiatric Association (1987). Diagnostic and Statistical Manual of Mental Disorders (3th Edition). Washington, DC: APA.

Bandura, A. (1969). Principles of Behavior Modification. New York: Holt, Rinehart & Winston.

Bandura, A. (1965). Vicarious processes: A case of no trial learning. In: Berkowitz (Ed.), Advances in Experimental Social Psychology (Vol. 2). New York: Academic Press.

Bandura, A., Blanchard, E. B. and Ritter, B. (1969). Relative efficacy of desensitization and modelling approaches for inducing behavioral, affective and attitudinal changes. Journal of Personality and Social Psychology, Vol. 13, No. 3, 173-199.

Bard, P. and Rioch, D. McK. (1937). A study of four cats deprived of neocortex and additional portions of the forebrain. Bulletin of John Hopkins Hospital, 60, 73.

Beck, A. T. (1976). Cognitive Therapy and the Emotional Disorders. New York: International Universities Press.

Bertino, E. 1985). Design issues in interactive user interfaces. Interfaces in Computing, 3, 37-53.

Bootzin, R. R., Herman, C. P. and Nicassio, P. (1976). The power of suggestion: Another examination of misattribution and insomnia. Journal of Personality and Social Psychology, 34, 673-679.

Brodal, A. (1981). Neurological Anatomy, in Relation to Clinical Medicine (3rd Ed.). New York: Oxford University Press.

Cannon, W. B. (1927). The James-Lange theory of emotion: A critical examination and an alternative theory. American Journal of Psychology, 39, 106-124.

Carr, A. C. and Ghosh, A. (1983a). Response of phobic patients to direct computer assessment. British Journal of Psychiatry, 142, 60-65.

Carr, A. C. and Ghosh, A. (1983b). Accuracy of behavioral assessment by computer. British Journal of Psychiatry, 142, 66-70.

Carr, A. C., Ghosh, A. and Ancill, R. J. (1983). Can a computer take a psychiatric history? Psychological Medicine, 13, 151-158.

Chambliss, C. and Murray, E. J. (1979). Cognitive procedures for smoking reduction: Symptom attribution versus efficacy attribution. Cognitive Therapy Research, 3, 91-95.

Cotton, J. L., Baron, R. S. and Borkovec, T. D. (1980). Caffeine ingestion, misattribution therapy, and speech anxiety. Journal of Res. Pers., 14, 196-206.

Diamond, S. J. (1980). Neuropsychology, A Textbook of Systems and Psychological Functions of the Human Brain. London: Butterworth.

Eysenck, H. J. (1987). Behavior Therapy. In: H. J. Eysenck and I. Martin (Eds.), Theoretical Foundations of behavior Therapy. New York: Plenum Press.

Fitter, M. J. and Cruickshank, P. J. (1982). The computer in the consulting room: A psychological framework. Behavior and Information Technology, Vol. 1(1), 81-92.

Foa, E. B. and Kozak, M. J. (1985). Treatment of anxiety disorders: Implications for psychopathology. In: A. H. Tuma and J. Maser (Eds.), Anxiety and the Anxiety Disorders. Hillsdale, NJ: Lawrence Erlbaum Associates.

Gray, J. A. (1982). The Neuropsychology of Anxiety: An enquiry into the functions of the septo-hippocampal system. New York: Oxford University Press.

Gray, J. A. (1990). Brain systems that mediate both emotion and cognition. In: J. A. Gray (Ed.), Psychobiological Aspects of Relationships Between Emotion and Cognition (A special Issue of Cognition and Emotion, 1990, 4(3), 289-302). Hove: Lawrence Erlbaum Associates,

Greenberg, L. S. and Safran, J. D. (1987). Emotion, cognition, and action. In: H. J. Eysenck and I. Martin (Eds.), Theoretical Foundations of Behavior Therapy. New York: Plenum Press.

Greist, J. H., Gustafson, D. H. and Stauss, F. F. (1973). A computer interview for suicide risk prediction. American Journal of Psychiatry, 130, 1327-1332.

Hassan, A. M. and ward, P. S. (1991). On the Primacy of the Brain. Current Psychology Research & Review, Vol. 10, No. 1&2, pp. 103-111.

Hugdahl, K. (1989). Simple phobias. In: G. Turpin (Ed.), Handbook of Clinical Psychophysiology. London: John Wiley & Sons.

Jacobson, N. S., Follette, W. C. and Revenstorf, D. (1984). Psychotherapy outcome research: Methods for reporting variability and evaluating clinical significance. Behavior Therapy, 15, 336-352.

Jacobson, N. S. and Truax, P. (1991). Clinical significance: A statistical approach to defining meaningful change in psychotherapy research. Journal of Counseling and Clinical Psychology, Vol. 59(1), 12-19.

James, W. (1950). Principles of Psychology. New York: Dover (Original work published 1890).

Kendall, P. C. and Norton-Ford, J. D. (1982). Therapy outcome research methods. In: P. C. Kendall and J. N. Butcher (Eds.), Handbook of Research Methods in Clinical Psychology. New York: Wiley.

Landauer, T. K. (1988). Research Methods in Human-Computer Interaction. In: M. Helander (Ed.), Handbook of Human-Computer Interaction. Amsterdam: North-Holland.

Lang, P. J. (1971). The application of psychophysiological methods to the study of psychotherapy and behavior modification. In: A. E. Bergin and S. L. Garfield (Eds.), Handbook of Psychotherapy and Behavior Change: An empirical analysis. New York: Wiley.

Lang, P. J., Melamed, B. and Hart, J. D. (1970). A psychophysiological analysis of fear modification using an automated desensitization procedure. Journal of Abnormal Psychology, 76, 220-234.

Lange, C. G. (1967). The emotions: A physiological study. In: C. G. Lange and W. James, The Emotions. New York: Hafner (Originally published 1885).

Lazarus, R. S. (1982). Thoughts on the relations between emotion and cognition. American Psychologist, 37, 1019-1024.

Lazarus, R. S. (1984). On the primacy of cognition. American Psychologist, 39, 124-129.

Leventhal, H. (1984). A perceptual motor theory of emotion. In: K. R. Scherer and P. Ekman (Eds.), Approaches to Emotion. Hillsdale, NJ: Lawrence Erlbaum Associates.

Leventhal, H. and Tomarken, A. J. (1986). Emotion: Today's problems. Annual Review of Psychology, 37, 565-610.

Leventhal, H. and Tomarken, A. J. (1988). A perceptual motor theory of emotion. In: K. R. Scherer and P. Ekman (Eds.), Approaches to Emotion. Hillsdale, NJ: Lawrence Erlbaum Associates.

Lewis, G., Pelosi, A. J., Glover, E., Wilkinson, G., Stansfeld, S. A., Williams, P. and Sheferd, M. (1988). The development of a computerized assessment for minor psychiatric disorder. Psychological Medicine, 18, 737-745.

Lucas, R. W., Mullin, P. J., Luna, C. B. and McIlroy, D. C. (1977). Psychiatrists and a computer as interrogators of patients with alcohol-related illnesses: A comparison. British Journal of Psychiatry, 131, 160-167.

MacLean, P. D. (1950). Psychosomatic disease and the 'visceral brain', recent developments bearing on the Papez theory of emotion. Psychosomatic Medicine, 11, 338-353.

Marshal, G. D. and Zimbardo, P. G. (1979). Affective consequences of inadequately explained physiological arousal. Journal of Personality and Social Psychology, 37, 970-985.

Maslach, C. (1979). Negative emotional biasing of unexplained arousal. Journal of Personality and Social Psychology, 37, 953-969.

Ost, L. G., Johansson, J. and Jerremalm, A. (1982). Individual response patterns and the effects of different behavioural methods in the treatment of claustrophobia. Behaviour Research and Therapy, 20, 445-460.

Panksepp, J. (1988). Brain emotional circuits and psychopathologies. In: M. Clynes and J. Panksepp (Eds.), Emotions and Psychopathology. New York: Plenum Press.

Panksepp, J. (1990). Gray zones at the emotion/cognition interface: A commentary. In: J. A. Gray (Ed.), Psychobiological Aspects of Relationships Between Emotion and Cognition (A special Issue of Cognition and Emotion, 1990, 4(3), 289-302). Hove: Lawrence Erlbaum Associates, Papez, J. W. (1937). A proposal mechanism of emotion. Archives of Neurology and Psychiatry, 38, 725-743.

Rachman, S. J. (1977). The conditioning theory of fear-acquisition: A critical examination. Behavior Research and Therapy, 15, 375-387.

Rachman, S. J. (1978). Human fears: A three-systems analysis. Scandinavian Journal of Behavior Therapy, 7, 237-245.

Rachman, S. J. (1981). The primacy of affect: Some theoretical implications. Behavior Therapy and Research, 19, 279-290.

Rachman, S. J. (1990). Fear and Courage (2nd Edn.). New York: W. H. Freeman.

Rachman, S. J. and Hodgson, R. (1974). Synchrony and desynchrony in fear and avoidance. Behavior Research and Therapy, 12, 311-318.

Rasmussen, J. A. (1986). Information Processing and Human-Machine Interaction: An Approach to cognitive engineering. New York: North-Holland.

Rogers, R. W. and Deckner, C. (1975). Effects of fear appeals and physiological arousal upon emotions, attitudes, and cigarette smoking. Journal of Personality and Social Psychology, 32, 222-230.

Sartory, G., Rachman, S. J. and Grey, S. J. (1977). An investigation of the relation between reported fear and heart rate. Behaviour Research and Therapy, 15, 435-438.

Schachter, S. (1964). The interaction of cognitive and physiological determinants of emotional state. Advances in Experimental and Social Psychology, 1, 49-80.

Scherer, K. R. (1984). On the nature and function of emotion: A component process approach. In: K. R. Scherer and P. Ekman (Eds.), Approaches to Emotion. Hillsdale, NJ: Lawrence Erlbaum Associates.

Sines, J. O. (1980). The use of computers in the delivery of mental health care: The necessary background conditions. In: J. B. Sidowski, J. H. Johnson and T. A. Williams (Eds.), Technology in Mental Health Care Delivery Systems. Norwood, NJ: Ablex Publishing Corporation.

Slack, W. V., Hicks, G. P., Reed, C. E. and Van Cura, L. J. (1966). A computer-based medical history system. New England Journal of Medicine, 274, 194-198.

Slack, W. V. and Van Cura, L. J. (1968). Patient reaction to computer-based medical interviewing. Computers and Biomedical Research, 1, 527-532.

Wall, P. D. and Pribram, K. H. (1950). Trigeminal neurotomy and blood pressure responses from stimulation of lateral cortex of macaca mulatta. Journal of Neurophysiology, 25, 258-263.

Watts, F. N. and Sharrock, R. (1984). Questionnaire dimensions of spider phobia. Behaviour Research and Therapy, 22(5), 575-580.

Watts, F. N., McKenna, F. P., Sharrock, R. and Trezise, L. (1986). Colour naming of phobia related words. British Journal of Psychology, 77, 97-108.

Williams, J. G., Watts, F. N., MacLeod, C. and Mathews, A. (1988). Cognitive Psychology and Emotional Disorders. Chichester: John Wiley.

Wilson, G. T. (1978). Cognitive behavior therapy: Paradigm shift or passing phase? In: J. P. Foreyt and D. P. Rathjen (Eds.), Cognitive Behavior Therapy: Research and Application. New York: Plenum Press.

Wolpe, J. (1958). Psychotherapy by Reciprocal Inhibition. Stanford, California: Stanford University Press.

Woods, D. D. and Roth, E. M (1988). Cognitive systems engineering. In: M. Helander (Ed.), Handbook of Human-Computer Interaction. Amsterdam: North-Holland.

Wright, A. F. (1990). A study of the presentation of somatic symptoms in general practice by patients with psychiatric disturbance. British Journal of General Practice, 40, 459-463.

Zajonc, R. B. (1980). Feeling and thinking: Preferences need no inferences. American Psychologist, 35, 151-175.

Zajonc, R. B. (1984). On the primacy of emotion. American Psychologist, 39, 117-123.

Zoltan, E. and Chapanis, A (1982). What do professional persons think about computers? Behavior and Information Technology, 1(1), 55-68.

15

Home Visits to Mothers with Children Between the Ages 0 to 4 Years: A Mental Health Intervention Strategy in Emerging Countries

Marcela Aracena, Consuelo Undurraga, Esteban Gómez, Loreto Leiva, Ariela Simonsohn and Pilar Navarro
Pontificia Universidad Católica De Chile, Chile

1. Introduction

According to recent investigations both in Chile and other countries, mental health of mothers show a special vulnerability during the post-partum period. This is an especially disturbing knowledge, because of the relevance of the first three years of life in the posterior development of children. The connection between the mental health of the mother (→ mother-son/daughter relationship→ attachment style→ regulation of the child experience→ development of the brain cyto-architecture→) and the present and future mental health of the child is solidly established, based on a large amount of empirical and multidisciplinary evidence (Shore, 2001). Strengthening and parental skills of the mother, especially in the first upbringing stages are then a priority focus of action for health policies in every country.

This chapter focuses on linking the need of support that many families require in terms of the mental health of parental figures -especially the mother- and mental health of infants, with a promising intervention strategy in natural context, the home visit. So, it is a chapter with an emphasis on the practical side of supporting mental health, that intend to communicate an analysis both from an investigational view and an implementation of Home Visiting generated by a research team of Pontificia Universidad Católica de Chile starting 2003, in three consecutive projects financed by the "Fondo Nacional de Desarrollo Científico y Tecnológico" (National Fund for Scientific and Technologic Development) - FONDECYT, a national institution responsible for financing investigation in Chile.

This work is useful in two different aspects: (a) it provides a systematization of our knowledge regarding home visits, and effect on health and early childhood in an emerging country; and (b) it is a reflection regarding the challenges of implementing this type of programs.

2. Home Visits to mothers with children between the ages 0 to 4 years

Home Visiting is an ecologically sensitive strategy for the delivery of various services, aimed at supporting and strengthening families in their own home, through regular meetings with a home visitor (Aracena et al., 2011).

The focus of home visits are diverse, including the prevention of child abuse and neglect, Promotion of child development, strengthening parenting skills and a secure attachment and knowledge and use of formal/informal networks (Kotliarenco, Gómez, Muñoz & Aracena, 2010). Interventions in home visits are also diverse (McNaughton, 2004): information delivery, evaluation, promotion of breastfeeding and child development, counseling, referrals, monitoring, social support and family therapy.

Home visiting is considered an experience involving actors from different functional areas such as information provision, direct support and/or practical aid to the family. Participating educational agents (professionals or non-professionals) can play different roles such as friend, teacher, role model, among others (Gracia, 1997).

In Chile, the Ministry of Health [MINSAL] (2008) proposed that the home visit should be developed according to four categories: (a) reproductive cycle of the family, (b) risk factors and protective factors, (c) contingent health problems, (d) family crisis. But currently, there is not a unified model of home visitation that guided the practice, and in fact, that is precisely one of the most important challenges for the future.

In the last decade, it has been published several systematic reviews and meta-analysis about the effectiveness of home visiting (Elkan et al., 2000, 2001; Kearney, York & Deatrick, 2000; Kendrick et al., 2000; Sweet & Appelbaum, 2004; Russell et al., 2007; Lagerberg, 2000; Nievar, Van Egeren & Pollard, 2010), which have generally proved effective for various purposes, but with a range from low to moderate effect size. Among the findings of these reviews, notes that home visits delivered by nurses impact the psychological well-being, perceived social support, repeated pregnancies rates and alcohol use, mother-infant interaction (in various outcomes), and in parenting skills (such as parental discipline, attitudes related to child abuse, parental expectations about parenting and child behavior and learning stimulation), with mixed results, as rates of real child abuse and neglect have proven very difficult to change.

On the other hand, there are fewer results in social skills, employment, re-education, health and child development, and use of health services (Kearney, York & Deatrick, 2000; Lagerberg, 2000; Kendrick et al., 2000). Cognitive development in children with low birth weight or preterm may be positively influenced by home visiting programs, particularly when performed in combination with a program of early stimulation in the neonatal unit.

Regarding postpartum depression, it appears that significant improvements can be achieved in home visits by nurses using counseling once a week, for 6-8 weeks (Lagerberg, 2000). These results showed by reviews, have been partially supported by the meta-analysis of Sweet and Appelbaum (2004). Also, in a systematic review and meta-analysis of 12 studies using the HOME instrument (Caldwell & Bradley, 2001), there was a highly significant effect, suggesting that home visitation is effective in improving the quality of home environment as assessed by this instrument (Kendrick et al., 2000).

In the field of mental health care, international research have shown the effectiveness of home visits as an intervention strategy of mothers and infants within highly vulnerable environments. A recent review of this issue (Kotliarenco, et.al., 2010), summarizes the characteristics of the most effective programs of home visits around the following axis: (a) building a trust relationship between the visiting agent and the mother; (b) focusing on modeling the mother-infant interaction; (c) start during pregnancy; (d) extensive duration; (e) specific training for visiting agents.

Regarding, who perform these visits; it is possible to identify different educational agents: professionals and non-professionals. Even when the favourable effects of home visits have been recognized, there are still divergences regarding the characteristics considered as adequate for the agents participating in such programs since different profiles are needed depending on the objectives of the intervention. The role of the educational agent has great importance since it helps build a space for support and control for the mothers, fathers or care providers and validates a space for the experience of maternity. The educational agent therefore acts as a cultural and social mediator and constitutes a model which facilitates the vicarious learning for the mother (Olds, 1997). Therefore, it is really important to discuss the inclusion of professional vs. non-professional visitors, their training, experience, skills and supervision (Elkan et al., 2000, Olds, et al., 2004, Nievar et al., 2010).

Research carried on by Olds and his team in the United States, has concluded that home visit has different effects depending on the characteristics of the visiting agent. The women visited by community monitors, compared with a control group, showed better mental health and more parental sensitivity to their children. On the other side, women visited by nurses presented a longer interval between the birth of their first and second child, lower level of family violence, and their children showed a better level of language and behavioral adaptation. In both cases, women visited achieved a better learning environment for their daughters and sons (Olds et al., 2004). Additionally, a review on the subject showed that outcomes obtained by paraprofessionals are similar to professionals (Kendrick et al., 2000).

A recently published meta-analysis on moderators of improvements in maternal behavior using home visiting programs, with 35 studies and a N = 6.453 (Nievar et al., 2010), reveal that programs with more frequent visitation had higher success rates, with two visits per month predicting a small, substantive effect, while intensive programs (with at least three visits per month) were more than twice as effective as were less intensive programs. It is interesting for the discussion on the professional/paraprofessional controversy, the finding of this meta-analysis that home visiting programs using nurses or mental health professionals as providers were not significantly more effective than were programs using paraprofessionals.

The literature on cost-effectiveness of home visiting in early childhood has shown preliminary findings indicating that it is cost-effective, with net income at rates ranging between $6,000 and $17,200 per child, in the United States (Aos et al., 2004). In Chile, there are indications that the home visit implemented by community workers (non-professionals) would be cost-effective with respect to mental health outcomes of mothers. Thus, Aracena et al. (2009) reported that the incremental cost compared with the effectiveness of a program for teenage mothers using home visit, gives a cost of $13.5 per unit of effectiveness (measured as a decrease of one point in the Goldberg questionnaire). The study concludes that significant gains are obtained investing $40 per teen in a total period of 15 months.

3. Interventions

In the this section, we describe in some detail the results of two research projects about home visit in Chile, seeking to illuminate some of the topics that constitute the frontier of knowledge about the relation between intervention and outcomes in vulnerable families using this strategy.

Both investigations evaluate the cost-effectiveness of home visiting performed by community monitors to young women under 20 years old. In the first case, research focused on Centros de Salud de Chile (Chilean Health Centers), a State organization. In the other hand, in the second case, the investigation was framed in a non-governmental organization managed by the Church as opposed to an intervention provided by a Health Care Center. Methodology details of every investigation can be reviewed in the Figure 1 which follows.

	Cost-effectiveness of Home Visiting to teenage mothers associated to Health Centers (2003-2005)	**Cost-Effectiveness of Home Visiting of teenage others associated to Health Centers and NGOs (2007-2009)**
Objective	Evaluate cost-effectiveness of a home visit program compared to the regular program in two health centers in Santiago, Chile oriented to teenage mothers.	Evaluate the maintenance of effects in time and without additional intervention and also the cost-effectiveness of two home visit programs to teenage mothers by comparing them with each other and with regular programs in Health Centers for mothers with children younger than 4 years old, in Santiago, Chile.
Design	Experimental, clinical trial type controlled and randomized.	Mixed, quasi-experimental: a study for the evaluation of the maintenance effect in a group under intervention previously compared to other groups under intervention and all of them with a control group.
Sample	Control Group: 50 pregnant young women. Experimental Group: 50 pregnant young women.	Control Group: 140 pregnant young women. Experimental Group: 123 pregnant young women.
Intervention	Control Group: standard intervention of health centers. Experimental Group: they also received home visits from the 3rd trimester of pregnancy up to the 12th month of life of the child. Experimental Group: The program targeted young women who conceived their first child between 14 and 19 years of age. It involved community participation in the implementation of the program through health educators who conducted the home visits under the guidance of nurse-midwives from the local health center. The program sought to: (a) encourage the young woman's development of her identity as a woman, adolescent, and mother, (b) help her develop life plans, (c) reinforce her parenting skills, (d) promote basic health care practices for both mother and child, and (e) strengthen the adolescent's relationships with those around her.	Control Group: standard intervention of health centers. Experimental Group 1: highly standardized home visit program, edited in a manual and intensive (average of 12 annual visits). Experimental Group 2: low standardized and low intensity home visit program, non-edited in a manual (6 annual visits average). Experimental Group 1 The program targeted young women who conceived their first child between 14 and 19 years of age. It involved community participation in the implementation of the program through health educators who conducted the home visits under the guidance of nurse-midwives from the local health center. The program sought to: (a) encourage the young woman's development of her identity as a woman, adolescent, and mother, (b) help her develop life plans, (c) reinforce her parenting skills, (d) promote basic health care practices for both mother and child, and (e) strengthen the adolescent's relationships with those around her.

		Experimental Group 2 The core component were voluntary monitors linked to the Catholic Church NGOs who participated in training processes and support to pregnant young women or women with infants between 0 to 2 years old. This work was developed around three components: home visiting, training workshops and communication actions, being the first one our principal axis. Visits were performed according to needs established jointly with the mother from the pregnancy until the child reached 2 years old. All mother-child pairs received routine assistance from all traditional programs performed by the primary medical assistance system of Chile.
Instruments	Evaluation of the mothers 1. Evaluation of physical health. Made by the medical team throughout the adolescent's pregnancy, in the post-partum period and during lactation, with prenatal check-ups and treatment for illness. 2. Evaluation of mental health. The Chilean adaptation of the Goldberg's General Health Questionnaire was used. This test allows for the detection of mental disorders of a neurotic origin as well as some personality and psychophysical disorders, indicating the presence and severity of symptoms (Araya, Wynn, & Lewis, 1992). 3. Evaluation of family function. This evaluation was carried out using the questionnaire 'What's YOUR family like?' developed by the Pan-American Health Organization (1992) and validated in Chile by Rodríguez et al. (1995). It includes 25 questions containing 132 items measuring family function, structure, processes of interaction, stressful events and potentially risky behaviors for the adolescent's health (Rodriguez, et al., 1995 en Hidalgo & Carrasco, 2002).	Evaluation of the mother 1. Evaluation of physical health. Made by the medical team throughout the adolescent's pregnancy, in the post-partum period and during lactation, with prenatal check-ups and treatment for illness. 2. Evaluation of mental health. The Chilean adaptation of the Goldberg's General Health Questionnaire was used. This test allows for the detection of mental disorders of a neurotic origin as well as some personality and psychophysical disorders, indicating the presence and severity of symptoms (Araya, Wynn, & Lewis, 1992). 3. Evaluation of family function. This evaluation was carried out using the questionnaire 'What's YOUR family like?' developed by the Panamerican Health Organization (1992) and validated in Chile by Rodríguez et al. (1995). It includes 25 questions containing 132 items measuring family function, structure, processes of interaction, stressful events and potentially risky behaviors for the adolescent's health (Rodriguez, et al., 1995 en Hidalgo & Carrasco, 2002). 4. Satisfaction with life: the satisfaction with life scale was taken from the questionnaire developed by the Panamerican Health Organization (1992) and validated in Chile by Rodríguez et al. (1995). 5. Psychosocial welfare: it was measured through the inclusion of the educational system after the delivery.

	Evaluation of the children 1. Evaluation of physical health. The medical team's examination of the children included: (a) regular well-baby checks; (b) visits for illnesses; and (c) kinesthetic consultations. The frequency of key illnesses among the children (and their mothers) was determined by examining the health center's medical records. 2. Evaluation of psychomotor skills children younger than two years old. As part of the periodic control within the health centers, nurses evaluated children using the Psychomotor Development Scale (EEDP). This scale, designed in Chile by Rodríguez, Arancibia and Undurraga (1974), measures the psychomotor development of children aged 0-2, showing a general score that differentiates between normal development and children at risk. It also allows for the establishment of a profile of development in relation to the chronological age, including 4 areas: motor, language, social skills and coordination. 3. Evaluation of indicators for child abuse. These evaluations were completed by the health center's social workers throughout the duration of the program.	Evaluation of the children 1. Evaluation of physical health. The medical team's examination of the children included: (a) regular well-baby checks; (b) visits for illnesses; and (c) kinesthetic consultations. The frequency of key illnesses among the children (and their mothers) was determined by examining the health center's medical records. 2. Evaluation of psychomotor skills (children younger than two years old): It was measured through the Psychomotor Development Evaluation Scale from 0 to 24 months. This scale, designed in Chile by Rodríguez, Arancibia and Undurraga (1974), measures the psychomotor development of children aged 0-2, showing a general score that differentiates between normal development and children at risk. It also allows for the establishment of a profile of development in relation to the chronological age, including 4 areas: motor, language, social skills and coordination. 3. Evaluation of indicators for child abuse. These evaluations were completed by the health center's social workers throughout the duration of the program. 4. Evaluation of psychomotor skills (children older than 2 years): It was measured through the Battelle tool (Newborg et al., 1988). This tool evaluates 5 domains of development: motor, cognitive, adaptive, communicational and social development. It has also a Spanish version and standardization for the Spanish speaking US population.
	Cost measurement. Costs related to health care, as well as administrative and logistical costs, were taken into account. To identify and measure these expenditures, the registries of both health centers were consulted regarding any costs related to the adolescents and their children. The cost of primary care services in the neighborhood in which the study was carried out was used as the point of reference for standard expenditures.	Cost measurement. 1. Use of micro-costing technique for each intervention. 2. Interview to know about the program, group meeting for the determination of unitary costs, frequency of use. 3. Estimation of different calculation scenarios through the awareness criteria (a) cost discount rate, (b) Results discount rate, (c) Intervention standardization: only home visiting in both groups (excluding all other components of the program associated to the NGO (d) Calculation of incremental cost in regard to control.

Effectiveness Analysis	Results were recorded in descriptive terms, using frequency, percentages and measures of central tendency. Differences between the experimental and control groups were measured using inferential terms: (a) nonparametric tests, such as comparison of proportions, Fisher's Exact Test and Chi-square (with or without Yates' correction for continuity); (b) parametric tests, specifically ANOVA, Student's *t*-test and MANOVA, according to the levels of measurement and specifications required by each test.	Sets and every group were descriptively analyzed. Parametric tests were performed (ANOVA, Student's *t*-test and MANOVA, according to the levels of measurement and specifications required by each test) and also non-parametric tests (Chi-square test)
Cost-effectiveness analysis	In order to evaluate the cost effectiveness of home visits versus the standard treatment provided at the health centers, the following elements were analyzed: (a) unitary costs of each program, (b) effectiveness, and (c) an analysis of incremental cost-effectiveness.	As for the cost-effectiveness analysis, we use an incremental analysis approach which permits us to determine costs and incremental effects of interventions in the study and to compare them with those of the regular programs.

Fig. 1. Home visits to mothers with children between the ages 0 to 4 years old: Results.

3.1 Main results: Compared analysis

3.1.1 "The relationship between a non-professional home visitor and the mother is the key" (results of the research 2003-2005)

This project evaluated the cost-effectiveness of an implemented Home Visiting program compared to the regular program provided by Health Centers to teenage mothers in a high biopsychosocial risk district. The sample included 50 young women in the experimental group which received Home Visits from the third quarter of pregnancy until the 12 months of the child as an average along with the regular programs in Health Care Centers. Control Groups included 50 young pregnant women receiving only the State Health Care Centers programs of the State of Chile.

Among conclusions we can highlight: (a) a better level of mental and nutritional health and compatibility between maternity and the tasks proper of the stage of life cycle reached by the young women receiving home visits, compared to teenagers in the control group; (b) a higher level of development of language in children of teenagers in the experimental group compared to the children in the group who didn't receive visits. Finally, when evaluating cost-effectiveness, the home visits program turned out to be more cost-effective in terms of mental health (Aracena et al., 2009).

Achievements obtained by teenagers in the experimental group can be attributed to the interaction between the young women and the monitor. This interaction represented a space of dialogue, company and orientation where the experience was valued and the skills were recognized. All these tools permit the young women to put into words and elaborate their thoughts and emotions associated to the maternity and their teenage phase and lead them to gain control over the events of their life making them capable to handle difficulties and profit opportunities. It also translated not only into less anxious-depressive symptomatology but also in the incorporation of the maternity adequately in their life projects and their stage in the life cycle along with self-care behaviors which impact in a better nutritional status compared to those women in the control group. It also favoured the interaction between young women and significant people leading to a higher development of language in their children.

It is worth to mention this is the first experimental study, controlled and randomized clinical trial performed in Chile and South America to evaluate the cost-effectiveness of an educational strategy addressing the teenage pregnancy globally. Results supported the need to continue this line of work and also to work with cost-effective community agents, profiting the resources of the community and approaching the public health service to their members. We can also mention the improvements obtained in the levels of mental health of the young women who received home visits which translated into benefits both at personal and family levels and medium and long term savings for the Chilean health system.

3.1.2 "Non-professional staff can have significant outcomes on parents" (results of the research 2007-2009)

The objective of this project was to evaluate the persistence of effects over time, with or without additional intervention, and the cost effectiveness of two programs of Home Visiting (the first, associated to Health Centers and the second, associated with an NGO) for teenage mothers (with different psychosocial risks), comparing them against each other and with the regular programs of the health centers for mothers with children under 4 years. The sample consisted of 263 families referred to the different studies.

The results at 12 months of life for children indicate that in the first program, women have better mental health and nutrition and their children better indicators of language. For the second program, women have better adherence to the school when their child is 12 months old (Aracena, et al. 2011). In this study, the non-professional staff showed better outcomes on parental-family variables.

The results of this project are not surprising since international evidence have already shown the highest effect from the visits performed by non-professional staff in the variables associated to parents. On the contrary, a marginal effect is found in the children and we must highlight the role of health professionals in this area. A doubt arises in this point of the study. It is possible that the effect in the early child development was lower because of the nature of the intervention (not focused on a direct work with children) and the high impact of other variables associated to child development and that were not measured in the study. It is also possible this is an effect of the underpowered design of the study given the size of the sample.

Home visits performed by non-professionals have a direct impact on teenagers according to the content developed in every model (more mental health vs. more networks) and an indirect impact on their children. It poses a question regarding the indirect mechanisms more adequate to impact the development of children and the value of emphasizing such aspects in the visits or definitely propose a parallel visit model focused on working with children, which has demonstrated to be useful in other latitudes and performed by professionals.

These results show the effectiveness and importance of home visits as intervention strategies to improve the biopsychosocial welfare of teenage mothers and their children in a context of poverty. In the other hand, it demonstrates the relevance of including community (non-professional) resources as a potential value in countries with few professional resources to assist the children and families.

Results after 48 months indicate no differences can be observed between the experimental group and the control group or between women or children. Controversy exists about the meaning of an immediate effect than later dilutes in time. This dilution can reflect not a lack of effectiveness of the intervention but the sustained effect of other negative stimuli after the end of such intervention. It can happen when mothers finish an intervention and enter a poor environment. Ramey and Ramey (2006) propose the principle of continuity of educational support. This principle indicates that the effects of an intervention dilute in time if no educational support to maintain learned attitudes and behaviours are in place.

Considering the previously described effects, this intervention permitted the awareness of the importance of a stable protocol for every home visit and the need of continuity in such programs in order to maintain the effects found in children 12 months old.

3.1.3 Home visits and its contribution to mental health: two necessary premises to consider for an effective implementation

3.1.3.1 At a theoretical-empirical level

Regarding the theoretical-empirical background of Home Visiting, it is necessary that those evaluating the possibility of using this strategy as a prevention strategy in mental health must have updated information as the one we have previously presented.

From the point of view of our line of investigation there are two array lines that must be addressed at this level: (a) strengthening the relationship as a mechanism of change and (b) the figure of the community monitor as a possible alternative for Latin-American countries, need to be understood not only at a conceptual level, but also set into the characteristics and challenges of its implementation in the local reality. Otherwise, it is impossible to break the dichotomy between theory and practice, and the proposal to strengthen the home visit as a tool for the promotion and intervention in mental health is weakened.

3.1.3.2 At an implementation level

The experiences of research previously described have generated an endless source of learning, at an implementation level which will be described in detail using the ecological scheme of Bronfenbrenner (1987), because this knowledge has different levels and compromise different actors in each of these levels.

4. Principal lessons regarding the implementation of Home Visiting in an emerging country

4.1 The socio-political national context

The projects presented were implemented in different moments of national contingence, which determine the diverse possibilities and also the diverse limitations for each project. As an example, the current project (2010-2012) initiates in a context of government change, after being in power for 20 years another political coalition (the one that leaded the country into democracy). This event determines big changes in the social environment, and more concretly in the public administration, creating situations of uncertainty about the stability/change of political and technical responsible officers, the ones that will have influence on the work of implementation of home visiting; and a big public policy like this one, must count with the support of the national, regional and provincial health administration system. Everyone was needed, but no certainty was granted.

4.2 The institutional context, national level

Influenced by the dynamic of political change, the context of central administration shows a particular dynamic, in which important changes in political responsibility are observed, slowing down the access to local Health Centers in an institutional culture that follows the central guidelines dictated by the national central level.

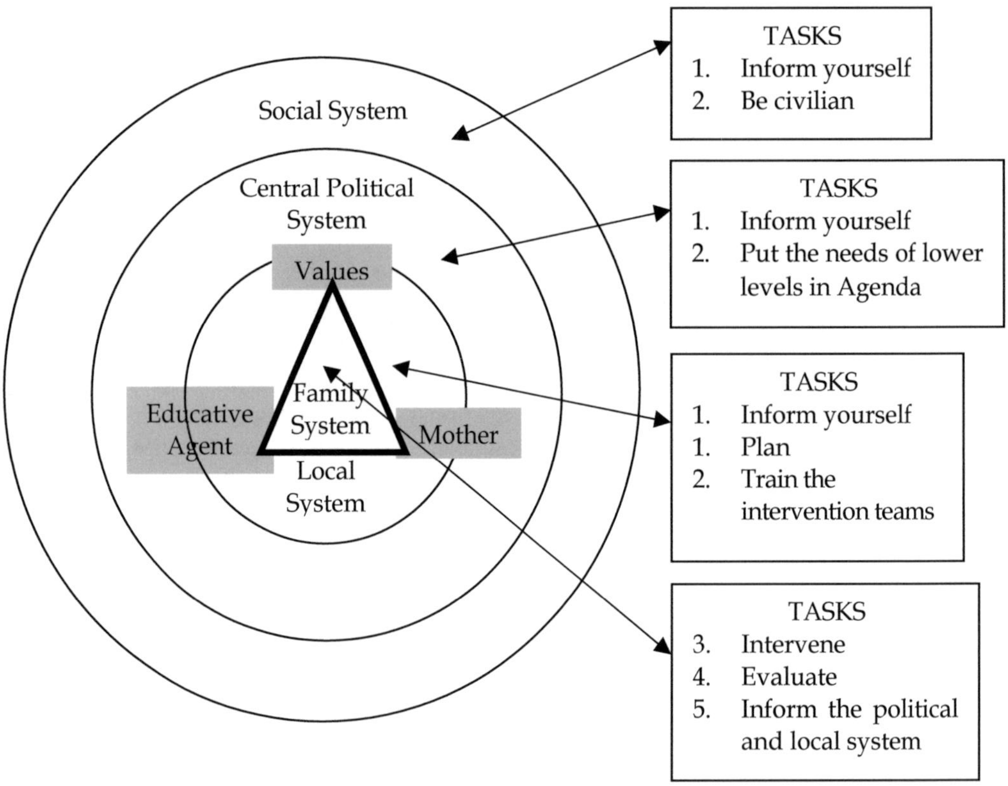

Fig. 2. Intervention Levels Diagram.

4.3 The institutional context, local level

In Chile, Health Centers depends -in terms of general guidelines- of central level, but in terms of administration, of "Municipalidades" that represents the local structure of government. The present research program has demonstrated that, although it is important, to enter the system, to count with the agreement and facilitation of central level, it is absolutely necessary to work with local responsible officers in their different levels ("Corporación municipal", directors of Health Centers). Although the officers of the central administration could facilitate the realization of the home visits if the officers of local government and the directors and operators of Health Centers are not receptive to the initiative (for different reasons, including overload of work, lack of staff, among others), it is impossible to implement home visits of quality.

It is in this context, at this level, that it is necessary a special care about the administrative aspects. These refer to the elements that allow the management of the project or intervention, partially or totally. Among the administrative aspects, it is important to consider the human, economics and material resources, beside the "time" resource -the most valuable and scarce one- to implement home visitation. Each one of these must be attended according to the specifics needs that home visits require in each local context.

The human resource must meet certain characteristics. For home visits, it is necessary to evaluate with whom will be possible to count on to implement the home visits in the institution. International literature reports that the professionals could have a differential response in contrast to paraprofessionals, but the evidence is controversial to date (Nievar et al., 2010; Kotliarenco et al., 2010). So, it is relevant that the human resource could be dimensioned considering the goals proposed for the home visiting intervention.

The economics and materials resources, such as the availability of a vehicle or money for the transportation to deliver the home visits, are important elements to consider when making a budget. It is important too, to document in the programs how and to whom these resources will be delivered, and how the staff directly involved in the intervention will access it.

About the "time" resource, it is necessary to consider the real amount of time of the implementation of home visits, in line with the specifications stipulated in the design of the program (objectives for the work with the families, distance to access the home). In the case of present visits that offers Health Centers in Chilean National Program of Health, this service consider -for each center- the meeting of an interdisciplinary staff, planning and schedule of the Visit, and its recording and evaluation. All of this, including the home visit itself, must be accomplished in a frame of 90 minutes (MINSAL, 2008).

The administrative considerations can be prioritized according to the clarity that it has of the service -in this case home visits- inside the institutional mission, allowing generating the required space.

In brief, and considering the elements previously explained, it can be stated that in order to successfully implement the home visits, it is necessary: to consider the reality of the national context; to contact and inform to national responsible officers about the advantages of the intervention and coordinate it with already existing policies; to solicit that they inform to local representatives, using the appropriated mechanisms, about the importance and meaning of the initiative.

At local level it is necessary, besides having the central authorization, to inform to each one of the persons responsible for the benefits of the initiative; to articulate it with the local policy; to assume administrative aspects and the training of the agents of intervention, by they professionals or persons of the community.

Everything that has been previously stated, as is evident, implies important resources, resources that are consequence not only from a technical and ethical compromise with the scientific evidence available, but also from a political compromise with the mission and vision, from a shared eagerness for the families, and the mental health and wellbeing of each one of their members.

4.4 Micro level intervention

Home Visits are performed at a level we can call micro level. Since it is inserted into a local and domestic context, it cannot be understood as an isolated unit but, according to Bronfenbrenner (1987), as receiving and providing mutual influence from and to such contexts. Home Visits are performed within the family environment, being generally present the pregnant woman/mother and the visiting agent. It is developed within the intimacy of a particular family with a family culture of its own. The visited family agrees to open the door and receive an agent it generally does not know whose function is to help it prepare for the delivery and raising of a son or daughter. To adequate the intervention to this reality is absolutely necessary to increase the possibility of success. In order to analyze this space more clearly we will be using the following axis concepts: Mission or Vision, Competences of the Visiting Agent and Quality of Service.

4.4.1 Mission and vision

Mission and vision are key elements of the strategic planning. Objectives determined derived from mission and vision to guide the intervention, Home Visits in this case (Stanton, Etzel & Walke, 2004). Thus, the mission provides a consistent guide to make important decisions.

In the other hand, the vision is defined as the future situation the institution desires to reach. Its purpose is guiding, controlling and encouraging the organization as a whole to reach the desired status (Quijado, 2003).

The strategic vision has the purpose of describing proposed future strategic scenarios according to the interests and objectives of an institution and with the purpose of obtaining evidence to determine the necessary projections to reach it through the protection of their freedom of action (op cit).

In such sense, Cuadra (2011) concludes it is necessary for the "sense of the intervention" to be transparent; it means that concepts or visions supporting the intervention are clearly stated both for the managers and the people performing the intervention and the users. According to the author, it permits a coherent and strategic look of the work to perform.

Cuadra also highlights the importance of providing technical and emotional support to the agents performing the intervention since it is an element favoring a responsible and effective practice (op cit).

It is important to point out that our research team focuses in the educational aspect of the Home Visiting, which considers the Visit as an educational situation, a privileged relationship between the woman (pregnant woman/mother or care giver) and the educator (visiting agent). The relationship between them is the privileged focus that triggers the expected changes. Therefore, this Home Visiting is a specific intervention centered in connections. It means, focused in the particular link between the pregnant woman/mother and the visiting agent. Evidently, it involves certain conditions.

4.4.2 Competences of the visiting agent

When defining in depth the competences necessary in a visiting agent, no matter it is a professional or not, Hodkinson and Issit (in Delamare Le Deist & Winterton, 2005) emphasized that the competences focus requires a perspective beyond the activities related to care services involving knowledge, comprehension, values and skills that: "live in the person performing an activity" (p. 39). Cheetman and Chivers (1996) identified five interconnected competences:

- Cognitive competences: theories and concepts, implicit knowledge obtained through experience. "The know-how".
- Functional competences: those aspects the person should be capable of doing or demonstrate.
- Personal competences: characteristics proper of a person and related to a good performance.
- Ethical competences: having a set of personal and professional values and the skills to make decision according to such set.
- Meta-competences: the skills to deal with uncertainty and also a constant learning and reflection. It is important to consider that every one of these competences must be put into practice since competences can only be defined in action, it means, cannot be reduced to resources (skills) but to the extent they move in contexts (Cuadra, 2011).

Since the relationship is the core element, the way the agent presents and establishes the relationship, it means how this agent privileges his/her "know how to be" (Cabello, 2008) is more important than its knowledge. Therefore, the way the agent sees itself and establishes a relationship determines to a great extent the construction of common meanings between the agent and the pregnant woman/mother. As Krause (2000) highlights, in the field of clinical interventions, it facilitates the work and lead to success. In this sense, when the agent is a member of the community, a common construction is easier since participants of Home Visits share the same daily world.

Monitors or community agents, in the other hand, have stated in studies performed by this team (Cabello, 2008; Cuadra, 2011), that cognitive competences are less relevant than interpersonal and instrumental competences. They have identified personal, interaction and organizational skills as the most relevant to achieve a significant relationship with the users (Cabello 2008; Cuadra 2011, Navarro, 2005).

As a resume, from the experience of our investigational team, it is possible to state that the competences necessary for the success of Home Visits point to certain personal characteristics of visiting agents that lead to an easier and significant relationship with the pregnant woman/mother (Simonsohn, 2011; Cuadra, 2011; Cabello, 2008). This relational context will be the lowest level to start a continuous training process with educational agents through regular supervisions, support manuals or didactic material that make learning easier. Opportunities of training and constant supervision are then essential in order to achieve such required competences and ensure the success of interventions (Cuadra, 2011).

4.4.3 Quality of service

Home Visiting is an intervention but is also a service provided to community. In such sense, it must be a service of quality and such quality must be evaluated. Quijado (2003) highlights that elements of quality of service being evaluated are subjective and depend on the diversity of people receiving such services. From this perspective, the author highlights five elements the users frequently evaluate:

- Tangible elements: the appearance of the premises of the organization, its staff and equipment being used. In the case of Home Visiting, there are no tangible assets. In the case of projects reported, tangible material involved educational worksheets the visiting agent gives the pregnant woman/mother. The report of the community agents clearly highlights its importance. For them, having support materials to deliver the pregnant woman/mother makes easier to have a specific reason to justify a visit. In the other hand, for the professionals, having these materials involves and is a benefit itself. (Simonsohn, 2011).
- Fulfilling promises: it involves to correctly and timely rendering the agreed service. In such sense, planning and making the visit turns into a form to validate the service by providing it the importance it deserves. In Home Visitis focused on a relational aspect, this is a fundamental issue since it makes possible to develop trust, the basis to establish an adequate relationship.
- Attitude of service: frequently users do not think the ones providing them a service are willing to listen to them and solve their problems or emergencies in a convenient way. This is a core aspect in relational Home Visits: the visited person must feel visible and listened and feel that she and her concerns are the ultimate objective of the service. These elements have turned to be the most relevant in projects developed in Chile according to the monitors and users evaluated (Cabello, 2008; Cuadra, 2011; Simonsohn 2011). In the other hand and considering Home Visiting as a service of the Comprehensive Child Protection System "Chile Crece Contigo"[1], and therefore a strategy connected to other services, when one person does not feel welcomed and supported, this situation can motivate a rejection to other experiences making more difficult to establish a relationship between the users and the Health Care Center (op cit).
- Competence of the staff: competences required by the educational agent must be different. For the users it is important the visiting agent is competent and can correctly assist it; if it is polite, if he/she knows its institution and the services it provides both tangible and not tangible. But for the user it is also important to trust the knowledge of the agent in order to receive an effective support if the visited mother so requires (Cuadra, 2011).
- Empathy: Quijado (2003) defines empathy as the capacity to be accessible for the other: ranging from the establishing an easy contact, to use a clear language and be empathetic with the other, making him/her feels pleasant and important. This characteristic has

[1] The Child Protection System "*Chile Crece Contigo*" is a local program offering a comprehensive system of high quality interventions and social services to support the child and the family and lead them to develop their potential, it involves children from 0 to 4 years old (Ministry of Health, 2008)

been already highlighted as essential for the visiting agent. In this sense, Hiatt et al. (1997), points out the importance of common experiences as an aspect permitting to establish and maintain a relationship with the users and increase the self-effectiveness feeling.

5. Conclusion

Home Visiting, as described previously, appears to be a valid intervention strategy and work in vulnerable sectors. It permits to approach the concrete reality these people lives into; it shows availability and access from agents working in this environment. We know both professional and non-professional agents are effective in different aspects.

It is important to highlight that according to advances in our knowledge, non-professional agents are most likely to open vulnerable families to the knowledge the system can provide (Nievar et al., 2010).

In order to be effective, these agents must have certain characteristics, mainly from a relational point of view but also in terms of commitment with the system and public policy.

Also, the relationship established between the educational agent and the pregnant woman/mother is fundamental. It is important to consider the relational aspect of Home Visits both for the selection of potential field worker and for training and support purposes (Simonsohn, 2011; Cuadra, 2011). It is necessary that visiting agents are not only competent in prevention or care services for the pregnant woman or the mother and child, but also in recognizing and developing competences that lead to the establishment of a positive relationship with the person they visit.

It is also fundamental that such educational agent is clearly convinced of the usefulness of the Home Visiting as a valid intervention to reach the proposed objectives and of course the support and same conviction by the institution offering this service.

Once people is convinced about the effectiveness of Home Visiting with clear objectives and they believe the visited person is capable of improving her conditions and the institution has political, administrative, methodological support and necessary materials and of course it shares this conviction, the first stage for a good development of the intervention is all set.

It is interesting to highlight the fundamental importance of incorporating a supervision based on reflection, an element not considered or left aside in most systems. As Cuadra (2011) points out, it permits to generate a space of technical and emotional support both to professionals and monitors, and favour a responsible and effective practice. This previous aspect makes the practice easier and also permits to level up cognitive competences, to detect training needs, to analyze cases, to promote self-care and team work among visitors, and others.

Within such context, supervision must be regular, collaborative and based on reflection. Regular as a part of the institution as a valid space; collaborative, in the sense of ensuring that all subjects participating in this type of supervisions are assuming responsibilities and finally, reflexive in the sense that it constitute a space for respect that incorporates the making, feeling and thinking and permit the system to observe and learn about itself (Cuadra, 2011).

Therefore, we can point out that within the context of an emerging country and an environment of vulnerable families, Home Visiting appears as an opportunity in the prevention and care of mental health when fulfilling certain specific characteristics. Home Visiting permits the system to intervene in hard access family environments, to directly know the reality of the family and to implement self-care strategies for the mother and child, a finding which has been reported by mothers in a study performed in Chile (Navarro, 2005).

Nevertheless, there are still many questions. The current investigation project implemented by Universidad Católica de Chile is trying to answer some of them. The areas where more information is needed regarding home visits and health and early childhood are: (a) an optimum number of visits connected to the expected results; (b) perceptions of the visiting agent about its role; (c) more effective practices when visiting mothers, especially those visits focused on building a work alliance; (d) theoretical framework, contents and models; (e) use of professional, paraprofessional and non-professional staff; (f) cost/effectiveness relation of home visit programs.

In emerging countries such as Chile, it is especially important to study different methods that could result pertinent both for the socio-cultural characteristics of the context and the low economic and technical resources available (Kotliarenco et al., 2010). Home visiting is therefore, a new, high impact strategy requiring not only a theoretical view regarding who, how and which model is necessary to perform such interventions but also a strategic view on how to implement this alternative in countries which intervention form in mental health is preferably associated to clinical-hospital environments.

The decision of working in Mental Health with Home Visiting requires at least two basic elements to start with. In one hand, a clear vision of the group and purpose to perform interventions with this strategy and in the other hand to size the political-administrative logistics such Home Visiting execution demands.

Home Visiting as a strategy for mental health is a great challenge but an excellent opportunity in emerging countries such as Chile.

6. Acknowledgment

Research funded by Chile's Fondo Nacional de Ciencias y Tecnología [National Fund for Science and Technology], project #1030476 , #1070836 and #1100762.

7. References

Aos S, Lieb R, Mayfield J, Miller M, Pennucci A. (2004). Benefits and Costs of Prevention and Early Intervention *Programs for Youth*. Olympia: Washington State Institute for Public Policy.

Aracena M, Krause M, Pérez C, Méndez MJ, Salvatierra L, Soto M, et al. (2009). A cost-effectiveness Evaluation of a Home Visit Program for Adolescent Mothers. *Journal of Health Psychology*; 14: 878-887.

Aracena, M.A., Leiva, L., Undurraga, C., Krause, M., Pérez, C., Cuadra, V., Campos, M.S. & Bedregal, P. (2011). Evaluación de la efectividad de programas de visitas domiciliarias para madres adolescentes y sus hijos/as. *Rev Med Chile*, 139, 60-65.

Araya, R., Wynn, R., & Lewis, G. (1992). Comparison of two self administered psychiatric questionnaires (GHQ-12 and SRQ-20) in primary care in Chile. Social Psychiatry and Psychiatric Epidemiology, 27, 168 - 173.

Bronfenbrenner, U. (1987). *La ecología del desarrollo humano.* Barcelona: Paidós.

Cabello, V. (2008). *Representaciones de las Monitoras de un programa de apoyo a la Maternidad Adolescente sobre facilitadores del aprendizaje y cambio.* Tesis para optar al grado de Magíster en Psicología. Escuela de Psicología, Pontificia Universidad Católica de Chile.

Caldwell, B. M., & Bradley, R. H. (2001). HOME inventory and administration manual. 3era ed. University of Arkansas for Medical Sciences and University of Arkansas at Little Rock, editor.

Cheetham, G. and Chivers, G. (1996). Towards a holistic model of professional competence, *Journal of European Industrial Training*, 20(5), pp. 20 - 30.

Cuadra, V. (2011). *Visitas Domiciliarias: Perfil de Competencias de Agentes no-profesionales en Intervenciones en Embarazo Adolescente.* Tesis para obtener el grado de Magíster en Psicología, mención Social Comunitaria. Pontificia Universidad Católica.

Delamare Le Deist & J. Winterton. (2005). What Is Competence?. In. *Human Resource Development International*, Vol. 8, No. 1, 27 - 46. Taylor & Francis. Extraído de: http://www.fse.provincia.tn.it/prgleonardo/leonardo/public/documentation/FinalSeminar/CompWintertonEN.pdf).

Elkan R, Kendrick D, Hewitt M, Robinson J, Tolley K, Blair M, et al. (2000). The effectiveness of Domiciliary Health Visiting: A systematic review of international studies and selective review of the British literature. *Health Technology Assessment* ; 4(13): pp.1-339.

Gracia, E. (1997). El apoyo social en la intervención comunitaria. Barcelona: Paidós.

Hiatt, S., Sampson, D. & Baird, D. (1997) Paraprofessional home visitation: conceptual and pragmatic considerations. *Journal of Comunity Psychology*, 25 (1): pp. 77 - 93.

Hidalgo, C. & Carrasco, E. (1999). Salud Familiar: *Un modelo de atención integral en la atención primaria. Santiago.* Ediciones Universidad Católica de Chile.

Hodkinson, P. and Issitt, M. (1995). *The Challenge of Competence.* London: Cassell Education.

Kearney M, York R, Deatrick J. (2000) Effects of Home Visits to Vulnerable Young Families. *Journal of Nursing Scholarship*; 32(4): pp. 369-376.

Kendrick D, Elkan R, Hewitt M, Dewey M, Blair M, Robinson J, et al. (2000). Does home visiting improve parenting and the quality of the home environment? A systematic review and meta analysis. *Archives of Disease in Childhood*; 82(6): pp. 443-451.

Kotliarenco, M.A., Gómez, E., Muñoz, M. & Aracena, M. (2010). Características, efectividad y desafíos de la Visita Domiciliaria en Programas de Intervención Temprana. *Revista de Salud Pública*, 12(2), pp. 184-196.

Krause, M. (2000). *Psicoterapia y cambio.* Dirección de Investigación y Postgrado de la Pontificia Universidad Católica de Chile.

Lagerberg D. (2000). Secondary Prevention in Child Health: effects of psychological intervention, particularly home visitation, on children´s development and other outcomes variables. *Acta Paediatrica Supplement*; 434: pp. 43-52.

McNaughton D. (2004). Nurse Home Visits to Maternal-Child Clients: A Review of Intervention Research. *Public Health Nursing*; 21(3): pp.207-219.

MINSAL. (2008). *Orientaciones Técnicas Visita Domiciliaria Integral para el Desarrollo Biopsicosocial de la Infancia.* Santiago : Gobierno de Chile, Ministerio de Salud.

Navarro, S (2005). *Satisfacción usuaria de un programa de educación para la salud realizado a través de Visitas Domiciliarias a adolescentes embarazadas.* Tesis para optar al grado de Magíster en Psicología. Escuela de Psicología, Pontificia Universidad Católica de Chile.

Newborg, J., Stock, J. R., & Wnek, L. (1996). Inventario de Desarrollo Battelle, Madrid: TEA.

Nievar, M.A. & Van Egeneren, L. (2010). A meta - análisis of home visiting programs: Moderators of improvements in maternal behavior. Infant Mental Health Journal, 31(5), 499- 520.

Olds D, Robinson J, Pettitt L, Luckey D, Holmberg J, Ng R. (2004). Effects of Home-visiting by paraprofessionals and by nurses: age 4 follow-up. Results of a randomized trial. *Pediatrics*; 114(6): pp. 1560-1569.

Quijado. (2003) ¿Qué es la calidad del Servicio?. En *Monografías.* 10.06.2011. Disponible en http://www.monografias.com/trabajos28/que-es-calidad-servicio/que-es-calidad-servicio.shtml.

Ramey, S. L. & Ramey, C. T. (2006). Early Educational Interventions: Principles of Effective and Sustained Benefits from Targeret Early Educations Programs. En D. K. Dickinson & S. B. Neuman (Eds). *Handbook of Early Literacy Research,* Vol. 2. Guilford Press: New York.

Rodríguez, S., Arancibia, V., & Undurraga, C. (1974). Escala de evaluación del desarrollo psicomotor de 0-24 meses. Santiago de Chile: Galdoc.

Russell B, Britner P, Woolard J. (2007). The Promise of Primary Prevention Home Visiting Programs: A Review of Potential Outcomes. *Journal of Prevention & Intervention in the Communit*; 34(1/2): pp. 129-147.

Shore, A. (2001) The effects of early relational trauma in right brain development, affect regulation and infant mental health. *Infant Ment Health* J 22: pp. 201–206.

Simonsohn, A (2011). *Aprendizajes y Desafíos para mejorar la Visita Domiciliaria. Una reflexión a partir de una línea de investigación en Chile.* Seminario para Institución Núcleo de Estudos da Violênca (NEV) Universidade de São Paulo.

Stanton, W., Etzel M., & Walker, B., (2004). Fundamentos de Marketing, Edición, Editorial McGraw Hill.

Sweet, M. Appelbaum (2004) M. Is Home Visiting an Effective Strategy? A Meta-Analytic Review of Home Visiting Programs for Families with Young Children. *Child Development*; 75(5): pp. 1435-1456.

16

Inter-Professional and Inter-Cultural Competence Training as a Preventive Strategy to Promote Collaboration in Encountering New-Coming Refugees in the Reception Programme – A Case Study

Solvig Ekblad and David Forsström
Karolinska Institutet, Department LIME, KI
Stockholm,
Sweden

1. Introduction

Every encounter with a patient/client in the mental health and social services constitutes a challenge for the responsible staff or organisation. Meeting a patient/client from a culture other than the one to which the caretaker/case manager belongs accentuates this challenge. The challenge will be even greater in the future because the number of refugees at mental health facilities is steadily increasing around the world. One of many aspects of the challenge is the language barrier. This may be a problem even when an interpreter makes the work of communication function smoothly (Farooq & Fear, 2003). A qualitative study by O'Donell et al. (2007) researched various aspects of health care for immigrants in the UK. Overall the participants were satisfied with the help they got from interpreters, but lacked help from them at key moments during their treatment. The participants also felt that the interpreters did not tell the GP what the patient had actually said and were not familiar with medical terminology, which impeded information sharing. This undermined trust. The participants stressed the importance of mental health services and the lack of care they received.

When the patient facing a clinician is a refugee from another culture (in some cases he/she could be a refugee from the clinician's own country of origin) the assessment or treatment will be even more complicated. Having access to the care to which the patient has a right is essential for refugees' mental health. Silove (2002) reports some of the consequences which the new Australian policy with detention centres had for refugees: an increase in self-harm behaviours, hunger strikes and riots at detention camps for refugees in Australia.

Regardless of the refugee's grounds for deciding to move from his/her country of origin to a reception country, the goal is to avoid death, secure a better future, avoid persecution and discrimination or leave a war zone to avoid being killed. The decision to move will have consequences for the refugee's entire life as well as for his/her family and will affect their health, economy and general welfare.

The migration process can be divided into two stages: pre- and post-migration. The pre-migration stage covers the time up to the decision to leave the place of residence as well as the journey to a new place in which to live; its duration will vary with the circumstances. Lindencrona, Ekblad and Hauff (2008) identified four dimensions of resettlement stress among recently resettled refugees from the Middle East in Sweden: social and economic strain, alienation, discrimination and loss of status, and violence and threats in Sweden. To remain where they came from would have exposed them to psychological and physical abuse.

The goal of this chapter is to prepare mental health and social service staff to cope with the challenges posed by the above at every level of the organization. An important part of this is to get tools to be able to assess and understand the inherent potential that refugees carry within the clinical and social service space. At the same time it is of significance to pay attention to resilience factors (Antonovsky, 1988); why some cope better than others, to bear in mind the strengths which these people possess. The chapter aims to provide an introduction to refugees' mental health and the challenges and gaps which health and social care staff meet in encounters with this target group. The topic is highly relevant as the world becomes increasingly globalised. Refugees' health, especially mental health, is thus a world problem. The competence training is presented as a Case from Sweden but it can be generalized to other countries in similar situations.

Keywords and definitions of key concepts are specified below.

1.1 Key words

Refugees, mental health, mental disorder, prevention strategies, resilience, SOC, mental health promotion, collaboration, inter-professional, inter-cultural communication

1.2 Definitions of key concepts

Collaboration: a fluid process whereby a group of diverse and autonomous actors undertakes a joint initiative, addresses shared concerns or otherwise achieves common goals (Fear & Barnett, 2003).

Health: according to WHO, as a state of complete physical, mental and social well-being, and not merely the absence of disease or infirmity (www.who.org).

Health promotion: the process of enabling people to increase control over their health and its determinants, and thereby improve their health. A core function of public health that contributes to the work of tackling communicable and non-communicable diseases and other threats to health (WHO, 1986).

Inter-cultural communication: occurs when two or more people with different backgrounds interact and communicate with each other. An optimal cultural communication means that those involved are affected; a real encounter is established where understanding arises despite different backgrounds in behaviour, perceptions and values/attitudes.

Inter-professional training: occurs when two or more professions learn with, from and about each other to improve collaboration and quality in health care (www.caipe.org).

2. Background

The process of globalization challenges our awareness of people's diverse backgrounds, especially for social service and health professionals. Human migration, voluntary or otherwise, has transformed Western countries into multicultural societies. This global phenomenon has significantly changed the number and nature of impacts on the health of individuals and populations (Zimmerman, Kiss and Hossain, 2011). Sweden as a case grants asylum, in accordance with the Geneva Convention, to those who have reason to fear persecution in their native country due to race, nationality, religious or political beliefs, gender, sexual orientation or membership of a particular social group (www.migrationsverket.se). Those who may qualify for asylum also include persons who have a well-grounded fear of suffering the death penalty or torture or who need protection due to an international or external conflict or a natural disaster in their native country. Further, family reunification is a possibility. In Sweden the proportion of immigrants, i.e. foreign born or born in Sweden to parents who are both foreign born (Statistics Sweden, 2011), has increased to 19 % in 2010 (December 31) of the nine million inhabitants. Until the mid-1970s this was primarily a matter of labour force immigration, mostly from elsewhere in Europe. More recently, increasing numbers of refugees and their relatives have come from non-European countries.

Up to now there has been a lack of coordinated policy approaches to deal with modern migration's impacts on health. This is an ethical responsibility in that all human beings have a right to autonomy, dignity and responsibility. Development, manifestations and illnesses vary with the context. An association between trauma and increased morbidity, lower life expectancy and higher risks of medical problems was identified more than fifteen years ago (Friedman and Schnurr, 1995). A systematic review and meta-analysis (Steel et al 2009) shows that pre-migration stress is associated with the diagnoses post traumatic stress disorder (PTSD, DSM-IV, APA 1995) and depression. Increasing levels of trauma lead to higher rates and severity of PTSD and depression, i.e. a dose-effect relationship (Mollica et al 1998, Sledjeksi et al 2008). Post-migration factors, e.g. the period of waiting for asylum, also have impacts on refugees' mental health (Carswell, Blackburn, and Barker, 2011). Vulnerable groups among migrants are refugees in general and, in particular, asylum seekers, temporary mass-evacuees, women and those with co-morbid PTSD and depression. A prospective study by Roth (2006) of mental health among mass-evacuated Kosvo Albanians in Sweden showed that the prevalence of PTSD was 37% at baseline and increased to an extremely high level (80%) at the 18 month follow-up and highest among those who decided to stay in Sweden; participants with PTSD had significantly lower cortisol levels. Depressive symptoms and aggression followed the same pattern as PTSD, while Sense of Coherence (SOC) was lower and aggression scores higher among participants with PTSD and co-morbid depression (Roth, 2006). Lindencrona, Ekblad and Hauff (2008) report that for many refugees the period after obtaining a permanent residence permit is extremely stressful as they may have a demanding social life with constant stress and perceived ill-health. According to a Swedish public health report (2009), foreign-born people have a lower rate of perceived health than the Swedish-born population. The literature shows that compared to age-matched general populations in western countries, refugees resettled in those countries could be about a tenfold greater risk of post-traumatic stress disorder (Fazel, Wheeler and Danesh, 2005) and social exclusion (Johansson Blight, Ekblad, Lindencrona and

Shahnavaz, 2009). Being a refugee is also associated with depression (Carta et al, 2005) and public health diseases, e.g. cardiac and vascular diseases, diabetes (Kinzie et al, 2008). Consequences of the disorder are not only a range of psychiatric symptoms but also individual suffering. There are also cognitive impairments that effect the everyday functioning of the patient/refugee. Several meta-analyses and reviews have been carried out regarding PTSD and changes in cognitive functioning. However, the conclusions that can be drawn are limited by co-morbidity and substance abuse and the level of individual functioning before the event that caused the onset of PTSD. A meta-analysis by Johnsen & Asbjorsen (2008) showed that patients had impairments in verbal memory. Brewin (2008) found that patients diagnosed with PTSD had memory impairments regarding neutral verbal and visual memory.

In a pilot study of whether neuropsychological impairments were alleviated after patients received trauma-focused treatment, Walter, Palmieri and Gunstad (2010) found that the patients improved in multiple aspects of executive functioning. Although the study needs to be replicated with a larger sample, the authors of this chapter suggest that patients' impairments can decrease with therapy, thereby contributing to a better everyday life. For refugees, this means better chances of establishing a functional life in the country of reception.

A register study of mental health differences between refugee and non-refugee immigrants, independent of the area of origin, assessed using purchase of prescribed psychotropic drugs as a proxy measure of mental ill health; it showed that refugee women who have lived in Sweden, a high-income country, for up to ten years have more mental ill health than other immigrant women and men, but do not seek health care (Hollander et al 2011). Refugees usually seek primary health care for their perceived illness, described as somatic complaints, as it is easier to communicate mental illness with somatic symptoms (Ekblad and Hollander, 2011). Further, cultural as well as language barriers, expectations of treatment and compliance between clinical staff and refugee patients may affect the outcome. Insufficient language entails a need for an interpreter, but the interpreter's competence and the patient's confidence in the interpreter are essential for an adequate inter-cultural health communication between the patient and the clinical staff (Fathai et al 2010, Farooq and Fear, 2003).

While the need for inter-cultural competence and the need for evidence-based practice in mental health services of patients with an immigrant background are complementary, there is little cross-fertilization in the literature (Whaley and Davis, 2007). A review reports that there is limited evidence of the effectiveness of inter-cultural competency training and service delivery (Bhui et al 2007). A public health report fourteen years ago from the Swedish National Board of Health and Welfare (Brisfjord, 1997) draws attention to the fact that training for health professionals allows little time for training in multicultural health care, including psychiatric care, and social service. Competence training in migration and health is constrained by sector silos, often with different goals. Thus, staff encountering new-coming refugees in the reception countries (mainly Western) are quite often unprepared to meet the refugees' needs, due to a lack of inter-professional and inter-cultural communication competence and collaboration in preventive strategies involving both health care and social service care (Ekblad, 2011). Collaboration is a recognized strategy in health promotion for dealing with this gap in health and social care, but not yet in the context of refugees. A health-promoting introduction model according to Lindencrona (2008, Abstract) "includes network building blocks, setting qualities, the health promoting spiral of personal capacities, outcomes and environmental facilitators and long-term health, social and economic outcomes at the individual, group and societal levels". According to WPA guidance, adequate resources for training, including competency training, should be available (Bhugra et al 2011). Training of both evidence based knowledge and collaboration strategies between mental health professionals as well as municipal staff in refugee reception must therefore be increased in order to improve the refugees' situation (Lindencrona, 2008). Results from a study among general practitioners in the management of mental health disorders highlight self-professed interest and prior training in mental health (Browne, Lee and Prabhu, 2007). A Danish study provides evidence that health professionals (doctors, nurses and assistant nurses) obtain their knowledge about immigrants mainly through the media and patient contact, and less through travel, courses and colleagues (Michaelsen et al 2004).

Screening and follow-up according to needs are vital when it comes to securing mental health among refugees. The common diagnoses among refugees, PTSD and Depression, impair the ability to function in everyday life in the new society. The complexity of the case demands collaboration. With the increasing demands on this group, it is important to assess the refugee's ability to perform. In Sweden, refugees are enrolled in classes to learn Swedish and are expected to be able to work shortly (within two years) after their permission to stay in Sweden. For most refugees, this may be an unattainable goal. For a refugee who is suffering from mental illness, the first part of the stay in Sweden can have a negative effect on his/her mental and physical health. Conclusion from a research study in Sweden is that collaboration between agencies leads to better care for new-coming refugees (Lindencrona, 2008).

During Spring 2010 the two authors conducted and evaluated a university course at Karolinska Institutet, Stockholm, Sweden, entitled *Refugee-related stress and mental health – local collaboration,* 7.5 ECT points, based on evidence and clinical experience. Details of the course are given in Table 1. One of the aims of the course was that the participants would establish a platform and produce new policy documents for their organization regarding encounters with refugees in the local context. The main question was whether inter-professional and inter-cultural competence training can promote collaboration in refugee reception?

2.1 Setting, participants and methodology

The explorative study concerns a Swedish refugee reception program and Södertälje municipality, not far from the capital, Stockholm, as a Case. Södertälje municipality and Stockholm county council commissioned competence training, 7.5 ECT (one week full-time course), from Karolinska Institutet (the first author was in charge of the course) during a one-year project entitled "Health promoting strategies in the reception of refugees with mental disorders and disabilities - a platform collaboration". The participants who encountered the target group were invited and participated voluntarily. The training took three full days and a half-day workshop, with homework in between. The participants had an obligatory list of references to read and homework during the course.

The syllabus was approved by the Board of Education at Karolinska Institutet under the provisions of Higher Education. The course was Commissioned by the Municipality of Södertälje and Stockholm County Council.

The course aimed to

- Introduce and provide guidance on mental health and its determinants from a refugee reception perspective
- Introduce theories of exclusion, segregation and discrimination processes and their relation to mental health for vulnerable groups (asylum seekers, refugees and their relatives)
- Introduce and develop an inter-cultural communication perspective to respond to, analyse, and propose actions to be quality-assured to promote mental health in a refugee reception perspective
- Make participants aware of their own and other's 'cultural spectacles'
- Provide opportunities to increase an understanding of their own and other's professional roles and to obtain information about the various actors' organizations, including the implementation of user organizations, their responsibilities, mission and values in a refugee reception perspective

The course would encourage co-education across professional boundaries in order to raise awareness and develop the ability to highlight and respond to mental illness/health and what promotes mental health in the given gender and diversity context. The course was designed to complement the knowledge the participants had received in their basic training.

Learning outcomes

After completing the course, participants will be able to:

Knowledge and understanding:

- explain the concept of mental health and its determinants from a refugee reception perspective
- orient themselves on different theories of exclusion, segregation and discrimination processes and their relation to mental health for vulnerable groups (asylum seekers, refugees and their relatives)
- describe how important organizational and inter-organizational strategies for collaboration can be developed to influence the determinants of mental health in vulnerable groups (asylum seekers, refugees and their relatives)

Skills and abilities:

- use an inter-cultural perspective to respond to, analyse, and propose actions to become quality-assured to promote mental health in a refugee reception perspective
- apply the principles of WHO Health Promotion to develop an overall strategy for the interaction of mental illness in the reception of refugees with mental illness and mental impairment
- apply the models to identify and plan for the relevant organizational and inter-organizational strategies for the development of refugee reception, which can promote

mental health • apply case-methodology under supervision Values and attitudes • critically examine their own 'cultural spectacles' • reflect on and consider the ethical implications of their professional conduct • discuss their own and other's roles in and around the mental health field Focus of education (pedagogics): Lectures, observation of the local context, and laboratory exercises in small and large groups according to the general and specific information related to their profession. Case-method according to the Harvard Model under supervision. Theme titles of the compulsory course days during Spring 2010: Day 1 (April 7) Introduction to local actors in asylum and refugee reception Day 2 (May 5) Primary health care perspective Day 3 (June 2) Specialist psychiatric care Participation: Participation in lectures and group work for three days, homework under supervision for 2 days and follow-up days, a total of 5 days is compulsory. In the event of absence, compensatory task discussed with course leaders. The prerequisite for getting the course certificate is to answer the evaluation questions before and after the course. Examination: Written examination and oral presentation. Grading: U/ G Course Evaluation: The course is evaluated in writing in accordance with guidelines established by the KI (survey sample) at the end of the course. Rationale for participation and open-ended questions about expectations before the course and follow-up after the course are planned. Course evaluation also retrieves relevant issues from the course leader's cooperation with the Harvard Program in Refugee Trauma (http://www.hprt-cambridge.org). The evaluation (pre- and post-evaluation) will guide the implementation of the future course of the report to the National Board of Health and Welfare. Reading List: Separate list to the participants

Table 1. Course: Refugee-related stress and mental health - local collaboration, 7.5 ECT points.

3. Methods

3.1 Evaluation methodology: quantitative and qualitative

The course was evaluated in several steps. A questionnaire was distributed to the participants at the onset and end of the course (Table 2). The course was evaluated, using an

11-item questionnaire (both quantitative and qualitative) which had been developed by the two authors (SE, DF). The quantitative questions covered how challenging the participants thought that the course would be and how challenging it actually was; also, how demanding the course would be and how demanding it actually was. Other items were about the demands and control which participants exercised over their work situation and how much knowledge they had acquired. Their responses were made on a standard Likert scale from 1 to 5, where 1 was "a little" and 5 was "a lot". The questionnaire was distributed to the course participants on the first day of the course before the course programme started and at the end of the last course day. Participation was voluntarily and responses were anonymous.

The qualitative questions from the questionnaire surveyed the participants' expectations of the course, their ability to gain new knowledge during the course, whether the course contained content relevant to the participants' work situation and how they were going to implement the new policy documents. In this chapter, the focus is on their expectations and whether the course contained relevant material. The ability to implement the new policy documents will also be discussed briefly.

Questions in the questionnaire distributed at the onset of the course	**Questions in the questionnaire distributed at the end of the course**
1) Have you attended a similar course before?	1) Were your expectations of the course fulfilled?
2) What are your expectations of the course?	2) What were your opportunities to learn during the course?
3) How do you view your opportunities to learn during the course?	3) Did the course contain relevant knowledge for you as a professional?
4) Does the course contain relevant knowledge for you as a professional?	4) What in the course material can you use in meetings with refugees?
5) Estimate how big a challenge you suppose the course will be?	5) Does your organization adhere to the policy documents?
6) Estimate how the competence you have enables you to apprehend the course material?	6) What can you do to enhance the use of the new policy documents in your organization?
7) How much control do you have over your work situation?	7) How much new knowledge did you gain during the course?
8) How do you regard the demands placed on you in your work situation?	8) How big a challenge was the course?
9) Other comments?	9) Estimate how the competence you had before the course enabled you to apprehend the course material?
	10) How much control do you have over your work situation?
	11) How do you regard the demands placed on you in your work situation?
	12) Other comments?

Table 2. Evaluation questions before and after the course.

The participants also had the opportunity to leave verbal commentaries on the course at the end of training. Also, each of the three sessions included in the course started off with a round among the participants to see if there were any questions regarding the course and its content. One of the aims of the course was that the participants would produce new policy documents for their organization regarding refugees. The documents were supposed to be created from the new knowledge derived during the course.

The results from the course evaluations will be presented below. Kirkpatrick's Evaluation Model (Alliger et al, 1997) will be presented to further clarify the results.

The two versions of the questionnaire had the same set of questions with the exception of questions 4, 5 and 6 in the questionnaire distributed at the end of the course. These questions focus on the results of the course as a whole for the participant and the organization the participants belong to.

Questions 5, 6, 7 and 8 in the questionnaire distributed at the onset of the course and questions 7, 8, 9, 10 and 11 distributed at the end of the course required the participants to rate their answer on a 5-point Likert scale ranging from "Very little" to "A lot". The other questions in both of the questionnaires were open-ended and the participants were supposed to write more extensive comments.

3.2 Data analysis

The quantitative answers from the questionnaires were analysed by descriptive statistics with PASW V.18. The quantitative analysis comparison of pre- and post-survey scores was conducted with a non-parametric test.

The basic categorization of the qualitative answers followed the items in the questionnaire. The responses to each question were summarized without knowledge of the participant's occupational background or sex. This content categorization yielded various themes. The frequency of the answers was categorized according to the system proposed by Hill et al. (2005). The term "general" is used when a majority of the participants answered the same way; "typical" is used when about half of the sample answered in that way and "variant" is used when about a quarter or less of the answers dealt with that topic. Revisions of the system proposed by Hill et al. (2005) were made to suit the questionnaire distributed to the participants. All written answers to each question were read through before any categorization was done. The field notes during the course days were read several times to obtain a sense of the whole. Citations will be reported as examples of exploring the results.

3.3 Ethical issue

The data from the study did not include information which according to law must have ethical approval. We got consent from the participants and answering the questions was voluntary and the results were on group level.

4. Results

4.1 Participants

Thirty-two participants took part in the course; twenty-eight (87.5%) passed it and received a diploma. Table 3 presents the number of participants in the course, in total and by profession, gender and workplace.

Participants' workplace	Profession	Total	Men	Women
Introduction/municipal	3 assistants, 1 counsellor	4		4
Income support/municipal	6 assistants	6	2	4
Swedish language course	1 teacher, 1 counsellor	2	1	1
Public employment service	Employment service officers	7	2	5
Primary care	1 nurse, 1 counsellor, 2 physicians, 1 social worker/psychotherapist	5	2	3
Speciality/county council	1 nurse assistant, 1 psychologist	2	1	1
Care/municipality	2 social workers, 2 assistants	4		4
NGO/Red Cross	2 NGOs	2		2
TOTAL		**32**		

Table 3. Number of students on the course, in total and by profession, gender and workplace.

4.2 Outcome

4.2.1 Before the course

1. Have you gone on a similar course before? If so, when, who organized it and what did you learn?

Twenty-three (82%) participants had not attended a similar course before, five responded that they had taken various courses in the field, such as previous courses the current course providers have given, courses at the Transcultural Centre, courses on migration at the Karolinska Institutet and Stockholm University.

2. What are your expectations of the course?

Some participants mentioned a number of things, so the answers are not representative of the whole group. Nine (42.9%) participants said they would create contacts/get a larger network. Twelve participants reported that they will get more knowledge. Two participants were hoping to refresh old knowledge. Two other participants stated that they will have more tools. In addition, a few more things were mentioned once only. They are related to the expectations set out. The following quotations illustrate how the participants formulated their expectations:

- to increase my competence regarding my and other people's work.
- networking and to gain better knowledge of how the situation for the refugee can be and what potential obstacles the refugee might need help with.

3. How do you see your opportunities for learning during the course (based on workload and other commitments)?

Eleven participants (39.3%) saw their learning opportunities as very good or good, while five (17.9%) wrote that they had to work in their leisure time to absorb the course content. Another five participants (17.9%) gave different answers about a high workload. A quarter of the participants (n=7) did not respond at all or gave an answer that cannot be understood on the basis of the question. Some quotes exemplify the participants' thoughts:

- I am interested in what the course has to offer, so I'll be fine, but the assignments for the course have to be prepared in my spare time.
- The possibilities for learning are not great if I don't use my spare time for preparations.

4. Does the course content include relevant knowledge from your work?

Twenty-five (89.3%) participants considered that the course contains relevant knowledge based on their work situation, while one each answered a bit, do not know or did not respond. The following quotes are examples of how students responded:

- Yes, absolutely since I work with newly arrived refugees who many times are stressed due to traumatic events.
- The content of the course seems very interesting and will help me a lot and make my teaching less difficult.

5. What challenge do you think the course will involve? Four participants did not answer. The mean was 3.3 "moderate challenge" (from 1-5, 1 = small challenge, 5 = very challenging)
6. How can you assimilate course content on the basis of the skills you possess? Two participants did not answer the question (from 1-5, 1 = little skill, 5 = very high level of expertise). The mean was 4. There seems to be a feeling that they have the skills to be able to integrate knowledge.
7. Based on your work situation, estimate (from 1-5, 1 = little control, 5 = much control) how much control you feel over your job? One participant did not answer. Group mean 3.9, meaning they feel they have relatively good control over their work.
8. Based on your work situation, estimate (from 1-5, 1 = low demands, 5 = very high demands) how much demand is there in your work situation? One participant did not respond. Group mean 3.8. The participants feel they have relatively high demands in their work situation.
9. Other comments: Twenty-two participants (78.6%) made no other comment. Two participants mentioned the importance of collaboration. Three participants referred to the course in positive terms, and one had a perspective on the course setup. Here are some comments:

- A major challenge is how to coordinate the management and political levels. Will there be room to develop and interact? Difficult to see that the opportunity will be given.
- The importance of cooperation cannot be emphasized enough! Prestige aside, and above all training to create an understanding of the work of others and focus on the individual.

4.2.2 After the course

A total of 26 (81.30%) of the 32 participants responded to the evaluation questionnaire at follow-up after the course. Table 3 summarizes the mean values of closed responses before and after the course.

1. Were your expectations of the course met?

Twenty-two (84.5%) of the 26 participants responded that their expectations were met. The following quotes from some participants illustrate the quantitative results:

- Yes, I have gained a better understanding of the problems that other vocational groups are working with and I have also had the opportunity to defend the organization that I represent.
- Yes! New thoughts and reaffirmation regarding collaboration between organizations.

2. Did you have your learning opportunities during the course (based on workload and other commitments)?

Just under half (46.1%) of the participants answered that their learning opportunities during the course were good. Three out of ten (30.8%) reported that they did not have time to do homework during working hours and were forced to do it in their spare time or were not able to spend time on the course because of heavy workloads. Here are some quotes that illustrate this:

- Have a big workload so I wish I had more time for this course. Asked my boss if I could do 2 days of study but that wasn't possible. During the course I participated in the group exercises.
- I learned a lot during the classes. Assignments in my spare time. The work load has been high or rather high. I can, however, say that the course has been educational and it was rewarding to meet other professionals working with the same clients.

3. Did the course contain relevant knowledge for your work?

The majority (80.8%) of the participants wrote that the course contained relevant knowledge based on their work situation. Here are some quotes that describe these responses:

- It certainly did. I come into contact with mental illness basically every day when I meet my clients.
- Yes, relevant to be able to guide individuals to the right service so they will receive adequate help.

4. What in the training can you use in responding to this target group?

The course participants' responses reflected their professions and work places but the following four themes dominated the responses: 1. How different organizations in the field work, 2. What resources are available, 3) How to improve the attempts of refugees, and 4) How to improve cooperation. These themes are mentioned four to five times. Further topics were presented in two responses: networking and to better understand refugees arriving in Sweden. The following quote substantiates the students' responses:

- The knowledge I have gained will help me to assess if a person suffers from psychiatric disorders or has been through a traumatic experience.
- A lot, since I now know much more regarding what differences mean and in which way different agencies work and with what groups they work. A lot of new knowledge.

5. What is your organization's policy document describing the process of the target group?

Just under a quarter (23.1%) of the participants answered that they follow current policy well or very well. Just over one in ten (15.4%) of the participants said they do not have a policy document in their organization. Four in ten (42.3%) misunderstand the question and responded about other aspects, such as working with the policy. The following quote illustrate the responses:

- We have no such documents, the aim is for our "new knowledge and method" received to be our policy.

6. How can you work to ensure that the new policy (Establishment Act as of December 1, 2010, when the Swedish Public Employment Service would take over the reception of refugees from the municipalities) becomes a reality in organizations?

A common response among four out of ten participants (38.5%) was that they intend to inform colleagues in their organization to improve the policy in their organization. One in ten of the participants (11.5%) wrote that they plan to increase cooperation with other organizations in the field. Four (15.4%) answered that they had policy documents in their organization. Some citations illustrate the results:

- To enhance collaboration between different agencies on different levels. We can work with specific cases on another day.
- To inform the management regarding what I encounter on an everyday basis, I try to influence the policy through that.

7. Estimate (from 1-5, 1 = some knowledge, 5 = much knowledge) how much knowledge you gained during the course?

The participants wrote that they have medium knowledge (mean 3.3). Table 4 shows the results from mean value before and after the course on challenge, competence, perceived control and perceived demands.

8. Estimate (from 1-5, 1 = small challenge, 5 = very great challenge) how challenging the course was?

The course posed a mediocre challenge (mean 3.0)

9. Estimate (from 1-5, 1 = low competence, 5 = very high level of expertise) how the competency you possessed made you able to assimilate the course content?

The participants estimated that they possessed great skills (mean 3.7) to be able to understand the course content.

10. Based on your work situation, estimate (from 1-5, 1 = little control, 5 = much control) how much control you feel you have over your work?

The participants considered that after the course they had more control (mean 4.1) of their duties.

11. Based on your work situation, estimate (from 1-5, 1 = low demands, 5 = very high demands) how great the demands are on your work situation.

After the course, the participants perceived that the requirements of their work situation were higher than before the start of the course (mean 4.3)

12. Other comments during the seminars

- I have received new information and also confirmed that a number of my thoughts and ideas are shared by several others.
- I have been strengthened in my profession because I realize that I am doing a good job with a strong client perspective.

- Good Reading! Key speakers! Good research rooted!
- What is important in everything we do is COLLABORATION, and not to work separately.
- A hope that the participants could be called to a follow-up meeting one year after the end of the course
- To discuss how the collaborative model developed. But it's certainly not money.
- The objective of 'good work on Health' increases an individual's participation in society, democracy and expression, which is the basis for a 'good and humane society'.

Question	Mean value before the course (N=28)	Mean value after the course (N=26)
Challenge	3.3	3.0
Competence	4.0	3.7
Perceived control	3.9	4.1
Perceived demands	3.8	4.3

Table 4. Mean values before and after the course.

In summary, the results were adapted to Kirkpatrick's Learning Evaluation Model (Table 5).

Level	Evaluation: what is measured	Evaluation: description and characteristics	Evaluation: tools and methods	Outcome
1	Reaction	To what the delegates felt about the training experience.	Verbal reactions from the course evaluation.	The participants expressed that they were pleased with the course during the training occasions.
2	Learning	Measurement of the increase in knowledge - before and after.	Questionnaire	The results from the questionnaire before and after training showed that the participants felt that their knowledge had expanded.
3	Behaviour	The extent of back-on-the-job implementation.	Questionnaire	The questionnaire showed that the participants thought that the content of the course was relevant for their work.
4	Results	The effect on the business or environment by the trainee.	Policy documents	New policy documents were supposed to be implemented after the course's completion.

Table 5. Adaptation to Kirkpatrick's Learning Evaluation Model (Alliger et al 1997).

5. Discussion

5.1 Results

The majority considered that the course included relevant and practical knowledge, prevention strategies that are evidence-based and learnt by experience. They wanted to implement the new knowledge from the course. The perception of demands and control seems to be similar, but increased during the course.

A majority of the participants answered that they expected to broaden their knowledge base and create new contacts and professional networks during the course. They also thought that the course contained relevant information that they could apply in their work situation. After the course the majority thought that their expectations of the course had been met and that the content of the course had been relevant for their work situation. The expectations mirrored the need among the participants to have more knowledge regarding refugees coming to Sweden. The fact that they thought that their expectations were met indicates that the participants actually gained new knowledge regarding refugees. This conclusion was confirmed during the rounds of verbal commentaries at the onset of every course day.

The participants also had new ideas about how to implement the new policy document in their organization. Before the onset of the training the participants had a vague idea of what was in the policy documents regarding refugees. Some even said that they did not know if they had policy documents regarding refugees. They also seemed to grasp the importance of having these policies as a guideline in their work.

Results were not only observed on an individual level. Due to the participants' enthusiasm and the organizations involved in the project, a new course was created to further build the participants' knowledge base and further enhance collaboration in the community.

Looking at the participants on a group level, they went from an understanding that their own work situation was related to working with refugees to a better understanding of how other professionals work with refugees. They also became more aware of the factors that influence the psychological and physiological wellbeing of refugees.

Further resources need to be allocated to study whether and how the situation for the refugees improved after the course in Södertälje. This is a difficult question to answer due to changes in directives for refugee care (a new from as of 1 December 2010). However, an established platform network with professionals working with refugees will provide the best chance of making transitions between different directives within refugee care.

5.2 Constraints, possibilities and lessons learnt

Despite the limitations of the study, such as that the data are based on a single course, a single context and a single group of mental health and social service staff, the results are promising for increasing inter-professional and cultural competence. On the path towards cultural competence, the review by Bhui et al (2007) showed that "a developmental process was proposed moving from cultural awareness to improved cultural knowledge and improved skills through encounters" (p.7). Reflexivity, i.e. practitioners looking within themselves, "is necessary to develop empathy through a better understanding of the patient's predicament, avoid assumptions and stereotypes, and to be aware of one's own attitudes and prejudices."

The majority of the participants mentioned in the evaluation that they had limited time to read the material during working hours and did this in their leisure time.

Due to the new law on introduction activities for certain newly arrived immigrants (2010:197) from December 1, 2010, when the organization of refugee reception moved from the municipalities to the Swedish Public Employment Service (www.arbetsformedlingen.se), the participants indicated that they wanted to continue with a new course in order to keep the platform alive as there were new actors.

Anyone between the ages of 20 and 64 (or 18 and 19 with no parents in Sweden) who has received a residence permit as a refugee or for reasons similar to being a refugee has the right to special support in order to get work as quickly as possible. This also applies to those who are in the same age group and came to Sweden because they have a relative who got a residence permit as a refugee or for reasons similar to being a refugee, provided that they have applied for a residence permit no later than two years after the relative was admitted to a municipality.

After the course, the participants and their superiors, a total of 40 persons, met on a workshop day and discussed the future collaboration model and what each actor/organisation needs to pay attention to in order to collaborate in the refugee reception in Södertälje.

The participants wanted to continue the course for the whole of 2011 (10.0 ECT points), which resulted in an application to the same funder and was approved. At present the majority of the participants are continuing and there are also new participants from the Swedish Public Employment Service. The participants have compulsory course days about once a month, with theory and discussion of Case from an inter-cultural communication and inter-professional training point of view. They also visit the actors' workplace. The development of a platform "Södertäljeplattormsanda" has started and is being stabilised. This process is not a quick fix; it takes time as the participants need to explore the settings and reflect.

5.3 Conclusions

Very few of the participants had experience of a course in the subject before this course started. The majority found that the new knowledge gained was relevant. They had the ambition to spread the knowledge to their colleagues in the respective organization. The participants had got to know "a face" of the other collaborators, which facilitated future contacts.

The participants' responses imply that the course made them more conscious of the issue, with an increased perception of workplace demands and control over their work. The most significant findings from the evaluation were that the participants had received preventive strategies, so inter-professional collaboration in the municipality's refugee reception could be improved, obtained information about which interventions are relevant, and had "faces" that created options for inter-professional exchanges with others in the refugee reception.

In inter-cultural communication training there is a need to achieve a balance between attention to "difference", attention to self and attention to power relations (Beagan, 2003).

A summary, presented below, of important aspects to treatment, learning and collaboration, as well as lessons learned from the study, can also be implemented in other reception settings.

Summary of important aspects

- Early screening and treatment are vital. For physical as well as mental illnesses, early screening is important for preventing the development of illness.
- Co-morbidity is prevalent among refugees. PTSD and depression are two common diagnoses among the refugee population. Treatment plans need to take this into account.
- PSTD and depression have major consequences for the patient's everyday functioning. Their ability to meet demands that they succeed depends on this and has consequences for learning and functioning and integration into society.
- Be aware of the complexity when meeting a refugee who seeks assistance. Language, culture, roles and expectations, both from the mental health professionals/public employment service and from the patient, can result in the loss of vital information.

Lessons learned from participation in the course

- Most of the participants thought that the course had been useful and that it had given them an opportunity to learn and network. Participants created a platform for future learning.
- To use local participants' own experiences of working with refugees as a tool for learning.
- Helping the participants to create a platform ensures future collaboration among agencies. You have a "face" at an agency to whom you can turn.
- Make sure that the participants are able to attend the course (anchor participation at all levels in the organization). To maximize learning, networking and future collaboration and evaluation, the participants need time to complete the course work.

Competing interests

None

6. Acknowledgements

The university course was funded by the National Board of Health and Welfare (Dnr 52-9291/2009); Södertälje municipality and Stockholm County Council had applied and got approval. Moreover, the authors thankfully acknowledge the contributions of Maria Stålgren, participant in the course, and a member of the steering group of the project, who wrote notes from the compulsory course days, and Clara Fagerlind, a student at KI who observed and made notes during the workshop.

Thanks to Mr Patrick Hort for language editing of the text.

7. References

Alliger, G.M., Tannenbaum, S.I., Bennet JR, W., Traver, H., Shotland, A. A meta-analysis of the relations among training criteria. *Personnel Psychology* 1997:50:341-358.

American Psychiatric Association. *Diagnostic and Statistical Manual of Mental Disorders.* 5th edition. Washington DC 1995.

Antonovsky, A. *Unrevealing the mystery of health. How people manage stress ands tay well.* San Francisco, California: Jossey-Bass Publishers, 1988.

Beagan, B. Teaching social and cultural awareness to medical students: "It's all very nice to talk about it in theory, but ultimately it makes no difference". *Academic Medicine* 2003:78(6):605-614.

Bhugra, D., Bupta, S., Bhui, K., Craig, R., Dogra, N., Ingleby, D.J., Kirkbride, J., Moussaoui, D., Nazroo, J., Qureshi, A., Stompe, T., Tribe, R. WPA guidance on mental health and mental health care in migrants. *World Psychiatry* 2011:10:2-10.

Bhui, K., Warfa, N., Edonya, P., McKenzie, K., Bhugra, D. Cultural competence in mental health care: a review of model evaluations. *BMC Health Services Research* 2007:7:15. doi:10.1186/1472-6963-7-15.

Brewin, C.R, Kleiner, J.S, Vasterling, J.J & Field, A.P. Memory for Emotionally Neutral Information in Posttraumatic Stress Disorder: A Meta-Analytic Investigation. *Journal of Abnormal Psychology* 2007:116(3):448-463.

Brisfjord, J. Högskoleutbildningar inom vård och omsorg kartlagda. Etnisk bakgrund saknas. *Invandrare & Minoriteter* 1997:4:36-38.

Browne, M.O., Lee, A., Prabhu, R. Self-reported confidence and skills of general practitioners in management of mental health disorders. *Aust J Rural Health* 2007:15:321-326.

Carswell, K., Blackburn, P., Barker, C. The relationship between trauma, post-migration problems and the psychological well-being of refugees and asylum seekers. *International Journal of Social Psychiatry* 2011:57:107-119.

Carta, M.G., Bernal, M., Hardoy, M.C., Hro-Abad, J.M. Migration and mental health in Europe (the state of the mental health in Europe) working group: appendix 1 *Clin Pract Epidemol Ment Health* 2005:1:13.

Ekblad, S. *Slutrapport till Socialstyrelsen. Hälsofrämjande strategier i mottagandet av flyktingar med psykisk sjukdom och psykisk funktionsnedsättning - plattformssamarbete mellan Södertälje kommun och landstinget - en redogörelse för bidragets användning samt effekter av genomförda åtgärder under år 2010.* Karolinska Institutet, Department of Learning, Informatics, Management and Ethics (LIME), Center for Medical Education (CME), 2011.

Ekblad, S., Hollander, A-C. Mental ill health among refugees and asylum seekers - differences between men and women (translation of the book chapter Psykisk ohälsa hos flyktingar och asylsökande - skillnader mellan män och kvinnor (sidor 103-121). In: S. Bergqvist Månsson (ed) *From Women's Health to Gender Medicine (Från kvinnohälsa till genusmedicin – en antologi: Stockholm: Forskningsrådet för arbetsliv och socialvetenskap*), 2011.

Farooq, S., Fear, C. Working through interpreters. *Advances in Psychiatry Treatment* 2003:9:104-109.

Fatahi, N., Nordholm, L., Mattsson, B., Hellström, M. Experiences of Kurdish war-wounded refugees in communication with Swedish authorities through interpreter. *Patient Education and Counseling* 2010:78:160-165.

Fazel, M., Wheeler, J., Danesh, J. Prevalence of serious mental disorder in 7000 refugees resettled in western countries: a systematic review. *The Lancet* 2005:365:April 9:1309-1314.

Fear, H. & Barnett, P. Holding fast: the experience of collaboration in a competitive environment. *Health Promotion International* 2003:18(1):5-13.

Friedman, M.J., Schnurr, P.P. The relationship between trauma, post-traumatic stress disorder, and physical health. Neurobiological and clinical consequences of stress:

From normal adaptation to posttraumatic stress disorder. In: Friedman, M.J., Charney, D.S:, Deutch, A.Y. (eds). *Neurobiological and clinical consequences of stress: From normal adaptation to post-traumatic stress disorder*. Philadelphia, PA: Lippincott Williams & Wilkins Publishers, 1995.

Hill, C. E., Knox, S., Thompson, B. J., Williams, E. N., Hess, S. A., & Ladany, N. Consensual qualitative research: An update. *Journal of Counseling Psychology* 2005:52:196-2005.

Hollander, A-C, Bruce, D., Burström, B., Ekblad, S. Gender-related mental health differences between refugees and non-refugee immigrants - a cross-sectional register-based study. *BMC Public Health* 2011:11:180 http://www.biomedcentral.com/1471-2458/11/180.

Johnsen, G.E & Asbjørnsen, A.E. Consistent impaired verbal memory in PTSD: A meta-analysis. *Journal of Affective Disorders* 2008:111:74-82.

Johansson Blight, S., Ekblad, S., Lindencrona, F., Shahnavaz, S. Promoting mental health and preventing mental disorder among refugees in Western countries. *International Journal of Mental Health Promotion* 2009:11(1):33-44.

Kinzie, J.D., Riley, C., McFarland, B., Hayes, M., Boehnlein, J., Leung, P., Adams, G. High prevalence rates of diabetes and hypertension among refugee psychiatric patients. *J Nerv Ment Dis* 2008:196(2):108-112.

Lindencrona, F. *Strategies for a health promoting Introduction for newly-arrived refugees and other immigrants*. Dissertation (PhD), Stockholm: Karolinska Institutet, 2008.

Lindencrona, F., Ekblad, S., Hauff, E. Mental health of recently resettled refugees from the Middle East in Sweden: the impact of pre-resettlement trauma, resettlement stress and capacity to handle stress. *Social Psychiatry and Psychiatric Epidemiology* 2008:43(2):121-131. DOI: 10.1007/s00127-007-0280-2.

Michaelsen, J.J., Krasnik, A., Nielsen, A.S., Norredam, M., Torres, A.M. Health professionals' knowledge, attitudes and experiences in relation to immigrant patients: A questionnaire study at a Danish hospital. *Scand J Public Health* 2004:32:287-295.

Mollica, R.F., McInnes, K., Poole, C., Tor, S. Does-effect relationships of trauma to symptoms of depression and post-traumatic stress disorder among Cambodian survivors of mass violence. *Br J Psychiatry* 1998:Dec;173:482-488.

O'Donell, C.A, Higgins, M., Cauhan, R. & Mullen, K. They think we're OK and we're not. A qualitative study of asylum seekers' access, knowledge and views to health care in the UK. *BMC Health Services Research* 2007:7:75.

Roth, G. *A prospective study of mental health among mass-evacuated Kosovo Albanians.* Dissertation (PhD), Stockholm: Karolinska Institutet, 2006.

Silove, D. *The asylum debacle in Australia: a challenge for psychiatric. Australian and New Zealand Journal of Psychiatry*, 2002: 36:290-296.

Sledjeski EM, Speisman B, Dierker L. Does number of lifetime traumas explain the relationship between PTSD and chronic medical conditions? Answers from the National Comorbidity Survey-Replication (NCS-R) *Journal of Behavioral Medicine* 2008:31:341-9.

Walter, K.H, Palmieri, P.A, Gunstad, J. More than Symptom Reduction: Changes in Executive Function Over the Course of PTSD treatment. *Journal of Traumatic Stress,* 2010:April; 23/2):292-295.

Whaley, A., Davis, K.E. Cultural competence and evidence-based practice in mental health services. A complementary perspective. *American Psychologist* 2007:62(6):563-574.

WHO. (1986) *Ottawa charter for health promotion*. Accessed 12 May 2011 from http://www.who.int/hpr/NPH/docs/ottawa_charter_hp.pdf

Zimmerman, C., Kiss, L., Hossain, M. Migration and health: A framework for 21st Century Policy-Making. *PLoS Med*, 2011:8(5):e1001034. doi:10.1371/journal.pmed.1001034.

Internet

www.arbetsformedlingen.se
www.caipe.org
www.hprt-cambridge.org
www.migrationsverket.se
www.scb.se
www.who.org

17

Development and Implementation of Suicide Prevention Activities – Report from Slovenia

Saška Roškar[1], Alenka Tančič Grum[2] and Vita Poštuvan[3]
[1]*National Institute of Public Health*
[2]*University of Primorska, Andrej Marušič Institute*
Slovenia

1. Introduction

On-going development and sustainable implementation of suicide prevention activities seem to be important factors that contribute to lower suicide rates over several years. In Slovenia, new programmes, initiatives and suicide prevention and research centres have emerged in the last decades. In our chapter we are presenting very well accepted project Let's Talk about Suicide and its impact on the society. The project is aimed to decrease suicidal behaviour among different high-risk groups. It integrates research, prevention and intervention through different activities targeting healthcare professionals, school counsellors and media.

2. Background

2.1 Suicide - a global public health problem

In 1984 the WHO's European Member States defined the reduction of suicide as one of their main health policy targets (WHO, 2002). Namely, every year more than 58,000 persons commit suicide/die by suicide within the European Union which is the highest rate for completed suicide in the world (WHO, 2003). Outside European Union the statistic is also devastating as almost 900,000 lives annually are lost worldwide through suicide, representing 1.5% of the global burden of disease (WHO, 2003). Closely related to completed suicide are non-fatal suicidal acts and their rate can be estimated to be even 10 times higher than that of completed ones. Given these facts, focusing on suicide, its prevention and appropriate interventions should be one of the key public mental health concerns.

2.2 Prevention/intervention programmes aimed at suicide reduction

In the past, many intervention programmes aimed at reducing suicide rates were launched, some of which proved more effective than others. In a simple way they can be divided into local (regional) and global (national, international level) prevention programmes of suicide (Marušič, 2008).

On the local level one of the most successful interventions to prevent suicide (which initially became global as it grew internationally) was the German Nuremberg Project/Nuremberg Alliance against Depression (NAD), which evolved into European Alliance against Depression (EAAD) (Hegerl and Schafer, 2007). Even though the EAAD was not directly aiming at reducing suicide (as it was focusing on depression) the project has had huge success in recognising and treatment of depression (and subsequently suicidality) and can without any doubt be regarded as an example of good practice (efficacy in terms of reduction in suicide and deliberate self-harm was not systematically investigated in EAAD, as was the case in NAD).

On the other hand, in addition to the EAAD approach, some European countries have also developed systematic national suicide prevention strategies. Regular evaluations and monitoring of progress of these strategies is a condition sine qua non as suicidologists need to be aware of what is working and what is not. Furthermore, policy makers must be provided with up to date and applicable data easy to translate into practice (Marušič, 2008).

The state of the art literature reveals that there are many papers listing appropriate divisions of suicide prevention activities. One of the most echoing systematic review on suicide prevention strategies is probably that of Mann and colleagues (Mann et al., 2005) where interventions for suicide preventions are divided in five broader areas:

1. interventions aimed at education and raising awareness among workers in primary health care, broader public and other gate keepers,
2. continuous care for persons and vulnerable groups at high risk,
3. treatment and rehabilitation of persons with mental health illnesses, with particular attention to suicidal risk,
4. restriction of lethal means and
5. guidelines for media on how to-report about suicides.

Recently, Cornelis van der Feltz and colleagues (2011) have conducted a systematic review of suicide prevention activities and have clustered intervention levels of suicide prevention into four groups:

1. focusing on primary health care workers,
2. focusing on general public and gatekeepers,
3. focusing on high-risk groups, and
4. focusing on restricting access to means of suicide.

As we can see, different resources suggest similar prevention and/or intervention activities for dealing with the issue of suicide. Further work on evaluating different kinds of suicide prevention is needed (Feltz-Cornelis et al., 2011; Mann et al., 2005) but we can classify suicide prevention activities into four groups (see Figure 1).

First intervention level is aimed at early recognition of depression and suicide risk in patients on the primary health care level, usually by their general practitioners. Second intervention level aims at raising awareness among the general public about suicide risk factors, signs of suicidality, underlying causes of suicidal behaviour and different forms of help. This level also focuses on gatekeepers training (individuals who have regular contact with suicide high risk groups and can potentially recognise the signs of mental health problems and suicidality, i.e. school counsellors, social workers, psychologists etc;

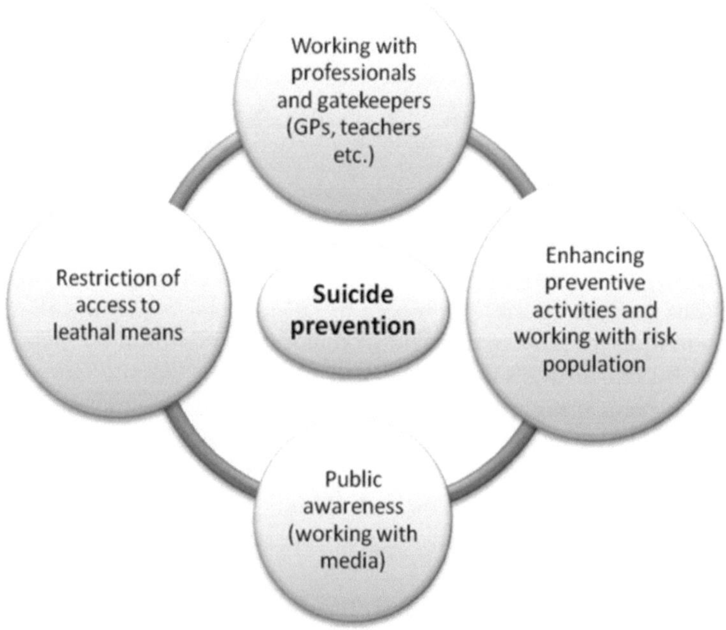

Fig. 1. Core elements of suicide prevention.

Rickwood et al., 2007). Third level of intervention aims at working with high-risk groups. Last but not least, forth level aims at restricting access to lethal means for suicide.

In addition, similar division of suicide prevention activities are listed in WHO strategy (2011b):

1. support and treatment of populations at risk,
2. reduction of availability of and access to means of suicide,
3. establishing and maintaining networks for survivors of suicide, and
4. trainings of primary health care workers and other sectors.

Regardless of different classification of suicide prevention strategies, the authors agree about that not all of listed intervention levels are equally effective in suicide prevention. In fact, rather than focusing on only one intervention level it turns out that focusing multi-level approach is the best way to efficient suicide prevention.

2.3 Suicide - a major public health problem in Slovenia

As stressed in the beginning of the chapter, suicide accounts for a great percentage of premature mortality in many European countries. However, suicide rates in Europe vary widely. They are higher in the northern and eastern part of Europe while southern European countries report lower suicide rates (Marušič, 1999). One European country which has traditionally been regarded as a high suicide rate country is Slovenia. With a population of something over 2 million, the average suicide rate for the whole population in Slovenia was 31 per 100 000 in the years 1985 - 1994, remaining more or less stable over the years

(Marušič, 1999). Speaking in absolute numbers this meant approximately 600 lives lost every year due to suicide. The overall male suicide rate for the period 1985 – 1994 was 48.5 and 14.4, for women, resulting in a male to female suicide ratio of about 3.4:1 (Marušič, 1999; National Mortality Database).

Some features of Slovenian suicide resemble suicide characteristics in other countries while others are unique for Slovenia. One such characteristic worthwhile mentioning is the regional distribution of suicides in Slovenia. As previously found by Marušič (1998), the distribution pattern of suicide rates in Slovenia resembles to that in Europe – i.e. suicide rates are highest in the north-eastern part of Slovenia and gradually decrease towards the south-east (Marušič, 1998). Differences in suicide rate between different regions in Slovenia are in some cases as high as are differences in suicide rate between different European countries. Also unique for Slovenia is the fact that hanging is used by majority of suicide victims, namely by two thirds of men and half of women. Usually hanging is a typical suicide method for men, who choose more violent methods (gases, firearms, hanging), while women more often choose poisoning by solid or liquid substances, drowning and jumping from high places (Marušič, 1999). As far as high risk groups are concerned they are similar as in other countries and include older, male, divorced, widowed and people with no formal education.

2.3.1 Challenges in suicide prevention activities in Slovenia

In terms of suicide prevention, Slovenia is up against many challenges, i.e. restriction of access to lethal means, improving the care for persons in suicidal crisis etc. The challenges most often pronounced can roughly be divided in following sections:

- under recognition of depression and suicide risk on the primary health care level,
- suicide in the elderly and suicidal behaviour in youngsters,
- the fact, that the subject of suicide is presented as a taboo and as something that is deeply embedded within the Slovenian nationality or national character.

In Slovenia, primary care physicians have a gatekeeping role as it is they who refer a patient to a specialist if needed, i.e. if a mental disorder is diagnosed which requires treatment from a specialist. A study conducted by Rodi et al. (2010) on a Slovenian sample of primary health care patients showed that 30 out of 77 suicide victims visited their primary health care physician in the last month before suicide (16/77 in the last week) whereas only 16 out of 77 controls did so before the index day (3/77 in the last week). In 30% of suicide victims, the reason for the last visit was mental health problems, while this was the case in only 3% in the control group. It remains to be investigated in how many cases the primary care physician was able to recognize mental health problems and potential sucidality. Given the fact, that many suicide victims seeks help from their GP prior to suicide speaks in favour of the statement that GP's are the first in the line of suicide prevention. Hence they need proper support in terms of identification of mental health disorders related to suicidality and suicide risk sign. Mental health disorder most often related to suicidal behaviour is depression. A better recognition of depression could thus subsequently lead to a reduction of suicide (as shown in the EAAD study). Roskar et al. (2010) found on a Slovenian sample that education of GP's on depression recognition and treatment of depression resulted in an increase of antidepressant prescription and a tendency of suicide rate drop.

As reported by Milton and colleagues (1999), the suicide risk is recognized in only 38% of cases, which is positively related to the presence of a psychiatric diagnosis and negatively with the diagnosis of physical illness. The later poses a particular danger in the elderly population where physical illness is rather a rule than an exception. According to the WHO HFA Database Slovenia is ranking third in the EU in mortality due to suicide in the age group 65 and more. Furthermore, the suicide rate in this age group is much higher than the overall suicide rate (figure 1) (Svetičič, 2010).

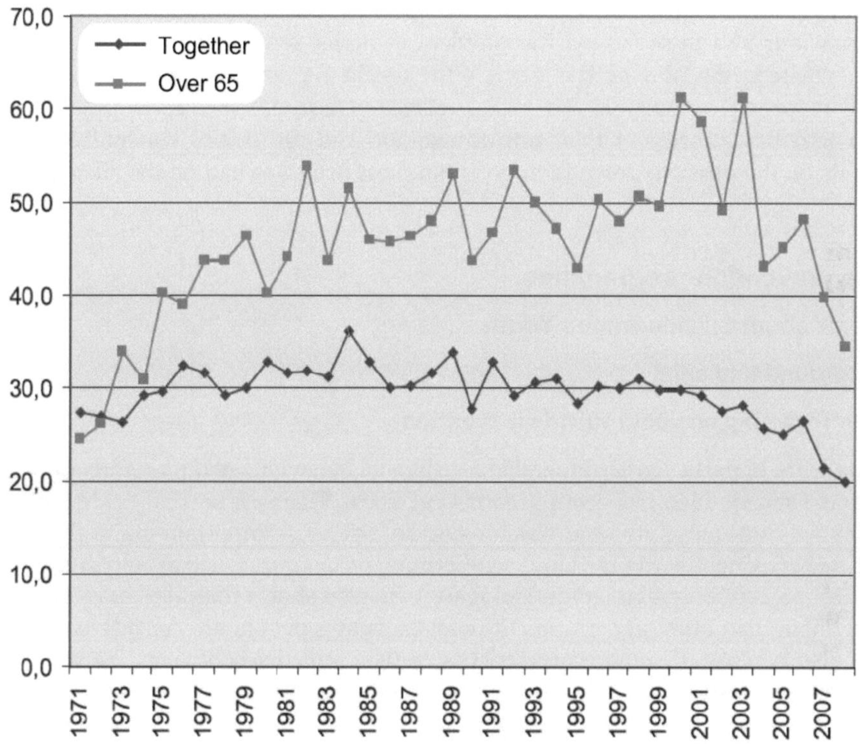

Fig. 2. The overall suicide rate in Slovenia and suicide rate in the age group 65+.

Similarly as in elderly, Slovenia is also above the EU average in terms of suicidality in young people (14 -25 yrs) (HFA MDB). What represents a special challenge in this age group is impulsivity of youngsters, under recognition of mental health problems and feelings of low competence to work with a suicidal individual in school workers. Annually, Slovenia loses on average 20 young lives due to suicide.

As stressed many times before, suicide prevention is the task of the society as a whole. If the society acknowledges the problem and is open to speak about it, the stigma is not so pronounced and persons needing help may feel less reluctant to seek help. And vice versa. One of the key gatekeepers in this regard are the media. In Slovenia the reporting on suicide was up until recently marked with sensationalism. The papers reported about all details of suicidal behaviour and showed little or no help possibilities. No guidelines on responsible reporting on suicide were complied.

The above mentioned difficulties called for action. In the last decade more effort was directed into suicide prevention in Slovenia. The aim of our chapter is to introduce three different suicide prevention activities in Slovenia that were launched in the last years with the aim to tackle challenges of suicidality in Slovenia:

- working with GP's,
- school counsellors and
- the media.

The goal of the first two programmes was to facilitate a better recognition and treatment of suicidal behaviour and to overcome the problem of under recognition of depression and suicidality, whereas the aim of the work with media representatives was to facilitate responsible reporting on suicide. We will particularly address the development of the prevention activities, process of their implementation and difficulties we confronted. We will elaborate on the possible prevention potential these activities had on the suicide rate in Slovenia.

3. Suicide prevention programmes

3.1 Let's Talk about Suicide among Youth

3.1.1 Background and aims

Reasons for focussing on youth suicide prevention

Young people are in particularly vulnerable for suicidal behaviour and therefore are widely recognised as a suicide-high risk group (Mann et al, 2005). There are several epidemiological reasons why we consider youth as at risk for suicide. The most important one is that young people are more frequently involved into self-harming behaviours (such as self-cutting) than other age groups. Not only that, epidemiological data also shows that they have also more suicidal attempts than other age groups. Moreover, young people are considered as high-risk group also because of some characteristics of their suicidal behaviour. Young people tend not to seek professional help in cases of distress mainly because of their attitude that *as they grow up, they need to know how to deal with their problems by themselves*. Often, they are also not seeking any professional help because of stigmatisation or peer pressure (Rickwood, Deane and Wilson, 2007). Besides, young people also have a tendency to commit suicides in a more impulsive nature than adults.

Young people have traditionally had relatively low suicide rate in Slovenia, but the number of suicides among youth is increasing globally, which is even more true for other suicidal- or self-harm behaviours (Tančič, 2009).

Reasons for focussing on gatekeepers

School counsellors have a direct access to young people in Slovenia, as each school is obliged to employ at least one psychologist, pedagogue, social worker or someone in similar profession as school counsellor. They collaborate with teachers and school staff among others also in order to help children with emotional problems (e.g. in distress, having mental disorders etc.). Often they educate teachers about mental health of youth and help them to help students. Besides, school counsellors also have individualised approach to students and can intervene in case of emergency. In this way they represent important gatekeepers for young people in detecting their suicidal ideations. They are both the gatekeepers that recognize suicidal behaviour among students and need the confidence to act upon cases, and also the ones that pass their skills and knowledge on to teachers and school staff.

The aims of *Let's Talk about Suicide among Youth* programme were to:

- educate school counsellors about suicidal and self-harming behaviour among youth,
- provide school counsellors tools for coping with suicidal youth,
- evaluate our activities through the changes in attitudes towards suicide, their competences and opinions before and after the intervention.

3.1.2 Development of the program

Let's Talk about Suicide among Youth started in 2008 and was the first in our series SoS. Within the span of two years we have run the pilot, evaluated it and prepared an improved program in line with the feedback from the field. Both, the pilot and the final programme consisted of the:

- Development and publishing of a manual with practical guidelines about working with suicidal youth.
- Development and facilitation of a 1-day educational programme covering the content of the manual for school counsellors.
- Evaluation of the program.

The programme was implemented in cooperation between the Institute of Public Health and Slovenian Centre for Suicide Research.

3.1.2.1 The pilot in 2008

The pilot version of the manual consisted of the following topics:

1. Shadow on the sunny part of Alps (chapter on suicide issues in Slovenia)
2. Do we know our youth? (chapter on characteristics of young people)
3. So young and already suicidal (chapter on suicide and young people)
4. Youngsters' help seeking
5. Suicide prevention in schools
6. Terminology dictionary

Besides the manual, the school counsellors of the Ljubljana region were invited to a 1-day education on the same topic. We evaluated the program with the pre-post changes of attitudes toward suicide, feelings of competence and with qualitative answers.

Attitudes towards suicide

Permissive attitudes toward suicide (these are attitudes that accept suicide more) usually correlate positively with suicidal behaviour and are therefore considered as one of the predictors for suicidal behaviour. People with lenient attitudes toward suicide more often have their own suicidal behaviour or are exposed to suicidal behaviour of others (for example relatives in family). Permissive attitudes might be considered also as the result of exposure to suicidal behaviour and as an attempt to socially justify this kind of behaviour.

These goes in line with the research that shows that the societies with higher suicide rates also have more permissive attitudes toward suicide (Kodaka et al., 2010).

Using the attitudes as evaluation tool was aimed to find how school counselling staff felt about suicide and to compare the level of functionality of attitudes. Namely, if the attitudes toward suicide are too permissive, they might be dysfunctional for preventing suicide.

Instruments

We used the Attitudes toward Suicide Questionnaire (ATTS) for our study. The ATTS was developed as an instrument to measure attitudes toward suicide in the general population (Renberg & Jacobsson, 2003). A recent review on scales that measure attitudes toward suicide (Kodaka et al., 2010) described it as one of the most widely used and more feasible to use.

When we tested the reliability of the previously suggested structure of ATTS, it was very low. Therefore we performed the principal component analysis by ourselves. We identified four dimensions with relatively good statistics. The content of first two dimensions describes the reason for suicidal behaviour. First one (*Illness;* α=0,81) justifies suicidal behaviour in cases of illness and the second one (*Isolation;* α=0,54) explains the effect of isolation on people with suicidal tendencies. Third and fourth dimension are more related to stigmatisation. The third one (*Impulsivity and revenge;* α=0,70) talks about the impulsivity and revenge (towards other people) as the reasons of suicidal behaviour. The last one (*Ability to prevent;* α=0,53) describes the preventability of suicidal behaviour and reveals the attitudes toward the determination of suicidal thoughts and to what level the society should intervene when preventing.

Procedure and sample

The 44 school counsellors involved in the education were tested before and three months after the education. The data collection was anonymous and the data was used only in an aggregated way. The data were paper-pencil and computer-based, both of which is very common for this profile of people.

Results and discussion

The overall average on the first dimension was just a bit lower than 3 that was (on a 5-grade scale) the middle value or the neutral value (where people didn't decide whether they agree or disagree) on the scale. According to this result people do not justify suicide because of illnesses. This didn't change a lot after the workshop. The average on the second dimension was again very neutral. There was also no significant differences between the first and second testing. The average on the third dimension is the lowest among dimensions and suggests that people do not consider suicide as an act of impulsivity of revenge. This lowered a bit after the workshop. Participants agreed the most with the last dimension that suggests that we are able and obliged to prevent suicide.

The results revealed that school counselling staff does not justify suicide in cases of illness, have neutral opinions about how isolation might trigger suicidal behaviour, do not find suicide as an impulsive and revengeful act and most importantly, feel it is possible and also necessary to prevent it. The pre-post changes were not statistically significant but showed that there was a bigger variance in the attitudes after the education. This implies that the concept of attitudes cannot be changed easily, but even non-intensive 1-day workshop

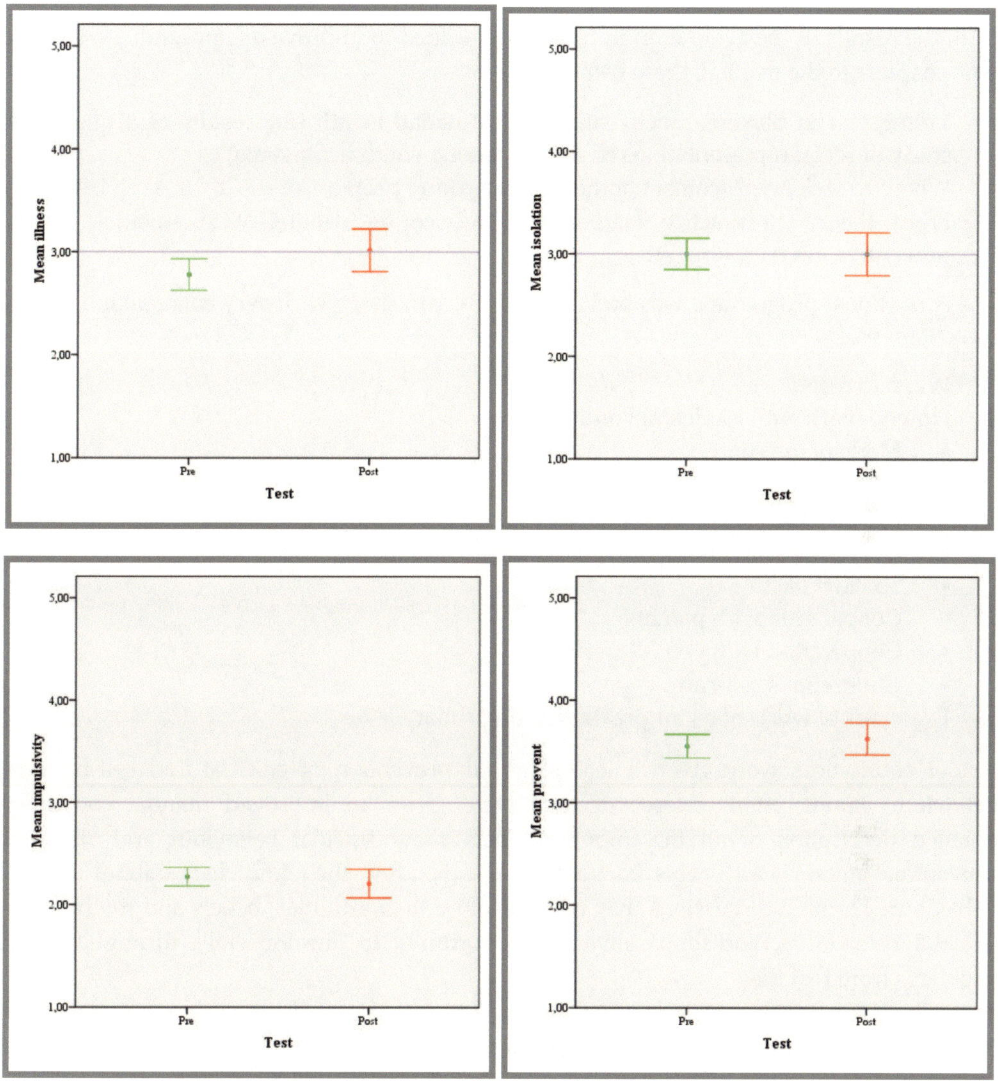

Fig. 3. Pre-post *attitudes toward suicide* changes.

showed some changes. The bigger variance is important because it shows that the attitudes started to be changed.

Feelings of competence and qualitative answers

When assessing the feelings of competence, there was a statistically significant improvement of the competence *When working with youngsters I recognize signs of suicidal behaviour* after the programme. The evaluation of qualitative questions and personal feedbacks at the end of the education revealed high need to address the issues of suicide prevention in the future. The main concern that participant expressed were the lack of concrete information on how to approach a young person in distress and where to refer him/her.

3.1.2.2 The 2009 program

With the results of the evaluation in mind, we decided to improve our program. We added new chapters to the manual, these were:

- Youngsters in Slovenia about suicide and mental health (the results of a qualitative study of social representations of suicide among youth in Slovenia)
- Where to seek help? (contact points to refer young people)
- From theory to practice (step-by-step advice on dealing with suicidal person, preventive interventions, etc.)

The educational programme was backed up with workshops with very concrete guidelines. Its content was:

1. When to react?
2. How to work with a suicidal youth?
   - Mode of questioning
   - Mode of listening
   - Confidentiality
   - Counselling or reference to an expert?
   - Suicidal pact
   - Cooperation with parents
   - Cooperation with youth's peers
   - Counsellor's self-care
3. Examples of workshops for prevention on primary level

School counsellors were given a lecture about prevention of suicidal and self-harming behaviour among youth. Moreover they were given an improved manual containing detailed description of all the important facts about suicidal behaviour and about its prevention among youth. This part aimed at expanding their knowledge about suicidal behaviour. Through discussions they could explore their attitudes, beliefs and myths about suicidal behaviour. Workshops gave the opportunity to develop skills through solving problems from real life.

3.1.3 Implementation and evaluation of the program

We have used the train the trainer principle to disseminate our knowledge. We had a central training and presentation for regional public health representatives on 10th September 2009. After that, they have organized regional educations for the school counsellors. Besides, we followed up and made sure that the manual was distributed to every primary or secondary school in Slovenia.

In the second round of the evaluation, the results showed that the programme was well accepted among professionals. The overall evaluation feedback showed very high scores. One of the reviewers of the manual stated: "*The authors have prepared a systematic and practical manual, which will be an important educational and supporting tool for school counselling staff and others, who work with youths.*" Besides, the programme also got positive public response and a lot of media coverage.

3.2 Let's Talk about Depression and Suicide among Elderly

3.2.1 Background and aims

According to comparable data on mortality due to suicide in the age group above 65 years, Slovenia ranks among the highest in the world (Svetičič, Marušič & Kravanja, 2006), as we have already mentioned in the section 2.3.1. Data from the WHO database (HFA Database) shows that the suicide rate for Slovenian elderly is at least two times higher than the total average of all 27 EU member states - between 1985 and 2007 the average in Slovenia was 52/100,000 whereas in the EU the suicide rate was considerably lower (23/100,000). In Slovenia, as well as elsewhere in the world, the suicide risk increases with age. The group with the highest suicide risk consists of men over 65 years. Compared with the overall Slovenian population, suicide risk is much higher among the elderly. Suicide rate among the age group above 65 is much higher than Slovenian average - between 1971 and 2008 the suicide risk in that age group was 45 whereas the Slovenian average was as low as 29/100,000 (Grad, Kogoj & Trontelj, 2001).

Suicidal behaviour among elderly thus presents a serious public health problem in Slovenia. We decided to address the issue with a specific prevention - intervention programme, which we named *Let's Talk about Depression and Suicide among Elderly*. The field of depression was included in the programme because depression is the most important risk factor for the development of suicidal behaviour in older age (De Leo & Scocco, 2002).

Also already mentioned in the section 2.3.1, family doctors represent the most important gatekeepers for the identification of depression and suicidal behaviour in the elderly population. Based on the results of foreign studies (Simon et al., 1999; Kohn, Saxena, Levav et al., 2004, Ani, Bazargan, Hindman et al., 2008) which established that more than half of depression cases are not discovered and consequently not treated, we anticipated a similar situation in Slovenia. Therefore we decided a significant portion of the programme should focus on the education of family doctors.

Programme *Let's Talk about Depression and Suicide among Elderly* started in January 2010 and will conclude in the end of December 2011. The programme was implemented in cooperation between the Institute of Public Health and Slovenian Centre for Suicide Research. As the programme presents a novelty in Slovenia and because it was co-funded by the Municipality of Ljubljana, we wanted to perform a pilot of the programme in the central Slovenian region.

Most important aims of the programme were:

- to increase competence of family doctors of central region of Slovenia in recognition and treatment of depression and suicidal behaviour among elderly patients,
- to support pilot groups of elderly patients with depression in dealing with their illness through psychoeducation.

3.2.2 Development

The first 6 months in 2010 were devoted to the developmental phase of the programme. It required the following three steps:

- Development of a manual with practical guidelines about working with depressed and suicidal elderly patients for family doctors.
- Development of a 1-day pilot educational programme covering the content of the manual for family doctors.
- Development of psychoeducational workshops for elderly patients with depression.

Development of the manual

Our first activity was focused on developing and publishing a manual with guidelines for recognizing and treating depressed and suicidal elderly patients. The manual was designed for family doctors in primary care setting, but it can be a useful tool for other professionals who work with elderly as well.

Experts who cooperated in the preparation of the manual were: three psychologists from the Institute of Public Health and Slovenian Centre for Suicide Research, a gerontopsychiatrist who leads the Unit for gerontopsychiatry at the Psychiatric Hospital Ljubljana and a family doctor who is a professor at the Medical Faculty and also a researcher in the field of care for elderly.

The manual is divided into two parts. The first part of the manual focuses on the theoretical presentation of the field and consists of six chapters. The first chapter treats older age as a developmental phase and describes its characteristics. The next two chapters present diagnostic criteria for depression and suicidal behaviour according to DSM IV and ICD 10 and the epidemiology of depression and suicide among the elderly in Slovenia and in other states. An extensive chapter is devoted to the risk factors which we divided in four groups: biological (genetic predisposition, physical changes and disease, sleep disorders), psychological (personality characteristics, mental disorders), social (socio-economic status, social support) and others (stress factors, medicine). The first part of the manual also delineates three groups of protective factors: appropriate support resources, effective strategies to cope with stressors and involvement in the activities. The last theoretical chapter is devoted to the characteristics of depression and suicidal behaviour among the elderly. The second part of the handbook represents a practical guide for working with older patients with depression or signs of suicidal behaviour in primary care setting. The first chapter describes general approaches to working with older patients and challenges in dealing with them. In the chapter to follow there are guidelines for screening, diagnosis and treatment of depression and suicidal behaviour in the elderly. Guidelines are also given for referring patients to other specialists. The final chapter sets out proposals for preventive activities that can help older people to maintain good mental health. The manual also includes attachments with important practical value: examples of step-by-step treatment of patients with depression in the outpatient clinic, myths about depression and suicide, together with the explanation, useful contacts for elderly assistance and two screening questionnaires for identifying depression in the elderly - Geriatric Depression Scale and Patient Health Questionnaire 9.

Before publishing the manual, we asked two experts for its review: a family doctor, who is the President of Gerontological Society of Slovenia, and Professor of Medical faculty.

Development of the educational programme for family doctors

We wanted to cover the content of the manual in a one-day (8-hour) educational programme, therefore we invited the co-authors of the manual to participate in the development of the programme as well.

In the first part of the educational programme we intended to present the problem of depression and suicidal behaviour among the elderly, focusing on Slovenia. Therefore, we included in it the following topics: the prevalence of depression and suicidal behaviour, the most important risk factors for developing mental disorders and description of the characteristics of depression and suicidal behaviour among older people.

The second part of the educational programme was set on a very practical level. The guidelines for the identification of signs of depression and suicidal behaviour among the elderly and all the steps in the treatment were to be presented through concrete examples from practice and discussion. We also added descriptions on how to approach the older patients, and what the family doctor should be aware of.

The last part of the educational programme was designed in form of a workshop, in which the participants first learn about psychological treatments and options that we have in Slovenia. Then the participants through working in groups try some simple cognitive behavioural techniques that help in coping with depression and suicidal ideation, and contribute to improving mental health.

Development of psychoeducational workshops for elderly patients with depression

As the Psychiatric Hospital in Ljubljana, already performs workshops for patients with depression and their families, which have proved to be successful, we did not need to develop an entirely new model of workshops. We adapted the existing workshops to elderly population especially in terms of comprehension, so we included simple explanations and anticipated more time for questions. All of the workshop leaders were first trained to conduct the workshops.

A brief description of the workshop (Dernovšek Tavčar, 2005): The workshop consists of four meetings to be conducted once a week. Individual meeting lasts an hour and a half. At the workshop, patients and their relatives receive workbooks, which contain a summary of the programme and tasks aimed at increasing awareness of depression symptoms and how to deal with them. Workshop can be conducted by a graduate nurse, psychologist, physician or other healthcare professional, who concluded the training and is regularly supervised.

Individual parts of the workshop:

1. The first meeting is devoted to identifying factors that influenced the development of depression in an individual. The participants learn about the symptoms and signs of depression.
2. The second meeting focuses on familiarizing the participants with different types of depression treatment, including treatment with antidepressants. Much emphasis is given to the activation of the participants with the support of their relatives.

3. The third meeting is devoted to the identification of specific thought patterns in depression and to the increase in the flexibility of thinking.
4. The fourth meeting is aimed at the prevention of exacerbations and relapses of depression.

3.2.3 Implementation

The implementation phase took place in the second half of 2010 and the first half of 2011 and involved three steps:

- Performing a 1-day educational programme for family doctors in the central region of Slovenia.
- Performing a few psychoeducational workshops for elderly patients with depression.
- Dissemination of the manual to all family doctors in the central region of Slovenia.

In September 2010, in the week the World Suicide Prevention Day took place an educational programme for family doctors was conducted. Through written invitation, through mailing lists and through the publication of the invitation on relevant websites, we invited all of the family doctors from the central Slovenian region to participate in the programme. About a third of the invited, attended the educational programme. The programme was performed by five experts and in accordance with the structure described in the developmental phase. In the scope of the educational programme, a great deal of time was devoted to practical questions of the participants and to discussion. The participants received the manuals and were presented with the other parts of the project. We emphasized the possibility of the psychoeducational workshops for elderly patients and we encouraged the participants to include their patients in the workshops as well.

This was followed by the dissemination of the manuals to all family doctors in the central Slovenian region by mail. When sending the manuals, we encouraged all the family doctors to include their patients in the psychoeducational workshops.

The last part of the implementation phase included conducting the pilot psychoeducational workshops for the elderly with depression and their families, which lasted until the end of June 2011 and was carried out by two psychologists. Four groups, consisting of 15 patients and their relatives were included in this part of the programme. Each psychoeducational workshop was held for four weeks and in accordance with the structure that is described in the developmental phase. At the last meeting the participants were presented with other forms of help which they can use after concluding the workshop.

3.2.4 Evaluation

Evaluation phase took place throughout the entire programme; in particular, we focused on the evaluation of three main parts of the programme:

- Manual
- Education for family doctors,
- Psychoeducational workshops for elderly patients with depressive disorder.

We had two important criteria for the evaluation of the manual: the expert opinion of manual containing expert knowledge on depression and suicide among elderly and family doctors' and other users' opinion of manual's usefulness in their daily work. As already mentioned, the manual was given in review to the President of Gerontological Society of Slovenia and to Professor of Medical faculty. Manual received positive reviews from both experts; they recommended it for usage to their colleagues - family doctors. Manual evaluation of its applicability in the work of family doctors was obtained through an evaluation questionnaire, which had been completed by every participant at the end of the educational programme. The average score on usefulness of the manual (on 5-level scale) was 4.5. The same question about usefulness of the manual had been included also in the questionnaire which was sent to all participants 1 year after the educational programme (the questionnaire described below). We are still in the process of collecting and analysing these questionnaires, the evaluation of the manual will be concluded at the end of the year 2011.

For the evaluation of the educational programme for family doctors there were again two criteria: participants' opinion about the educational programme itself and the impact educational programme had on participants' attitudes about depression. Participants' opinions about educational programme were acquired through an evaluation questionnaire that was distributed to all participants at the end of training. The questionnaire included questions about usefulness of content of the educational programme, organization and manual's usefulness, and we asked participants for other comments as well. The average score on usefulness of content of the educational programme was 4.6, on the organisation 4.4 and on the manual 4.5. The impact of educational programme on participants' attitudes about depression we wanted to measure through comparison their attitudes before the educational programme and 1 year after it. For this purpose, all participants completed The Depression Attitude Questionnaire (DAQ) before the lectures of the educational programme started. DAQ (Dowrick et al., 2000) is a self-completion questionnaire which assesses health workers knowledge and attitude towards the causes, consequences and treatment of depression. Each question has four possible responses: strongly disagree, moderately disagree, moderately agree and strongly agree. One year after the educational programme we have again sent one questionnaire to participants. The questionnaire included DAQ, but also questions about the usefulness of the manual and the content of educational programme in their daily work. We do not have the results yet, since we are still in the process of collecting and processing questionnaires - the evaluation concludes at the end of 2011.

Psychoeducational workshops for elderly patients with depressive disorder were evaluated from participants' view and workshop leaders' view. All participants completed an evaluation questionnaire at the end of the last meeting. Through the questionnaire we asked them if the workshop was helpful in their dealing with the depression, how useful was content of the workshop and how they felt in the group. All participants responded that the workshop was of help to them, the average score of usefulness was 4.4, and of their feeling in the group 4. Since the workshops were conducted as a pilot, we also asked workshop leaders about their suitability. They agreed that the content of the workshop is suitable for wider implementation but as the elderly need more time for understanding the topics, they proposed the extension of the workshop for one meeting.

3.3 Let's Talk about Suicide and Media

3.3.1 Background and aims

There is evidence that the media plays a significant role in both suicide risk and suicide prevention. On the one hand, vulnerable individuals may be influenced to engage in imitative behaviours by reports of suicide. Systematic reviews of studies on media impact on suicide risk have consistently drawn the same conclusion: media reporting of suicide can lead to imitative suicidal behaviours (Pirkis, Blood, 2001; Stack, 2000 and 2005 ...). According to these reviews imitation is more evident when the coverage is extensive, prominent, sensationalist and/or explicitly describes the method of suicide. Repeated coverage and 'high impact' stories are being most strongly associated with imitative behaviours (Etzersdorfer, Voracek and Sonneck, 2004), especially when person described in the story and the reader or viewer are similar in some way, or when the person described in the story is a celebrity and is held in high regard by the reader or viewer (Cheng et al., 2007). Specifically vulnerable to engaging in imitative suicidal behaviours are particular subgroups in the population (e.g., young people, people suffering from depression) (Phillips, Carstensen, 1988). The study from Fu and Yip (2007) also showed that imitation of suicide after media reporting varies as a function of time, usually peaking within the first three days and levelling off by about two weeks, but sometimes lasting longer. Along with described characteristics of media reporting, which can influence the imitative suicidal behaviour we have to mention another one - overt description of suicide by a particular method may lead to increases in actual suicidal behaviour employing that method (Hawton et al., 1996).

On the other hand, responsible reporting may serve to educate the public about suicide, and may encourage those at risk of suicide to seek help. There is also some evidence regarding the potential for the media to exert a positive influence, which comes from a study which considered whether 'best practice' media reporting of suicide could lead to a reduction in completed and attempted suicide rates. The study by Etzersdorfer and colleagues (1998) showed that the introduction of media guidelines regarding reporting suicides on the Vienna subway had an important result. There was a reduction in sensationalist reporting of these suicides and, which lead to a 75% decrease in the rate of subway suicides and a 20% decrease in the overall suicide rate in Vienna. After that they repeatedly distributed the guidelines nationwide, which resulted in a great success - a trend change in national Austrian suicides. Specially regions with strong media collaboration were more prone to this positive impact in and it is important that the impact was largely maintained over time.

Even though there was no study on media reporting and its impact on suicide conducted in Slovenia, above mentioned studies gave us enough evidence about how media reporting of suicide can lead to imitative behaviours, resulting in statistically significant increases in completed and attempted suicide rates, and on the other hand that responsible reporting can have very positive impact and serve as suicide prevention. And since suicide is such great problem in Slovenia and since noticing the reporting on suicide in Slovene media was marked with sensationalism, with no guidelines on responsible reporting on suicide to rely on, we decided develop a programme *Let's Talk about Suicide and Media.*

Most important aim of the programme was:

- To increase awareness of journalists and other media representatives about responsible reporting about suicide and suicidal behaviour in media.

Programme *Let's Talk about Suicide and Media* started in January 2009 and will conclude in the end of December 2012. The programme was implemented in cooperation between the Institute of Public Health and Slovenian Centre for Suicide Research.

3.3.2 Development

The first year of the project was devoted to the development of the programme and guidelines. It consisted from the following steps:

- Translation and adaptation of WHO/IASP guidelines.
- Discussion on the content of guidelines with an expert group of journalists (focus group format).
- Preparation and publication of the final version of guidelines.
- Development of the workshop for journalists and editors.

International Association of Suicide Prevention (IASP) and WHO have published the media guidelines on responsible media reporting in the year 2008. The guidelines were first published in English, but in the following years they have already been translated in several other languages and adapted to different cultures. As IASP members we have gotten the approval from WHO to translate and adapt the guidelines to Slovene language. The initial step of the *Let's Talk about Suicide and Media* project was therefore the translation of the WHO/IASP guidelines which was done in a consortium of a journalist involved in mental health topics and three psychologists working in the field of suicidology (from the Institute of Public Health and Slovenian Centre for Suicide Research). The outcome was a first draft of the Slovene guidelines on responsible media reporting on suicide.

Afterwards, we wanted to evaluate the draft with our target group (journalists, editors). Therefore, we invited journalists from all major media houses in Slovenia to read the draft and to participate in a focus group. A group of twelve journalists and editors discussed the guidelines content and format with us. The data collected were qualitative responses and opinions about our draft guidelines. The main suggestions on the content from the participants of the focus group were to include some concrete examples for specific guidelines (e.g. what is an appropriate and inappropriate title of the article) and vignettes about how to write an optimal article covering suicide event.

In line with the results, the cultural adaptation of the guidelines was prepared and the final version of the guidelines was published. Besides incorporating the journalists' suggestions (concrete examples and vignettes) we also included other extra chapters in the guidelines:

- Contacts of professionals in field of suicidology.
- Contacts of professional help for people in need (according to guidelines these should be essentially included in any reporting about suicide).
- Most important myths about suicidal behaviour and their explanations.
- Guidelines on how to respond to a call of a suicidal person in a life-broadcasting radio or TV show.

Final stage of the development of the programme was preparation of the workshops for journalist and editors. The length of the workshop was 2 hours and included presentation of all important guidelines with concrete examples from Slovene media and questions for discussion.

3.3.3 Implementation

The implementation began in the September 2010 and is still on going. The parts of the implementation are:

- Dissemination of the manual to all registered journalists in Slovenia.
- Presentations and informative workshops on the content of guidelines for journalists and interested media houses in all the regions of Slovenia.

The beginning of the dissemination of the guidelines was marked with a big national opening ceremony on the World Suicide Prevention Day in 2010, where published guidelines were first time presented to the public. Afterwards we disseminated the guidelines to interested journalists and editors in Slovenia, with the help of Slovene Journalists' Association. Not only that, the guidelines are also available free of change online (webpage of Institute of Public Health).

The presentations and informative workshops on the content of guidelines for journalists and interested media houses were conducted in all nine regions of Slovenia with the help of regional public health representatives. All local and regional journalists from different types of media were invited to participate in the workshops free of charge. Participants represented all main media houses of Slovenia and were from newspapers, online media, radio and television. Among them, there were also a few editors. They all received a paper version of guidelines.

3.3.4 Evaluation

The evaluation of the programme consists of:

- pre-post questionnaire on attitudes toward suicide and reporting on suicide
- pre-post qualitative and quantitative analysis of media reporting on suicide.

In the first phase, editors and journalists, who participated at the educational workshops, took part. Before the workshop they filled in a paper version of two questionnaires: Attitudes Toward Suicide Questionnaire (ATTS, Renberg & Jacobsson, 2003) and a questionnaire on reporting about suicide (the questionnaire was developed by the editors of the guidelines). The post-evaluation will be done in the beginning of year 2012 by sending the same questionnaires to journalists who participated in the workshops.

In the second evaluation phase, we will use qualitative and quantitative analysis of the contents of the reporting of suicide in selected media (particularly newspapers and online media). The number of suicide reports after the education period will be followed up and the content of the report will be analysed. This evaluation will enable us to compare the effect of the implemented guidelines and workshops on the reporting of Slovene media on the subject of suicide. These second evaluation will take place in the second half of the year 2012.

4. Conclusion - making progress in suicide prevention activities in Slovenia

In the last two decades, Slovenia has acknowledged the high prevalence and problem of suicide. The taboo has loosened up a little bit and the topic becomes easier to talk about. Many preventive activities and initiatives arouse, aimed at reducing suicide, raising awareness and aimed at different professionals.

Let's Talk about Suicide programme was one of the initiatives. What is very important about this programme is that it has used the train the trainer approach, by which a broad public was affected. People trained by the facilitators have used this knowledge in their direct work with high risk groups. Besides, they were encouraged to further educate their colleagues and were also the resource of knowledge for them. It was also important that the educational meetings created the opportunity to create networks of people and encourage the exchange of experiences, knowledge and ideas not only from the suicidologists, but also among gatekeepers themselves.

Programmes *Let's Talk about Suicide among Youth and Let's Talk about Depression and Suicide among Elderly* directly addressed the feelings of competence and self-confidence in dealing with suicidal persons. What seems to be a very useful tool are the manuals, which can help the gatekeepers to refresh their knowledge. All of them were accepted in a very good manner and are also widely used by different lay and professionals all over Slovenia.

We can say from the first impressions from conducting the programme *Let's Talk about Suicide and Media* that we still need to target journalists in specific fields. It seems that so far the chronicle-section journalists were most eager to join the educational workshop, but not many journalists from sports- or culture-sections participated. This clearly is a lack, as it was seen from the case studies that in cases of suicide of specific sports celebrities, journalists from the sports-sections prepare the articles and they lack the understanding of responsible reporting. So, in this manner, the dissemination of the guidelines needs to be broader. Nonetheless, we have also encountered changes of media reporting, in particular including information of the helplines and other contacts of help for the people in need in numerous articles on the topic of suicide (but only the evaluation phase will give us the more exact results).

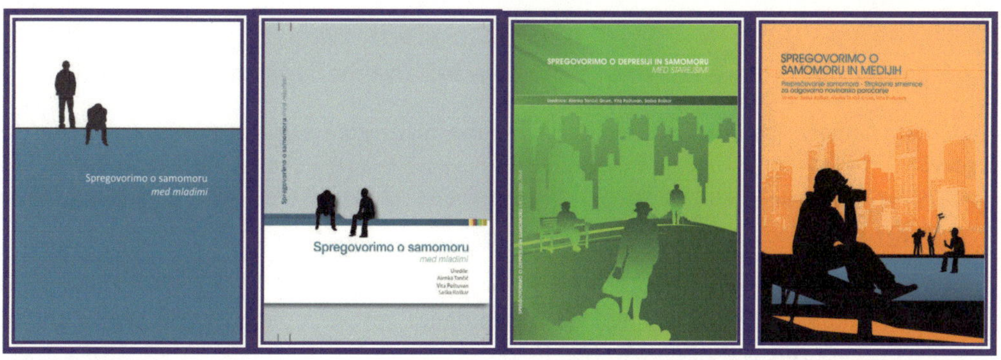

Fig. 4. Front pages of the manuals (first two: Let's Talk about Suicide among Youth, third: Let's Talk about Depression and Suicide among Elderly and last: Let's Talk about Suicide and Media).

The limitations of the project are at the first in the limited funding. So far, we were not able to provide the sustainability of the educations or to repeat them. We would wish that the topics of suicidal behaviour would become a part of the system (e.g. education of GPs, nurses ...), which is at this moment done only in part. What is more, we have encountered a problem of low response rate in some gatekeepers and in some regions of training. Probably the reason for this is on the one hand still in the lack of awareness about the importance of these topics or on the other hand the lack of time (e.g. for GPs).

Nonetheless, in the last decade (1997 – 2010) we noticed a 14% decline in the overall suicide rate, 11.4% decline for men and 19% decline for women (see figure 5). The decline was noticed in all age groups. This probably means that the initiatives that were launched in Slovenia were designed in such a manner that they targeted the before mentioned challenges of suicidality in Slovenia and furthermore followed the guidelines on successful suicide prevention strategies (as outlined by Mann et all, 2005; van der Feltz et al., 2011).

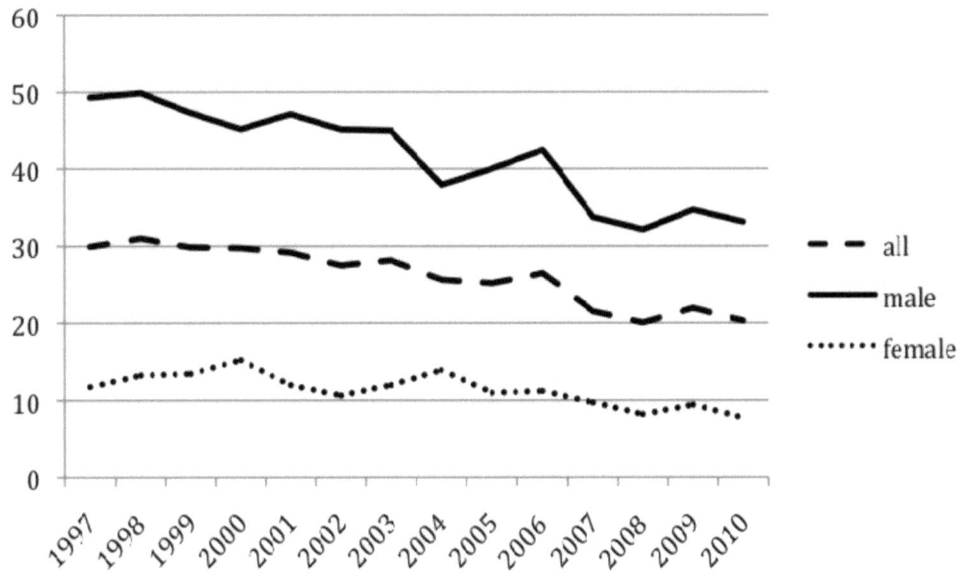

Fig. 5. Suicide rate in Slovenia in the years 1997 – 2007 (National Mortality Database, IVZ).

And that, namely the suicide prevention, is the main goal our programs are trying to achieve.

5. References

Ani C, Bazargan M, Hindman D, Bell D, Farooq MA, Akhanjee L et al. (2008). Depression symptomatology and diagnosis: discordance between patients and physicians in primary care settings. *BMC Fam Pract*; 9:1.

Cheng ATA, Hawton K, Chen THH, Yen AMF, Chang J-C, Chong M-Y, et al. (2007). The influence of media reporting of a celebrity suicide on suicidal behaviour in patients with a history of depressive disorder. *Journal of Affective Disorders*, 103, pp. 69-75.

De Leo D, Scocco P. Treatment and Prevention of Suicidal Behaviour in the Elderly. (2002). In: Hawton K. in van Heeringen K, editors. *The International Handbook of Suicide and attempted suicide.* West Sussex: Willey, pp. 553-570.

Dernovšek MZ, Tavčar R. (2005). *Prepoznajmo in premagajmo depresijo: priročnik za osebe z depresijo in njihove svojce.* Ljubljana: IVZ RS.

Dowrick, C., Gask, L., Perry, R., Dixon, C. and Usherwood T. (2000). Do general practitioners' attitudes towards depression predict their clinical behaviour? *Psychological Medicine,* 30, pp. 413-419.

Etzersdorfer E, Sonneck G. (1998). Preventing suicide by influencing massmedia reporting: The Viennese experience 1980-1996. *Archives of Suicide Research;*4(1), pp. 64-74.

Etzersdorfer E, Voracek M, Sonneck G. (2004). A dose-response relationship between imitational suicides and newspaper distribution. *Archives of Suicide Research,* 8(2), pp. 137-145.

Fu KW, Yip PSF. (2007). Long-term impact of celebrity suicide on suicidal ideation: Results from a population-based study. *Journal of Epidemiology and Community Health,* 61(6), pp. 540-546.

Grad TO, Kogoj A, Trontelj J. (2001). Elderly suicide in Slovenia. In: de Leo D, editor. *Suicide and euthanasia in older adults: A transcultural journey.* Seattle: Hogrefe & Huber Publishers, pp. 77 - 88.

HFA Database. 5th July 2010. Available from: http://www.euro.who.int

Hawton K, Simkin S, Deeks J, O'Connor S, Keen A, Altman DG, et al. (1996). Effects of a drug overdose in a television drama on presentations to hospital for self poisoning: Time series and questionnaire study. *British Medical Journal;* 318(7189), pp. 972-977.

Hegerl, U. and Schafer, R. (2007). From the Nuremberg Alliance Against Depression to a European network (EAAD) - Extending community-based awareness-campaigns on national and European level. *Psychiatrische Praxis,* 34, pp. S261-5.

Kodaka, M., Poštuvan, V., Inagaki, M., Yamada, M. (2010). *A Systematic Review of Instruments measuring attitudes toward suicide.* International Journal of Social Psychiatry, ePub..

Kohn R, Saxena S, Levav I,3 & Saraceno B. (2004). The treatment gap in mental health care. *Bulletin of the World Health Organization,* 82, pp. 858-66.

Mann JJ, et al. (2005). Suicide Prevention Strategies. *Journal of the American Medical Association,* 294 (16), pp. 2064-74.

Marušič A. (1999). Suicide in Slovenia: lesson for cross-cultural psychiatry. *International Review of Psychiatry,* 11, pp. 212-218.

Marušič A. (1998). Suicide mortality in Slovenia: Regional variation. *Crisis,* 19, pp. 159-167.

Marušič, A. (2008). Seven steps to Integrating Suicidology. *Crisis,* 29 (3), pp. 115-117.

Milton, J., Ferguson, B. & Mills, T. (1999). Risk assesment and suicide prevention in primary care. *Crisis,* 20(4), pp.171–177.

Phillips DP, Carstensen LL. (1988). The effect of suicide stories on various demographic groups, 1968-1985. *Suicide and Life Threatening Behavior;*18(1), pp. 100-114.

Pirkis J, Blood RW. (2001). Suicide and the media: (1) Reportage in nonfictional media. *Crisis,* 22(4), pp. 146-154.

Rickwood, D. J., Deane, F. P., & Wilson, C. J. (2007). When and how do young people seek professional help for mental health problems? *Med J Aust,* 187, pp. 35-39.

Renberg, E.S. & Jacobsson, L. (2003) Development of a questionnaire on attitudes towards suicide (ATTS) and its application in a Swedish population. *Suicide & Life-Threatening Behavior*, 33, 52–64.

Rodi PM, Roskar S, Marusic A. (2010) Suicide Victims Last Contact With the Primary Care Physician: Report From Slovenia, *Int J Soc Psychiatry* 56, 280.

Roskar S, Podlesek A, Zorko M, Tavcar R, Dernovsek MZ, Groleger U, Mirjanic M, Konec N, Janet E, Marusic A. (2010). Effects of training program on recognition and management of depression and suicide risk evaluation for Slovenian primary-care physicians: follow-up study. *Croat Med J.*, 51 (3), pp. 237-42.

Simon GE, Goldber D, Tiemens BG, Ustun TB. (1999). Outcomes of recognized and unrecognized depression in primary in an international primary care study. *Gen Hosp Psych*, 21, pp. 97-105.

Stack S. (2000). Media impacts on suicide: A quantitative review of 293 findings. *Social Science Quarterly*, ;81(4), pp. 957-972.

Stack S. (2005). Suicide in the media: a quantitative review of studies based on non-fictional stories. *Suicide and Life Threatening Behavior*, 35(2), pp. 121-33.

Svetičič J, Marušič A, Kravanja M. (2006). Slovenija z najvišjim količnikom samomorov med starejšimi na svetu. *Zbornik strokovnih prispevkov srečanja: Izobraževalni program iz javnega zdravja IV: socialne determinante zdravja "Zdravo staranje, iluzija ali realnost?"*. Maribor: ZZV Maribor in IVZ RS,.

Tančič, A. (2009). Tako mlad pa že samomorilen. In *Spregovorimo o samomoru med mladimi.* Ljubljana: IVZ.

Van der Feltz-Cornelis, C. M., Sarchiapone, M., Postuvan, V., Volker, D., Roskar, S., Tancic Grum, A., Carli, V., McDaid, D., O'Connor, R., Maxwell, M., Ibelshäuser, A., Van Audenhove, C., Scheerder, G., Sisask, M., Gusmão, R., & Hegerl, U. (2011). Best practice elements of multilevel suicide prevention strategies: A review of systematic reviews. *The Journal of Crisis Intervention and Suicide.*

WHO. (2002). *The World Health Report 2003. Shaping the Future.*

WHO. (2003). *Suicide prevention in Europe. The WHO European monitoring survey on national suicide prevention programmes and strategies.*

WHO (2011b). SUPRE Prevention of suicidal behaviours: a task for all. 29th September 2011. Available on:
http://www.who.int/mental_health/prevention/suicide/information/en/index.html

18

Factors Contributing to Enrollment in Treatment Programs for Adults

Joanne M. Cannavo[1] and Thomas H. Nochajski[2]
[1]Social Work & Sociology Department, Daemen College;
[2]School of Social Work, University at Buffalo,
USA

1. Introduction

The concept of enrollment can mean different things to different groups. For purposes of the current chapter, it specifically refers to treatment entry only. It does not address treatment retention or completion. In general, treatment tends to refer to formal treatment programs. However, we will also include findings from research on enrollment into drug courts. While enrollment in mental health treatment or mental health courts will be discussed, the extent is limited by the lack of extensive literature on mental health treatment entry. Thus, the major focus of the current chapter will be on enrollment into substance abuse treatment. Furthermore, the chapter focuses on adult entry into treatment; adolescent treatment entry is not discussed.

2. Factors related to enrolling in substance abuse treatment

Overview

While there has been some research into factors that influence whether an individual will enroll into substance abuse treatment programs, there is a need to consider the research in an aggregate form to better understand how we might better serve individuals who might benefit from formal treatment but for various reasons never seek it out. In terms of the current chapter, this is not a meta-analysis, nor is it a critical review; rather, it is a summary of what we know influences treatment entry. As such, we first discuss reasons why individuals may not seek treatment for substance use problems. We then consider factors associated with treatment entry. As we present this information, we will also consider various groups, where factors may differ, including individuals mandated to treatment, injection drug users, and drug court participants. Finally, we propose a model for substance abuse treatment entry.

3. Reasons for not seeking treatment

In general, the main reason that individuals do not seek treatment is that they see no need for it. Within the general population, Schmidt and Weisner (1999) found that many individuals who were identified as problem drinkers did not consider themselves as such. Specifically, Schmidt and Weisner (1999) found that 11.3% of the individuals in a general population sample met objective problem drinking criteria, whereas only 5.4% of respondents labeled themselves as a problem drinker or alcoholic. Furthermore, Hedden and Gfroerer (2011) point out that only 3.3% of individuals in need of treatment for an alcohol use disorder who did not receive treatment actually perceived a need for treatment. While the percentage increases for drug use disorders to 8.3% and for drug and alcohol disorders combined to 12.5%, the numbers are still very low. Another study that considered illicit stimulant users in rural areas of the United States found that those who had a perceived need for substance abuse treatment were positively associated with enrolling in drug treatment (Carlson et al., 2010). Furthermore, consistent with other research examining one's perception or personal state of readiness, a form of perceived need, opiate-using IDUs recruited from the street who were in the contemplation or determination stage of change were also associated with enrollment in the drug treatment program (Corsi et al., 2007).

Given the large number of individuals who meet criteria for a substance use disorder but see no need for treatment, the next aspect to consider is the reason that might be the case, and what the ramifications of this lack of perceived need are. The one group that has had some research with respect to why the perception of a need for treatment is lacking is the DWI area. A primary problem is that a large portion of DUI offenders do not want to change their substance use behavior, especially if the intended outcome is abstinence. As a result, they are disinclined to admit they have problems (Lapham, C'de Baca, McMillan, & Hunt, 2004; Lapham, C'de Baca, Chang, Hunt, &Berger; 2002; Lincourt, Kuettel, & Bombardier, 2002; Nochajski & Wieczorek, 1998; Nochajski &Stasiewicz, 2001; Vingilis, 1983). Additionally, DUI offenders tend to be angry about the arrest and what has occurred to them; they may be even angrier if referred for an evaluation and fearful of the consequences for failing to comply with the treatment provider's recommendations (Cavaiola & Wuth, 2002; Wieczorek, Callahan, & Morales, 1997). Another potential reason for use of discretion in following treatment referrals or seeking treatment is that many of these individuals do not meet criteria for dependence as determined by a structured interview (Lapham et al., 2001; Stasiewicz & Nochajski, 2003; Stasiewicz, Nochajski, & Homish, 2007). Thus, when mandated for an evaluation and then told to go for treatment, these individuals may remain unconvinced about the necessity of formal treatment.

Stigma is also a major reason that individuals may not seek treatment (Corrigan, 2004; Corrigan, Kuwabara, & O'Shaughnessy, 2009; Corrigan, Larson, & Rusch, 2009; Corrigan & Penn, 1999; Corrigan & Wassel, 2008; Gibbs et al., 2011; McFarling, D'Angelo, & Drain, 2011). There has been a large amount of research on the effects of stigma and a thorough review of this topic is beyond the scope of the current chapter. However, because of the relationship with treatment entry, it is prudent to point out that Corrigan and his colleagues have done extensive work with the stigma of mental health problems showing how it may influence the decision to seek out formal treatment. They suggest that because of the stigma associated with mental illness, individuals may feel shame and guilt, and low self-esteem and self-efficacy towards the ability to change their life. The low self-efficacy can then lead to beliefs that nothing will help them, resulting in a belief that formal treatment will not work; thus, it raises the reasoning of why one would seek out help. Additionally, Gibbs et al. (2011) and McFarling et al. (2011) consider stigma associated with mental health and substance abuse in the military, pointing out that many in need of help never seek it out because of the stigma that the military culture has imposed on these problems.

Another reason for not seeking treatment is a lack of resources, or treatment availability. Appel et al.'s (2007) study with injection drug users (IDU) validated the presence of individual client factors that serve as barriers to enrollment, such as readiness to begin treatment or denial of having a substance problem; however, they also found that treatment accessibility is essential for all addiction treatment clients, suggesting that a larger concentration on accessibility may be more economical and efficient than on individualized treatment motivation interventions. The findings of Appel et al. on treatment accessibility may begin to explain realistic systematic constraints in society instead of solely focusing on individualized limitations, traits or factors of substance abusers seeking treatment. Ravarino et al. (2008) notes that dwindling state and federal budgets have contributed to deficiencies in funds allotted for public health for substance abuse and mental health treatment programs to assist towards recovery from substance abuse. Such decreases in funds have resulted in waiting lists for treatment programs that are subsidized by the government, and when services are finally made available to persons on the lists, many do not appear to receive such services. Limitations in funding, management information systems, and staffing have been the main perceived barriers to the linkage of services (Wenzel, Longshore, Turner, & Ridgely, 2001).

Possibly related to the issue of a lack of resources for treatment is transportation (Evans, Li, & Hser, 2008). This is especially true for rural areas, where the distance to and from the treatment agency may be such that public transportation is unreliable or unavailable. Additionally, even when public transportation is available, the individual may not have sufficient income to allow for use of the transportation system. Furthermore, when the individual has multiple problems, or a dual diagnosis (substance use and mental health), the treatment agencies may be housed in different places, adding further to the transportation issue. As with resources for treatment services, transportation is another area that needs consideration.

Type of insurance or whether the individual has insurance coverage is also a factor when looking at treatment enrollment (Lundgren, Amaro, & Ben-Ami, 2005; Schmidt &Weisner, 2005). The relationship between drug court completion and structural-level barriers is particularly strong, ranging from barriers such as 'the system' and insurance requirements (Wolf & Colyer, 2001). When individuals have private insurance or are covered by Medicaid, they are more likely to enter treatment then those covered by Medicare. However, it is also known that dropout from treatment is associated with insurance coverage. Individuals will generally maintain treatment for as long as the insurance they have pays for it. Once the insurance provider will no longer cover treatment, the odds of dropping out increase significantly. The number of sessions covered by private insurance and what Medicaid and Medicare will cover are areas to consider when evaluating how to get more people in need to enroll in treatment.

Summary. In summary, individuals with substance use or mental health problems elect not to seek treatment for a variety of reasons. Some of these, such as lack of availability, transportation, and insurance, are systemic in nature. Having influence in these areas means working within systems to create sufficient resources for individuals in need of treatment. In contrast, perceived need for treatment and stigma can be construed as individually based, although some systemic issues may also play a role in how these factors influence treatment seeking. Nonetheless, individual focused interventions can be utilized to help improve rates for treatment entry among those in need of treatment. With respect to stigma, In Our Own Voice and Cognitive Behavioral Therapy have been used to decrease the impact of stigma (Corrigan, Rafacz, Hautamaki et al., 2010; Corrigan & Wassel, 2008). For the perceived need for treatment, Motivational Interviewing (Miller & Rollnick, 2002) has shown some promise in helping individuals recognize the severity of their problems and the need for treatment (Wain, Wilbourne, Harris et al., 2011).

4. Factors associated with treatment entry

The information provided in the previous section focused on possible barriers or reasons why individuals may not seek treatment. This section now considers factors that have shown either a positive or negative relationship with treatment entry.

Demographics. A number of characteristics have been associated with entry into substance abuse treatment. These include demographic characteristics. Gender is one element that seems to influence treatment entry. Jakobson, Hensing, and Spak (2008) compared treatment entry factors for men and women. Their findings indicated that women showed greater stigma over substance use problems than men, which hindered their entrance into formal treatment. Additionally, men entered treatment because they had a belief they could change and were looking to the future. In contrast, women entered treatment because of pressure from someone close and a need to talk to someone about their problems. Tuchman (2010) also indicates that stigma of a substance use disorder appears to be greater for women than men. She also goes on to suggest that women are more likely to face greater barriers to treatment access than men, pointing out the differences in biological vulnerabilities as a potential issue for women. Hernandez-Avila, Rounsaville and Kranzler (2004) considered differences in men and women with regard to age of substance use onset and time to treatment entry. Their findings show that women showed less time between onset of substance use and entry into treatment. Likewise, women and men did not differ in severity of substance use problems; however, women reported more severe psychiatric, medical, and employment complications. In addition, Greenfield et al. (2007) noted that the collective evidence related to substance disorders supports that women with substance use disorders have less of a likelihood, across the lifespan, to enroll in treatment, compared to males with substance use disorders. The above information suggests that gender can influence the types of problems experienced, the severity of those problems, as well as self-efficacy and readiness to change.

Age may also influence treatment entry. Shin, Lundgren, and Chassler (2007) considered admissions to all state-licensed drug treatment programs, looking at differences between younger (18-25) and older injection drug users (IDUs). Results showed that the younger IDUs were more likely to use only detoxification and not enter additional treatment. Additionally, they point out that the younger individuals were less likely to use methadone maintenance and more likely to use residential treatment services than the older group of IDUs. These findings might suggest that the younger individuals have different sets of perceived needs and that clinicians may need to consider age as a critical factor when determining treatment.

Ethnicity, race and culture may also influence entry into treatment. Cannavo and Nochajski (2011) found that African Americans were more likely to enroll in a Family Treatment Court than Caucasians. With regard to AIDS care, findings suggest that African Americans and Latinos were more likely to be highly engaged in services than were Caucasians (Bastaa, Shachamb, and Reecec, 2008). Culture may play a significant role in subsequent treatment seeking behavior. Depending on cultural beliefs with respect to mental illness and substance abuse, individuals may be more or less likely to seek out treatment. While there has been some work on treatment dropout and treatment outcomes, studies are limited for treatment entry. More work in this area could help define interventions for specific subgroups to get people in need to treatment services.

It is also interesting to note that employment at the time of drug court enrollment was found to be predictive of successful completion of the drug court treatment program (Roll, Prendergast, Richardson, Burdon, & Ramirez, 2005); this court was mostly methamphetamine abusers. Logistic regression analysis by Cannavo (2008) for a study of a Family Treatment Court found that unemployment showed a marginal trend for significance to identify those individuals who may be more likely to enroll in the FTC program.

Substance Abuse Behaviors. Various substance use behaviors were also predictors of enrollment. Cannavo & Nochajski (2011) found that substance users who shared needles were less likely to enroll in an FTC; however, as the number of drugs used in the last six months increased, the likelihood of enrolling in the FTC also increased. Prior treatment for substance abuse also led to a greater likelihood of enrolling in an FTC. In addition, Corsi et al. (2007) found that having fewer problems with alcohol yet more problems with opiate drugs were associated with enrolling in drug treatment among IDUs recruited from the street. In a study of illicit stimulant users in rural United States, those who had higher Addiction Severity Index (ASI) legal problem composite scores were positively associated with enrollment into treatment; having had a history of experiencing substance abuse treatment as well as tranquilizer use were also positively associated with enrolling into treatment. Those who did not use crack cocaine or marijuana on a daily basis were less likely to enter treatment (Carlson et al., 2010).

Also among the limited enrollment literature related to substance abuse enrollment, Booth et al. (2004, 1996) studied enrollment in the form of treatment entry and retention on the IDU population. Booth et al. (2004) examined factors associated with methadone maintenance retention, which the authors defined as remaining in treatment for a minimum of 90 days, and the injection drug users (IDUs) was again examined. A sum of 577 IDUs were randomly assigned to either a risk reduction intervention, focusing on safer injection and sex behaviors, or motivational interviewing, addressing more sweeping lifestyle changes including drug treatment. All persons who wanted treatment were given transportation, expedited intake process and a waiver of the intake fee. In addition, 50% were randomly assigned a voucher for ninety days of treatment free of cost. In total, 33% entered treatment and 60% of those who entered treatment remained for at least ninety days. Factors associated with retention that are relevant to enrollment included higher methadone dose, treatment at no cost, as well as greater contacts with the clinic. Interestingly, although desire for treatment, or motivation, was associated in univariate analyses with greater retention, no differences were noted between motivational interviewing and risk reduction interventions (Booth et al., 2004). In addition, in an earlier study, Booth et al. (1996) studied the same population. Factors positively correlated with treatment entry included having had the experience of prior treatment, outreach intervention by community workers, not injecting cocaine, and injecting opiates. Sites where the enhanced intervention included an active referral achieved significantly higher treatment entry rates than sites where the enhanced intervention did not include an active referral. The addition of staff assistance to facilitate clients' entry into treatment and the involvement of community outreach workers were both noted in achieving treatment entry.

Consistent with such findings related to enrollment and community outreach, Coviello et al. (2006) studied outreach case management for post-discharged methadone patients. Heroin dependence is a chronic relapsing disease often requiring multiple treatment experiences; however, a minimal number of methadone programs follow-up with clients who have been discharged. At 6 months following the start of intervention, 29% of the outreach case management clients had successfully re-enrolled in drug treatment compared to 8% of former participants who had received the standard referral for services. A logistic regression analysis showed that outreach case management clients were almost six times more likely than standard referral clients to re-engage in methadone maintenance treatment. In addition, outreach case management clients had fewer opiate and cocaine positive toxicologies at the 6-month follow-up compared to standard referral participants. The findings demonstrate the significance in engaging former clients in treatment and actively supporting them towards treatment re-entry (Coviello et al., 2006). In addition, support for professional outreach was also found in a study of 491 opiate-using IDUs recruited from the street, where more outreach contacts increased the likelihood of treatment entry (Corsi et al., 2007). There has been much support for outreach case management, as it is a straightforward approach to reduce the number of out-of-treatment drug users. The previous data reinforce the need for active referral processes, good follow-up with referrals, and available resources to allow for timely treatment entry. The issue seems to be one of increasing the load on an individual who may already be at capacity. Asking them to perform another task, or wait for available spots in treatment programs, may push them towards avoiding treatment. These findings also underscore the limited enrollment opportunities due to the often compromised availability of treatment funding (Coviello et al., 2006)

Alcohol Use. In terms of potential predictors of help-seeking for alcohol problems, studies have found that entering treatment is related to various demographic characteristics (Kaskutas, Weisner, & Caetano, 1997; Weisner, Matzger, Tam, & Schmidt, 2002), environmental contexts (Tucker, Vuchinich, & Pukish, 1995), perceived barriers to treatment (Cunningham et al., 1993), and history of prior treatment (Freyer et al., 2007; Weisner & Matzger, 2002; Wieczorek & Nochajski, 2005). Although greater problem severity predicts treatment entry (Bannenberg, Raat, & Plomp, 1992; Freyer et al., 2007; Hingson, Mangione, Meyers, & Scotch, 1982; Weisner & Matzger, 2002; Weisner et al., 2002; Wieczorek & Nochajski, 2005), help-seeking is less influenced by amount of alcohol consumed, and more by the degree to which drinking contributes to adverse health, relationship, and work-related consequences (Beckman & Amaro, 1986; Hingson et al., 1982; Simpson & Tucker, 2002; Tucker & Gladsjo, 1993; Tucker & King, 1999). In one study, individuals who had 3 or more lifetime drinking-related consequences were 4.5 times more likely to seek help during an 8-year follow-up than those who had less than three drinking-related consequences (Kaskutas et al., 1997). In a study looking at treatment engagement and treatment readiness or motivation, Knight, Hiller, Broome, and Simpson (2000) found that the best predictor of engagement and outcomes was the individual's readiness or motivation for treatment. When comparing individuals entering treatment with individuals in the general population, Storbjork and Room (2008) found that previous treatment, unemployment, age, problem severity, and consumption were related to treatment entry. Finally, in a study involving DUI offenders, Wells-Parker, Dill, Williams and Stoduto (2006) found that depression was related to a willingness to seek treatment.

Therapeutic Courts. A study by Cannavo and Nochajski (2011) on enrollment in a Family Treatment Court found that African Americans were marginally more likely than all others to enroll in the FTC. In addition, if the individuals received more than $3000 in government assistance over the previous year, they were 2.4 times more likely to refuse to enroll in the FTC. Prior treatment for substance use showed a marginal trend, indicating that individuals who had prior treatment for substance use were over twice as likely to enroll than those who did not have prior treatment for substance use. There was a significant effect for the total number of drugs used in the 6 months prior to the FTC assessment, reflecting that for every unit increase in the number of drugs, there was a 49% increase in the likelihood that the individual would enroll in the FTC. There was also a significant effect for sharing needles, indicating that those who shared needles were approximately 76% less likely to enroll in the FTC than those who did not share needles. Finally, the motivation to change substance use behavior showed a marginal trend reflecting an increase in the likelihood of enrollment of approximately 5% for every unit increase in motivation to change. Regarding aspects of parenting factors, for every unit increase in the number of activities parents engaged in with their children, there was a 21% increase in the likelihood they would enroll in the FTC. Of specific interest, in terms of the activities, were reading and doing chores. Parents who engaged in reading activities with their children, were over 3 times more likely to enroll in the FTC than parents who did not engage in this activity with their children. Those parents who engaged in chores with their children were almost 3 times more likely than parents who did not do so to enroll in the FTC. In regards to recognizing the impact of substance use on parenting, relative to the individuals who did not recognize that drug and alcohol use had an impact on their parenting, those who did recognize this were over twice as likely to enroll in the FTC. While some of the variables noted here play a role in the decision to enroll in the FTC, there are other factors that also contribute to the decision-making process that were not included in the study which suggest various other reasons to enroll that exist and supports the needs for further study in this area (Cannavo & Nochajski, 2011).

5. Model for treatment entry

The information presented thus far suggests that treatment entry may be a complex issue, with numerous elements to consider if we wish to increase treatment experience for those who need it. However, from a standpoint of actual development of intervention strategies to help increase treatment experience, it would suggest that we need to consider a range of things. In Figure 1, we propose a model of treatment entry that suggests the best point for interventions might be readiness for change. Let's consider the model in that context. Stigma would be represented as psychological distress in the current model. For substance use, we include the type of substance, type of use, severity of the problems, frequency of use, and expectancies related to the primary substances of use. Personal history would include any childhood or adult victimization, interpersonal relationships, peer-related issues, family-related issues, school-related issues, and work-related issues. For self-efficacy, we are focused on the confidence the individual has that they will be able to remain abstinent, or at a minimum reduce the risky use of substances to a less harmful consumption pattern. Within the mandates we are including only criminal justice and work-related referrals. Family referrals would fall under substance use problem severity.

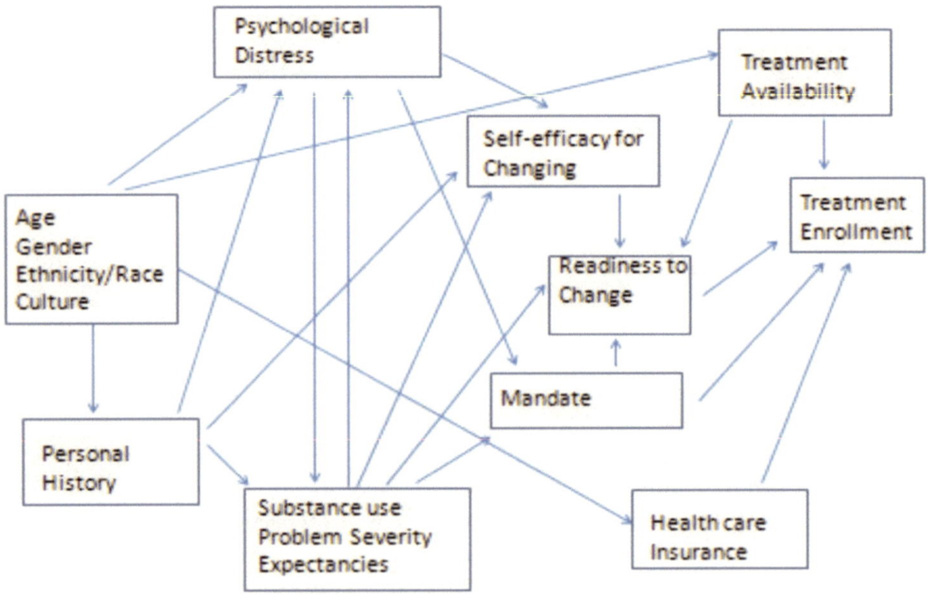

Fig. 1. Model for treatment enrollment in substance abuse treatment agencies.

With respect to readiness to change, there are two forms, readiness to change risky behavior, and readiness to enter treatment. While the readiness to enter treatment may reflect a readiness to change, that may not always be the case; as such, we have chosen to focus on treatment readiness. However, we use the Transtheoretical Model of Change for the purposes of this chapter, even though progression and tasks might differ between the two forms of readiness. The Transtheoretical Model of Change views motivation or readiness to change behavior as a multidimensional series of tasks or stages that are part of intentional behavior change processes (DiClemente, 2003; Prochaska & DiClemente, 1984). While the literature is mixed on the idea of whether intentional behavior change follows discrete stages or is more continuous in nature, the stage approach provides a good mechanism for understanding the underlying mechanisms for change that are needed to be in play as the person moves towards recovery or a better quality of life. The model proposes five stages that move from problem non-recognition to problem resolved and behavior change attained and stable. The first stage is that of precontemplation. This stage can be construed in two ways. One is when the individual does not see a need for changing their behaviors because they may not perceive sufficient evidence to suggest that change is necessary. A second group may know they have problems but elect not to change their behaviors for various reasons. Within the context of information we have presented thus far, stigma might result in the latter, where individuals recognize they have a problem but see no way to change their behavior. Likewise, individuals may recognize they have problems but not have the resources for formal treatment entry. As such, we need to consider these elements as we look at readiness to change.

The second stage is that of contemplation. In this stage, the individuals have recognized their vulnerability but are not yet completely swayed that they need treatment or that treatment will be effective in reducing their problems. Self-efficacy may enter into this decision process, as a lack of belief in the ability to successfully change behavior could result in a decision not to enter treatment and a move back to precontemplation status. Another way that self-efficacy may enter into the decision is when it is actually very high, where the individual may believe that 'I can quit anytime I want to,' which would lead to non-entry into treatment. However, Davey-Rothwell, Frydl, and Latkin (2009) showed that individuals who engaged in attempts at trying to change their behavior were more likely to engage in treatment. The authors suggested that it may have been due to the social networks they formed when attempting to quit, pointing out that research suggests that if the social network contains more individuals who are in treatment or attending AA or NA, the individual is more likely to engage in treatment. What this means is that the issue of self-efficacy is complex and needs to be understood within the context of other elements in the model.

The next stage in the process is preparation. If the individual moves towards making the behavioral change, they next need to make a commitment to the change and develop a plan. Here we might see the individual begin the process of making some of the changes that Davey-Rothwell and colleagues indicated in their study but from a treatment entry perspective. They may begin to think about how they will get to the treatment agency, and what they need to take care of prior to entry, especially if it is an inpatient or residential treatment setting. If they stay committed, they will then move into the action stage and begin to take the actual steps of entering treatment. The dynamic nature of the model allows for set-backs, such that individuals may return to prior stages for various reasons. If there is a wait list for treatment, the individuals' readiness may lessen and they may end up not entering treatment. Likewise, if something happens in the person's life, the individual may shift again towards an earlier stage where treatment entry is not an option. If the individual has a dual diagnosis, this may be a significant factor. How is the mental health treatment being handled? Is it in a different agency from that where the substance abuse is being treated? If yes, there may be a chance for the individual to not enroll in one or the other treatment programs, increasing the likelihood for relapse. Insurance payments, or lack of economic ability to pay for treatment, is another factor that may result in relapse, as the individual may drop out of treatment before the positive benefits have been attained.

The final stage is that of maintenance, where the task is to sustain the behavior change. Here the individual should normalize the new behavior so that it becomes second nature. However, as with the other stages, the dynamic nature of the model allows for regression to occur. Until the individual has completely incorporated the new behavior into his/her lifestyle, there is always the potential for a relapse. Considering the model, this may occur if new life events unfold that result in trauma for the individual, which may trigger old cues for substance use, which result in the increase of use until it becomes hazardous, increasing the psychological distress, decreasing the belief that change can occur, and deflating the readiness to change the risky behavior which they make an everyday experience. Thus, the model we propose has the flexibility to handle the varied situations that may arise concerning treatment entry.

Summary. In summary, the model recognizes that demographic factors such as age, gender, race/ethnicity, education, income, employment and culture can influence the personal history of the individual, as well as the development of psychiatric problems and substance use issues, and treatment availability. We also recognize that personal characteristics like childhood sex abuse or other forms of traumatic exposure can result in psychological distress that persists into adulthood. Similarly, we also recognize that trauma of any type may influence the psychological distress of the individual. Additionally, we recognize that personal factors like family relations, interpersonal relations, and work relations, may result in specific mental health or substance use patterns. The model also recognizes that psychological distress both influences and is influenced by substance use. Personal history also shows a relationship with self-efficacy, as patterns of substance use in the family, family history of mental illness, family functioning, and interpersonal relationships may all influence the development of self-efficacy.

Mandates show both a direct path to treatment entry, as well as an indirect pathway through readiness to change. This gives recognition to the fact that many individuals may be mandated to treatment but not all enroll and many who do enroll never fully engage in the process, suggesting that readiness to change may be low. We expect a similar effect for treatment entry. In the model that is presented (Figure 1), we also show direct paths to treatment entry for insurance and treatment availability. For treatment availability we show an indirect path through readiness to change. This reflects the effects of time delays on an individual's motivation level for treatment entry. The longer the period of time between the initial attempt at treatment entry, or the more energy an individual needs to expend to enter treatment, the less likely they are to enroll in treatment.

In essence, the model gives credence to all the factors that have shown a relationship with treatment entry but places them in a context where potential associations between factors may be identified. While placing emphasis on readiness to change, the model gives recognition to all factors of importance; but basically it is suggesting that when we consider how to increase treatment entry for those in need, an area that may provide more cost-effective outcomes is readiness to change. Within that context we can consider the influence of gender on personal history, psychological distress, and substance use and how those factors may interact to produce specific levels of readiness to enter treatment, which will inform the approaches used to increase the motivation to change of the individual. Similar statements can be made for ethnicity and culture.

The underlying point is that one can consider how all other factors may relate to readiness to enter treatment and then develop a plan to increase the entry into treatment for those who are in need.

6. References

Appel , P.W., Ellison, B.S., Jansky, M.A. & Oldak, R. (2004). Barriers to enrollment in drug abuse treatment and suggestions for reducing them: Opinions of drug injecting street outreach clients and other system stakeholders. *The American Journal of Drug and Alcohol Abuse, 30* (1), 129-153.

Appel, P.W., & Oldak, R. (2007). A preliminary comparison to enrolling in substance abuse treatment (AOD) reported by injecting street outreach clients and other stakeholders. *The American Journal of Drug and Alcohol Abuse, 33*, 699-705.

Ashford, J. (2004). Treating substance-abusing parents: A study of the Pima County family drug court approach. *Juvenile and Family Court Journal, 55*(4):27-37.

Bastaa, T. Shachamb, E., and Reecec, M. (2008). Psychological distress and engagement in HIV-related services among individuals seeking mental health care. *Aids Care, 20,* 969-976.

Ball, S. A., Martino, S., Nich, C., Frankenforter, T. L., Van Horn, D., Crits-Christoph, P., Woody, G. E., Obert, J. L., Farentinos, C., & Carroll, K. M. (2007). Site matters: Multisite randomized trial of motivational enhancement therapy in community drug abuse clinics. *Journal of Consulting and Clinical Psychology, 75,* 556-567.

Bandura, A. (1977). *Social Learning Theory. Englewood Cliffs,* N.J: Prentice-Hall.

Bandura, A. (1998). Health promotion from the perspective of social cognitive theory. *Psychology and Health, 13,* 623-649.

Bannenberg, A. F. I., Ratt, H., & Plomp, H. N. (1992). Demand for alcohol treatment by problem drinkers. *Journal of Substance Abuse Treatment, 9,* 59-62.

Beckman, L. J. & Amaro, H. (1986). Personal and social difficulties faced by women and men entering alcoholism treatment. *Journal of Studies on Alcohol, 47,* 135-145.

Boles, S., & Young, N.K. (2006). Sacramento County dependency drug court: Year three summary report. Sacramento County Juvenile Drug Court Committee: Children and Family Futures, Irvine, CA.

Booth, R.E., Crowley, T.J., Zhang, Y. (1996). Substance abuse treatment entry, retention, and effectiveness: Out-of-treatment opiate injection drug users. *Drug Alcohol Dependence (Ireland), 42* (1), 11-20.

Booth, R.E. Corsi, K.F., & Mikulich-Gilbertson, S.K. (2004). Factors associated with methadone maintenance treatment retention among street-recruited injection drug users. *Drug and Alcohol Dependence, 74* (2), 177-185.

Brisbane, F., Marmo, R., Cohen, S., Nichol, P., Finch, J., Golbin, J., Vidal, C., McKay, A., Graziano, F. (2000). Evaluation of the Suffolk County Family Treatment Court. Child Welfare Training Program: SUNY Stony Brook School of Social Welfare, Stony Brook, NY.

C'de Baca, J., Miller, W. R., & Lapham, S.C, (2001). A multiple risk factor approach for predicting DWI recidivism. *Journal of Substance Abuse Treatment, 21*(4), 207-215.

Cannavo, J.M. (2008). Evaluation of the Erie County Family Treatment Court. Dissertation Abstracts International Section A: Humanities and Social Sciences; 68(9-A):4068.

Cannavo, J.M., & Nochajski, T.H. (2011). Factors contributing to enrollment in a family treatment court. *The American Journal of Drug and Alcohol Abuse, 37*, 54-61.

Carey, K. B., Purnine, D. M., Maisto, S. A., & Carey, M. P. (1999). Assessing readiness to change substance abuse: A critical review of instruments. *Clinical Psychology: Science and Practice, 6*(3), 245-266.

Carlson, R.G., Sexton, R., Wang, J., Falck, R., Leukefeld, C.G., & Booth, B.M. (2010). Predictors of substance abuse treatment entry among rural illicit stimulant users in Ohio, Arkansas, and Kentucky. *Substance Abuse, 31,* 1-7.

Carroll, K. M., Ball, S. A., Nich, C., Martino, S., Frankforter, T. L., Farentinos, C., Kunkel, L. E., Mikulich-Gilbertson, S. K., Morgenstern, J., Obert, J.L., Polcin, D., Snead, N, & Woody, G. (2006). Motivational interviewing to improve treatment engagement and outcome in individuals seeking treatment for substance abuse: A multisite effectiveness study. *Drug and Alcohol Dependence, 81,* 301-312.

Cavaiola, A. A., Strohmetz, D. B., Wolf, J. M., & Lavender, N. J. (2003). Comparison of DWI offenders with non-DWI individuals on the MMPI-2 and the Michigan Alcoholism Screening Test. *Addictive Behaviors, 28,* 971- 977.

Cavaiola, A., & Wuth, C. (2002). *Assessment and treatment of the DWI offender*. New York: Haworth Press.

Chang, I., & Lapham, S. C. (1996). Validity of self-reported criminal offences and traffic violations in screening of driving-while-intoxicated offenders. *Alcohol and Alcoholism, 31,* 583- 590.

Corrigan, P.W. (2004). How stigma interferes with mental health care. *American Psychologist, 69,* 614-625.

Corrigan, P. W., Kuwabara, S. A., & O'Shaughnessy, J. (2009). The public stigma of mental illness and drug addiction: Findings from a stratified random sample. *Journal of Social Work, 9,* 139–147.

Corrigan, P. W., Larson, J. E., & Rusch, N. (2009). Self stigma and the "why try" effect: Impact on life goals and evidence-based practices. *World Psychiatry 8,* 75–81.

Corrigan, P. W., & Penn, D. L. (1999). Lessons from social psychology on discrediting psychiatric stigma. *American Psychologist, 54*(9), 765–776.

Corrigan, P.W., Rafacz, J.D., Hautamaki, J., Walton, J., Rusch, N., Rao, D., Doyle, P., Obrien, S., Pryor, J., & Reeder, G. (2010). Changing stigmatizing perceptions and recollections about mental illness: The effects of NAMI's In Our Own Voice. *Journal of Community Mental Health,* 46, 517–522.

Corrigan, P.W. & Wassel, A.(2008). Understanding and influencing the stigma of mental illness.*Journal of Psychosocial Nursing , 46* (1), *42-48.*

Coviello, D.M., Zanis, D.A., Wesnoski, S.A., & Alternam, A.I. (2006). The effectiveness of outreach case management in re-enrolling discharged methadone patients. *Drug and Alcohol Dependence, 85* (1), 56-65.

Cunningham, J. A., Sobell, L. C., Sobell, M. B., Agrawal, S., & Toneatto, T. (1993). Barriers to treatment: Why alcohol and drug abusers delay or never seek treatment. *Addictive Behaviors, 18,* 347-353.

Davey-Rothwell, M., Frydl, A., &Latkin, C. (2009). Does taking steps to control one's drug use predict entry into treatment? *The American Journal of Drug and Alcohol Abuse,* 35, 279–283.

Davey, M. A., Latkin, C.A., Hua, W., Tobin, K.E., Strathdee, S. (2007). Individual and social network factors that predict entry to drug treatment. *American Journal of Addiction, 16*(1), 38–45.

Dill, P.L., Wells-Parker, E., Cross, G.W., Williams, M., Mann, R. E., Stoduto, G., & Shuggi, G. (2007). The relationship between depressed mood, self-efficacy and affective states during the drinking driving sequence. *Addictive Behaviors, 32*, 1714-1718.

Evans, E., Li, L., & Hser, Y. (2008). Treatment entry barriers among California's Proposition 36 offenders. *Journal of Substance Abuse Treatment, 35*, 410-418.

Freyer, J., Coder, B., Bischof, G., Baumeister, D. E., Rumpf, H., John, U., & Hapke, U. (2007). Intention to utilize formal help in a sample with alcohol problems: A prospective study. *Drug and Alcohol Dependence, 87*, 210-216.

Fromme, K. & Corbin, W. (2004). Prevention of heavy drinking and associated negative consequences among mandated and voluntary students. *Journal of Consulting and Clinical Psychology, 72*(6), 1038-1049.

Gentilello, L.M., Rivara, F. P., Donovan, D. M., Jurkovich, G. J., Daranciang, E., Dunn, C. W., Villaveces, A., Copass, M., & Ries, R. R. (1999). Alcohol interventions in a trauma center as a means of reducing the risk of injury recurrence. *Annals of Surgery, 230*, 473-483.

Gibbs, D.A., Olmsted, K.L.R., Brown, J.B., Clinton-Sherrod, A.M. (2011). Dynamics of stigma for alcohol and mental health treatment among army soldiers. *Military Psychology, 23*(1), 36-51

Ginsburg, J. I. D., Mann, R. E., Rotgers, F., & Weekes, J. R. (2002). Using motivational interviewing with criminal justice populations. In W. R. Miller & S. Rollnick (Eds.), *Motivational interviewing: Preparing people for change* (pp. 333-346). New York: Guilford Press.

Gossop, M., Stewart, D. & Marsden, J. (2006). Readiness for change and drug use outcomes after treatment. *Addiction, 102*, 301-308.

Green, B.L., Furrer, C., Worcel, S., Burrus, S., & Finigan, M.W. (2007) How effective are family treatment drug courts? Outcomes from a four-site national study. *Child Maltreatment. 12*(1):43-59.

Green-Hennessy, S. (2002). Factors associated with receipt of behavioral health services among persons with substance dependence. *Psychiatric Services, 53*, 1592– 1598.

Greenfield, S.F., Brooks, A.J., Gordon, S.M., Green, C.A., Kropp, F., McHugh, R.K., Lincoln, M., Hein, D., & Miele, G.M. (2007). Substance abuse treatment entry, retention, and outcome in women: A review of the literature. *Drug and Alcohol Dependence, 86*, 1-21.

Haack, M., Alemi, F., Nemes, S., & Cohen, J.B. (2004). Experience with family drug courts in three cities. *Substance Abuse, 25*(4), 17-25.

Hedden, S.L. &Gfroerer, J.C. (2011). Correlates of perceiving a need for treatment among adults with substance use disorders: Results from a national survey. *Addictive Behaviors, 36*, 1213-1222.

Hernandez-Avila, Rounsaville, & Kranzler (2004). Opioid-, cannabis- and alcohol-dependent women show more rapid progression to substance abuse treatment. *Drug and Alcohol Dependence, 74*, 265–272.

Hiller, M. L., Knight, K., Broome, K. M., & Simpson, D. D. (1998). Legal pressure and treatment retention in a national sample of long-term residential programs. *Criminal Justice and Behavior, 25,* 463-481.

Hingson, R., Scotch, N., Day, N., & Culbert, A. (1980). Recognizing and seeking help for drinking problems: A study in the Boston metropolitan area. *Journal of Studies on Alcohol, 41,* 1102-1117.

Hingson, R., Mangione, T., Meyers, A., & Scotch, N. (1982). Seeking help for drinking problems: A study in the Boston metropolitan area. *Journal of Studies on Alcohol, 43,* 273-288.

Hoffman, N. G., Ninonuevo, F., Mozey, J., & Luxenberg, M. G. (1987). Comparison of court-referred DWI arrestees with other outpatients in substance abuse treatment. *Journal of Studies on Alcohol, 48,* 591-594.

Innovation Research & Training, Inc. Durham family treatment court process evaluation report. Durham, NC, 2005.

Jakobsson, A., Hensing, G., and Spak, F. (2008). The role of gendered conceptions in treatment seeking for alcohol problems. *Scandinavian Journal of Caring Sciences, 22,* 196-202.

Kaskutas, L. A., Weisner, C., & Caetano, R. (1997). Predictors of help seeking among a longitudinal sample of the general population, 1984-1992. *Journal of Studies on Alcohol, 58,* 155-161.

Kirchner, J. E., Booth, B. M., Owen, R. R., Lancaster, A. E., & Smith, G. R. (2000). Predictors of patient entry into alcohol treatment after initial diagnosis. *Journal of Behavioral Health Services & Research, 27,* 339–346.

Knight, K., Hiller, M. L., Broome, K. M., & Simpson, D. D. (2000). Legal pressure, treatment readiness, and engagement in long-term residential programs. *Journal of Offender Rehabilitation, 37,* 101-115.

Lapham, S. C., C'deBaca, J., McMillan, G. P., & Hunt, W.C. (2004). Accuracy of alcohol diagnosis among DWI offenders referred for screening. *Drug and Alcohol Dependence, 76*(2), 135-141.

Lapham, S. C., C'de Baca, J., Chang, I., Hunt, W. C., & Berger, L. R. (2002). Are drunk-driving offenders referred for screening accurately reporting their drug use? *Drug and Alcohol Dependence, 66,* 243– 253.

Litell, J. H. & Girvin, H. (2002). Stages of change: A critique. *Behavior Modification, 26,* 223-273.

Lincourt, P., Keuttel, T. J., & Bombardier, C. H. (2002). Motivational interviewing in a group setting with mandated clients: A pilot study. *Addictive Behaviors, 27,* 381-391.

Lundgren, L.M., Amaro, H., & Ben-Ami, L. (2005). Factors associated with drug treatment entry patterns among Hispanic women injection drug users seeking treatment. *Journal of Social Work Practice in the Addictions, 5*(1-2), 157-174.

MacDonald, S., DeSouza, A., Mann, R., & Chipman, M. (2004). Driving behavior of alcohol, cannabis, and cocaine abuse treatment clients and population controls. *American Journal of Drug and Alcohol Abuse, 30,* 429-444.

McCammon, K. (2001). Alcohol-related motor vehicle crashes: Deterrence and intervention. *Annals of Emergency Medicine, 38,* 415-422.

McConnaughy, E. A., Prochaska, J. O., & Velicer, W. F. (1983). Stages of change in psychotherapy: Measurement and sample profiles. *Psychotherapy: Theory, Research, and Practice, 20,* 368-375.

McFarling, L., D'Angelo, M., & Drain, M. (2011). Stigma as a barrier to Substance Abuse and mental health treatment. *Military Psychology, 23, 1-5.*

McMillian, H.E. (2008). Process and outcome evaluation of the Spokane County Meth Family Treatment Court, 2003-2005. *Dissertation Abstracts International Section A: Humanities and Social Sciences, 69* (2-A): 767.

Miller, W.M. & Rollnick, S. (2002). *Motivational interviewing: Preparing people for change* (2nd ed.). New York, NY, US: Guilford Press.

Monti, P. M., Colby, S. M., Barnett, N. P., Spirito, A., Rohsenow, D. J., Myers, M., Woolard, R., & Lewander, W. (1999). Brief intervention for harm reduction with alcohol-positive older adolescents in a hospital emergency department. *Journal of Consulting and Clinical Psychology, 67,* 989-994.

Nochajski, T. H. (1999). Alcohol program completion: Does it matter for DWI recidivism? *Alcoholism: Clinical and Experimental Research, 23*(5), 239.

Nochajski, T. (2006). The Research Institute on Addictions Self Inventory: A screening instrument for convicted drinking-drivers. Unpublished revised manual.

Nochajski, T. H., & Stasiewicz, P. R. (2001). Under-reporting by DWI offenders: Implications for motivational interviewing. *Alcoholism: Clinical and Experimental Research, 25,* 277.

Nochajski, T. H. & Stasiewicz, P. (2005). Assessing stages of change in DUI offenders: A comparison of two measures. *Journal of Addictions Nursing, 16,* 57-67.

Nochajski, T. H. & Stasiewicz, P. R. (2006). Relapse to driving under the influence (DUI): A review. *Clinical Psychology Review, 26,* 179-195.

Nochajski, T. H. & Wieczorek, W. F. (1998). Identifying potential drinking-driving recidivists: Do non-obvious indicators help? *Journal of Prevention and Intervention in the Community, 17,* 69-83.

Nochajski, T. H. & Wieczorek, W. F. (2000). Driver characteristics as a function of DWI history. In H. Laurell & F. Schlyter (Eds.), Alcohol, drugs and traffic safety. Stockholm: Ekonomi.

Peck, R. C., Arstein-Kerslake, G. W., & Helander, C. J. (1994). Psychometric and biographical correlates of drunk-driving recidivism and treatment program compliance. *Journal of Studies on Alcohol, 55,* 667-678.

Prochaska, J. O. & DiClemente, C. C. (1982). Transtheoretical therapy: Toward a more integrative model of change. *Psychotherapy: Theory, Research, and Practice, 19,* 276-288.

Prochaska, J. O. and DiClemente, C. C. (1984). The transtheoretical approach: Crossing traditional boundaries of therapy. Homewood, Ill., Dow Jones-Irwin.

Prochaska, J.O., DiClemente, C.C., & Norcross, J. (1992). In search of how people change: Applications to addictive behaviors. *American Psychologist, 47,* 1102-1114.

Roll, J.M., Prendergast, M., Richardson, K., Burdon, W., & Ramirez, A. (2005). Identifying predictors of treatment outcome in a drug court program. *The American Journal of Drug and Alcohol Abuse, 31,* 641-656.

Saunders, S.M., Zygowicz, K. M., and D'Angelo, B. R. (2006). Person-related and treatment-related barriers to alcohol treatment. *Journal of Substance Abuse treatment, 30,* 261-270.

Schmidt, L.A. &Weisner, C.M. (2005). Private insurance and the utilization of chemical dependency treatment.*Journal of Substance Abuse Treatment, 28,* 67-76.

Schmidt, L. A. & Weisner, C. M. (1999). Public health perspectives on access and need for substance abuse treatment. In J.A.Tucker, D. M. Donovan, & G. A. Marlatt (Eds.), *Changing addictive behavior: Bridging clinical and public health strategies* (pp. 67-96). New York: Guilford.

Shin, S.H., Lundgren, L., & Chassler, D. (2007). Examining drug treatment entry patterns among young injection drug users. *The American Journal of Drug and Alcohol Abuse, 33,* 217-225.

Simpson, C. A. & Tucker, J. A. (2002). Temporal sequencing of alcohol-related problems, problem recognition, and help-seeking episodes. *Addictive Behaviors, 27,* 659-674.

Stasiewicz, P., Herrman, D. H., Nochajski, T. H., & Dermen, K. (2006). Motivational interviewing - engaging highly resistant clients in treatment. *Counselor, 7*(1), 26-32.

Stasiewicz, P. R. & Nochajski, T. H. (2003). Determining alcohol use disorders in DWI offenders. *Alcoholism: Clinical and Experimental Research, 27*(5), 432.

Stasiewicz, P., Nochajski, T. H., Smith, K., & Bradizza, C. (2000, November). *Assessment of alcohol problems in DWI offenders: The sooner the better?* Presented at The Association for Advancement of Behavior Therapy annual convention in New Orleans, LA..

Stasiewicz, P. R., Nochajski, T. H., & Homish, D. L. (2007). Assessment of alcohol use disorders among court-mandated DWI offenders. *Journal of Addiction and Offender Counseling, 27*(2), 102-112.

Stein, L. A. R. & Lebeau-Craven, R. (2002). Motivational interviewing and relapse prevention for DWI: A pilot study. *Journal of Drug Issues, 32*(4), 1051-1070.

Storbjork, J. & Room, R. (2008). The two worlds of alcohol problems: Who is in treatment? *Addiction Research Theory, 16*(1), 67-84.

Tucker, J. A. & Gladsjo, J. A. (1993). Help-seeking and recovery by problem drinkers: Characteristics of drinkers who attended alcoholics anonymous or formal treatment or who recovered without assistance. *Addictive Behaviors, 18,* 529-542.

Tucker, J.A. & King, M. P. (1999). Resolving addictive behavior problems: influences on addictive behavior change and help-seeking processes. In J.A. Tucker, D. M. Donovan, & G. A. Marlatt (Eds.), *Changing addictive behavior: Bridging clinical and public health strategies (pp. 96-126).* New York: Guilford Press.

Tucker, J. A., Vuchinich, R. E., & Pukish, M. M. (1995). Molar environmental contexts surrounding recovery from alcohol problems by treated and untreated problem drinkers. *Experimental and Clinical Pharmacology, 3,* 195-204.

Tuchman, E. (2010). The importance of gender issues in substance abuse research. *Journal of Addictive Diseases, 29,* 127–138.

Vingilis, E. (1983). Drinking drivers and alcoholics: Are they from the same population? In R. G. Smart, F. B. Glaser, Y. Israel, H. Kalant, R. E. Popham, & W. W. Schmidt (Eds.), Research advances in alcohol and drug problems. Vol. 7 (pp. 299–342) . New York: Plenum Press.

Wain, R.M., Wilbourne, P.L., Harris, K.W., Pierson, H., Teleki, J., Burling, Lovett. S. (2011). Motivational interview improves treatment entry in homeless veterans. *Drug and Alcohol Dependence, 115,* 113–119.

Washousky, R., & Pirowski, H. (2003). Erie County Family Treatment Court Evaluation. Erie Community College: Department of Alcohol and Substance Abuse.

Weisner, C. & Matzger, H. (2002). A prospective study of the factors influencing entry to alcohol and drug treatment. *Journal of Behavioral Health Services and Research, 29,* 126-137.

Weisner, C., Matzger, H., Tam, T., & Schmidt, L. (2002). Who goes to alcohol and drug treatment? Understanding utilization within the context of insurance. *Journal of Studies on Alcohol, 63,* 673-682.

Wells-Parker, E., Bangert-Drowns, R., McMillen, R., & Williams, M. (1995). Final results from a meta-analysis of remedial interventions with drink/drive offenders. *Addiction, 90,* 907-926.

Wells-Parker, E., Dill, P., Williams, M., & Stoduto, G. (2006). Are depressed driving/driving offenders more receptive to brief intervention? *Addictive Behaviors, 31,* 339-350.

Wells-Parker, E., Dill, P., Cross, G, Mann, R.E., Stoduto, G, & Nochajski, T.H. (2007). An integrated theoretical model for matching DUI offenders to intervention options: Negative cognitive/affective patterns, dissonance, and motivation. In B. Logan, D. Isenschmid, J. Walsh, D. Beirness, & J. Morland (Eds.), *Alcohol, drugs and traffic safety*, Seattle, Washington.

Wells-Parker, E., Kenne, D., Spratke, K. L., and Williams, M. (2000). Self-Efficacy and motivation for controlling drinking and drinking/driving: An investigation of changes across a driving under the influence (DUI) intervention program and of recidivism prediction. *Addictive Behaviors, 25*(2), 229-238.

Wells-Parker, E. and Williams, M. (2002). Enhancing the effectiveness of traditional interventions with drinking drivers by adding brief individual components. *Journal of Studies on Alcohol, 63,* 655-664.

Wells-Parker, E., Williams, M., Dill, P., & Kenne, D. (1998). Stages of change and self-efficacy for controlling drinking and driving: A psychometric analysis. *Addictive Behaviors, 23* (3), 361-363.

Wenzel, S.L., Longshore, D., Turner, S., Ridgely, M.S. (2001). Drug courts: A bridge between criminal justice and health services. *Journal of Criminal Justice, 29,* 241-253.

Wieczorek, W. F., Callahan, C. P., & Morales, M. A. (1997). Motivation for change among DWI offenders. In C. Mercier-Guyon (Ed.), *Alcohol, drugs and traffic safety.* (pp. 1069–1075). Annecy, France: CERMT.

Wieczorek, W. F., & Nochajski, T. H. (2005). Characteristics of persistent drinking drivers: comparisons of first, second and multiple offenders. In D. A. Hennessey & D. L. Wiesenthal (Eds.), Contemporary issues in traffic research and road user safety. Hauppauge, NY: Nova Science.

Williams, D. J., Simmons, P. and Thomas, A. (2000). Predicting DUI recidivism following an alcohol safety action program. *Journal of Offender Rehabilitation, 32*(1/2), 129-145.

Worcel, S., Furrer, C., Green, B.L., Rhodes, B. (2006). Family treatment drug court evaluation final phase I study report. NPC Research: Portland, OR.

Young, D. & Belenko, S. (2002). Program retention and perceived coercion in three models of mandatory drug treatment. *Journal of Drug Issues, 32,* 297-328.

Yu, J. & Williford, W. R. (1993). Alcohol and risk/sensation seeking: Specifying a causal model on high-risk driving. *Journal of Addictive Diseases, 12,* 79-96.

Yu, J. & Williford, W. R. (1995). Drunk-Driving recidivism: Predicting factors from arrest and case disposition. *Journal of Studies on Alcohol, 56,* 60-66.

Zweben, A. & Fleming, M. F. (1999). Brief interventions for alcohol and drug problems. In J. A. Tucker, D. M. Donovan, & G. A. Marlatt (Eds.), *Changing addictive behaviors* (pp. 251–282). New York: Guilford Press

Section 4

Psychosocial Factors in the Development of Mental Disorders in Children

19

Maternal Depression, Mothering and Child Development

Douglas M. Teti[1], Bo-Ram Kim[1], Gail Mayer[1],
Brian Crosby[1] and Nissa Towe-Goodman[2]
[1]*The Pennsylvania State University*
[2]*University of North Carolina – Chapel Hill*
USA

1. Introduction

Depression is a highly prevalent disorder of affect characterized by persistent sadness or anhedonia (an inability to experience pleasure), typically accompanied by additional symptoms such as negative cognitions (self- perceptions of failure, feelings of guilt, and/or suicidal thoughts), somatic dysfunction (fatigue, loss of appetite, fatigue, disturbances in sleep), and impairment in daily functioning (e.g., indecisiveness) (Gelfand & Teti, 1990). When such a symptom pattern persists for at least two consecutive weeks and is not accompanied by period manic swings, the American Psychiatric Association's Diagnostic and Statistical Manual (DSM-IV-TR; American Psychiatric Association, 2000) identifies it as a major depressive episode (MDD). A formal DSM-IV-TR diagnosis of MDD can be given for a single major depressive episode, or for multiple, recurring episodes over time, which is common. Other depressive disorders identified in DSM-IV-TR include dysthymic disorder, and adjustment disorder with depressed mood.

Depression is more likely to occur under adverse circumstances, such as poverty, single parenthood (Gallagher, Hobfoll, Ritter, Lavin, 1997; Grant, Jack, Fitzpatrick, & Ernst, 2011), and chronic illness (Davidson, Echeverry, Katon, Lin, & Von Korff, 2011), and it may also be co-morbid with other psychiatric disorders. It is common to find, for example, that depression co-occurs with anxiety (Balta, & Paparrigopoulos, 2010) and that chronic depression is a salient feature of some personality disorders (Brieger, Ehrt, Bloeink, & Marneros, 2002). Because of the ubiquity of depressed mood as a feature of psychiatric, medical, and psychosocial conditions, researchers frequently focus on the severity and chronicity of depressive symptoms as a predictor of behavior in different contexts, using well-established, validated questionnaires that tap directly into participants' level of sadness, anhedonia, negative dysfunctional cognitions, somatic complaints, and impairments in daily living. Such measures include the Beck Depression Inventory (Beck, Steer, & Garbin, 1988), the Center for Epidemiological Studies - Depression scale (Radloff, 1977), and the Hamilton Rating Scale for Depression (Hamilton, 1960). These assessments tap the frequency and severity of depressive symptoms and provide overall scores and cut points that, when exceeded, identify individuals with clinical levels of symptom severity.

This chapter focuses on the impact of maternal depression on the mother-child relationship, writ large, and then specifically on maternal and infant behavior in infant sleep contexts. We begin with a discussion of family and child risks associated with maternal depression, and then turn to linkages between maternal depression and dysfunctional parental cognitions and the putative impact of maternal depression on the mother-child relationship and child development at different developmental stages. We then turn to empirical data linking elevations in maternal depressive symptoms and infant night waking, and present new data on relations between maternal depressive symptoms, dysfunctional cognitions about infant sleep behavior, and parenting of infants at bedtime and during the night that can help explain these links.

2. Maternal depression, family functioning, and child outcomes

As several reviews attest (Radke-Yarrow, 1998; Gelfand & Teti, 1990; Wachs, Black, & Engle, 2009), the effects of maternal depression are broad-based, with consequences not only for individual functioning but also for the quality of the mother's relationships with other family members. Marital discord in families with depressed mothers is common, as are troubled relationships between the depressed mother and her children. Indeed, children of depressed mothers are at significant risk for maladjustment and cognitive delays. Infants of depressed mothers are more likely than are infants of nondepressed mothers to be fussy, irritable, or withdrawn; to deploy attention ineffectively and manifest developmental delays in significant cognitive milestones such as object permanence; and are at risk to become insecurely attached to their mothers. Among older children of depressed mothers, rates of psychiatric disorder are as much as 4-to-5 times those among their same-aged counterparts of non-depressed mothers. Although maternal depression appears to predispose children to become depressed, these children are also at elevated risk for the full spectrum of externalizing disorders, including oppositional-defiant disorder and conduct disorder. Not surprisingly, these children are also at risk for poor academic performance, and for difficulties in interpersonal relationships, anxiety disorders, substance abuse, and delinquency over the long term (Goodman & Gotlib, 2002).

Mechanisms for the transmission of psychopathology from depressed parent-to-child are poorly understood. Depression appears to be at least partially heritable (Franić, Middeldorp, Dolan, Ligthart, & Boomsma, 2010), which may account in part for the elevated psychiatric risk status among children of depressed women. Other biologically based influences may also be at work. Recurrent bouts of significant depression among women are common. It is not unusual that women suffering from postpartum depression have experienced depressive episodes during pregnancy and pre-pregnancy (Field, Diego, Hernandez-Reif, Figueiredo, & Schanberg, 2008). Interestingly, infants born to mothers suffering prepartum depression manifest a biochemical profile (i.e., levels of cortisol, catecholamines, and serotonin) similar to that of their mothers, but different from infants born to nondepressed mothers (Field, Diego, & Hernandez-Reif, 2006). The potential impact of genetically and biologically based factors on the psychiatric risk status of children of depressed women has been given relatively short shrift among researchers who study parental depression and its effects.

The lion's share of research examining mechanisms of transmission of psychopathology from depressed parent-to-child has focused on the kinds of environments depressed parents create for their children, and the impact such environments have on the developing child's interpersonal, cognitive, and emotional life (Goodman & Gotlib, 2002; Wachs et al., 2010). Depressed mothers appear to create pathogenic child-rearing environments to which even very young (3-4 months old) infants are reactive (Cohn & Tronick, 1983). Importantly, the degree to which maternal depression singly influences child outcomes, however, depends on the chronicity and severity of the mothers' illness (Campbell & Cohn, 1995; Teti, Gelfand, Messinger, & Isabella, 1995). A single, isolated, non-recurrent bout of major depression, albeit debilitating to the mother while it occurs, is much less likely to affect children's adjustment over the long term than is chronic, severe depression, involving multiple, recurrent bouts of depression during the early postpartum period and beyond. Unfortunately, a woman who experiences postpartum depression is likely to experience at least one additional depressive episode sometime during her child's first five years of life (Campbell, Matestic, von Stauffenberg, Mohan, & Kirchner, 2007).

3. Depression, dysfunctional cognition, and mothering

Depression is common among women of childbearing age. Approximately 13% of women can be expected to experience at least one bout of significant depression during the early postpartum period (Leahy-Warren, McCarthy, & Corcoran, 2011). In most cases, elevations in depressive symptoms during the postpartum period resolve during the early months following delivery. In other cases, symptom levels are higher and persist, which can pose problems for the developing mother-child relationship from infancy onward (Campbell, Cohn, & Meyers, 1995).

Cognitive distortion is a central feature of depression (Abramson, Metalsky, & Alloy, 1989; Beck, 1987; Nolen-Hoeksema, 1990), and thus it is not surprising that mothers who are depressed harbor distorted perceptions about themselves as parents and about their children. Compared to nondepressed mothers, mothers with elevated depressive symptoms are more likely to perceive themselves as less adequate and less competent in the parenting role, to be less satisfied as parents, and to view their children and their children's behavior in more negative terms (Cornish et al., 2006; Fleming, Ruble, Flett, & Shaul, 1988; Teti & Gelfand, 1991, 1997; Whiffen & Gotlib, 1989). The degree to which depressed mothers are at risk for negative attributions about themselves and their children is likely to be directly proportional to the severity of their depressive symptoms.

A depressed mother's tendency to dwell on the negative (e.g., to interpret a perfectly normal, developmentally appropriate behavior or accomplishment as problematic), may have its own impact on a developing child's emotional well-being and in turn help explain why children of depressed mothers are at developmental risk. A child whose mother repeatedly labels her/him in negative terms is likely, at the least, to be at risk for low self esteem, and possibly for a host of internalizing and externalizing problems (Teti & Gelfand, 1997). The negative affect and negative cognitions that define depression, however, are intimately tied to action tendencies (Teti & Cole, 2011), and thus it is expected that depression would exact a toll on the quality of mother-child interactions, making it difficult for a mother to interact with her children in a developmentally supportive manner. Indeed, many studies describe depressed mothering as non-contingent and unresponsive, irritable and intrusive, insensitive, asynchronous, and incompetent (Goodman & Gotlib, 2002). Difficulties observed in depressed mothering may stem from deficiencies in the depressed mother's awareness and interpretation of her child's behavior (i.e., a "signal detection" deficiency). For example, a depressed mother's rumination and self-absorption can influence her attention to and awareness of her children's needs and social signals, and can also interfere with her ability to process social information efficiently and accurately. Her negative affective bias may create tendencies to misinterpret child behavior, and depressed mothers may be inclined to attribute negative intentions and motives to their children's behavior. Further, a depressed mothers' own need for support and comfort may lead her to expect more support and comfort from her child than the child is able to provide. Parenting difficulties among depressed mothers may also stem from the general slowing effect depressed affect has upon one's capability and motivation to act. Lack of energy and indecisiveness are hallmark features of depression, which in turn would be expected to influence a mother's motivation to respond promptly and contingently to child signals that she does prehend. Thus, the problems observed in depressed parenting may arise from the debilitating effect depression has on mothers' capacities for processing social information (awareness and interpretation of child cues), and from the dampening effect of depression on a mother's capacity and motivation to respond contingently (Gelfand & Teti, 1990).

Importantly, depression is highly co-morbid with anxiety, and it is very common for depressed individuals to harbor excessive worries about their own behavior and that of others (Beck et al., 2001). Thus, we might also expect that depressed mothers may worry excessively about their children's behavior, perhaps leading to misinterpretations about child behavior that could lead to maladaptive maternal responses. We will re-visit this point later in this chapter.

Depressed mother-infant interactions. The emotional climate of parent-infant interactions is particularly important for the development of self-regulation, secure attachments, and the promotion of other social and emotional competencies (Cole, Michel, & Teti, 1994; Radke-Yarrow, 1998). As several reviews attest, the disturbances associated with depression have a clear impact on the emotional quality of early mother-child interactions (Goodman & Gotlib, 2002; Radke-Yarrow, 1998; Teti & Towe-Goodman, 2008). Depressed mothers interact less with their infants, are less aware of their infants' signals, and are less contingently responsive to their infants' bids for attention. The joint attention, shared positive affect, and appropriate scaffolding that characterizes warm, nurturant parent-child relationships are often missing in depressed mother-infant dyads. Further, depressed mothers show less emotional availability and affection toward their infants, display less pleasure and positive emotion during interactions, and express more negative affect overall. Some depressed mothers may alternate between being disengaged and then overly stimulating, that latter of which can be so intrusive that they appear disorganizing to the infant. In turn, their infants' behavior is conspicuously devoid of positive affect, and is also characteristically high in distress or protest, unresponsiveness to maternal bids, avoidance, and withdrawal, and this behavior sometimes generalizes to other, non-depressed adults. The infant's distress and unresponsiveness in turn may increase the mother's feelings of inadequacy or rejection, thus creating a vicious cycle of negative, dysregulated affect in the mother-infant relationship.

Depressed mothering and infant-mother attachments. Attachment theory (Ainsworth, Blehar, Waters, & Wall, 1978) would predict that depressed mothers' interactional difficulties with their infants, if prolonged, will predispose infants to become insecurely attached. Indeed, maternal sensitivity during infancy, which can be defined as an empathic awareness of and appropriate responsiveness to infant needs and social cues, is taken by attachment theory as the single most important predictor of attachment security in infancy (Teti & Huang, 2005). Research that has examined linkages between maternal depression and infant-mother attachment security typically employs the Ainsworth Strange Situation procedure (Ainsworth et al., 1978), a brief, 21-24 minute 7-episode procedure used for infants between 12 and 18 months of age. The procedure, which almost always takes place in a small room that is novel to the infant, puts the infant through a series of 3-minute episodes of separations and reunions with the mother, a (typically) female stranger, and one episode in which the infant is alone.

Specific attention is given to the infant's behavior during the two Strange Situation reunion episodes with the mother. Secure infants typically greet the mother during infant-mother reunions, approach the mother and seek her out for comfort (if the infant experiences separation distress), and are ultimately able to return to toy play and exploring their environment in the mothers' presence. Sensitive mothering during the infant's first year would be expected to promote secure infant-mother attachments, which, as many studies now attest, predicts healthy adjustment in the preschool years and beyond in terms of empathic awareness, child compliance, and peer relations. Insecure-avoidant infants, by contrast, typically do not greet the mother during reunions. They do not approach the mother except in the context of toy play, and it is not uncommon for insecure-avoidant infants to prefer to play with toys rather than interact with their mothers. Theoretical accounts of specific linkages between parental insensitivity and insecure attachment (Cassidy & Berlin, 1991; Cassidy & Kobak, 1988) suggests that maternal insensitivity characterized by intrusiveness and rejection would be expected to predict insecure-avoidant infant-mother attachments, which some attachment theorists propose is develops as a defense against maternal rejection. Insecure-ambivalent/resistant infants direct overt expressions of anger toward their mothers during reunions and typically do not soothe in response to maternal attempts to do so. Mothering characterized by unresponsiveness and/or inconsistency in responsiveness would be expected to predict insecure-ambivalent (resistant) infant-mother attachments. Both insecure-avoidant and insecure-ambivalent/resistant attachments, albeit not adaptive to the infant over the long term, are viewed as "strategies" the child has developed to maintain access to the attachment figure (the mother) in times of stress. Insecure-avoidant infants learn not to seek out their mothers because doing so in the past has led to rejection. Thus they employ a "close, but not too close" strategy to maintain some degree of proximity to the mother. Insecure-ambivalent/resistant infants have learned that overt expressions of anger and prolonged distress is "what works" to keep their mothers focused on them. This "strategy", although maladaptive to their development over the long run, is functional in the short-term to maintain access to their mothers. Both insecure-avoidance and insecure-resistant/ambivalent infants are at risk for difficulties in later mother-child relationships and peer relationships, compared to secure infants (Sroufe, 2005).

Elevations in insecure infant-mother attachments (i.e., insecure-avoidant and insecure-ambivalent attachments) have been reported in several studies of depressed mother-infant dyads (Teti et al., 1995; Campbell & Cohn, 1995; Carter, Garrity-Rokous, Chazan-Cohen, Little, & Briggs-Gowan, 2001; Lyons-Ruth, Connell, Grunebaum, & Botein, 1990). Further, when mothers' depression is chronic and severe over the infant's first year, infants are at risk for developing insecure-disorganized attachment to their mothers, which some attachment theorists cite as the most "insecure" of all of the insecure attachment classifications (Teti et al., 1995). Unlike the insecure-avoidant and insecure ambivalent attachment patterns, which appear to be governed by clear-cut "strategies" (albeit not ideal) for accessing the attachment figure, insecure-disorganized attachment is identified by conspicuous absence of a clear-cut strategy (Main & Solomon, 1990). Disorganized attachment is instead hallmarked by fear and confusion about how to access the attachment figure (the mother) at times when it is in the infant's best interests to do so (Hesse, 2008). In the Strange Situation, insecure-disorganized infants are identified by any of a variety of behavior patterns signifying fear and/or confusion during the infant-mother reunion episodes (Main & Solomon, 1990). For example, disorganization is identified when the infant manifests clear-cut expressions of fear (e.g., infant brings hand to mouth and has a fearful expression) of the mother when she enters the room to begin the reunion episode. It is also identified when the infant freezes or stills in the mother's presence for a substantial period of time, or when the infant, upon approaching the mother, repeatedly veers away from her. These are but a few of a variety of indicators of disorganized attachment, all of which reflect a state of fear or confusion about how to access the attachment figure in times of stress. Rates of disorganized infant-mother attachment are found to be elevated among infants of alcoholic parents, substance abusing parents, and parents with significant psychopathology (Hesse, 2008). Of the three insecure infant-parent attachment classifications, children identified as insecure-disorganized are at highest risk for the development of behavior problems in the preschool years (Guttmann-Steinmetz, & Crowell, 2006).

Attachment theory proposes that, over time, children develop "working models" of relationships that spawn from their early attachments with their caregivers, models that are carried forward and applied in subsequent relationships (Bowlby, 1969; Bretherton, 2005). Such models can be thought of as a set of affectively laden cognitions or expectations about relationships that develop as a result of repeated interactions with attachment figures and that guide behavior and the processing of social information. Attachment theory (Bretherton, 2005) predicts that children with secure working models develop expectations that their caregivers will be appropriately responsive to them when needed, and such children in turn come to believe that they are worthy of love and support. Such expectations are consistent with a history of sensitive, responsive caregiving. Children who develop insecure working models, by contrast, do not expect their caregivers to be appropriately responsive, and insecure working models may serve as a foundation for low self-worth. Attachment theory also proposes that children internalize not just the child's role in their early attachment relationships, but the role of the parent as well, and that they are likely to carry forward and enact the parent's side in subsequent relationships with others (Sroufe, 2005). Indeed, it is the development of these working models that provides the theoretical link between the insecure attachment patterns infants develop to their depressed mothers and the adjustment problems these children present later in development (Teti et al., 1995).

It is important to emphasize, however, that the link between maternal depression and insecure infant-mother attachment is most clear when mothers' depression during the infants' first year is prolonged. A single maternal depressive episode during the post-partum period that resolves and does not recur is unlikely to have long-term negative effects on security of infant-mother attachment, nor on other aspects of infant and preschool child functioning (Campbell & Cohn, 1995).

Depressed mother-toddler relationships. A number of studies demonstrate that toddlers of depressed mothers experience significant emotional and behavioral regulatory problems (Dietz, Jennings, Kelley, & Marshal, 2009; Gartstein et al., 2010; Leckman-Westin, Cohen, & Stueve, 2009), including reduced positive affect, prolonged bouts of sadness and emotional volatility, and high levels of aggression. Emergent social, emotional, and cognitive capabilities in the toddler years create new opportunities for change and growth, but may also place new demands on the depressed mother. The affective connection between the toddler and mother and the need for parents to emotionally support their children in response to stress is still quite important during the toddler years (Cole et al., 1994). Because of the debilitating effects of depression on attentional and processing capacities, depressed mothers may be less able than nondepressed mothers to follow the child's interests or facilitate joint attention, making mutual engagement in activities challenging. Further, depressed mothers' lack of verbal communication and reduced responsiveness in interactions with their toddlers may impact the acquisition of linguistic and cognitive skills, important developmental tasks during this time. The inability of mothers to provide adequate emotional support to their toddlers in stressful contexts can in turn lead to the significant increases in internalizing or externalizing behavior observed among toddlers of depressed mothers.

Additionally, toddlers' growing desire to assert their independence (i.e., the onset of the "terrible twos") can increase parent-child conflict during this period, and depressed mothers may be less able to provide the gentle guidance and limit setting necessary to successfully negotiate these conflicts (Gelfand & Teti, 1990). Some mothers experiencing depression may be more likely to avoid confrontation with their toddlers, expressing fears over their child's willful behavior and their inability to assert appropriate authority. Other mothers with depression may resort to harsh discipline (Gelfand & Teti, 1990; McLoyd, 1998), showing greater hostility towards their children and utilizing more physical punishment than their non-depressed counterparts. Maternal feelings of helplessness and lack of control over their children's behavior may increase the likelihood that they will employ coercive or punitive tactics in disciplinary encounters (Bugental & Happaney, 2004). In fact, maternal depression may be considered a risk factor for physical abuse and maltreatment of young children (Arnow, Blasey, Hunkeler, Lee, & Hayward, 2011). In either case, these ineffective socialization techniques employed by depressed mothers are often met with dysfunctional behavior on the part of the toddler. In some cases, children of depressed mothers show more frequent defiance, hostility, aggression and externalizing behavior. Alternatively, the toddlers of depressed mothers may show more depressed affect and withdrawal themselves, as well as helplessness in the face of challenges. Notably, the behavior of these toddlers often matches that of their mother, such that the affect and symptoms of the mother are mirrored in her child's actions (Gelfand & Teti, 1990).

Interestingly, disorganized attachment in infancy is predictive of two rather sophisticated yet very maladaptive preschool behavior patterns directed toward the mother, and both of these patterns have been linked to chronic maternal depression (Main & Cassidy, 1988; Teti, 1999). One of these is characterized by the child's repeated attempts to take care of and nurture the mother (i.e., a role-reversing "caregiving" pattern). Such a pattern, on the surface, does not present with any outward signs of trouble or hostility between the child and mother. However, a role-reversed caregiving pattern that develops in a child at such an early developmental stage has been identified by some as representing attempts on the part of the child to repair a damaged relationship, with consequences for the child's emotional well-being (Crittenden, 1992). Insecure-disorganized infant-mother attachment is also associated with a second maladaptive preschool behavior pattern, characterized by repeated, overt attempts by the child to embarrass and punish the mother. These "coercive" child behavior patterns are thought to develop in response to a caregiving history characterized by unresponsiveness and inconsistency, perhaps particularly in the area of appropriate limit-setting (Teti, 1999). The coercive and caregiving preschool patterns may be different manifestations of an overarching "controlling" strategy of accessing mothers in times of stress. Not surprisingly, these caregiving and coercive patterns have straightforward links to child behavior problems (Moss, Cyr, Dubois-Comtois, 2004).

4. Maternal depression and children in middle childhood and adolescence

There tend to be fewer studies of the effects of maternal depression on developmental outcomes of school-aged children and adolescents, but available evidence indicates that such children are at high risk for externalizing and internalizing disorders (particularly depression), deficits in social competence, lower self-esteem, attentional deficits, and academic failure (Gross, Shaw, Burwell, & Nagin, 2009). Similar to younger children with depressed mothers, interactional difficulties are common between children of depressed mothers and their parents (Foster, Garber, & Durlak, 2008), with sadness, withdrawal, poor limit setting, and criticism being central features of depressed mothering for children in this age range. School aged children and adolescents develop stable representations of themselves in relation to others, and they are more likely than are children of nondepressed mothers to develop negative attributional styles and low self-worth (Smith, Calam, & Bolton, 2009). Peer relations may also suffer, with children of depressed mothers being more likely to suffer peer isolation, loneliness, and rejection (Zimmer-Gembeck, Waters, & Kindermann, 2010).

5. Individual differences in depressed mother-child relationships, and child outcomes

The role of maternal self-efficacy. Despite the well-documented associations between maternal depression and difficulties within the mother-child relationship, it is important to emphasize that problematic interactions are not seen in all cases in which the mother is experiencing depression. One important source of individual differences in depressed mothering may be variations encountered in maternal self-efficacy, or a mother's beliefs in her own competencies as a parent. Bandura (1986) defines self-efficacy as a set of beliefs or judgments about one's competency at a particular task or setting. Self-efficacy beliefs are viewed as the final common pathway in predicting the degree of effort one expends to succeed at a particular task. Self-efficacious individuals are strongly motivated to marshal whatever resources (personal, social, economic, etc.) that are available to them to succeed at a given task. Self-inefficacious individuals, by contrast, are likely to give up prematurely, despite the fact that success may be within reach. Whereas the strongest predictor of self-efficacy is the degree of prior success at that task, self-efficacy beliefs are also sensitive to social persuasion, vicarious experiences, (e.g., modeling), and affective state (Bandura, 1986).

Given the link between self-efficacy and affect, it would not be surprising to find that depressed mothers feel less efficacious in the parenting role than non-depressed mothers. At the same time, social-cognitive theory would predict that maternal self-efficacy should also be sensitive to support for their mothering provided by intimate support figures (social persuasion), by previous learning experiences about mothering by watching other competent mothers (modeling), and by mothers' perceptions of how "easy" or "difficult" their infants are to care for (perceptions of infant temperament, which should be linked with mothers' histories of prior successes and failures with the infant). Thus, variation in maternal self-efficacy is not a simple, direct function of variations in maternal depression, but also of variations in other social influences in the environment. Self-efficacy theory would also predict, however, that any influences of mothers' affective state, social persuasion, or prior experiences with their infants on parenting should be mediated by maternal self-efficacy, which is the final common pathway in the prediction of behavioral competence.

Teti and Gelfand (1991) tested this hypothesis in a study of 86 mothers (48 with clinical depression, and 38 non-depressed) of first-year infants. Maternal self-efficacy was assessed with a scale developed by the authors that tapped mothers' self-efficacy beliefs in nine parental domains relevant to mothering an infant in the first year of life (e.g., soothing; maintaining infant attention; diapering, feeding, changing), with a tenth item asking mothers to report on their overall feelings of competence in the mothering role. Ratings of mothers' behavioral competence (e.g., sensitivity, warmth, disengagement) with their infants were conducted from observations of feeding and free play by "blind", highly reliable observers. Standard, well-established measures were used to assess severity of maternal depressive symptoms, social and marital supports, and infant temperament.

As expected, mothers' parenting efficacy beliefs were negatively associated with maternal depressive symptoms and perceptions of infant temperament, such that mothers felt less efficacious in the maternal role when they were more depressed and when they perceived their infants as more difficult. Mothers' self-efficacy beliefs, by contrast, were positively associated with perceived quality of social-marital supports and with observer judgments of maternal behavioral competence with their infants. In addition, as expected, mothers' behavioral competence was significantly related to perceptions of infant temperamental difficulty (negatively) and with social-marital supports (positively). Importantly, self-efficacy beliefs continued to predict maternal behavioral competence even after depressive symptoms, social-marital supports, and infant temperamental difficulty were statistically controlled. Further, when maternal self-efficacy was statistically controlled, the linkages between maternal behavioral competence and depression, infant temperament, and social-marital supports were substantially reduced in magnitude. Taken together, these findings identified maternal self-efficacy beliefs as a central mediator of relations between mothers' behavioral competence with their infants and the severity of maternal depressive symptoms, perceptions of infant temperamental difficulty, and social-marital supports.

These findings indicate that depression is more likely to debilitate parenting quality when maternal self-efficacy is also compromised. This is likely to be the case in many depressed mothers because of the strong linkage between affective state and self-efficacy beliefs. However, maternal self-efficacy is also sensitive to infant temperament and social-marital supports, and thus it is possible for depressed mothers to have more positive self-efficacy beliefs about parenting, and in turn to parent more effectively, when their infants are temperamentally easy and when they receive consistent encouragement from intimate support figures. Conversely, the combination of significant depression and difficult infant temperament and/or inadequate social-marital supports may be particularly devastating in their joint effects on maternal self-efficacy beliefs. In their 1991 study, Teti and Gelfand (1991) found this to be the case when examining the single vs. joint impact of maternal depression and infant temperamental difficulty on mothers' parenting efficacy beliefs. Maternal self-efficacy was much more compromised among mothers who had high levels of depressive symptoms and who also perceived their infants to be difficult. Further, the joint "impact" of severe maternal depression and infant temperamental difficulty on maternal self-efficacy was significantly greater than what would have been expected from an additive model of effects.

6. Maternal depression and infant night waking

The conclusions drawn about the putative impact of maternal depression on mother-child interactions and relationship outcomes has relied almost exclusively on observations of depressed mother-child behavior during the day. We have found, however, that the negative influence of depressed mothering may extend into the nighttime hours (Teti & Crosby, in press), from data drawn from a larger, NIH-sponsored study of parenting, infant sleep, and infant development currently underway (Project SIESTA, or the Study of Infants' Emergent Sleep TrAjectories; R01HD052809).

The Teti and Crosby examination of depressed mothering at night drew from a host of earlier studies reporting significant linkages between elevated depressive symptoms in mothers and infant night waking (Armitage et al., 2009; Armstrong, O'Donnell, McCallum, & Dadds, 1998; Bayer, Hiscock, Hampton, & Wake, 2007; Gress-Smith, Luecken, Lemery-Chafant, & Howe, 2011; Hiscock & Wake, 2001, 2002; Dennis & Ross, 2005; Diego, Field, & Hernandez-Reif, 2005; Field et al., 2007; Mindell, Telofski, Wiegand, Kurtz, 2009; O'Connor et al., 2007; Warren, Howe, Simmens, & Dahl, 2006; Zuckerman, Stevenson, & Bailey, 1987). The nature of these associations was not clear. At least some of the variance appears to be biologically-based. Armitage et al. (2009), for example, found that, as early as 2 weeks of age and later at 6 months, infants of mothers ever diagnosed (past or present) with major depressive disorder took longer to fall asleep and spent more time awake during the night than infants of mothers with no depression. Field et al. (2007) reported that newborns of mothers who were depressed during pregnancy spent less time in deep sleep, more time in indeterminate sleep, and more time fussing and crying than newborns of non-depressed mothers. Finally, in a large community study relying exclusively on maternal report data, O'Connor et al. (2007) found prenatal maternal depression and anxiety to predict sleep disturbances in children at 18 and 30 months of age (but not at 6 months), even after controlling for postpartum maternal symptoms. O'Connor et al. proposed that infants of prenatally distressed mothers may be exposed to higher levels of maternal glucocorticoids, which in turn affects infants' postnatal diurnal cortisol patterns and, in turn, infants' propensity to establish a normal diurnal sleep cycle. Additional studies report predictive relationships, from assessments of maternal depressive symptoms at earlier points in time to assessments of infant night waking made later (Gress-Smith, Luecken, Lemery-Chafant, & Howe, 2011; Zuckerman et al., 1987), suggesting that maternal depression is causally linked to infant night waking. Other studies, suggest that maternal dysphoria is the result of, rather than the cause of elevations in infant night waking (Hiscock & Wake, 2001, 2002; Mindell et al., 2009). Finally, Warren et al. (2006) found maternal depressive symptoms to be predicted by infant night waking from 15-to-24 months, but predictive of infant night waking throughout the first three years of life, suggesting bidirectional, mutual influences (see also Sadeh, Tikotzky, & Scher, 2010).

There is general agreement that infant sleep patterns are dynamic and co-regulated, and that both infants and parents contribute to this dynamic (Mindell, Kuhn, Lewin, Metzer, & Sadeh, 2006). In addition, as suggested above, "mother-driven" and "infant-driven" models of influence may be at play, although any support for a mother-driven model would require on-site observations of maternal behavior at infant bedtimes and throughout the night. Stated differently, the viability of a mother-driven model of influence would depend on (a) the discovery that depressed mothers' behavior with their infants at night differed in some substantial way from nondepressed mothers' nighttime behavior with their infants, (b) finding that these differences were predictive of differences in infant night waking, with infants of depressed mothers showing more night waking than infants of nondepressed mothers. Some direction, in terms of what maternal behaviors at bedtime and during the night might be relevant to this question, was provided by studies that addressed relations between specific parental behaviors during infant sleep contexts and infant sleep disturbance. These studies revealed that specific practices used by parents with infants at night were predictive of infant night waking. These practices included parental presence at bedtime (Adair, Bauchner, Phillip, Levenson, & Zuckerman, 1991; Mindell, Meltzer, Carskadon, & Chervin. 2009), inconsistency in where the infant slept at night (Atkinson, Vetere, & Grayson, 1995), putting the infant down in her/his bed after, rather than before, s/he fell asleep (Burnham, Goodlin-Jones, Gaylor, & Anders, 2002; DeLeon & Karraker, 2007), short latency of response to nighttime crying (Burnham et al., 2002), infant sleeping with the parent (Burnham et al., 2002; DeLeon & Karraker, 2007; Johnson, 1991; Mao, Burnham, Goodlin-Jones, Gaylor, & Anders, 2004; Mindell, Sadeh, Kohyama, & How, 2010), breastfeeding (DeLeon & Karraker, 2007; Johnson, 1991; Mindell, Sadeh, Kohyama, & How, 2010; Tikotzky, Sadeh, & Glickman-Gavrieli, 2010), and active physical comforting and close contact (Morrell, & Cortina-Borja, 2002; Morrell & Steele, 2003).

Two working hypotheses emerge from this literature with regard to maternal depressive symptoms and parenting practices with infants at night. The first, which articulates a mother-driven model of influence, is that depressed mothers may be more likely than nondepressed mothers either to engage in close physical contact or spend increased time with their infants, either during bedtime or during the night, which disturbs infant sleep and leads to increases in night waking. The second, which outlines an infant-driven model, is that chronic infant night waking leads to high levels of maternal intervention at night (and, as a result, maternal sleep loss), which in turn predisposes mothers to become dysphoric. Teti and Crosby (in press) examined both mother- and infant-driven paths of influence between maternal depressive symptoms and infant night waking. Both models are theoretically defensible and have received support from prior work. Beyond assessing mothers' depressive symptoms, however, Teti and Crosby also took into consideration the likely link between maternal depressive symptoms and mothers' dysfunctional cognitions about infant sleep behavior, and the possibility that maladaptive maternal cognitions about infant sleep could relate uniquely to infant night waking. Such linkages are predicted by cognitively-based theories of depression (Abramson et al., 1989; Beck, 1987; Nolen-Hoeksema, 1990) and from earlier work indicating that mothers of infants with sleep problems worry more about their parenting competence, their ability to set limits at night, and about their infants' physical and emotional well-being (Morrell, 1999; Sadeh, Flint-Ofir, Tirosh, & Tikotsky, 2007). These cognitions in turn are associated with mothers' attempts to soothe infants to sleep and to co-sleep with them (Morrell & Steele, 2003; Tikotsky & Sadeh, 2009; Tikotzky, Sharabany, Hirsch, & Sadeh, 2010).

7. SIESTA I (Study of Infants' Emergent Sleep TrAjectories)

Data for Teti and Crosby's (in press) investigation came from a larger study, Project SIESTA I, a cross-sectional investigation of parenting and infant sleep during the first two years of life (Teti, Principal Investigator). In their study, Teti and Crosby examined several theoretically defensible paths of influence involving maternal depressive symptoms, maternal dysfunctional cognitions about infant sleep behavior, and infant night waking. The first (see Figure 1) was a mother-driven model in which both maternal depressive symptoms and dysfunctional cognitions about infant sleep jointly and uniquely predicted maternal behavior (at bedtime or during the night), which in turn predicted infant night waking. The second (Figure 2) was an infant-driven model in which infant night waking predicted maternal behavior with infants at night, which in turn predicted maternal depressive symptoms. The third (Figure 3) was another infant-driven model in which infant night waking predicted maternal behavior with infants at night, which in turn predicted mothers' dysfunctional cognitions about infant sleep. In all models, the mediating role of maternal behavior (either maternal presence, or mother-infant close physical contact) was directly assessed from video-recorded observations of bedtime and nighttime parenting.

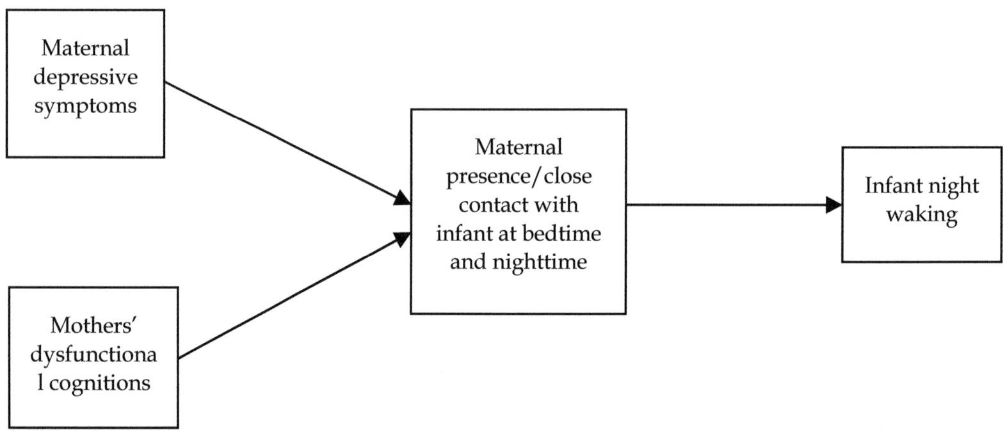

Fig. 1. Mother-driven model in which mothers' depressive symptoms and dysfunctional cognitions about infant sleep affect infant night waking indirectly, via their direct influence on bedtime and nighttime parenting.

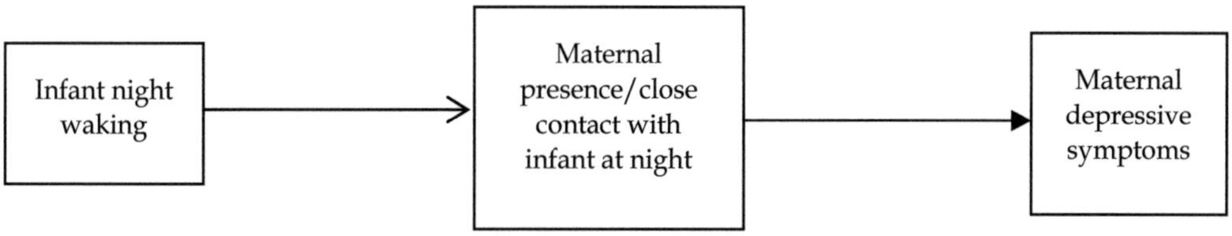

Fig. 2. Infant-driven model in which infant night waking predicts maternal depressive symptom levels indirectly, via its direct influence on nighttime parenting.

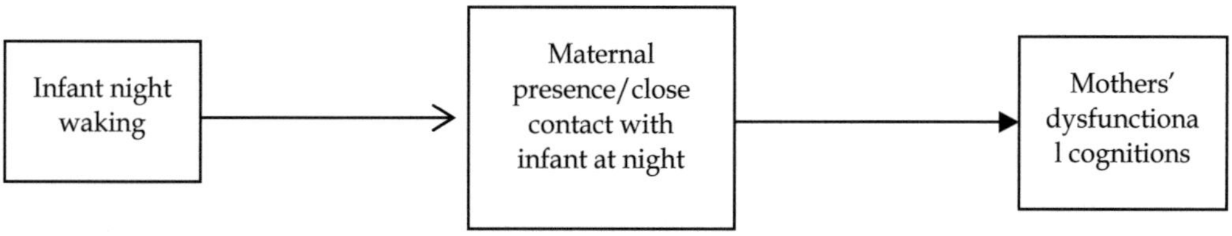

Fig. 3. Infant-driven model in which infant night waking predicts mothers' dysfunctional cognitions about infant sleep indirectly, via its direct influence on nighttime parenting.

Sample characteristics. Teti and Crosby's participants were 45 socioeconomically diverse mothers and their healthy infants who ranged in age from 1 to 24 months of age. Five age cohorts of infants were recruited: 1 month (n = 9, 5 girls), 3 months (n = 8, 3 girls), 6 months (n = 8, 4 girls), 12 months (n = 12, 7 girls), and 24 months (n = 4 girls). Recruitment of families with 1- and 3-month infants took place at a local hospital, and recruitment of the remaining families was done using a data base of local birth announcements or newspaper advertisements. Infant gender was evenly split within each cohort. The sample was largely White (91%), with the remaining 9% composed of Asian and African American families. Mothers were 22 to 42 years old (M = 30.5, SD = 4.9), 93% were married, and 73% had completed some post-secondary education. Family income was wide-ranging ($20,000/year to $200,000/year) and did not vary by cohort. Twenty infants were firstborn, and birth order was found to be unrelated to infant cohort and infant gender. Almost half (45%) of the infants were being breastfed at least part of the time and most of these (80%) were 6 months of age or younger. Breastfeeding, however, was not associated with infant night waking after infant age was statistically controlled, and mothers' age, educational level, and yearly income were not associated with infant night waking. Although most infants slept in a separate room from their parents, 13 shared the same room with parents at night, and 5 of these infants shared the same bed with parents. Not surprisingly, there was significantly more close contact between mothers and room-sharing infants than between mothers and infants who slept in separate rooms.

Study protocol and measures. Data were collected during home visits to each family, across seven consecutive days. Measurements included an assessment of mothers' depressive symptoms (on Day 1 of data collection), mothers' dysfunctional cognitions about infant sleep behavior (also on Day 1), a digital video recording of parent-infant interactions beginning at bedtime and continuing throughout the night until morning wake-up (on Day 6), and a daily diary of infant sleep behavior (to assess frequency of infant night waking), which was collected on the morning of each day across the 7-day data collection window. The depressive symptom measure used was the Depression subscale of the SCL-90-R

(Derogatis, 1994), which is composed of 13 items asking mothers to report on such symptoms as "loss of sexual interest or pleasure", "feeling hopeless about the future", and "feelings of worthlessness". Each item used a 5-point Likert-type scale, ranging from 0 (not at all) to 4 (extremely). The final overall depressive symptom severity score for each mother was obtained by summing the 13 item scores. Mothers' dysfunctional cognitions about infant sleep was assessed with the Maternal Cognitions about Infant Sleep Questionnaire (MCISQ; Morrell, 1999), which was composed of 20 items asking mothers to report on their thoughts about their infants' behavior during the night. Sample items included "When my child doesn't sleep at night, I doubt my competence as a parent," and "My child will feel abandoned if I don't respond immediately to his/her cries at night". Mothers respond to each item on a 6-point scale (0 = strongly disagree, 5 = strongly agree). Using principal components analysis, Teti and Crosby identified two factors, each of which measured a conceptually coherent dimension of mothers' thoughts about infant sleep. The first factor (alpha = .89), labeled "worries about infant physical/emotional needs", included 9 items, each of which related to maternal anxieties about infant night waking and how to deal with them (e.g., "My child might go hungry if I don't give him/her a feed at night", "I should be getting up during the night to check that my child is still all right", "If I give up feeding at night, then he/she will never sleep"). The second factor (alpha = .77), labeled "helplessness/loss of control", was composed of three items pertaining to mothers' doubts about their parenting competencies in dealing with infant night wakings, worries about losing control and harming the infant, and regrets about having a child in the first place. Mothers received a score on each factor by summing the individual item scores.

Finally, digital video was used to record mothers' bedtime parenting with their infants, using a video setup based on parental input about where the infant was put to bed, where the infant slept at night, and whether or not the parents took their infants to a separate room for night feedings. In most cases, camera setup involved suspending one camera directly above the infant using an overhanging boom stand, a second camera in the corner of the room where the infant slept that was trained on the doorway of the room to identify who (mother, father) entered and exited the room, and a third camera trained on any location parents said they typically took if/when they responded to infant night waking. This location was sometimes in the same room where the infant slept, or in a separate room. Each camera generated its own screen on the TV monitor and thus one could get clear recordings of where the infant was, who was with the infant, who entered and exited the room, and any parent-infant interactions that took place. Video setup was done in such a way that the parent could flip just one switch on a surge protector to activate the entire system. Parents were asked to turn on the system at the point they began putting their infants to bed.

Infant and parent behavior during bedtimes and infant night wakings were coded using an interval sampling (30 second) procedure, in which the presence or absence of specific behaviors was documented in each interval. Separate summary variables were derived for bedtimes and night times. The end of bedtime (and the beginning of night time) was defined by 10 consecutive intervals of the infant being asleep (i.e., 5 minutes of continuous infant sleep). Video data were coded by two coders, trained by the first author, both of whom were blind to other data on the families. Two maternal behaviors were coded from bedtime and nighttime videos: (1) maternal presence, or the total number of intervals mothers spent in proximity to the infant (i.e., by the infant's bedside, in the infant's same room), and (2) close mother-infant physical contact. Total scores for these two variables were obtained by summing the number of intervals in which each occurred and then dividing by the total number of intervals for either bedtime or night-time. Inter-rater reliability (between two coders) on summary behavior codes, based on 10 videos that were equally distributed across the 1, 3, 6, 12, and 24-month age groups, was quite adequate (bedtime: mean intraclass correlation = .89; night-time: mean intraclass correlation = .91).

8. Results

This study yielded a number of linkages between maternal depressive symptoms, dysfunctional cognitions about infant sleep, maternal behavior, and infant night waking. To begin, after first controlling for infant age, mothers' depressive symptoms were correlated with mothers' worries about infant nighttime needs, r (40) = .41, $p < .01$, and with mothers' feelings of helplessness/loss of control, $r(42) = .47$, $p < .01$. Interestingly, mothers' worries about infant nighttime needs and feelings of helplessness/loss of control were not associated. Consistent with earlier reports (Armitage et al., 2009; Meltzer & Mindell, 2007; Morrell & Steele, 2003; Tikotsky & Sadeh, 2009), maternal depressive symptoms and maternal worries about infant nighttime needs were each associated with infant night waking, $r(42) = .40$, $p < .01$ and $r(40) = .36$, $p < .05$, respectively, and each was also associated with mothers' presence and close physical contact with infants during the night (rs ranged from .33 to .45, all $p < .05$), but not during bedtime. By contrast, maternal reports of helplessness/loss of control were not associated with infant night waking and correlated with only one measure of maternal behavior, close physical contact with infant at night, r(37) = .32, $p < .05$. Thus, the bulk of associations involving mothers' depressive symptoms and dysfunctional cognitions about infant sleep behavior were with nighttime (not bedtime) infant and maternal behavior, and of the two dimensions of dysfunctional cognitions, mothers' worries about infant nighttime needs was the stronger predictor. Finally, although measures of maternal behavior at bedtime did not correlate with infant night waking, both maternal presence with infants at night, and close mother-infant physical contact during the night, were associated with infant night waking [$r(37) = .61$, $p < .001$ and $r(37) = .37$, $p < .05$, respectively].

Criteria outlined by Baron and Kenny (1986) and MacKinnon (2008) were used to test the mediational models depicted in Figures 1, 2, and 3. Preliminary criteria to be satisfied for mediation include (a) the predictor variable(s) must correlate with the putative mediator variable, (b) the predictor variable(s) must correlate with the "criterion" variable, and (c) the mediator variable must correlate with the criterion variable. These criteria were satisfied for one variable tetrad: maternal depressive symptoms, mothers' worries about infant nighttime needs, maternal presence with infants at night, and infant night waking. Full mediation is supported if (a) specific tests of the mediated pathway are statistically significant, and (b) the link between the predictor and criterion variable is no longer significant after statistically controlling for the mediator variable. If the predictor-criterion variable link remains significant after statistically controlling for the mediator, partial mediation can still be supported if the mediated pathway is still found to be significant. The significance of the mediated pathways was assessed using a regression-based bootstrapping procedure outlined by MacKinnon (2008).

Support was obtained for the mother-driven, mediation model depicted in Figure 1. The specific mediational path from maternal depressive symptoms to maternal presence with infants at night to infant night waking was significant, as was the specific mediated path from maternal worries about infant nighttime needs to maternal presence to infant night waking. In addition, when maternal presence with infants at night was statistically controlled, the links between maternal depressive symptoms and infant night waking, and between maternal worries about infant nighttime needs and infant night waking, were no longer statistically significant. However, support for each of the infant-driven models of influence, depicted in Figures 2 and 3, was not obtained, although we note that the mediated paths in both approached significance (p = .08 and p = .06, respectively).

Thus, when comparing mother-driven vs. infant-driven models of influence in accounting for associations between maternal depressive symptoms and infant night waking, Teti and Crosby (in press) found more robust support for mother-driven paths of influence. Stronger support was obtained for the mediated pathway in which maternal depressive symptoms predicted maternal presence with infants at night, which in turn predicted infant night waking, and for the mediated pathway in which mothers' worries about infant nighttime needs predicted maternal presence with infants at night, which in turn predicted infant night waking. Importantly, additional qualitative observations of maternal behavior with their infants at night lent support to the premise that mothers with elevated depressive symptoms may be predisposed to spend more time with their infants at night and possibly engage in behaviors with them that disrupts infant sleep. Teti and Crosby used a cutoff SCL-90 Depression subscale score of 11 to differentiate mothers with high (M = 16.75) vs. low (M = 4.77) depressive symptom levels and examined their behavior with their infants throughout the night. Although most mothers (88%) engaged in calming bedtime routines with their infants (typically feeding younger infants and activities such as reading with those who were older), mothers reporting higher depressive symptoms represented a majority (75%) of those who did not have a calming bedtime routine for their infant. During infant bedtimes, these mothers had the television on, allowed older children to play rough/make loud noises near the infant, appeared insensitive to the infant's needs (e.g., hunger), and kept their infants awake after the infant appeared ready for sleep.

Teti and Crosby (in press) reported on several specific behaviors observed among mothers with higher depressive symptoms that seemed to impact infants' ability to maintain sleep and/or soothe themselves back to sleep during the night. Mothers who reported higher depressive symptoms were observed responding very quickly to infant vocalizations. For example, one mother of a 12-month-old infant appeared to be hyper-attentive to her infant during the night. She responded to non-distressed vocalizations very quickly throughout the night (sometimes <40 seconds) and nursed her infant three times in a period of less than 10 hours. Two other mothers were observed waking their sleeping infants unexpectedly during the night. One mother of a 1-month-old infant, for example, woke her non-distressed, sleeping infant during the night (i.e., not for the purposes of feeding) and brought the baby to the parents' bed for the rest of the night. This behavior was only observed among mothers reporting higher symptoms of depression. A final behavior observed included mothers' inability to set appropriate limits with their children after bedtime and during the night, especially among older children. Although most mothers were able to establish effective limits, a majority (60%) of those who were not able to were those who reported higher symptoms of depression. The most striking example of this was a mother who appeared unable to structure bedtime for her 24-month-old infant. As the rest of the family went to sleep, this infant remained awake until 2:00 a.m. watching a TV that remained on in the bedroom, occasionally wandering out of the bedroom to other areas of the home. This mother eventually brought her infant close to her and held her until she fell asleep.

In sum, although most mothers implemented a calming bedtime routine, ignored non-distressed vocalizations, and had children who sleep through the night (aside from expected night feedings for younger infants), Teti and Crosby (in press) found that mothers reporting more depressive symptoms displayed much more variability in nighttime interactions with their infants, intervened with their infants when there did not appear to a clear need for intervention (e.g., going to the infant when the infant was awake but not distressed, or when the infant was sound asleep), and had difficulty setting limits with their infants during bedtime and at night. Caution must be exercised in drawing conclusions about causality in this cross-sectional data set. Although statistical support was obtained for depressed mother-driven influences on infant night waking, the mediated paths in the two infant-driven models tests approached significance, and we propose that both mother- and infant-driven influences are at work in accounting for links between maternal depression and infant night waking. In some cases, mothers with high depressive symptom levels or excessive worries about their infants' well-being at night (which were strongly correlated with depressive symptoms) may be more likely than low-distress mothers to seek out their infants and engage in behaviors that increase infant wake time at night. In other cases, infants with chronic night waking problems (e.g., night waking accompanied by signaled distress) could lead to increased maternal intervention and, over time, increased maternal distress.

This data, however, suggest that mother-driven models of influence are worthy of further study, because very little is currently known about the effects of maternal depression on parenting at night, and on the consequences of depressed maternal nighttime parenting on infant development. Mothers with elevated depressive symptoms may be more likely than nondepressed mothers to seek out and spend more time with their infants at night, perhaps to satisfy unmet maternal emotional needs. Further, mothers who worry excessively about their infants' well-being at night (and such mothers tend to have elevated depressive symptom levels) may similarly seek out and intervene with their infants, regardless of whether or not intervention is needed, in order to reduce mothers' anxieties about their infants' physical and emotional needs. What is clear from these data is that parent-infant sleep patterns are complexly co-regulated and that more observational studies need to be conducted to determine what parenting looks like in child sleep contexts, how depressed parenting at night differs from nondepressed parenting, and what these differences portend for child development long-term.

9. Conclusions

Maternal depression can have serious consequences for children in social, emotional, and cognitive developmental domains, and children of depressed parents are 4-to-5-times as likely as children of nondepressed mothers to be at risk for behavior problems. Children's risk for behavioral disturbances appears to be directly proportional to the chronicity and severity of mothers' depression. Even very short bouts of maternal depression appear to have an emotionally dysregulating effect on infants as young as three months of age, and postpartum depression that is recurrent places infants at risk for insecure attachment. Children who grow up in households with depressed mothers are at risk for elevated psychiatric symptoms, both internalizing and externalizing, and to develop psychiatric disorders along a broad spectrum, including depressive and anxiety disorders, oppositional defiant disorder, and conduct disorder. Mechanisms of parent-to-child transmission have focused primarily on the impact of depressogenic mothering, although there is also evidence that depression is partially heritable. Importantly, depression's effects on mothering, and on children's development, are heterogeneous and may be buffered or exacerbated by a variety of additional parent, child, and environmental influences. Understanding the effects of maternal depression in the context of other risk and protective factors is a worthy goal for the field.

Happily, depression ranks as one of the more treatable psychiatric disorders. Women who suffer from postpartum depression can avail themselves of a variety of treatment approaches, including pharmacological, psychotherapeutic (e.g., cognitive-behavioral, psychodynamic, and support-based "talking" therapies), or some combination. In addition, approaches that target mother-child interactions have also been successful, in particular when maternal depression co-occurs with skill deficits in mothering. All of these treatment approaches have been effective, to varying degrees, in reducing symptom severity and improving quality of mothering. Pediatricians are likely to be the first health professionals to identify postpartum depression. It is thus important to equip pediatricians with the training and assessment tools to screen for postpartum depression, and to refer mothers to the appropriate mental health facilities for further evaluation and treatment.

Mothers who suffer from depression clearly need help, not just for themselves but for their children. Continued research is needed to understand more clearly the heterogeneous nature of maternal depression and its effects, what role maternal, child, spousal, and family characteristics play in this regard, and to develop effective interventions. Efforts to increase public awareness of postpartum depression and its effects on children are also critically important, if only because such awareness could lead to more mothers seeking treatment.

10. Acknowledgments

In press, in V. Olisah (Ed.), *Mental Health*, InTech Open Access Publisher

This chapter was supported by NIH Grant # R01HD052809. We wish to express our appreciation to all families who have participated in this project, and to the many graduate and undergraduate assistants who have assisted in data collection, coding, and analysis.

11. References

Abramson, L. Y., Metalsky, G. I., & Alloy, L. B. (1989). Hopelessness depression: A theory-based subtype of depression. *Psychological Review, 96(2)*, 358-372. DOI: 10.1037/0033-295X.96.2.358

Adair, R., Bauchner, H., Phillip, B., Levenson, S., & Zuckerman, B. (1991). Night waking during infancy: Role of parental presence at bedtime. Pediatrics, 87, 500-504.

Ainsworth, M.D.S., Blehar, M. C., Waters, E., & Wall, S. (1978). Patterns of attachment: A psychological study of the Strange Situation. Hillsdale, NJ: Erlbaum.

American Psychiatric Association (2000). Diagnostic and Statistical Manual of Mental Disorders (4th ed., text revision). Washington, DC. Author.

Armitage, R., Flynn, H., Hoffman, R., Vazquez, D., Lopez, J., & Marcus, S. (2009). Earlydevelopmental changes in sleep in infants: The impact of maternal depression. Sleep: Journal of Sleep and Sleep Disorders Research, 32(5), 693-696.

Armstrong, K. L., O'Donnell, H., McCallum, R., & Dadds, M. (1998). Childhood sleep problems: Association with prenatal factors and maternal distress/depression. Journal of Paediatrics and Child Health 34(3), 263-266.

Arnow, B. A., Blasey, C. M., Hunkeler, E. M., Lee, J., & Hayward, C. (2011). Does gender moderate the relationship between childhood maltreatment and adult depression? *Child Maltreatment, 16(3)*, 175-183.

Atkinson, E., Vetere, A., & Grayson, K. (1995). Sleep disruption in young children. The influence of temperament on the sleep patterns of pre-school children. Child: Care, Health and Development, 21, 233-246. doi:10.1111/j.1365-2214.1995.tb00754.x

Balta, G., & Paparrigopoulos, T., (2010). Comorbid anxiety and depression: Diagnostic issues and treatment management. *Psychiatriki, 21(2),* 107-114.

Bandura, A. (1986). Social foundations of thought and action: a social cognitive theory. Englewood Cliffs, NJ: Prentice-Hall, 1986.

Baron, RM, & Kenny, DA (1986). The moderator-mediator variable distinction in social psychological research: Conceptual, strategic, and statistical considerations. Journal of Personality and Social Psychology, 51, 1173-1182. DOI: 10.1037/0022-3514.51.6.1173

Bayer, J. K., Hiscock, H., Hampton, A., & Wake, M. (2007). Sleep problems in young infants and maternal mental and physical health. Journal of Paediatrics and Child Health, 43(1-2), 66-73. DOI: 10.1111/j.1440-1754.2007.01005.x

Beck, A. (1987). Cognitive models of depression. *Journal of Cognitive Psychotherapy, 1(1),* 5-37.

Beck, R., Perkins, T. S., Holder, R., Robbins, M., Gray, M., & Allison, S. H. (2001). The cognitive and emotional phenomenology od depression and anxiety: Are worry and hopelessness the cognitive correlates of NA and PA? *Cognitive Therapy and Research, 25(6),* 829 – 838.

Beck, A. T., Steer, R. A., & Garbin, M. G. (1988). Psychometric properties of the Beck Depression Inventory: Twenty-five years of evaluation. *Clinical Psychology Review, 8(1),* 77-100.

Bowlby, J. (1969). *Attachment and loss. Volume 1: Attachment.* New York, NY: Basic Books.

Brieger, P., Ehrt, U., Bloeink, R., Marneros, A. (2002). Consequences of comorbid personality disorders in major depression. Journal of Nervous and Mental Disease, 190(5), 304-309.

Bretherton, I. (2005). In pursuit of the internal working model construct and its relevance to attachment relationships. In K. E. Grossmann, K. Grossmann, & E. Waters (Eds.), *Attachment from infancy to adulthood: The major longitudinal studies* (pp. 13-47). New York, NY: Guilford.

Bugental, D. B., & Happaney, K. (2004). Predicting infant maltreatment in low-income families: The interactive effects of maternal attributions and child status at birth. *Developmental Psychology, 40(2),* 234-243.

Burnham, M.M., Goodlin-Jones, B.L., Gaylor, E.E., & Anders, T.F. (2002). Nighttime sleep-wake patterns and self-soothing from birth to one year of age: A longitudinal intervention study. Journal of Child Psychology and Psychiatry, 43, 713-725. doi:10.1111/14697610.00076

Campbell, S. B. Cohn, J. F. (1995). The timing and chronicity of postpartum depression: Implications for infant development. In L. Murray & P. J. Cooper (Eds.), Postpartum depression and child development (165-197). New York, NY, Guilford.

Campbell, S. B., Cohn, J. F., & Meyers, T. (1995). Depression in first-time mothers: Mother-infant interaction and depression chronicity. *Developmental Psychology, 31(3),* 349-357.

Campbell, S. B., Matestic, P., von Stauffenberg, C., Mohan, R., & Kirchner, T. (2007). Trajectories of maternal depressive symptoms, maternal sensitivity, and children's functioning at school entry. *Developmental Psychology, 43(5),* 1202-1215.

Carter, A. S., Garrity-Rokous, F. E., Chazan-Cohen, R., Little, C., & Briggs-Gowan, M. J. (2001). Maternal depression and comorbidity : Predicting early parenting, attachment security, and toddler social-emotional problems and competencies : Assessment of Infant and Toddler Mental Health : Advances and Challenges. *Journal of the American Academy of Child and Adolescent Psychiatry, 40(1),* 18-26.

Cassidy, J., & Berlin, L. (1994). The insecure/ambivalent pattern of attachment: Theory and research. Child Development, 65, 971-991

Cassidy, J., Kobak, R. R. (1988). Avoidance and its relation to other defensive processes. In J. Belsky & T. Nezworski (Eds.), Clinical implications of attachment (pp. 300-323). Hillsdale, NJ: Erlbaum

Clark, D. A. (2001). The persistent problem of negative cognition in anxiety and depression: New perspectives and old controversies. *Behavior Therapy,* 32, 3-12.

Cohn, J. F., & Tronick, E. Z. (1983). Three-month-old infants' reaction to simulated maternal depression. *Child Development, 54(1),* 185-193.

Cole, P. M., Michel, M. K., & Teti, L. O. (1994). The development of emotion regulation and dysregulation: A clinical perspective. Monographs of the Society for Research in Child Development, 59(2-3), 73-100.

Cornish, A. M., McMahan, C. A., Ungerer, J. A., Barnett, B., Kowalenko, N., & Tennant, C. (2006). Maternal depression and the experience of parenting in the second postnatal year. *Journal of Reproductive and Infant Psychology, 24(2),* 121-132. DOI: 10.1080/02646830600644021

Crittenden, P. M. (1992). Quality of attachment in the preschool years. *Development and Psychopathology, 4(2),* 209-241.

Davidson, M. B., Echeverry, D., Katon, W. J., Lin, E., & Von Korff, M. (2011). Collaborative care for depression and chronic illnesses. *The New England Journal of Medicine, 364 (13),* 1278-1279.

DeLeon, C.W. & Karraker, K.H. (2007). Intrinsic and extrinsic factors associated with night waking in 9-month-old infants. Infant Behavior & Development, 30, 596-605. doi:10.1016/j.infbeh.2007.03.009

Dennis, C-L., & Ross, L. (2005). Relationships among infant sleep patterns, maternal fatigue, and development of depressive symptomatology. Birth, 32(3), 187-193. DOI: 10.1111/j.0730-7659.2005.00368.x

Derogatis, L. R. (1994). SCL-90 Symptom Checklist-90-R: Administration, scoring, and procedures manual. Minneapolis, MN: National Computer Systems.

Diego, M. A., Field, T., & Hernandez-Reif, M. (2005). Prepartum, postpartum and chronic depression effects on neonatal behavior. Infant Behavior and Development, 28, 155-164.

Dietz, L. J., Jennings, K. D., Kelley, S. A., Marshal, M. (2009). Maternal depression, paternal psychopathology, and toddlers' behavior problems. *Journal of Clinical Child and Adolescent Psychology, 38(1)*, 48-61.

Field, T., Diego, M., & Hernandez-Reif, M. (2006). Prenatal depression effects on the fetus and newborn: A review. *Infant Behavior and Development, 29(3)*, 445-455.

Field, T., Diego, M., Hernandez-Reif, M., Figueiredo, B., Schanberg, S., & Kuhn, C. (2007). Sleep disturbances in depressed pregnant women and their newborns. Infant Behavior and Development, 30(1), 127-133. DOI: 10.1016/j.infbeh.2006.08.002

Field, T. Diego, M., Hernandez-Reif, M., Figueiredo, B., & Schanberg, S. (2008). Chronic Prenatal depression and neonatal outcome. *International Journal of Neuroscience, 118(1)*, 95-103.

Fleming, A. S., Ruble, D. N., Flett, G. L., & Shaul, D. L. (1988). Postpartum adjustment in first-time mothers: Relations between mood, maternal attitudes, and mother-infant interactions. *Developmental Psychology, 24(1)*, 71-81. DOI: 10.1037/0012-1649.24.1.71

Foster, C. J. E., Garber, J., & Durlak, J. A. (2008). Current and past maternal depression, maternal interaction behaviors, and children's externalizing and internalizing symptoms. *Journal of Abnormal Child Psychology: An official publication of the International Society for Research in Child and Adolescent Psychopathology,* 36(4), 527-537.

Franić, S., Middeldorp, C. M., Dolan, C. V., Ligthart, L., & Boomsma, D. I. (2010). Childhood and adolescent anxiety and depression: Beyond heritability. *Journal of the American Academy of Child & Adolescent Psychiatry, 49(8)*, 820-829.

Gallagher, R. W., Hobfoll, S. E., Ritter, C., Lavin, J. (1997). Marriage, intimate support and depression during pregnancy: A study of inner-city women. *Journal of Health Psychology, 2(4)*, 457-469.

Gartstein, M. A., Bridgett, D. J., Rothbart, M. K., Robertson, C., Iddins, E., Ramsay, K., & Schlect, S. (2010). A latent growth examination of fear development in infancy: Contributions of maternal depression and the risk for toddler anxiety. *Developmental Psychology, 46(3)*, 651-668.

Gelfand, D. M., & Teti, D. M. (1990). The effects of maternal depression on children. Clinical Psychology Review, 10, 329-353.

Goodman, S. H., & Gotlib, I. H. (2002) (Eds). *Children of depressed parents: Mechanisms of risk and implications for treatment.* Washington, DC, US: American Psychological Association.

Grant, T. M., Jack, D. C., Fitzpatrick, A. L.& Ernst, C.C. (2011). Carrying the burdens of poverty, parenting, and addiction: Depression symptoms and self-silencing among ethnically diverse women. *Community Mental Health Journal, 47 (1)*, 90-98.

Gress-Smith, J. L., Luecken, L. J., Lemery-Chafant, K. & Howe, R. (2011). Postpartum depression prevalence and impact of infant health, weight, and sleep in low-income and ethnic minority women and infants. Maternal and Child Health Journal. DOI 10.1007/s10995-011-0812-y

Gross, H. E., Shaw, D. S., Burwell, R. A., & Nagin, D. S. (2009). Transactional processes in child disruptive behavior and maternal depression: A longitudinal study from early childhood to adolescence. *Development and Psychopathology, 21(1),* 139-56.

Guttmann-Steinmetz, S., & Crowell, J. A. (2006). Attachment and externalizing disorders: A developmental psychopathology perspective. *Journal of the American Academy of Child & Adolescent Psychiatry, 45,* 440-451.

Hamilton, M. A. (1960). A rating scale for depression. *Journal of Neurology, Neurosurgery, and Psychiatry, 23,* 56-62. doi: 10.1136/jnnp.23.1.56

Hesse, E. (2008). The Adult Attachment Interview: Protocol, method of analysis, and empirical studies. In Handbook of attachment: Theory, research, and clinical applications (2nd ed.) (J. Cassidy & P. R. Shaver, Eds..) (pp. 552-598). New York, NY: Guilford.

Hiscock, H., & Wake, M. (2001). Infant sleep problems and postnatal depression: A community-based study. Pediatrics, 107(6), 1317-1322.

Hiscock, H., & Wake, M. (2002). Randomised controlled trial of behavioural infant sleep intervention to improve infant sleep and maternal mood. British Medical Journal, 324(7345), 1062-1065. DOI: 10.1136/bmj.324.7345.1062

Johnson, C.M. (1991). Infant and toddler sleep: A telephone survey of parents in one community. Developmental and Behavioral Pediatrics, 12, 108-114.

Leahy-Warren, P., McCarthy, G., & Corcoran, P. (2011). Postnatal depression in first-time mothers: Prevalence and relationships between functional and structural social support at 6 and 12 weeks postpartum. Archives of Psychiatric Nursing, 25(3), 174-184.

Leckman-Westin, E., Cohen, P. R., & Stueve, A. (2009). Maternal depression and mother-child interaction patterns: association with toddler problems and continuity of effects to late childhood. *Journal of Child Psychology and Psychiatry, 50(9),* 1176-1184.

Lyons-Ruth, K., Connell, D. B., Grunebaum, H. U., & Botein, S. (1990). Infants at social risk: Maternal depression and family support services as mediators of infant development and security of attachment. Child Development,61(1), 85-98.

MacKinnon, D. P. (2008). Introduction to statistical mediation analysis. New York: Erlbaum.

Main, M., & Cassidy, J. (1988), Categories of response to reunion with the parent at age 6: Predictable from infant attachment classifications and stable over a 1-month period. Developmental Psychology, 24, 415-426.

Main, M.; Solomon, J. (1990). Procedures for identifying infants as disorganized/disoriented during the Ainsworth Strange Situation. In M. T. Greenberg, D. Cicchetti, & E. M.

Cummings (Eds.), Attachment in the preschool years: Theory, research, and intervention. The John D. and Catherine T. MacArthur Foundation series on mental health and development (pp. 121-160). Chicago, IL: University of Chicago Press.

Mao, A., Burnham, M.M, Goodlin-Jones, B.L., Gaylor, E.E., & Anders, T.F. (2004). A comparison of the sleep-wake patterns of cosleeping and solitary-sleeping infants. Child Psychiatry and Human Development, 35, 95-105. doi:10.1007/s10578-004-1879-0

McLoyd, V. C. (1998). Socioeconomic disadvantage and child development. American Psychologist, 53, 185-204.

Mindell, J. A., Kuhn, B., Lewin, D. S., Meltzer, L. J., & Sadeh, A. (2006). Behavioral treatment of bedtime problems and night wakings in infants and young children. *Sleep: Journal of Sleep and Sleep Disorders Research, 29*, 1263-1276.

Mindell, J. A., Meltzer, L. J., Carskadon, M. A., & Chervin, R. D. (2009). Developmental aspects of sleep hygience: Findings from the 2004 National Sleep Foundation Sleep in America poll. Sleep Medicine, 10(7), 771-779. DOI: 10.1016/j.sleep.2008.07.016

Mindell, J. A., Sadeh, A., Kohyama, J., & How, T.H. (2010). Parental behaviors and sleep outcomes in infants and toddlers: A cross-cultural comparison. Sleep Medicine, 11, 393-399.

Mindell, J. A., Telofski, L. S., Wiegand, B., Kurtz, E. S. (2009). A nightly bedtime routine: Impact on sleep in young children and maternal mood. Sleep: Journal of Sleep and Sleep Disorders Research, 32(5), 599-606.

Morrell, J., & Cortina-Borja, M. (2002). The developmental change in strategies parents employto settle young children to sleep, and their relationship to infant sleeping problems, as assessed by a new questionnaire: The parental interactive bedtime behavior scale. Infant and Child Development, 11, 17-41. doi:10.1002/icd.251

Morrell, J. M. B. (1999). The role of maternal cognitions in infant sleep problems as assessed by a new instrument, the Maternal Cognitions about Infant Sleep Questionnaire. *Journal of Child Psychology and Psychiatry, 40(2)*, 247-258. DOI 10.1111/1469-7610.00438

Morrell, J., & Steele, H. (2003). The role of attachment security, temperament, maternal perception, and care-giving behavior in persistent infant sleeping problems. Infant Mental Health Journal, 24, 447-468. doi:10.1002/imhj.10072

Moss, E., Cyr, C., Dubois-Comtois, K. (2004). Attachment at early school age and developmental risk: examining family contexts and behavior problems of controlling-caregiving, controlling-punitive, and behaviorally disorganized children. *Developmental Psychology, 40(4)*, 519-532.

Nolen-Hoeksema, S. (1990). *Sex differences in depression.* Stanford University Press.

O'Connor, T. G., Caprariello, P., Blackmore, E. R., Gregory, A. M., Glover, V., & Fleming, P. (2007). Prenatal mood disturbance predicts sleep problems in infancy and toddlerhood. Early Human Development, 83(7), 451-458. DOI: 10.1016/j.earlhumdev.2006.08.006

Radke-Yarrow M. (1998). Children of depressed mothers. New York, NY: Cambridge University Press.

Radloff, L. S. (1977). The CES-D scale: A self-report depression scale for research in the general population. *American Psychological Measurement, 1*, 385-401.

Sadeh, A., Flint-Ofir, E., Tirosh, T., Tikotzky, L. (2007). Infant sleep and parental sleep related cognitions. *Journal of Family Psychology, 21*, 74-87. DOI: 10.1037/0893-3200.21.1.74

Sadeh, A., Tikotzky, L., & Scher, A. (2010). Parenting and infant sleep. Sleep Medicine Reviews 14 (2), 89-96. DOI: 10.1016/j.smrv.2009.05.003

Smith, M., Calam, R., & Bolton, C. (2009). Psychological factors linked to self-reported depression symptoms in late adolescence. *Behavioural and Cognitive Psychotherapy, 37(1)*, 73-85.

Sroufe. L. A. (2005). Attachment and development: A prospective, longitudinal study from birth to adulthood. Attachment and Human Development, 7, 349-367.

Teti, D. M. (1999), Conceptualizations of disorganization in the preschool years: An integration. In J. Solomon & C. George (Eds.), Attachment disorganization (pp. 213-242). New York, NY: Guilford.

Teti, D. M., & Cole, P. M. (2011). Parenting at risk: New perspectives, new approaches.*Journal of Family Psychology, 25(5)*, 625-634.

Teti, D. M., & Crosby, B. (in press). Maternal depressive symptoms, dysfunctional cognitions, and infant night waking. The role of maternal night-time behavior. *Child Development.*

Teti, D. M., & Gelfand, D. M. (1991). Behavioral competence among mothers of infants in the first year: The mediational role of maternal self-efficacy. *Child Development, 62(5),* 918-929. DOI: 10.2307/1131143

Teti, D. M., & Gelfand, D. M. (1997). Maternal cognitions as mediators of child outcome in the context of postpartum depression. In L. Murray and P. J. Cooper (Eds.), *Postpartum depression and child development.* (pp. 136-164). New York: Guilford.

Teti, D. M., Gelfand, D. M., Messinger, D., & Isabella, R. (1995). Maternal depression and the quality of early attachment: An examination of infants, preschoolers, and their mothers. *Developmental Psychology*, 31, 364-376.

Teti, D. M., & Huang, K.Y. (2005). Developmental perspectives on parenting competence. In D. M Teti (Ed.), *Handbook of research methods in developmental science.* (pp. 161- 182). Malden, MA: Blackwell.

Teti, D. M., & Towe-Goodman, N. (2008). Post-partum depression, effects on child. In M. Haith & J. Benson (Eds.), Encyclopedia of infant & early child development. Oxford, UK: Elsevier.

Tikotzky, L., & Sadeh, A. (2009). Maternal sleep-related cognitions and infant sleep: A longitudinal study from pregnancy through the 1st year. *Child Development, 80(3),* 860-874. DOI: 10.1111/j.1467-8624.2009.01302.x

Tikotzky, L., Sadeh, A., & Glickman-Gavrieli, T. (2010). Infant sleep and paternal involvement in infant caregiving during the first 6 months of life. Journal of Pediatric Psychology, 36, 36-46.

Tikotzky, L., Sharabany, R., Hirsch, I., & Sadeh, A. (2010). "Ghosts in the nursery": Infant sleep and sleep-related cognitions of parents raised under communal sleeping arrangements. Infant Mental Health Journal, 31(3), 312-312-334. doi:10.1002/imhj.20258

Wachs, T. D., Black, M. M., & Engle, P. L. (2009). Maternal depression: A global threat to Children's health, development, and behavior and to human rights. *Child Development Perspectives, 3(1),* 51-59.

Warren, S. L., Howe, G., Simmens, S. J., & Dahl, R. E. (2006). Maternal depressive symptoms and child sleep: Models of mutual influence over time. Development and Psychopathology, 18(1), 1-16. DOI: 10.1017/S0954579406060019

Whiffen, V. E., & Gotlib, I. H. (1989). Stress and coping in martially distressed and nondistressed couples. *Journal of Social and Personal Relationships, 6(3),* , 327-344. DOI: 10.1037/0021-843X.98.3.274

Zimmer-Gembeck, M. J., Waters, A. M., & Kindermann, T. (2010). A social relations analysis of liking for and by peers: Associations with gender, depression, peer perception, and worry. Journal of Adolescence, 33(1), 69-81.

Zuckerman, B., Stevenson, J., & Bailey, V. (1987). Sleep problems in early childhood: Continuities, predictive factors, and behavioral correlates. Pediatrics, 80(5), 664-671.

20

Developmental Aspects of Parental Mental Health and Child Development

For-Wey Lung[1,2] and Bih-Ching Shu[3]
[1]*Taipei City Psychiatric Center, Taipei City Hospital, Taipei*
[2]*Department of Psychiatry, National Defense Medical Center, Taipei*
[3]*Institute of Allied Health Sciences and Department of Nursing, National Cheng Kung University, Tainan, Taiwan*

1. Introduction

Scientists and parents alike have pondered the development of infants in the first few months of life: their physical growth, motor development, ability to think, language development, and building of social relationships. More importantly, does their early relationship with their parents shape their development? An important factor which may influence the parent-child relationship and interaction is the mental health condition of the mother. A study has shown that although mothers with and without depressed symptoms both show the same concern for their children's safety and feeding, differences can be found in the finer interactions with their children (McLearn et al., 2006). Mothers who do not have a healthy mental state may not provide a positive environment or interaction, which can diminish the children's motivation and interest in communication. Tough and colleagues (2008) further found that a mother's poor emotional health is a predictor for her child's developmental delay. Mothers need to have the ability to detect the needs of their children and respond positively to them. This positive interaction can then motivate the children to communicate, which stimulates their cognitive development (Sohr-Preston & Scaramella, 2006). Thus, maternal mental health plays an important role in child development.

Fathers have a moderating effect on the influence of the mothers on children's development. With the increase in the number of mothers entering the workforce, the roles fathers play in children's lives are also greater. Mezulis et al. (2004) found that paternal involvement can reduce the effect of maternal depressive symptoms on their children. The father's better mental health may decrease the negative influence that maternal poor mental health has on children's behavioral and emotional problems (Kahn et al., 2004). However, when both parents have poor mental health, the children will develop more severe behavioral and emotional problems (Kahn et al., 2004).

In addition, as early as seven months, infants are able to react to mood regulation and social interaction and can attempt to influence their parents (Kochanska & Akasan, 2004). Mothers of children who are born premature with autism spectrum disorder or other chronic illnesses experience higher parenting stress (Davis & Carter, 2008; Mussatto, 2006; Singer et al., 1999). Thus, not only does parental mental health affect children's development, but children's development can in turn affect maternal mental health.

Many other factors in the environment in which children grow up can also influence children's development. The triad of parental mental health, children's development and child-rearing context is important in understanding children's development. Of most importance, since this interaction is continuous, continuous follow-up is necessary to understand the possible reciprocal effect among these factors.

Both prospective and retrospective studies have been used to investigate the influence of parents on their children. Retrospective studies have generally used recollections of the influence of parental mental health on children, including adult recall of parenting skills on their personality characteristics and mental health state. On the other hand, prospective studies generally are longitudinal cohort studies, which have the advantage of no recall bias. A previous study found that in the investigation of lifetime prevalence of mental disorders, the number of prospective studies was double that of retrospective studies (Moffitt et al., 2010). This was due to the participants' underreporting of past disorder symptoms (Simon & VonKorff, 1995). However, since cohort studies are costly and time-consuming, and may have the problems of possible bias due to loss to follow-up (Cesar & Carvalho, 2011), both retrospective and prospective studies can provide valuable information regarding the effect of parents on their children.

2. Retrospective studies: the effect of parental attachment and mental health

The mental health condition of parents can affect their parenting style, for when mothers are in a state of emotional distress, or do not have the time and energy to care for their children, they may not be able to provide the positive interaction or environment that the child needs (Stein et al., 1991), which may increase children's distress and arousal and diminish their interest and motivation in communication (Field, 1995; Gauvain, 2001). It is well established that parenting style has an influence on children's later development, including the children's psychosocial development, academic achievement, and social competence, and the development of mental disorders (Lung, 2011; U.S. Census Bureau, 2004). Using Parker et al.'s theory (1979), parental bonding can be separated into the two dimensions of care and protection. A high level of care indicates warmth, and a low level implies neglect. On the other hand, a high level of protection implies over-protection and control, and a low level indicates encouragement of autonomy and independence. Thus, a parenting style with a high level of care and a low level of protection has generally been found to be better for the mental health of children (Huppert et al., 2010; Lung, 2011). A series of studies have found that the influence of parental bonding on mental health is mediated by personality characteristics (see review in Lung, 2011). Parenting rearing behaviors can influence children's development in terms of behavior, personality, interpersonal relationships and the ability to adjust (Parker & Gladstone, 1996). Lung et al. (2002) and Chen et al. (2011) both found that males who were overprotected by their mothers had higher neuroticism and lower extraversion, which increased their risk of developing adjustment disorder. Similarly, maternal overprotection can lead to a greater tendency to develop neurotic personality characteristics, which may affect the individual's mental health status and contribute to the development of hyperventilation syndrome (Shu et al., 2007; Lung et al., in press). This is understandable, since mothers are the main caregivers.

Thus, the molding of an individual's personality and that person's ability to adjust psychologically are influenced by their attachment to their parents (Bowlby, 1977). Besides mental illnesses, parenting style has also been found to contribute to the tendency to commit offenses, and to develop antisocial behavior and poor interpersonal relationships (Clifford, 1959). The above-mentioned retrospective studies all found parental rearing style to play a vital role in the development of children's mental health and behavior.

3. Prospective cohort studies

As stated earlier, retrospective studies have the possibility of recall bias, but cohort studies or even birth cohort studies can provide us with a longitudinal understanding of how conditions develop overtime and how exposures in childhood can influence outcomes later in life (Thompson et al., 2010). For instance, the British cohort study, which started in 1970, is one of the longest-standing birth cohort studies with the largest existing sample (Thompson et al., 2010) showing that parental style affects children well into adulthood (Huppert et al., 2010). However, secular changes have caused differences in family structures. In the British cohort study, mothers are generally stay-at-home moms and the rate of separation and divorce is much lower (Huppert et al., 2010). In addition, the mean maternal and paternal age has also increased (Bray et al., 2006). In fact, most of mental disorders are emotional disorders. Categorical diagnoses have to pay attention to environmental factors (Horwitz & Wakefield 2007). On the other hand, Anna Freud (1965) argued against adopting a symptomatological diagnostic system for psychopathology, advocating instead the evaluation of disturbances in children based on their abilities to perform age-appropriate developmental tasks. For instance, the studies of serotonin related polymorphism associated with depression vulnerability and suicide (Chen et al., 2011; Hung et al., in press; Hung et al., 2011; Lin et al, 2009; Lung & Lee, 2008; Lung et al., 2011c). Genes interact with life events to create mental disorder (Caspi et al., 2003). The body is not a machine that built from a plan. Bodies are resilient as a product of natural selection overtime (Nesse & Stearns, 2008).

In the following sections we present recent findings from recent cohort or birth cohort studies regarding the relationship between parental mental health and children's development, and the factors mediating or confounding this relationship in Taiwan. Along with results from cohort studies worldwide, the results from the Taiwan Birth Cohort Study and the Taiwan Birth Cohort pilot Study were also presented. The Taiwan Birth Cohort Study is a national household study, which randomly sampled 21,648 infants and their family at birth, and followed up their development, parental health and environmental context factors (as shown in Appendix I). General population birth cohort studies can eliminate the bias from high risk populations and help us understand the phenomenon of common sporadic cases. For example, previous medical-center based studies have shown that taking care of children with autism spectrum disorder increases stress on both parents (Davis & Carter, 2008), and especially affects the mental health condition of the mothers (Shu et al., 2000). However, in the household probability sample database of the Taiwan Birth Cohort pilot Study, mothers who had perceived better physical health quality of life had increased concern regarding their children being at risk for autism spectrum disorder (as described in Lung et al., 2011b). We hypothesized this increased concern might be due to children who are brought to medical centers exhibiting more disruptive symptoms, and creating greater maternal distress, which is why their parents chose to seek help. However, since most studies on autism spectrum disorder are medical center-based samples, a health worker effect bias is shown in these studies, and the results may not be generalizable to all mothers of children with autism spectrum disorder. Thus, a household probability sample is important in understanding community-based factors which effect child development (Lung et al., 2011b).

3.1 The effect of parental mental health vs. education and age at childbirth on children's development

As mentioned in the introduction, the mental health of both parents has been found to have a vital impact on children's development. However, other important parental characteristics have also been found to impact children's development, and one of these is the parental level of education (Kolobe, 2004). The educational level of the mother has been found to impact the mother's dietary practices (Wachs et al., 2005), childbearing style (Kolobe, 2004) and breastfeeding, which affects children's cognitive development (Angelsen et al., 2001). Furthermore, the parental level of education has been found to be a stronger predictor for child well-being than family income, single parenthood or family size (Zill, 1996). Parental age at childbirth is another important factor which has been found to influence children's development. Parents who are either too young or too old at childbirth can have a potentially detrimental effect on children's development. Both teenage pregnancies and elder paternal age have been found to increase the rate of low birth weight (Li & Chang, 2005; Reichman & Teitler, 2006), which is associated with an increased risk of motor developmental delays (Liu et al., 2001).

The Taiwan Birth Cohort Study found the mental health of both parents had an effect on children's development, with maternal mental health having a more persistent and pervasive effect than paternal mental health (Lung et al., 2009b). Paternal mental health was not associated with children's six months' development, and was associated only with children's fine motor development at 18 months (Lung et al., 2009b). This may be because mothers are generally the main caregiver at infanthood, and paternal involvement in children's development increases over time (Bailey, 2004).

However, when the covariates of parental education and age were added, parental education had a more pervasive and persistent effect than parental mental health, showing that parental level of education is a vital confounding factor in children's development (Lung et al., 2009b). Lung et al. (2010b) further found the impact of maternal education on child development increases with time, and the effect of maternal mental health on child development decreases with time. This may be because the maternal level of education is a variable that does not change with time; however, the mother's own perceived mental health may change with time. Parents who are highly educated may have more access to up-to-date information regarding childcare and make better use of family and community resources (Guldan et al., 1993), thus promoting child development.

With regards to parental age, children of mothers who were older had better development, but children of fathers who were older had worse development at six months; however, this association dissipated at 18 months, showing only slower language development (Lung et al., 2009b). This is consistent with the results of the US Collaborative Perinatal Project, also a general population birth cohort study, which found an opposing effect of older paternal and maternal age on children's behavioral outcomes (Saha et al., 2009). In that study, advanced paternal age increased the risk of adverse externalizing behaviors, and advanced maternal age was found to be protective of adverse externalizing behaviors, but carried a risk of internalizing behavior outcomes (Saha et al., 2009). Furthermore, a New Zealand birth cohort study also found advanced maternal age to be associated with declining risks of educational underachievement, juvenile crime, substance misuse, and mental health problems (Fergusson & Woodward, 1999). In previous studies, older parental age has generally been shown to be a risk factor for children's development (Li & Chang, 2005; Liu et al., 2001; Reichman & Teitler, 2006), since older age is associated with a higher risk of low birth weight (Li & Chang, 2005; Reichman & Teitler, 2006), which is associated with motor developmental delay (Liu et al., 2001). One of the risks of being an older parent is the increase in the children's mortality rate (Donoso & Carvajal, 1999; Zhu et al., 2008), and if the mother's age at first birth was over 40, the rate of maternal health problems and birth complications was greatly increased (Gilbert et al., 1999). However, since birth cohort studies only included children who survived the birth mortality risk, we hypothesized that since older parents have had more time to build their wealth, establish a more stable marriage, and provide their children with better, more supportive nurturing and a stable home environment, the socioeconomic advantage would seemingly overtake the biological limitation of parental age.

A British and American cohort study investigated the association between women's young age at first childbirth and their mental health in midlife, and found that poorer mental health persisted in those who experienced early motherhood long after the birth itself (Henretta et al., 2008). Although young mothers from both Britain and the United States were from lower socioeconomic backgrounds, the association between mental health at midlife and early motherhood remained significant, even after the factor of socioeconomic background was controlled; however, this association became non-significant after the level of education was controlled (Henretta et al., 2008). Again, this showed the importance of controlling for the level of education and age at childbirth when investigating the mental health condition of the parents.

In conclusion, although parental mental health plays an important role in children's development, parental education and age at childbirth are vital confounding factors, which should be considered in future studies. Since the association of paternal mental health had a delayed effect on children's development (Lung et al., 2009b), follow-up of the long-term effect of parents on children's development is necessary. Health care workers should screen for the mental health condition of parents and provide appropriate treatment when necessary to prevent a future impact on children's development. Furthermore, special attention should be paid to young parents or those with a lower level of education. Health care workers should provide these parents with additional resources and childrearing skills when necessary to advance the children's development and prevent delays.

3.2 Reciprocal association between parental mental health and child development

In the previously mentioned study (Lung et al., 2009b), the uni-directional effect of parental mental health on children's development was investigated. However, we hypothesized that a bi-directional or reciprocal effect may exist in the relationship between parental mental health and children's development, since children may also affect the mental health of their parents. For instance, children of low birth weight are at higher risk of motor developmental delay (Cheung et al., 2001), which can potentially augment maternal distress (Singer et al., 1999). To adjust for the possible effect of the children's own characteristics of low birth weight or short gestational age on their development (Cheung et al., 2001), we included gestational age and weight at birth in our investigation of the reciprocal association of parental mental health and children's development (Lung et al., 2009a).

The Taiwan Birth Cohort pilot Study showed that parental mental health did not affect children's development until 36 months (Lung et al., 2009a). On the other hand, children's development affected maternal mental health at 6 months, and this effect expanded to the mental health of both parents at 18 and 36 months (Lung et al., 2009a). Parental mental health at 6 months had a delayed effect on children's development at 36 months (Lung et al., 2009a), implying that as early as 6 months, children were able to detect the emotional changes of their parents. A study found that as early as 3.5 months, infants were able to differentiate their mother's expressions (Montague & Walker-Andrews, 2002). Specifically, maternal mental health at 6 months affected children's 36 months' development, and paternal mental health at 6 months affected children's 36 months language development (Lung et al., 2009a). The stages of emotional development proposes that children learn to express emotions through modeling how others around them express their emotions with words, thus language is closely linked with children's ability to express emotion (Thomasgard & Metz, 2004). Furthermore, when children fail in an attempt to verbally express their emotions, they will express them by action (Thomasgard & Metz, 2004); therefore, children of mothers with mental symptoms are at higher risk of developing emotional and behavioral problems (Kahn et al., 2004). On the other hand, the Providence, Rhode Island birth cohort study found that a high level of maternal affection when the infants were 8 months old was associated with fewer symptoms of distress in the offspring 30 years later (Maselko et al., 2011).

In conclusion, increasing attention has been paid to the effect of parental mental health on their children (Kahn et al., 2004; Lung et al., 2009b; Ramchandani et al., 2005). However, we found that besides the effect of parental mental health on the children's development, a reciprocal effect of the children's developmental state on parental mental health was found (Lung et al., 2009a). In addition, the effect of parental mental health had a postponed effect on children's language and social development. Thus, future research should consider reciprocal effects when investigating the relationship between parental mental health and children's development. Clinicians should also take notice of the stress and mental health condition of the parents of children with developmental delay to prevent possible development of mental health symptoms. Intervention should be provided to these parents to alleviate their stress and mental health problems when necessary.

3.3 The relationship of paternal and maternal mental health

Lung et al. (2009a, 2009b) found that the mental health states of the father and mother were positively correlated with each other, and that when mothers had better mental health, fathers did too, and vice versa. This is consistent with previous studies which found that depression in one partner is correlated with depression in the other (Ballard et al., 1994; Ramchandani et al., 2008; Soliday et al., 1999). In further investigation, we found that the mental health of parents with children at high risk of autism spectrum disorder was not affected by the children's developmental condition, but rather, by maternal mental health. This is supported by a previous qualitative study showing that stress perceived by fathers of children with autism spectrum disorder was not associated with the children's characteristics but with their partner's mental health condition (Hastings et al., 2005). Along the same line, fathers of children with autism spectrum disorder were not affected by their children's condition (Gray, 2003), but the children's condition was associated with the mothers' condition, which in turn would affect the fathers (Gray, 2003). Mothers carry the main burden in the care-giving role, thus they are closely connected with the conditions of the children, while fathers serve more as backup support for the mothers (Gray, 2003).

3.4 Factors which can exacerbate or alleviate maternal mental health related to childcare

There are several factors which can alleviate or exacerbate maternal mental health conditions. Factors that have been found to be associated with maternal mental health included a perception of more family support, which led to better maternal mental health conditions (Wills, 1998). On the other hand, working mothers had worse mental health (Grice et al., 2007; Walker & Best, 1991). Nowadays, a higher percentage of mothers have entered the work force (U.S. Census Bureau, 2004), thus women have to take on multiple social roles, including the primary roles of employee, spouse, and parent (Repetti, 1998). These roles interact with each other, positive characteristics in one role have been found to reduce the impact of the strain of another role, and in turn, stressful experiences in one role can also cause a vulnerability to negative experiences in another role (Repetti, 1998). For instance, a study has shown that working mothers have the tendency to neglect their own health (Walker & Best, 1991), and dissatisfaction with the work-family balance has been found to result in negative mental health outcomes (Grice et al., 2007), showing that multiple roles can potentially drain the mother's energy, leading to a lower level of life satisfaction (Grice et al., 2007).

In contrast, social support is a health-promoting resource, and has a direct, positive effect on mental and physical health (Grice et al., 2007). Social support has been found to have a buffering effect on both the mental and physical health of women, lowering their risk of depression and mortality, and giving them a greater likelihood of recovery from clinical illnesses (Wills, 1998).

The spouse is an important source of support, thus a marriage of poor quality or the end of a marriage can also have an influence on the mental health of the mother (Dehle & Weiss, 1998; Whisman & Bruce, 1999). An Australian population birth cohort study found that a marital relationship of poor quality was associated with increased depressive symptoms in both mothers and children 7 years later (Clavarino et al., 2011). However, the mothers' depressive symptoms alleviated if they became single, although the children experienced an increase in depression (Clavarino et al., 2011).

Therefore, although mothers experience stress from childcare and this stress may increase if they are working at the same time, other factors can minimize this stress. Factors such as emotional and social resources, including positive marital adjustment, a sense of accomplishment in parenting, social support, and higher educational achievement can all serve as protective factors against stress-related somatic symptoms (Weiss, 2002).

4. Conclusion

These studies show that the mental health of both parents can impact children's development (Lung et al., 2009a, 2009b). Furthermore, mother's mental health is more closely tied to children's development, and fathers act more as a support for maternal mental health. All these studies show that parental mental health may have a delayed effect on children's development, showing the importance of longitudinal studies in the investigation of children's development.

Since social support has been shown to be an important factor alleviating mother's mental health (Grice et al., 2007), parent support programs for parents with greater stress could be implemented. An interesting phenomenon found in our studies is that the parental level of education has a great and enduring impact on children's development. Furthermore, since a sense of accomplishment in parenting can also ameliorate maternal mental health (Weiss, 2002), parental educational programs may be of assistance to parents with a lower level of education and help prevent the development of mental symptoms in the parents.

On the other hand, children's development has a reciprocal effect on parental mental health. Thus, besides focusing on parental mental health, early screening of children's development and providing effective intervention is also vital in preventing the future development of parental mental symptoms.

These retrospective and prospective birth cohort studies have provided us with a wealth of information regarding the relationship between parental mental health and the development of children, including the importance of confounding factors such as parental age at childbirth, level of education, support system, family structure, etc. However, existing birth cohort studies provide us only with limited information regarding the full range of factors which may contribute to the development of mental illnesses (Thompson et al., 2010). Through continuous follow-up of the Taiwan Birth Cohort Study and future nested-controlled studies, we hope to continually investigate the association between parents and children, and provide ongoing information regarding the predisposing and maintaining factors which predict the long-term outcome of parental mental health and children's development.

5. Appendix I. The Taiwan birth cohort study

The Taiwan Birth Cohort Study is a national household probability sampled study of randomly sampled children born between January 1st and December 31st of 2005 with no exclusion criteria, so the study was designed to represent the Taiwanese Community. Since the aim was to select a sample which incorporated rare illnesses with a prevalence of less than 4%, 12% of the original sample was selected, resulting in the final sample size of 21,248 babies selected at 6 months (response rate of 87.8%). The sampling process is mentioned in detail in Lung et al. (2011b). A pilot sample was collected and conducted prior to the Taiwan Birth Cohort Study. The response rate of the Taiwan Birth Cohort pilot Study and Taiwan Birth Cohort Stud is shown in Figure 1.

In the Taiwan Birth Cohort Study, parental characteristics and environmental factors which may have a potential impact on children's health, growth or development were all collected. Within these factors, an important factor was parental mental health. Parental mental health

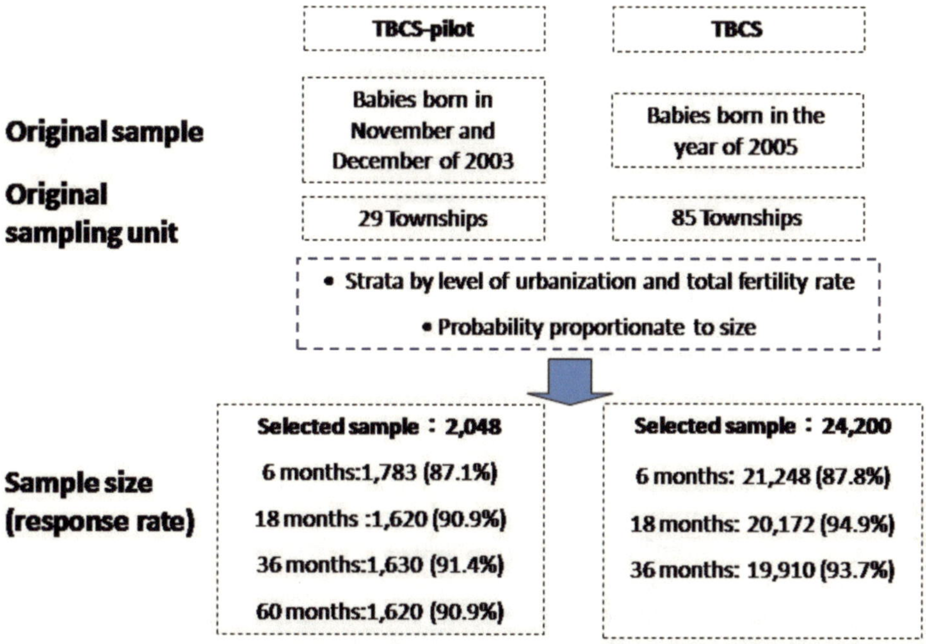

Fig. 1. The sampling process and response rate in each stage of the Taiwan Birth Cohort (TBCS) and Taiwan Birth Cohort Study-pilot (TBCS-p).

was measured using the Taiwanese version of the 36-Item Short Form Health Survey (Ju et al., 2003; Tseng et al., 2003) and children's development using the parent-report Taiwan Birth Cohort Study Developmental Instrument (Lung et al., 2010a; Lung et al., 2011a). It should be noted that the SF-36 does not measure mental health symptoms; instead it is a self-perceived instrument of the overall assessment of quality of life in relation to the mental health conditions.

6. References

Angelsen, N. K., Vik, T., Jacobsen, G., & Bakketeig, L. S. (2001). Breast feeding and cognitive development at age 1 and 5 years. *Archives of Disease in Childhood*, 85, 183-188.

Bailey, W. T. (2004). A longitudinal study of fathers' involvement with young children: Infancy to age 5 years. *The Journal of Genetic Psychology*, 155, 331-339.

Ballard, C. G., Davis, P. C., Cullen, P. C., Mohan, R. N., & Dean, C. (1994). Prevalence of psychiatric morbidity in mothers and fathers. *The British Journal of Psychiatry*, 164, 782-788.

Bowlby, J. (1977). The making and breaking of affectionate bonds: An etiology and psychopathology in the light of attachment theory. *The British Journal of Psychiatry*, 130, 201-210.

Bray, I., Gunnell, D., & Davey Smith, G. (2006). Advanced paternal age: how old is too old. *Journal of Epidemiology and Community Health*, 60, 851-853.

Caspi, A., Sugden, K., Moffitt, T. E., Taylor, A., Craig, I. W., Harrington, H., McClay, J., Mill, J., Martin, J., Braithwaite, A., & Poulton, R. (2003). Influence of life stress on depression: moderation by a polymorphism in the 5-HTT gene. *Science*, 301, 386-389.

Cesar, C. C., & Carvalho, M. S. (2011). Stratified sampling design and loss to follow-up in survival models: evaluation of efficiency and bias. *BMC Medical Research Methodology*, 11, 99.

Chen, P. F., Chen, C. S., Chen, C. C., & Lung, F. W. (2011). Alexithymia as a screening index for male conscripts with adjustment disorder. *The Psychiatric Quarterly*, 82, 139-150.

Chen, W. J., Chen, C. C., Ho, C. K., Chou, F. H. C., Lee, M. B., Lung, F. W., Lin, G. G., Teng, C. Y., Chung, Y. T., Wang, Y. C., & Sun, F. C. (2011). The relationships between quality of life, psychiatric illness, and suicidal ideation in geriatric veterans living in a Veterans' Home: A structural equation modeling approach. *The American Journal of Geriatric Psychiatry*, 19, 597-601.

Cheung, B., Yip, P. S. F., & Karlberg, J. P. E. (2001). Fetal growth, early postnatal growth and motor development in Pakistani infants. *International Journal of Epidemiology*, 30, 66-74.

Clavarino, A., Hayatbakhsh, M. R., Williams, G. M., Bor, W., O'Callaghan, M., & Najman, J. M. (2011). Depression following marital problems: different impacts on mothers and their children? A 21-year prospective study. *Social Psychiatry and Psychiatric Epidemiology*, 46, 833-841.

Clifford, E. (1959). Discipline in the home: A controlled observational study of parental practices. *The Journal of Genetic Psychology*, 95, 45-82.

Davis, N. O., & Carter, A. S. (2008). Parenting stress in mothers and fathers of toddlers with autism spectrum disorders: associations with child characteristics. *Journal of Autism and Developmental Disorders*, 38, 1278-1292.

Dehle, C., & Weiss, R. L. (1998). Sex differences in prospective associations between marital quality and depressed mood. *Journal of Marriage and the Family*, 60, 1002-1011.

Donoso, E., & Carvajal, J. A. (1999). Maternal age and educational and psychosocial outcomes in early adulthood. *Journal of Child Psychology and Psychiatry*, 40, 479-489.

Fergusson, D. M., & Woodward, L. J. (1999). Maternal age and educational and psychosocial outcomes in early adulthood. *Journal of Child Psychology and Psychiatry*, 40, 479-489.

Field, T. (1995). Infants of depressed mothers. *Infant Behavior & Development*, 18, 1-13.

Freud, A. (1974). *Normality and Pathology in Childhood: Assessments of Development 1965*. The Writings of Anna Freud (Vol. 6). New York: International Universities Press.

Gauvain, M. (2001). *The Social Context of Cognivitve Development*. Guilford, New York.

Gilbert, W. M., Nesbitt, T. S., & Danielsen, B. (1999). Childbearing beyond age 40: pregnancy outcomes in 24032 cases. *Obstetrics and Gynecology*, 93, 9-14.

Gray, D. E. (2003). Gender and coping: the parents of children with high functioning autism. *Social Science & Medicine*, 56, 631-642.

Grice, M. M., Feda, D., McGovern, P., Laexander, B. H., McCaffrey, D., & Ukestad, L. (2007). Giving birth and returning to work: the impact of work-family conflict on women's health after childbirth. *Annals of Epidemiology*, 17, 791-798.

Guldan, G., Zeitlin, M., Beiser, A., Super, C., Gershoff, S., & Datta, S. (1993). Maternal education and child feeding practices in rural Bangladesh. *Social Science & Medicine*, 36, 925-935.

Hastings, R. P., Kovshoff, H., Ward, N. J., degli Espinosa, F., Brown, T., & Remington, B. (2005). Systems analysis of stress and positive perceptions in mothers and fathers of pre-school children with autism. *Journal of Autism and Developmental Disorders*, 35, 635-644.

Henretta, J. C., Grundy, E. M. D., Okell, L. C., & Wadsworth, M. E. J. (2008). Early motherhood and mental health in midlife: A study of British and American cohorts. *Aging and Mental Health*, 12, 605-614.

Hung, C. F., Lung, F. W., Hung, T. H., Chong, M. Y., Wu, C. K., Wen, J. K., & Lin, P. Y. (in press). Monoamine oxidase A gene polymorphism and suicide: An association study and meta-analysis. *Journal of Affective Disorders*.

Hung, C. F., Lung, F. W., Chen, C. H., O'Nions, E., Hung, T. H., Chong, M. Y., Wu, C. K., Wen, J. K., & Lin, P. Y. (2011). Association between suicide attempt and a tri-allelic functional polymorphism in serotonin transporter gene promoter in Chinese patients with schizophrenia. *Neuroscience Letters*, 504, 242-246.

Huppert, F. A., Abbott, R. A., Ploubidis, G. B., Richards, M., & Kuh, D. (2010). Parental practices predict psychological well-being in midlife: life-course associations among women in the 1946 British birth cohort. *Psychological Medicine*, 40, 1507-1518.

Ju, J. F. R., Tseng, H. M., & Tsai, Y. J. (2003). Assessment of health-related quality of life in Taiwan (I): development and psychometric testing of SF-36 Taiwan version. *Taiwan Journal of Public Health*, 22, 501-511.

Kahn, R. S., Brandt, D., & Whitaker, R. C. (2004). Combined effect of mothers' and fathers' mental health symptoms on children's behavioral and emotional well-being. *Archives of Pediatrics &Adolescent Medicine*, 158, 721–729.

Kochanska, G., & Akasan, N. (2004). Development and mutual responsiveness between parents and their young children. *Child Development*, 75, 1657-1676.

Kolobe, T. H. (2004). Childbearing practices and developmental expectations for Mexican-American mothers and the developmental status of their infants. *Physical Therapy*, 84, 439-453.

Li, Y. M., & Chang, T. K. (2005). Maternal demographic and psychosocial factors associated with low birth weight in eastern Taiwan. *The Kaohsiung Journal of Medical Sciences*, 21, 502-510.

Lin, C. H., Chang, Y. Y., & Lung, F. W. (2009). Sex-specific interaction between MAOA promoter polymorphism and Apo ε2 allele in major depressive disorder in the Chinese population. *Psychiatric Genetics*, 19, 337.

Liu, X., Sun, Z., Neiderhiser, J. M., Uchiyama, M., & Okawa, M. (2001). Low birth weight, developmental milestones, and behavioral problems in Chinese children and adolescents. *Psychiatry Research*, 101, 115-129.

Lung, F. W. (2011). Developmental aspects of parental attachment and mental health in structural equation modeling. *Taiwanese Journal of Psychiatry*, 25, 63-75.

Lung, F. W., Chiang, T. L., Lin, S. J., Lee, M. C., & Shu, B. C. (2010a). Child developmental screening instrument from six to thirty-six months in Taiwan Birth Cohort Study. *Early Human Development*, 86, 17-21.

Lung, F. W., Chiang, T. L., Lin, S. J., & Shu, B. C. (2009a). Parental mental health and child development from six to thirty-six months in a birth cohort study in Taiwan. *Journal of Perinatal Medicine*, 37, 397-402.

Lung, F. W., Chiang, T. L., Lin, S. J., & Shu, B. C. (2011a). Autism-risk screening in the first 3 years of life in Taiwan Birth Cohort Pilot Study. *Research in Autism Spectrum Disorders*, 5, 1385-1389.

Lung, F. W., Chiang, T. L., Lin, S. J., Shu, B. C., & Lee, M. C. (2011b). Developing and refining the Taiwan Birth Cohort Study (TBCS): Five years of experience. *Research in Developmental Disabilities*, 36, 2697-2703.

Lung, F. W., & Lee, M. B. (2008). The five-item Brief-Symptom Rating Scale as a suicide ideation screening instrument for psychiatric inpatients and community residents. *BMC Psychiatry*, 8, 53-60.

Lung, F. W., Lee, T. H., & Huang, M. F. (in press). Parental bonding in males with adjustment disorder and hyperventilation syndrome. *BMC Psychiatry*.

Lung, F. W., Lee, F. Y., & Shu, B. C. (2002). The relationship between life adjustment and parental bonding in military personnel with adjustment disorder in Taiwan. *Military Medicine*, 167, 678-682.

Lung, F. W., Shu, B. C., Chiang, T. L., & Lin, S. J. (2009b). Parental mental health, education, age at childbirth and child development from six to 18 months. *Acta Peadiatrica*, 98, 834-841.

Lung, F. W., Shu, B. C., Chiang, T. L., & Lin, S. J. (2010b). Maternal mental health and childrearing context in the development of children at 6, 18 and 36 months: a Taiwan birth cohort pilot study. *Child: Care, Health and Development*, 37, 211-223.

Lung, F. W., Tzeng, D. S., Huang, M. F., & Lee, M. B. (2011c). Association of the MAOA promoter uVNTR polymorphism with suicide attempts in patients with major depressive disorder. *BMC Medical Genetics*, 12, 74-84.

Maselko, L., Kubzanksy, L., Lipsitt, L., & Buka, S. L. (2011). Mother's affection at 8 months predicts emotional distress in adulthood. *Journal of Epidemiology and Community Health*, 65, 621-625.

McLearn, K. T., Minkovitz, C. S., Strobino, D. M., Marks, E., & Hou, W. (2006). Maternal depressive symptoms at 2 to 4 months postpartum and early parenting practices. *Archives of Pediatrics &Adolescent Medicine*, 160, 279–284.

Mezulis, A. H., Hyde, J. S., & Clark, R. (2004). Father involvement moderates the effect of maternal depression during a child's infancy and child behaviour problems in kindergarten. *Journal of Family Psychology*, 18, 575–588.

Moffitt, T. E., Caspi, A., Taylor, A., Kokaua, J., Milne, B. J., Polanczyk, G., & Poulton, R. (2010). How common are common mental disorders? Evidence that lifetime prevalence rates are doubled by prospective versus retrospective ascertainment. *Pscyhological Medicine*, 40, 899-909.

Montague, D. R., & Walker-Andrews, A. S. (2002). Mothers, fathers, and infants: the role of person familiarity and parental involvement in infants' perception of emotional expressions. *Child Development*, 73, 1339-1352.

Mussatto, K. (2006). Adaptation of the child and family to life with a chronic illness. *Cardiology in the Young*, 16, 110-116.

Nesse, R. M., & Stearns, S. C. (2008). The great opportunity: Evolutionary applications to medicine and public health. *Evolutionary Applications*, 1, 28-48.

Parker, G., & Gladstone, G. (Eds.). (1996). *Parental characteristics as influences on adjustment in adulthood*. Plenum Press, New York.

Parker, G., Tupling, H., & Brown, L. B. (1979). A Parental Bonding Instrument. *The British Journal of Medical Psychology*, 52, 1-10.

Ramchandani, P. G., Stein, A., Evans, J., & O'Connor, T. G. (2005). Paternal depression in the postnatal period and child development: a prospective population study. *Lancet*, 265, 2201-2205.

Ramchandani, P. G., Stein, A., O'Connor, T. G., Heron, J., Murray, L., & Evans, J. (2008). Depression in men in the postnatal period and later child psychopathology: a population cohort study. *Journal of the American Academy of Child and Adolescent Psychiatry*, 47, 390-398.

Reichman, N. E., & Teitler, J. O. (2006). Paternal age as a risk factor for low birthweight. *American Journal of Public Health*, 95, 862-866.

Repetti, R. L. (Ed.). (1998). *Multiple roles*. Guilford Press, New York.

Saha, S., Barnett, A. G., Buka, S. L., & McGrath, J. J. (2009). Maternal age and paternal age are associated with distinct childhood behavioural outcomes in a general population birth cohort. *Schizophrenia Research*, 115, 130-135.

Shu, B. C., Chang, Y. Y., Lee, F. Y., Tzeng, D. S., Lin, H. Y., & Lung, F. W. (2007). Parental attachment, premorbid personality, and mental health in young males with hyperventilation syndrome. *Psychiatry Research*, 153, 163-170.

Shu, B. C., Lung, F. W., & Chang, Y. Y. (2000). The mental health in mothers with autistic children: a case control study in southern Taiwan. *The Kaohsiung Journal of Medical Sciences*, 16, 308-314.

Simon, G. E., & VonKorff, M. (1995). Recall of psychiatric history in cross-sectional surveys: implications of epidemiologic research. *Epidemiology Review*, 17, 211-227.

Singer, L. T., Salvator, A., Guo, S., Collin, M., Lilien, L., & Baley, J. (1999). Maternal psychological distress and parenting stress after the birth of a very low-birth-weight infant. *JAMA*, 281, 799-812.

Sohr-Preston, S. L., & Scaramella, L. V. (2006). Implications of timing of maternal depressive symptoms for early cognitive and language development. *Clinical Child and Family Psychology Review*, 9, 65-83.

Soliday, E., McCluskey-Fawcett, K., & O'Brien, M. (1999). Postpartum affect and depressive symptoms in mothers and fathers. *The American Journal of Orthopsychiatry*, 69, 30-37.

Stein, A., Gath, D. H., Bucher, J., Bond, A., Day, A., & Cooper, P. J. (1991). The relationship between postnatal depression and mother child interaction. *The British Journal of Psychiatry*, 158, 46-52.

Thomasgard, M., & Metz, W. P. (2004). Promoting child social-emotional growth in primary care settings: using a developmental approach. *Clinical Pediatrics*, 32, 119-127.

Thompson, L., Kemp, J., Wilson, P., Pritchett, R., Minnis, H., Toms-Whittle, L., et al. (2010). What have birth cohort studies asked about genetic, pre- and perinatal exposures and child and adolescent onset mental health outcomes? A systemic review. *European Child & Adolescent Psychiatry*, 19, 1-15.

Tough, S. C., Siever, J. E., Leew, S., Johnston, D. W., Benzies, K., & Clark, D. (2008). Maternal mental health predicts risk of developmental problems at 3 years of age: follow up of a community based trial. *BMC Pregnancy Childbirth*, 8, 16-26.

Tseng, H. M., Lu, J. F., & Tsai, Y. J. (2003). Assessment of health-related quality of life in Taiwan (II): norming and validation of SF-36 Taiwan version. *Taiwan Journal of Public Health*, 22, 512-518.

U.S. Census Bureau. (2004). *Women in the labor force*. U.S. Census Bureau, USA.

Wachs, T. D., Creed-Kanashiro, H., Cueto, S., & Jacoby, E. (2005). Maternal education and intelligence predict offspring diet and nutritional status. *The Journal of Nutrition*, 135, 2179-2186.

Horwitz, A., & Wakefield, J. (2007). *The loss of sadness: how psychiatry transformed normal sorrow into depressive disorder*. New York: Oxford University Press.

Walker, L. O., & Best, M. A. (1991). Well-being of mothers with infant children: a preliminary comparison of employed women and homemakers. *Women Health*, 17, 71-89.

Weiss, M. J. (2002). Hardiness and social support as predictors of stress in mothers of typical children, children with autism, and children with mental retardation. *Autism*, 6, 115-130.

Whisman, M. A., & Bruce, M. L. (1999). Marital dissatisfaction and incidence of major depressive episode in a community sample. *Journal of Abnormal Psychology*, 108, 674-678.

Wills, T. A. (Ed.). (1998). *Social Support*. Guilford Press, New York.

Zhu, J. L., Vestergaard, M., Madsen, K. M., & Olsen, J. (2008). Paternal age and mortality in children. *European Journal of Epidemiology*, 23, 443-447.

Zill, N. (1996). Parental schooling and children's health. *Public Health Reports*, 111, 34-43.

21

Children's Mental Health in the Era of Globalisation: Neo-Liberalism, Commodification, McDonaldisation, and the New Challenges They Pose

Sami Timimi
University of Lincoln
United Kingdom

1. Introduction

Children and families across the world face a multitude of ever changing challenges that will affect their sense of emotional well-being. Dilemmas for children in the first world include: competition, consumerism, individualism, narcissism and family breakdown contributing to children as consumers, the erosion of collective (social) responsibility, dislocation, alienation, inequality, relative poverty, and crime. Dilemmas for children in the third world include: regional wars and conflict, ecological catastrophe - man-made and natural contributing to material poverty, lack of state resources (e.g. medical), migration, fragmentation of communities, disease, malnutrition, and crime. Each society has its own mechanisms to promote the natural resilience of children and families in the face of each individual, family and society's unique challenges. The era of globalisation has resulted in the global exchange of not only goods, but also ideas and values, resulting in new challenges. Aggressive free market global economic systems contribute to the creation of new dangers. The development of universalised therapeutic approaches has inadvertently replicated colonial dynamics by imposing Western notions of self, childhood, and family onto non-Western populations. Globalisation also brings new opportunities for new identities, fusions and creative solutions.

A variety of economic, political, and cultural pressures shape beliefs and practices around children and families. Policies that promote a particular form of aggressive capitalism lead to a narcissistic value system that permeates social institutions, including those that deal with children. Not only does this impact children's emotional well-being, but it also shapes the way we conceptualise children and their problems. These beliefs and practices have facilitated the rapid growth of child psychiatric diagnoses and the tendency to deal with aberrant behaviour or emotions in children through technical – particularly pharmaceutical – interventions, a phenomenon I refer to as the 'McDonaldization' of children's mental health. Diagnoses do not yet reveal the causes of mental difficulties or provide clear differentiators for treatment. As subjective constructs they are thus vulnerable to 'commodification' processes. Commodification can distance people from a more considered in-depth understanding of the problems being experienced. Thus, unlike diagnoses that are attached to a pathophysiological aetiology and/or differential treatment indicators that effect outcomes, there is little evidence to support the contention that long-term prognosis for child mental health problems have improved.

The present chapter seeks to challenge many of the cultural assumptions regarding childhood embedded within the narrow biomedical frame currently dominant in mainstream child and adolescent psychiatry and explores the connections between economy, politics, culture, globalisation, and children's mental health. Implications for child and adolescent mental health practice and suggestions for adopting a more context rich perspective will be outlined.

2. Contrasting beliefs

Teachers in an inner London school become concerned about a fourteen-year-old girl whose parents come from the Indian sub-continent. She has been behaving, in their opinion, 'bizarrely' for some days now, laughingly inappropriately at times; appearing preoccupied, and has stopped mixing with her peers. An urgent psychiatric assessment is arranged and the psychiatrist concludes that this young adolescent is suffering from a psychotic illness and requires admission to a psychiatric unit for treatment with anti-psychotic medication. However, her parents and the young adolescent herself disagree, claiming that, in their opinion she is not 'ill' but suffering the manifestations of a spiritual problem as they consider it is likely that she has become possessed by evil spirits. What they feel she needs is a consultation with a local 'priest' to ascertain the nature of the current spiritual crisis.

Cases such as the above, increasingly encountered in clinical practice in multi-cultural societies such as those in modern Europe and North America, raise clinical and ethical dilemmas. Whose version should we believe? Can either version (that she is mentally ill or that she is possessed by bad spirits) claim any objective evidence to support its case? Should the beliefs of the more powerful party (in this case the psychiatrist and to a lesser extent the teachers) impose their view of the problem on this young lady and her family? To what extent should the professionals take into account the young lady and her family's beliefs about the nature of her problems, and how might they work with this? Indeed, do scenarios such as the above present new opportunities for professionals to learn new ways of working from communities considered in many ways to be culturally inferior and whose belief systems professionals therefore often dismiss? Whilst clinicians may rightly assert that they need more information in order to come to a pragmatic conclusion on how to proceed, the advantage of stripping away extra details is that it exposes starkly opposing views that don't disappear within the extra layers of complexity surrounding any case. These questions are of more importance than just that of passing philosophical and academic interest as incompatible belief systems between users and professionals have been shown to have potentially fatal consequences (Smith, 2003). Further, these clinical, ethical, and philosophical questions are not limited to those with the most 'extreme' presentations, but are relevant across the spectrum of mental health in the young, including our approaches to child development and child protection (Maitra, 1996; Timimi, 2002; 2005a; 2005b; Timimi & Maitra, 2006).

A psychiatric trainee of Nigerian origin starting her second year of psychiatry training in the UK commences in her first placement in a child and adolescent mental health service. She observes her supervising consultant psychiatrist conducting the first three assessments she has witnessed. She later confesses in a private conversation with a sympathetic colleague that she could not see anything 'abnormal' in the referred children's behaviour, and could not understand why these children needed to be dealt with by the medical profession and why each received a psychiatric diagnosis.

The easiest way for a professional to deal with the ambiguities in the two scenarios above, is to avoid questioning the basis on which the assumptions of the dominant ideology is based and instead side with the moral certainties that a universalising approach to problems of mental health the psychiatric belief system provides. However, the problematic nature of such an approach can be found in even what might seem areas where certain cultural beliefs and practices appear clearly unethical and unacceptable. For example, Kaplan (1997) in her discussion of the film Warrior Marks (a film that is a graphic critique of clitoridectomies in Africa, dramatising the pain and terror involved), noted that the adult African woman in the film, defend clitoridectomies as a necessary part of their tradition and sacred practices. Kaplan makes the point that the film argues against clitoridectomy at the expense of African women's (in the film) beliefs, reproduces the imperialist tradition of teaching Africans a better way of living, relies on established stereotypes of Africans as exotic and potentially savage, and finally assumes a global women's rights approach. Whilst it is important to acknowledge that many Africans in a variety of countries are actively working toward abolishing this procedure (e.g., Cook et al., 2002), it is also vital not to frame these complex issues in a one-sided manner by imposing the value system of one culture upon another. After all one wonders what many of these African women might think about the ease with which women in the West use a variety of cosmetic surgeries to make them more attractive and appealing. Premature closure of on-going debates is likely to result in entrenched positions rather than meaningful dialogue.

Similar problems with a universal approach to children's rights can also be found. For example Segal (1992) found that health and social work professionals in India and America saw child abuse in very different terms. Indian professionals' more than American ones considered a wider range of adult sexual behaviours and media images seriously abusive to children. However, Indian professionals did not consider physical 'maltreatment' to be as seriously abusive as their American counterparts did.

Certain writers have tried to resolve some of these issues, for example Finkelhor and Korbin (1988) argue that certain cultural practices such as scarification which confers identity in tribal groups can be viewed as non-abusive as opposed to others such as clitoridectomy which can be viewed as abusive because the latter increase morbidity and certain ethical/moral/human rights standards are violated. This argument still remains suspect, however, as it draws on an ethical framework to make this separation and the question then becomes who is it that sets these standards and decides what is acceptable morbidity (Maitra, 1996). If we are to apply such standards universally, how much of current Western psychiatric practices could then be viewed as unethical? After all there is known morbidity, including fatalities, associated with the use of psychiatric medication for childhood behaviours that other cultures may not see as being at all problematic or abnormal amongst the young (Timimi, 2005a; 2008a).

3. Contrasting childhoods

Whilst the immaturity of children is a biological fact, the ways in which this immaturity is understood and made meaningful is a fact of culture (Prout & James, 1997). Members of any culture hold a working definition of childhood, its nature, limitations and duration based on a network of ideas that link children with other members of society and with the social ecology (Harkness & Super, 1996). While they may not explicitly discuss this definition, write about it, or even consciously conceive of it as an issue, they act upon these assumptions in all of their dealings with, fears for, and expectations of, their children (Calvert, 1992). In addition, different social practices of different cultures produce different childhoods each of which are 'real' within their local regime of truth (Prout & James, 1997; Stephens, 1995). As a result it has been argued that in any culture, children and then adults come to acquire their subjective selves through incorporation of values, beliefs and practices that sustain the desired social relationships of that culture (Althusser, 1969).

People, 'know' themselves through the mediation of ideological institutions and some of the most important of these institutions, such as schools, focus their attention on children. As Rose (1999) points out, "*Individuals act upon themselves and their families in terms of the languages, values and techniques made available to them by professions, disseminated through the apparatuses of the mass media or sought out by the troubled through the market.*" (Rose, 1999: 88) The implication is that we cannot just take at face value that individual actions evolve only from innate desires. Desires grow from norms and regulations. At the same time there is a danger in such a perspective of falling into a socially deterministic ideology; thus even though a person's experience depends on the prescriptions of the day, agency does play its part. As Martin & Sugarman (2000) claim, that "*While never ceasing to be constructed in sociocultural terms, psychological beings, as reflection-capable, intentional agents, are able to exercise sophisticated capabilities of memory and imagination, which in interaction with theories of self can create possibilities for present and future understanding and action that are not entirely constrained by past and present sociocultural circumstances.*" (Martin & Sugarman, 2000: 401).

Such an ecological framework, that includes an appreciation of the intentional person making sense of the reality from within their broader social, political and cultural context, makes it difficult to pass a value or scientific judgment about whether children are better or worse off in any particular culture or society, as the idea that there are universal ideals or natural unfolding process that all children should be able to achieve, becomes suspect. Nonetheless, this position also understands that children are socialised by belonging to a particular culture at a certain stage in that culture's history, so certain differences in children's behaviour can be seen as a result of different child rearing philosophies, socialisation processes, and political realities. We can, therefore, make some comparisons, whilst keeping in mind the above caveats and indeed using them to help us 'interrogate' any naïve or romanticised assumptions.

4. Western childhoods

The space of childhood in contemporary Western culture has witnessed rapid changes that effect children. Well-documented changes include (Timimi, 2010):

1. Children's diets (which have increased in sugar, saturated fats, salt, chemical additives and decreased in certain essential fatty acids and fresh fruit and vegetables);
2. Family structure (which has seen the demise of the extended family, increase in separation and divorce, increase in working hours of parents, and a decrease in the amount of time parents spend with their children);

3. Family lifestyle (there has been an increase in mobility, decrease in 'rooted' communities, and an increasing pursuit of individual gratification);
4. Children's lifestyle (which has witnessed a decrease in the amount of exercise, the 'domestication' of childhood due to fears about the risks for children resulting in more indoor pursuits such as computers, virtual socialisation through 'Facebook' and the like, and TV);
5. The commercialisation/commodification of childhood (increase in consumer goods targeted at children and the creation of new commercial opportunities in childhood, for example the 'parenting' industry and the pharmaceutical industry) and;
6. Changes in the education system (modern teaching ideology is rooted in methods such as continuous assessment and socially orientated worksheets that some argue favour the learning style of girls over boys (e.g. Burman, 2005)).

These changes are occurring at a time when our standards for what we consider to be acceptable behaviour in the young and acceptable child rearing methods are both narrowing. It is now harder than ever to be a 'normal' child or parent (Timimi, 2005a; 2009a).

4.1 Rising rates of mental disorders in the young

In parallel with this, evidence from longitudinal studies show rising rates of 'mental' disorders among the young (such as emotional, anxiety, eating, and behavioural disorders) in the past few decades (British Medical Association, 2006) despite the perception that recent generations have 'never had it so good'. Cross-cultural research finds considerable differences in prevalence rates for psychiatric disorder, with children, particularly boys, in politically stable developing countries appearing to have considerably lower rates of behavioural disorders than in Western societies (e.g., Cederblad, 1988; Pillai et al., 2008). Figures for prescriptions of psychotropic medication to children and adolescents both illustrate the depth of this problem and our peculiar cultural style of responding to it.

Of particular concern is the increase in rate of stimulant prescription to children. By 1996 over 6% of school-aged boys in America were taking stimulant medication (Olfson et al, 2002) with children as young as two being prescribed stimulants in increasing numbers (Zito et al., 2000). Surveys in the late 1990s showed that in some schools in the US over 17% of boys were taking stimulant medication (LeFever et al, 1999) and recent estimates suggest that about 10% of school boys in the US have been or are being prescribed a stimulant (Sharav, 2006). Between 1991 and 2010, prescriptions in the USA of stimulants increased from 5 million to 45 million, a 9-fold increase (National Institute of Drug Abuse, 2011). In the UK prescriptions for stimulants have increased from about 6000 prescriptions a year in 1994 to over 450,000 by 2004; a staggering 7000% rise in one decade (Department of Health, NHSE, 2005) with figures continuing to increase, reaching over 800,000 by 2009 (NHS Information Centre, 2010). These trends are being replicated across other psychotropic medications too (Timimi, 2009b).

These rapid changes in practice in the area of children's mental health have not come about as a result of any major new scientific discovery (see Timimi, 2002; 2004; 2005a; 2009; Timimi & Maitra, 2006). There are two other possibilities that could explain these increases. The first is that there has been a real increase in emotional and behavioural disorders in children leading to greater public scrutiny and concern about such behaviours which, in turn, has resulted in a greater professional effort to understand and alleviate these behavioural and emotional problems. The second possibility is that there has not been a real increase in emotional and behavioural disorders in the young but there has been a change in the way we think about, classify, and deal with children's behaviour – in other words our perception of and the meaning we ascribe to children's emotions and behaviour. Both possible causes for the rapid increase in our identification of and treatment for mental health disorders in the young require an examination of contexts. Indeed the third, and in my opinion, most likely possibility that explains the increase is an interaction between the aforementioned two possibilities. In other words, it could be that changes in our cultural/environmental contexts are causing increases in certain emotional and behavioural problems and these, in turn, are changing our perception of and the meaning we give to childhood behaviour. For example, an increase in certain behaviours will lead to increasing levels of anxiety about the long term consequences of these behaviours leading to greater scrutiny, study, and attempts at intervening to change these behaviours. This process then changes the way view childhood behaviour and our common cultural practices around children (such as child rearing and education), and by further increasing our anxieties and scrutiny of these behaviours we begin to 'pathologise' behaviours that previously would not have aroused such anxieties.

In examining these trends, two aspects of the Western value system that have become embedded in our daily discourse due, at least in part, to our reliance on rather aggressive forms of neo-liberal free market principles, deserve further scrutiny. These are the problems of 'narcissism' and 'commodification'. Narcissism describes the character trait of 'self love' or in the more everyday sense 'looking after number one'. The spread of narcissism has left many children in a psychological vacuum, pre-occupied with issues of psychological survival and lacking a sense of the emotional security that comes through feeling you are valued and thus have an enduring sense of belonging. The growth of narcissism contributes to the growth of behavioural and emotional problems in the young. Commodification refers to the process by which goods, ideas, indeed anything can become a 'thing' with a commercial value that can be bought and sold, and subject to the influence of the market, which then makes it available for exploitation. Childhood, parenting, children's distress and professional approaches to intervening in this have, I will argue, all become subjects of 'commodification'. The growth of commodification contributes to both an increase in certain behavioural problems and the continual expansion of the repertoire of behaviours and emotional states found in children that are considered to be 'abnormal'.

4.2 The impact of growing up in a narcissistic value system

One of the dominant themes used by advocates of neo-liberal free market economy ideology is that of 'freedom'. At the economic level this is a core requirement of free market ideology. Companies must be as free from regulation as possible to concentrate on competing with others, with maximizing of profits the most visible sign of success. There is little to gain from social responsibility (only if it increases your 'market share'). At the emotional level the appeal to freedom can be understood as an appeal to rid us of the restrictions imposed by authority (such as parents, communities and governments) (Richards, 1989). By implication this value system is built around the idea of looking after the wants of the individual – narcissism. Taking this a step further, once the individual is freed from authority they are (in fantasy at least) free to pursue their own individual self-gratification desires, free from the impingements, infringements and limitations that other people represent. The effect of this on society is to atomise the individual and insulate their private spaces to the degree where obligations to others and harmony with the wider community become obstacles rather than objectives. In this 'look after number one' value system, other individuals are there to be competed against as they too chase after their personal desires. This post second world war shift to a more individualistic identity was recognized, as early as the mid-1950s, by commentators who first spoke about how the new 'fun based morality' (Wolfenstein, 1955) was privileging fun over responsibility - having fun was becoming obligatory (the cultural message becoming that you should be ashamed if you weren't having fun). With the increase in new possibilities for excitement being presented, experiencing intense excitement was becoming more difficult, thus creating a constant pressure to push back the boundaries of acceptable and desirable experiences, and lifestyles, opening the doors, amongst other things, to sub-cultures comfortable with drinking to excess, violence (for pleasure), sexual promiscuity, and drug taking.

In this value system others can more easily become objects to be used and manipulated wherever possible for personal goals and thus social exchanges become difficult to trust as the better you are at manipulating others the more financial (and other narcissistic) rewards you will get. Such a value system, which ultimately seeks to eradicate or at least minimize social conscience as a regulator of behaviour, cannot sustain itself without the moral conscience beginning to feel guilty (Richards, 1989). Thus it is no coincidence that those who are the most vociferous advocates of free market ideology tend also to advocate the most aggressive and punitive forms of social control. Thus another hallmark of Western culture's increasing psychological reliance on developmentally immature impulses that encourages it to avoid taking responsibility for its beliefs and practices, is the so called 'blame culture', which fills the media and contemporary discourse more generally. In addition, Western politicians, who act as advocates for this system, repeatedly use childhood, the family and 'traditional values' as rhetorical devices to shore up the 'free' market ideology. Throughout the past few centuries, at regular intervals and particularly at times of economic uncertainty and social unrest, calls are made by the ruling classes to 'return' to traditional values (Harvey, 2010), passing responsibility for addressing the behavioural problems away from the structural inequalities necessary for a market economic system to successfully compete in the global market, back to parents who are criticised for not doing a better job of disciplining their children.

With narcissistic goals of self-fulfilment, gratification and competitive manipulation of relationships so prominent, together with the discouragement of the development of deep interpersonal attachments from which a sense of social responsibility arises, it is not difficult to see why so-called narcissistic disorders (such as anti-social behaviour, substance misuse, and eating disorders) are on the increase (Dwivedi, 1996). A heightened concern for the self can be both 'liberating' and simultaneously oppressive.

Children are cultured into this value system by virtue of living within its institutions and being exposed daily to its discourse. Although none of us are one dimensional in our experiences or our interpretation of them, a narcissistic value system helps create an environment of winners and losers, a kind of survival of the fittest where compassion and concern for social harmony contradicts the basic goal of the value system. As this system is showing itself to be bad for children's happiness a similar process as above works to try and distance us from the anxiety arising from the guilt thus produced. Instead of asking ourselves painful questions about the role we may be playing in producing this unhappiness, we can view our children's difficulties as being the result of biological diseases that require medical treatments (we can blame their genes) (Timimi, 2008b). This gives governments new ways of regulating the population, with biological models of psychiatry providing convenient ways to subcategorise discontent and behavioural deviance making 'divide and rule' easier (Moncreiff, 2008).

4.3 Surveillance, commodification, and McDonaldisation

The dynamics involved in concepts of self being shaped in a narcissistic direction, interacting with the collective guilt and fear of retribution and becoming a loser in the competition, means that governments feel the need to police potentially dangerous selves that may thus emerge, in an increasing variety of ways. Thus, one other feature that has changed dramatically over the past century of Western society is the amount of surveillance to which parents and their children are subjected. The state has all sorts of mechanisms of surveillance and an 'army' of professionals tasked with monitoring and regulating family life. This is not to say that we do not need surveillance as the effects of, for example, uninterrupted traumatic events such as child abuse can be many and far reaching, thus robust child protection services and legislation are vital in any society that wishes to claim that it takes childhood welfare seriously. But we must also ask questions about the what we chose not to notice (such as structural and social inequalities) in carrying out such surveillance, at the same time as understanding the potential impact of how we decide to do this on children, families and our culture more generally.

The increase in levels of anxiety amongst parents who may fear the consequences of their action, has reached the point where the fear for many is that any influence that is discernible may be viewed as undue influence. This increases the likelihood that parents will leave essential socialising and guidance to the expertise of professionals as, surrounded by a discourse that paints childhood and child rearing as loaded with risk, they lose confidence in their own abilities (Maitra, 2006). The increase use of medical explanations for behavioural problems has far reaching effects changing our ideas about free will, choice and personal responsibility for our behaviour. For example, if impulsive and aggressive behaviour by a child is viewed as being caused by a brain disorder called Attention Deficit Hyperactivity Disorder (ADHD), then it is considered to be behaviour that a child or their parent cannot consciously control and one that requires medical assistance to remedy (assuming of course it has been decided that the behaviours need to be changed), thus shifting activities previously considered pedagogic and the remit of parents and teachers into the medical arena (Tait, 2006).

Into this anxiety loaded, narcissistically pre-determined vision of childhood and practices of child rearing, new diagnoses (such as childhood depression, ADHD, Aspergers syndrome) appear to provide a temporary relief to the beleaguered, intensely monitored child carers. Viewing children's poor behaviour and distressed emotional state as being caused by an 'illness' apparently spare all from further scrutiny. The result however, fits into another aspect of our 'fast culture'. With the widespread application of the techniques of medicine to manage our children's behaviour and emotional state, particularly through use of drugs, we have achieved what I call the 'McDonaldisation' of children's mental health. Like fast food, recent medication centred practice came from the most aggressively consumerist society (USA), feeds on peoples desire for instant satisfaction and a 'quick fix', fits into a busy lifestyle, requires little engagement with the product, requires only the most superficial training, knowledge and understanding to produce the product, creates potential lifelong consumers of their products, and has the potential to produce damage in the long term to both the individuals who consume these products as well as public health more generally.

It is no accident that such forms of practice have emerged most prominently in those countries, such as the USA, that are the strongest advocates of the neo-liberal market system. Such societies are characterised by a consumer culture. As such the culture is driven by the social arrangement in which the buying and selling of goods and services is not only the predominant activity of everyday life but is also an important arbiter of social organisation, significance and control. Slater (1997: 101) has commented that today *"more of social life is produced in a thing-like form"* and this notion of a 'thing-like form' fits well as a way of thinking about how diagnosis and professional practice in mental health often views mental distress and behavioural deviance. Commodification entails processes of abstraction that not only creates a 'thing', but, specifically, a commoditised 'thing' that can enter into the market. Castree (2003: 281) describes abstraction as the process by which *"the qualitative specificity of any individualised thing (a person, a seed, a gene or what-have-you) is assimilated to the qualitative homogeneity of a broader type or process."* Thus diagnostic categories relegate markers of individual differences to ones of lesser significance and instead promote a more uniform and standardised 'type', which is clearly easier to 'package', promote and sell. Robertson (2000) developed the concept of 'functional abstraction' to refer to circumstances where individual cases are considered as 'instances' of the generic category, which stands over and above them. For example, Robertson (2000:472) in exploring the formal assessment methodologies and taxonomic systems which work to commodify 'wetlands', comments: *"Taxonomic classification systems provide both an imposed order and a common language for scientists [...] assessment methodologies involve paper forms, filled out on a brief visit to a site, which allow the assessor to total up a 'score' for a given site"* (Robertson (2000: 473), an observation that could just as easily be applied to diagnostic practice.

As psychiatric diagnostic categories are built on a subjective basis and have as yet not been found to attach to any physical markers to support their existence as 'natural' biologically congruent entities, they are ripe for exploitation as a commodity. Childhood distress was once the remit of parents and families to deal with and in most parts of the world this remains the case. However, once this responsibility begins to migrate into being the remit of a professional class whose livelihood is based on an 'expertise' in alleviating childhood distress and preventing behavioural deviance, and when this occurs in a 'free' market context, then commodification is just around the corner. Once we have categorised states of emotional and behavioural deviance and these categories enter the market, they become the equivalent of brands. Each brand will develop a market including professionals (with expertise in the brand) and treatments (such as a particular medication or a particular form of psychotherapy). Consumers will be largely made of parents, who (partly as a result of the dynamics mentioned above) have come to be concerned that their child has a problem and that this problem is beyond their capability to resolve. However, it is not just parents, but layers of social pressures and cultural beliefs (in the shape of, for example, politicians, family practitioners, social workers, teachers) that play an important role directly as consumers for children under their authority or as consumer advocates encouraging parents to become consumers. These consumers now seek out a product (a diagnosis, an expert, a treatment) based on the information they receive (from advocates, media and a variety of marketing sources) in the hope that the product will offer a form of 'validation' (of the struggles and anxieties being experiencing) and/or a sense of 'promise' (having the 'product' or brand such as a diagnosis will lead to an improvement in their life). Like all commodities the appeal is more at the emotional/desire level than the rational one.

Once this system is set in motion we can predict a number of things will happen. Commodities tend to give only temporary experiences of satisfaction as markets must keep selling to keep the monetary flow going and so must keep convincing consumers that there is a better 'brand' waiting for them. In other words, once an area of life has been subject to market commodification, we should predict that the market will grow in volume as new products and competitors enter the fray. Thus the number of available psychiatric diagnostic categories has continued to expand, both in the 'official' manuals and in everyday practice. Not only do new categories emerge but so do new subcategories, number of professionals providing services, the number of professionals with specialisations and sub-specialisations, the number of treatment models (for example we have well over 400 systematised models of psychotherapy), and so on (Double, 2002). There is now a bewildering array of commodities out there for the concerned parent to try and access. Yet, unlike the rest of medicine where diagnostic categories have largely developed around an aetiological basis and where treatments have demonstrated sustained improvements in outcomes for patients, there is little encouraging news for long term mental health outcomes and some potentially discouraging ones (Whitaker, 2010). Like any market there are periods of over-consumption resulting in cut-backs and a pruning off of some competitors. Likewise commodities can be subject to the changing whims of the producers and consumers as certain products go in and out of 'fashion' (such as 'autism' is the new 'ADHD'!). However, as a relatively young market the globalisation of this 'McDonalisation' of children's mental health has only just started. The owners of these new products (largely institutional psychiatry and psychology based in the West and in partnership with the financial and marketing prowess of the Pharmaceutical industry) are only just beginning the mass export and globalisation of this market and all the ideological implications this contains (Timimi, 2009c).

4.4 Family life and children's rights

The increase in working hours, increased inequality in incomes, greater job insecurity, and the breakdown of contacts with extended family in the context of a cultural drive toward individual aspirations and consumerism also has a direct impact on the mental health of children. Many studies have documented an association between poverty, marital disruption, and a wide range of deleterious effects on children's behaviour and emotional state (e.g. McMunn et al, 2001). Children, who live with a lone parent, with unemployed parents, parents on low incomes, and families living in public sector housing, are at higher risk of developing emotional and behavioural disorders (Dodds, 2005). Pressures on working mothers can be particularly intense with those who strive to be so-called 'super-mums' expecting to be able to seamlessly blend their working life and parenting, being most at risk of depression (University of Washington, 2011). Parental stress and depression is known to adversely impact infants and children in a variety of ways including, interpersonal communication, emotional expressiveness and responsiveness, withdrawal, and disengagement with their children, with social adversity compounds these effects (Timimi & Dwivedi, 2010).

Social inequality seems a powerful mediator of mental distress and dissatisfaction. In the last few generations, we have seen many changes in the way we interact with each other - both within and without our atomized family units. Increasingly, mental well-being seems closely linked to how well one is able to compete in highly inegalitarian societies. Thus a recent World Health Organization (Friedli, 2009) report concluded: "*It is abundantly clear that the chronic stress of struggling with material disadvantage is intensified to a very considerable degree by doing so in more unequal societies. An extensive body of research confirms the relationship between inequality and poorer outcomes, a relationship, which is evident at every position on the social hierarchy and is not confined to developed nations. The emotional and cognitive effects of high levels of social status differentiation are profound and far reaching: greater inequality heightens status competition and status insecurity across all income groups and among both adults and children. It is the distribution of economic and social resources that explains health and other outcomes in the vast majority of studies.*" (Friedli, 2009: III)

Surveys for childhood well-being consistently put those countries that pursue the most aggressive neo-liberal policies (such as the UK and the USA) at the bottom of league tables for the developed world (e.g. UNICEF, 2007). A recent report of an in-depth comparison of children's experiences across three developed countries - the UK, Sweden and Spain - emphasised the impact of consumerism and economic inequality. It found that children in the UK (bottom of the 2007 UNICEF table on childhood wellbeing) feel 'trapped' in a materialistic culture and don't spend enough time with their families. Children in all three countries told researchers that their happiness is dependent on having time with a stable family and plenty of things to do, especially outdoors, rather than on owning material goods. Despite this, parents in the UK said they felt pressure from society to buy goods for their children with this pressure felt most acutely in low-income homes. As UK parents often felt they lose out on time together as a family, due in part to long working hours, they often tried to make up for this by buying material things for their children (UNICEF, 2011).

The guilt that all this causes, both at the individual level and societal level, spurs on an industry of 'child savers', campaigning for greater protection of children and ever-greater surveillance of family life. In recent years, advocates of this 'children's rights' movement have focussed their campaigns on trying to get governments to outlaw the physical punishment of children, often citing Sweden as a positive example. Yet an examination of various morbidity and mortality figures shows Swedish children to be somewhere in the middle of league tables for rich countries (Beckett, 2005). For example, rates of death from child maltreatment in Sweden at 0.6 per 100,000 children is much higher than countries who fare best in these tables, namely Spain (at 0.1) and Greece and Italy (at 0.2) (UNICEF, 2001) who have not outlawed corporal punishment (but who interestingly have family orientated cultures). The problem with this approach to protecting children is that the focus on individual perpetrators permits complacency about the collective responsibility of governments and their institutions, for allowing environments that cause other forms of harm to develop. Children's rights have regularly emerged as an issue in the history of the developed/industrialised nations. Exploitation for profit is the guiding rule of a market led economy and children have often been the subjects of such exploitation. Children's rights movements then appear at regular intervals with the focus of protest shifting, from child labour to the commercialisation of childhood to child abuse. However, whilst the focus is on saving the individual child, important as this is, it can distract from appreciating the degree to which children's rights are intertwined with the political and social pressures of that society and the degree to which the economic system may exploit them.

Thus, many children in the West grow up with an experience of childhood that is shaped by emotional insecurity and unhappiness, conflict, and competitiveness, in a context where their (and their families) behaviour is subject to a great deal of surveillance, exploitation of emotional desires, and insidious social control. Of course such generalisations need qualifying as they are just that – generalisations – arising from a particular interpretation of the current challenges facing children growing up in what psychologist Oliver James calls 'selfish capitalism' (James, 2007). We must remember that Western societies are not one homogenous mass, but encompass large diversities of ethnicity, class, location, social capital, climate, and services to name but a few. Whilst understanding the 'general' may help to understand the 'particular' it is no substitute for this, as staying at the level of the general, risks falling into unhelpful stereotypes.

5. Non-western childhoods

Any attempt to encompass the history, politics, and religion, not to mention psychology, of any culture or region is always going to be only partially successful. It would also be wise to be cautious of an analysis of cultural difference that relies on attractive and convenient polarized dichotomies that gloss over enormous intra-cultural differences and problematic local beliefs that cause suffering to their populations such as female infanticide and self-immolation (Lari et al, 2005; Banhatti et al, 2006).

As with generalisations about the impact of neo-liberal market dominated philosophies on children and families, there are also obvious limitations when making generalised statements about cultural beliefs and practices in the non-Western world. Nonetheless it is possible to note that some general differences can be found. Broadly speaking the predominant differences between non-Western and Western approaches to children is visible in the prolonged indulgence accorded to infants, and in the earlier acceptance of certain adult responsibilities in the children of many non-Western cultures. Thus, in many Western cultures the search for evidence of independence, self-reliance, and self-control starts more or less as soon as the child is born, while many non-Western cultures promote emotional dependence through immediate gratification of an infant's perceived needs. As the child grows older in Western culture independence is encouraged in thinking style, verbal communication, and emotional expression. Physical labour and the acceptance of duties and responsibilities do not occur until much later in Western than many non-Western cultures. In many non-Western cultures adolescence as a clear life stage with its own sub-culture is not so readily apparent, while a movement into adult duties and responsibilities (that include the products of a child's physical labour, as well as an early introduction to spiritual duties) may be already apparent before the onset of puberty. Many of these differences arise from a social orientation toward the 'individual' in Western cultures and toward the 'collective' in many non-Western cultures. This, at least in part, reflects the differing aims of many non-Western cultures where the ideologies behind parenting practices reflect the aim of helping the child transcend egotistic narcissism and toward the cultivation of dependability and interdependence, rather than towards independence as in the West (Timimi, 2005a; 2005b).

5.1 Models of child development

Long established theories and practices with regard child development have extensive histories in many non-Western traditions. For example, in traditional Indian thinking the human life cycle is conceptualised as unfolding in a series of stages each having unique tasks. Traditional Indian medicine and philosophy in the form of Ayurveda describes childhood Samskaras (which are expressive and symbolic performances) including rites and ceremonies that are held over the child to mark her/his transition from one stage to another (Kakar, 1994; 1997). Middle Eastern culture is heavily influenced by Islamic ideas on child development, which has been debated by Islamic scholars over many centuries (Gil'adi, 1992). Emphasis is placed on learning about the social values of Islam such as cooperation, truthfulness, helping the elderly, obeying parents, systems of spiritual purity and pollution, and the importance of cleanliness of the body. Various stages of cognitive development are identified, which revolve around sophisticated concepts such as Tamyiz (facility for discernment), Addab (respect/ public manners), and aql (mindfulness or social intelligence) the development of which in a child are seen as evidence of readiness to progress to the next developmental phase (Davis & Davis, 1989; Fernea, 1995; Gregg, 2005; Timimi, 2005a).

These models of child development, when coupled with early 'indulgence' of the infant and an orientation toward group identity and spiritual goals, lead to a high acceptance, low pressure, low competitiveness approach that fosters children's desire to show respect and obedience, as opposed to becoming preoccupied with self esteem as is often the case with children growing up in the Western tradition. Several social and anthropological studies have noted the positive impact this seems to have on children's mental health (Gregg, 2005; Hackett & Hackett, 1994; Kakar, 1994; Le Vine et al, 1994). There is good evidence that children growing up in such a value system show lower prevalence of mental disorder when compared to Western children (see for example Banhatti & Bhate, 2002; Banhatti et al, 2006; and Pillai et al, 2008 with regard children from the Indian Diasporas).

There is a general trend in many non-Western cultures toward the welcoming of children into society, greater acceptance of a range of childhood behaviours, and more consensual and hierarchical interpersonal relationships. This is mediated by value systems that place the child firmly in an ecological, spiritual and social context. Children grow up in an atmosphere where they are accepted for just being rather than for achieving certain 'developmental milestones'. Referring to Indian mothers Kakar (1994) and Roland (1980) have commented on the more relaxed attitude about the ages at which they expect children to develop skills. Furthermore, traditional Indian attitudes toward imperfection, disease, and misfortune, encourages an attitude of acceptance rather than seeking to blame, control, or redress; an attitude that can lead to resilience in the face of adversity (Banhatti et al, 2006). As Bhagwat (2002: iv) noted "*The child rearing practices and the childcare techniques have been practised over Indian subcontinents for thousands of years from generations to generations with minor changes in different regions and culture. However, no notable bad effects are observed. This has more importance in the light of behavioural disturbances found in children from the so-called developed countries*".

In many cultural settings the self is conceptualized as necessarily existing in a social context. For example, according to the concept of Ubuntu, prevalent in certain parts of Africa, "*a person is a person through other persons.*" In such cultures one can hardly be conceived of as existing as a human being in isolation. Such 'ethno-theories' contribute to shaping child rearing practices by helping to structure the goal of childrearing, its underlying developmental models, and hence the preferred methods and practices. For example, in comparative studies Japanese mothers are found to emphasize harmonious relations through cooperation, compliance, and empathy, while German mothers prefer the developmental goals of independence and individuality, reinforcing their child's autonomy. In case of conflicts, Japanese as compared to German mothers tend to empathize with their child's emotional state and attribute their child's behaviour to positive factors (such as 'a child is only a child'). These ethnotheories are linked to differing models of childhood, child development and child rearing. These models, in turn, lead to variations in childhood experiences. Thus Japanese mothers' approach seems to foster the establishment of a close emotional bond with their children, which helps the child control negative emotions more successfully than is the case for German children (Trommsdorff, 2002).

Thus many non-Western children grow up in contexts where a nurturing and, to many Westerners, an indulgent attitude towards the demands of an infant, is encouraged and where integration into wider society takes place earlier and with recognised stages marked by concrete rituals as they move from one stage to the next. This reflects on, not only their view of themselves as individuals and their aspirations, but also on the behaviour of those around them towards them. In 'collectivist' cultures (i.e. cultures whose value systems are orientated towards the importance of the group as opposed to the individual), people are, from birth onwards, integrated into strong, cohesive groups that continue to offer them protection in exchange for loyalty throughout that person's life (Hofstede, 1994). The sense of 'we' dominates over the sense of 'I' with obligations and duties often overriding personal preference in importance (Triandis, 1995).

When functioning well this way of life, provides sufficient emotional security, guidance, and a view of life that makes, for most, displays of defiant and aggressive behaviour less likely. With a greater number of adults available for care, nurturing, friendship, and physical affection and a greater number of peers readily available to entertain them, we have a good model of a system that is arguably better for the emotional nurturing of children than the increasingly fragmented and narcissistic models found in the West (Timimi, 2005a).

6. Globalisation

The ever-increasing abundance of global connections and our understanding of them constitute globalisation. This 'compression of the world' has led to an intensification of consciousness of the world and a shortening of distance and time across the globe. Many forces have been at play to bring about the globalisation we are so familiar with today, including the extension of world capitalist economy, industrialization, increasing surveillance (most notable through global information systems) and the world military order (Gidens, 1990; 1991). Global recessions have often hastened globalisation of world economic activity involving the speeding up of production and consumption turnover.

6.1 Globalisation from above and the problem of colonialism

One important aspect of globalisation is the neo-colonial character of the way the world economy has become organised. This economic system has resulted in glaring inequalities between the economically 'developed' and 'developing' worlds and, from a human rights perspective, it can be argued that the global economic system is guilty of on-going and systematic human rights violations and bears a large responsibility for many man made problems, such as poverty, starvation, lack of health care, militarization, and regional conflicts. It is notable that children are often disproportionately affected by famine and morbidity from lack of access to treatment for treatable diseases (such as malaria) and many of the issues above affect their lives directly (for example in many regional conflicts, child soldiers are involved in the fighting). These political, health, and social problems have a direct impact on children's mental health, as a result of factors such as trauma, chronic stress, loss of important people in their family, dislocation, and the effects of becoming accustomed to a life immersed in hardship and violence.

A more subtle impact of the neo-colonial nature of globalisation is the export of Western value systems to countries with value systems born out of different traditions. This can result in undermining the stability of traditional beliefs and practices that have served the children of many communities well, at the same time as producing points of conflict, antagonism and contradiction as the merits of different value systems clash (Ang, 1996). All too often these conflicts are resolved in favour of the more powerful and influential culture (i.e. that of the industrialized West).

These hierarchical dynamics can be found in our popularised visions of childhood. It is not only modern Western citizens whom Western professionals and governments feel should have a particular sort of childhood, but also worldwide populations who are often viewed as in need of civilisation and development (according to ideals derived from Western psycho-medicine). The export of Western notions of childhood, socialization, and education is inextricably connected to the export of modern Western constructions of gender, individuality, and family amongst other things (Comaroff & Comaroff, 1991; Stephens, 1995). As particular conceptions of 'normal' childhood are exported so are particular conceptions of 'deviant' childhoods. The perception that many third world children are living deviant childhoods can then be interpreted as local peculiarities and instances of backwardness and under-development thus justifying continued efforts to export Western visions of childhood around the world (Stephens, 1995).

We can see this dynamic occurring in the highest global political bodies. In 1989 the United Nations convention on the rights of the child was adopted by the United Nations general assembly (UN, 1989). The convention was not only a general statement of good intent, but also an instrument that is legally binding to those states that ratified it. More than previous treaties, the convention recognizes the child's capacity to act independently, bestowing not just protective but also enabling rights, such as the right to freedom of expression and association (Cantwell, 1989). According to Jo Boyden (1997) closer scrutiny of the convention shows that it has a strong interest in spreading to the poor countries of the South, the values and codes of practice devised in the public sector of the medico-psychological led visions of childhood of the industrialized North.

In the name of universal children's rights the UN convention asserts one dominant cultural, historical framework. For example, the language of the rights of 'the child' rather than the rights of 'children' suggests a universal freestanding individual child on a particular developmental trajectory. Caution is necessary when transplanting the concept of individual rights to societies where the family, not the individual, is considered the basic social unit. While the industrialized North places a high value on the development of the individual and their individuality, for many societies the desire to maintain group solidarity means that individual aspirations are not given the same level of importance. Therefore, what might be considered an abuse of rights in a Northern context (for example not giving a child free choice) may in other countries be perceived as a vital mechanism for maintaining the more highly valued aspiration of group cohesion.

Although raising children's rights as an international issue is potentially of great importance, greater account has to be taken of regional diversity – one universal standard risks causing further colonial oppression (Newman-Black, 1989). When this occurs important and often-conflicting conceptualizations of children's rights emerge. For example, when the Organization of African Unity drew up a charter on the rights and welfare of the child (Organisation of African Unity, 1990), much of the charter was framed in terms of responsibilities and duties of children and families rather than rights and needs of the child. Thus according to the Organization of African Unity's charter every child should have responsibilities towards their family and society, with children viewed as having a duty to work for the cohesion of the family, and to respect their parents, superiors and elders.

Just as problematic notions of child rearing are being imposed on countries of the South, so also are problematic notions of child mental health problems. As mentioned earlier, market economies need to continually expand markets has allowed drug companies to exploit new, vague, and broadly defined childhood psychiatric diagnoses, resulting in a rapid increase in the amount of psychotropic medication being prescribed to children and adolescents in the West. Globalisation means this trend is spreading to countries of the poorer South where growth in the prescribing of psychotropic medications to children is occurring (Wong et al, 2004). This suggests that the Western individualized biological/genetic conception of childhood mental health problems is spreading to the countries of the South and may be undermining more helpful indigenous belief systems (Timimi, 2005a; 2005b).

For the last few decades Western mental health institutions have been pushing the idea of 'mental-health literacy' on the rest of the world. Cultures are viewed as becoming more 'literate' about mental illness the more they adopt Western biomedical conceptions of diagnoses like depression, ADHD, and schizophrenia. This is driven by a belief that modern, 'scientific' approaches reveal the biological and psychological basis of psychic suffering and so provide a rational pathway to dispelling pre-scientific approaches that are often viewed as harmful superstitions. In the process of doing this, it is not only implied that those cultures that are slow to take up these ideas are therefore in some way 'backward', but also disease categories and ways of thinking about mental distress that were previously uncommon in many parts of the world are successfully exported. Thus conditions like depression, post-traumatic stress disorder, and anorexia appear to be spreading across cultures, replacing indigenous ways of viewing and experiencing mental distress (Summerfield, 2008; Watters, 2009). In addition to exporting these beliefs and values, Western drug companies see in such practice the potential to open up new and lucrative markets (Watters, 2009; Petryna et al, 2006).

Despite copious evidence from research in the non industrialised world, that shows the outcomes for major 'mental illnesses', is consistently better than in the industrialised world and particularly amongst populations who have not had access to drug based treatments, (Hopper et al, 2007; Whitaker, 2009) the World Health Organisation, together with the pharmaceutical industry, has been campaigning for greater 'recognition' of mental illnesses in the non-industrialised world, basing their assumptions on the idea that ICD/DSM descriptions are universally applicable categories (World Health Organisation, 2010). Like other marketing campaigns, this strategy has the potential to open up new markets for psychiatric drugs that maybe ineffective and can have serious side effects, at the same time as painting indigenous concepts of, and strategies to deal with, mental health problems, as being based on ignorance, despite their obvious success for these populations.

A subtler source of impact on cultural beliefs is due to psychiatric diagnoses inadvertently setting standards for 'normality', by categorising what emotional and behavioural traits and experiences should be considered 'disordered'. As the criteria for diagnoses are arrived at by subjective judgments rather than objective evidence (being literally voted in or out of existence by committees), they will have an automatic bias toward the cultural standards found in economically dominant societies (who also tend to control what counts as 'knowledge' globally). This sets in motion a diagnostic system vulnerable to institutional racism in the dominant societies and colonialism in others, as other standards of normality will, at least to some extent, come to be viewed as 'primitive', 'superstitious' etc. and their populations will be viewed as needing to be (psycho)educated. As a result then, for the majority of the world, all manner of complex somatic/emotional complaints have to be re-categorised, spiritual explanations have to be denounced, parenting practices viewed as oppressive and so on.

Thus imposing Western medical model DSM/ICD style psychiatry on non-Western populations risks a number of things including: adoption of Western psychiatric notions of 'psychopathology' to express mental distress, undermining of existing cultural strategies for dealing with distress, and the imposition of an individualistic approach that may marginalise family and community resources and divert attention from social injustice.

It is acknowledged by mainstream diagnostic manuals that cultural variations in psychopathology may be found in affective, behavioural, or linguistic expressions of distress, or in the content of disturbed cognitions and sensory experiences (e.g. American Psychiatric Association, 2000). However, the study of these variations in children and adolescents and how they change with increasing age has been largely ignored. Research is needed to investigate culture's role in the development and long-term course of emotional distress and behavioural deviance amongst children and adolescents. Prior to undertaking epidemiological studies, more work is needed to ascertain the ways psychopathology is defined in various cultures (Hoagwood & Jensen, 1997), including cultural variations in symptom expression and phenomenology (Manson et al, 1997). Despite its acknowledgment of culture's role in psychopathology, the nosological systems (i.e. DSM and ICD) applied currently in research still conceptualizes mental disorder as residing mainly in the individual. Such a nosological system itself emerged from an epistemology that is culturally constituted. The diagnostic criteria and measurement tools currently employed may thus restrict the likelihood of finding differences in prevalence, presentations and prognosis among differing cultural groups.

6.2 Stigma

One often cited reason for exporting Western model psychiatry to the rest of the world is the belief that societies in the developing world stigmatise those who have mental health problems (e.g. World Health Organisation, 2010). A review of the evidence however, shows that stigma maybe more of a problem for Western societies whose institutions support the mainstream medical model view of mental distress and behavioural deviance. Exporting Western psychiatry may thus result in more not less stigma for those in the developing countries who present with mental health problems.

Read et al (2006) carried out a comprehensive review of the literature on stigma and schizophrenia to assess whether the 'schizophrenia is an illness like any other' approach helps reduce prejudice towards those with the diagnosis. They found an increase in biological causal beliefs across Western countries in recent years, but also that biological attributions for psychosis were overwhelmingly associated with negative public attitudes. For example, Angermeyer & Matschinger (2005) subjected two representative population surveys of public attitudes to psychiatric patients conducted in Germany in 1990 and 2001 to a trend analysis. Over the period of the study an increase in public acceptance of biomedical explanations of psychosis was associated with a public desire for an increased distance from people with schizophrenia.

The 'medical model' of schizophrenia not only increases public stigma, but also contributes to patients internalising an explanatory model that can hinder recovery. For example, it has been found that the presence of 'insight' (in psychiatric terms, meaning accepting the medical model of having a brain illness) in schizophrenia lowers self-esteem, leads to despair and hopelessness, and also predicts higher levels of depression and risk of suicide attempts several years later (Crumlish et al, 2005). Hasson-Ohayon et al (2006) found that the presence of this sort of 'insight' was negatively correlated with emotional well-being, economic satisfaction, and vocational status. The conclusion we may draw from this body of research is that the empowerment of people with mental illness and helping them reduce their internalised sense of stigma are as important as helping them find insight into their illnesses (Warner, 2010). Accepting a diagnosis of schizophrenia means that the person must also accept the negative public attitudes and stigma associated the diagnosis. As this 'medical model' seems to increase internal and external stigma, exporting this worldwide seems like a counterproductive step. Some anthropological evidence supports this stance as it seems that part of the reason why the outcome is better for those who develop a psychotic episode in the developing world is less stigma.

For example, the anthropologist Juli McGruder spent a number of years in Zanzibar studying the families of those diagnosed with schizophrenia. Though the population is predominantly Muslim, Swahili spirit-possession beliefs are still prevalent and commonly evoked to explain the actions of those who violate social norms. McGruder found that far from being stigmatizing, these beliefs served certain useful functions. The beliefs prescribed a variety of socially accepted interventions and ministrations that kept the ill person bound to the family and kinship group. McGruder saw this approach in many small acts of kindness, watching family members use saffron paste to write phrases from the Koran on the rims of drinking bowls so the ill person could literally imbibe the holy words. The spirit-possession beliefs had other unexpected benefits. This way of viewing mental distress allowed the person a cleaner bill of health when the illness went into remission. An ill individual enjoying a time of relative mental health could, at least temporarily, retake his or her responsibilities in the kinship group. Since the illness was seen as the work of outside forces, it was understood as an affliction for the sufferer but not as an identity inscribed through unalterable internal factors such as his or her genes (Watters, 2009).

Although emotive images of unacceptable practice in developing countries are often used, such as pictures of persons deprived of their liberty by being tied to a tree or whatnot, we should remember that mental health systems in the West have institutionalised deprivation of liberty through legal means and that mental hospitals often use restraint and rapid tranquilisation, sometimes with fatal consequences - hardly evidence of a more 'humane' system.

6.3 Globalisation from below- new opportunities

The politics of neo-liberal globalisation also creates opportunities and paradoxes. Thus, neither the economic or cultural flow has been all one-way. Globalisation has arguably brought many aspects of non-Western cultures, from cuisine to medicinal, and from spiritual to aesthetic into the mainstream. Thus, the centre - periphery model of globalisation cannot account for these other complex, overlapping and disjunctive variations which result in differing regional concerns together with new forms of cultural hybridity and multiplicity (Appadurai, 1993).

Not only does globalisation create the space and possibilities for reverse cultural flow and thus new emerging fusions of identities, beliefs and practices, but, in addition, globalisation can produce resistance and, in some cases, a rediscovery of the importance of certain aspects of traditional culture. For example, despite prolonged attempts at influencing public opinion in Arab Middle East and North Africa, attitudes have, if anything, hardened against Western value systems and there has been a move to reaffirm and strengthen the regional, Muslim, identity (Fernea, 1995; Gregg, 2005). The rapid increase in exposure to global influences may indeed expose children and young people to conflict between contradictory values systems. This conflict can lead to vulnerability and mental health problems, but it can also lead to innovative solutions, and new cross- cultural identities both within the 'outsider' culture and the young of the host community (Banhatti et al, 2006).

7. Implications

There has been an increase in psychosocial disorders in children and adolescents in most Western societies. Childhood problems are increasingly medicalised resulting in an apparent 'epidemic' of emotional and behavioural disorders in children in the West and a rapid rise in the prescription of psychotropics to the young. I have summarised the problematic nature (in terms of lack of evidence for a biological substrate, high co-morbidity, lack of cross-cultural validity, boundary issues, marginalisation of certain types of evidence, and lack of evidence for effectiveness of medications used) of current popular child psychiatric diagnoses such as ADHD, autism and childhood depression elsewhere (Timimi, 2002; 2004; 2005a; 2008a; 2009b; Timimi & Maitra, 2006; Timimi et al, 2004; Timimi et al, 2010).

In this chapter I have explored how Western economic, political, and social conditions, often via its effects on the common value system, are contributing to increasing levels of poor mental health amongst children, and how potentially valuable alternative models can be found in non-Western traditions. The current professional response of medicalising these complex issues raises many practical, clinical and ethically dilemmas.

Whatever part of conditions such as ADHD are biological (all behaviour ultimately derives from a biological substrate), how we construct meaning out of this is a cultural process. Similarly, Western child protection systems also have problematic aspects. They have developed in the context of protecting the 'individual' child and often involve removal of the child from dangerous/abusive situations. Little legislative attention has been given to strengthening social cohesion and reducing inequality as an important avenue to improving child protection.

Our lack of engagement with alternative perspectives from non-Western traditions reflect a rather hidden form of institutionalized racism (or more accurately, institutionalized cultural hegemony) that has infected Western academic and political endeavours for several centuries. Not only does this present real dangers to the traditions and knowledge bases in existence in the non-Western world, but it also means that populations of the Western world are being denied the opportunity to benefit from the positive effects that giving serious consideration to non-Western knowledge, values and practices may bring.

Ethnographic or observational studies to identify and classify cultural variations in the expression of distress or psychopathology can provide data for hypothesis generation. Other exploratory studies using qualitative, ethnographic, and narrative methods can be used to generate ideas for construct definition and identification of culturally appropriate indices as well as correlates that, in turn, can serve as a basis for measurement construction and generation of alternative nosologies. Quantitative studies using larger, representative samples would follow. More careful consideration should be given to the following question: To what degree is what we find in cross-cultural research, the result of measures that are predicated on premises of the dominant, culturally constituted epistemology? If we have developed a measure with samples dominated by majority culture participants and then apply these measures cross-culturally, and find little difference in prevalence and little variability in the expression of, for example, anxiety, what does this finding mean? By defining, via the measurement instruments, what anxiety is in the majority European/American culture, there is likely to be a restriction of what we allow ourselves to find, and this will increase the likelihood that the disorder will look the same everywhere. For example, in an interesting paper by Jadhav (2007) the diagnostic criteria of an established South Asian culture specific neurosis, 'Dhat' syndrome (which revolves around a fear of semen loss), were deployed by a psychiatrist of South Asian origin, amongst white Britons in London, UK, presenting for the first time with a clinical diagnosis of Depression. Based on both narrative accounts and quantitative scores, Jadhav found a significant subset of white British subjects diagnosed with depression, may in fact be expressing a psychological variation of a previously 'unknown' local White British somatisation phenomena that he labels 'Semen Retention Syndrome'. Jadhav suggests that if you do the reverse of the usual procedure for categorizing mental distress in non-Western societies, substantial numbers of Western patients can be re-categorised into apparent culture bound syndromes, suggesting that Western derived mental health/illness categories commonly in use in psychiatry are just as culture bound.

Western professional's lack of knowledge about non-Western approaches to children is depriving the West of a rich source of alternative strategies. New ideas to help enrich theory and practice with regards children's mental health can be found in three key areas:

7.1 Defining problems

Different cultures see different behaviours as problematic. A model of child development that recognises that different cultures have different (and healthy) versions of child development has the potential to reduce the amount of pathologising of childhood in current Western medical practice and cultural discourse more generally. This requires Western professionals such as child psychiatrists, psychologists, paediatricians, psychotherapists, teachers, and social workers to question the universal validity of the concepts used in relation to children's development and mental health, and the rating questionnaires that accompany them and to accept a greater variety of childhood behaviours, child developmental trajectories, and parenting approaches as being 'normal' (Timimi, 2002; 2005a; 2005b; 2009a).

7.2 Solving problems

Western culture has many methods of treating childhood problems, including: family therapy, cognitive behavioural therapy, humanistic therapies, psychodynamic psychotherapy, and drugs. In addition, all communities have valuable resources, including spiritual/religious ones. For many non-Western cultures, the family not the individual is regarded as the basic social unit. Families' strengths and capacity to heal or comfort children can be recognised and promoted (Timimi, 2005a; Maitra, 2006, Banhatti et al, 2006).

Ideas from other systems of medicine may be useful. For example, Ayurvedic medicine sees illness as a disruption in the delicate somatic, climactic, and social system of balance. Causes are not located as such but seen as part of a system out of balance, with symptoms viewed as part of a process rather than a disease entity (Obeyesekere, 1977). Such an attitude based on balance with nature (as opposed to controlling it) has resonance with new approaches that include lifestyle interventions such as diet, exercise, mindfulness, family routines, and systemic psychotherapy all of which can help enhance and diversify clinical practice.

7.3 Cultural influences on behaviour

As socially respected practitioners, we have a responsibility to understand that we bring a cultural value system into our work. Our actions will ripple out into the wider local community. For example, if we calm a child's behaviour with drugs, the child's school may understandably refer more children for this treatment, resulting in a ripple effect into beliefs and practices around children's behaviour in that community, thus sparking off of a commodification process that can lead to a deskilling in the school staff and unnecessary exposure of children to potentially harmful medicines that do not improve outcomes in the long term. With regard policy we could support policies likely to promote a more pro-social value system, which limits opportunities for the commodification of children, and that supports stronger more cohesive families and communities. An exhaustive argument about what policies would produce such a change is not within the remit of this chapter. What we do need, however, is a wider debate that engages the public with politicians, in which knowledge about children's development, mental health, protection, and their relationship to culture should be included. Suggestions of policy areas that may promote a more pro-social set of values and consequently practices include: fighting global child poverty, support for community based services that use local resources and beliefs, limiting advertising aimed at the young, family friendly business practices such as flexible working hours, and criminalising wilfully absent parents.

8. Conclusion

Globalisation is happening in an era when the power relation between the world's rich and poor nations is glaringly unequal. We see this in the arena of health, with grossly disproportionate funds available to rich and poor countries. We also see it in the ideas that shape global approaches to health policy - for example, the World Health Organization continues to advocate the Western model of distress and mental illness as suitable for all countries and cultures– and to childhood.

The challenge for both the theory and practice in child and adolescent mental health is daunting, but there will be rich pickings if it can be met. We must critically re-examine the narrow basis on which current theory and practice has developed. This will help not only other culture's children but also children in the West. Increased knowledge will also make it easier to engage with multi-ethnic communities that have different faith traditions and cultural beliefs from the host society.

9. References

American Psychiatric Association. (2000). *Diagnostic and statistical manual of mental disorders (4th edition, text review)*, APA, Washington, DC.

Althusser, L. (1969). *For Marx*, Allen Lane, London.

Ang, I. (1996). *Living Room Wars*, Routledge, London.

Angermeyer, M.C., & Matschinger, H. (2005). Causal beliefs and attitudes to people with schizophrenia. Trend analysis based on data from two population surveys in Germany. *British Journal of Psychiatry*, 186, 331-334.

Appadurai, A. (1993). Disjuncture and difference in the global cultural economy. In: *Colonial Discourse and Post-Colonial Theory*, P. Williams & L. Chrisman (Eds.), Harvester Wheatsheaf, Hemel Hempstead.

Banhatti, R., & Bhate, S. (2002). Mental health needs of ethnic minority children. In: *Meeting the Needs of Ethnic Minority Children*, K.N. Dwivedi (Ed.), Jessica Kingsley, London.

Banhatti, R., Dwivedi, K., & Maitra, B. (2006) Childhood: An Indian perspective. In: *Critical Voices in Child and Adolescent Mental Health*, S. Timimi & B. Maitra (Eds.), Free Association Books, London.

Beckett, C. (2005). The Swedish myth: Corporal punishment ban and child death statistics. *British Journal of Social Work*, 35, 125-138.

Bhagwat, B.K. (2002). Foreword. In: *Child Care in Ancient India From the Perspectives of Developmental Psychology and Paediatrics*, M. Kapur & H. Mukundan, Sri Satguru Publications, Delhi.

Boyden, J. (1997). Childhood and the policy makers: a comparative perspective on the globalization of childhood. In: *Constructing and Reconstructing Childhood*, A. James & A. Prout (Eds.), Falmer Press, London.

British Medical Association. (2006). *Child and Adolescent Mental Health: A Guide for Professionals*, BMA, London.

Burman E. (2005). Childhood, neo-liberalism and the feminization of education. *Gender and Education*, 17, 351-367.

Calvert, K. (1992) *Children in the House: The Material Culture of Early Childhood, 1600-1900*, Northeastern University Press, Boston.

Cantwell, N. (1989). A tool for the implementation of the UN convention. In: *Making Reality of Children's Rights*, R. Barnen (Ed.), UNICEF, New York.

Castree, N. (2001). Commodity fetishism: Geographical imaginations and imaginative geographies. *Environment and Planning*, 33, 1519-1525.

Comaroff, J. & Comaroff, J. (1991). Africa observed: Discourses of the imperial imagination. In: *Of Revelation and Revolution: Christianity, Colonialism and Consciousness in South Africa, Vol.* 1, J. Comaroff & J. Comaroff (Eds.), University of Chicago Press, Chicago.

Cederblad, M. (1988). Behavioural disorders in children from different cultures. *Acta Psychiatrica Scandinavia*, 78(S344), 85–92.

Cook, R.J., Dickens, B.M. & Fathalla, M.F. (2002). Female genital cutting (mutilation/circumcision): Ethical and legal dimensions. *International Journal of Gynecology and Obstetrics*, 79, 281-287.

Crumlish, N., Whitty, P., & Kamali, M. (2005). Early insight predicts depression and attempted suicide after 4 years in first-episode schizophrenia and schizophreniform disorder. *Acta Psychiatrica Scandinavica*, 112, 449 - 455.

Davis, S.S., & Davis, D.A. (1989) *Adolescence in a Moroccan Town*, Rutgers University Press, New Brunswick.

Department of Health, NHSE (2005) *Prescription Cost Analysis England 2004*. Available at http://www.dh.gov.uk/PublicationsAndStatistics/Publications/PublicationsStatistics/PublicationsStatisticsArticle/fs/en?CONTENT_ID=4107504&chk=nsvFE0

Dodds, C. (2005). *Latest NICE Guidelines Sets New Standards for Treating Depression in Children and Young People*. Available http://www.nice.org.uk/pdf/2005_022_Depression_in_Children_Guideline.pdf

Double, D. (2002). The limits of psychiatry. *British Medical journal*, 324, 900-904.

Dwivedi, K.N. (1996). Culture and Personality. In: *Meeting the Needs of Ethnic Minority Children*, K.N. Dwivedi & V.P. Varma (Eds.), Jessica Kingsley, London.

Fernea, E.W. (Ed.) (1995). *Children in the Muslim Middle East*, University of Texas Press, Austin.

Finkelhor, D., & Korbin, J. (1988). Child abuse as an international issue. *Child Abuse and Neglect*, 12, 3-23.

Friedli, L. (2009). *Mental Health, Resilience and Inequalities: How Individuals and Communities are Affected*, World Health Organisation, Copenhagen.

Giddens, A. (1990). *The Consequences of Modernity*, Polity Press, Cambridge.

Giddens, A. (1991). *Modernity and Self-Identity*, Polity Press, Cambridge.

Gil'adi, A. (1992). *Children Of Islam: Concepts Of Childhood In Medieval Muslim Society*, MacMillan, Oxford.

Gregg, G.S. (2005). *The Middle East: A Cultural Psychology*, Oxford University Press, New York.

Hackett, L., & Hackett, R. (1994). Child rearing practices and psychiatric disorder in Gujarati and British children. *British Journal of Social Work*, 24, 191-202.

Hasson-Ohayon, H., Kravetz, S., Roe, D., David, A.S., & Weiser, M. (2006). Insight into psychosis and quality of life. *Comprehensive Psychiatry*, 47, 265-269.

Harkness, S., & Super, C. (Eds.) (1996). *Parents' Cultural Belief Systems: Their Origins, Expressions and Consequences*, Guilford Press, London.
Harvey, D. (2010). *A companion to Marx's Capital*, Verso, London.
Hoagwood, K., & Jensen, P. (1997). Developmental psychopathology and the notion of culture. *Applied Developmental Science*, 1, 108-1 12.
Hofstede, G. (1994). *Cultures and Organisations: Software of the Mind*, Harper-Collins, London.
Hopper, K., Harrison, G., Janka, A., & Sartorius, N. (Eds.) (2007). *Recovery from Schizophrenia: An International Perspective*, Oxford University Press, Oxford.
Jadhav, S. (2007). Dhis and Dhat: Evidence of semen retention syndrome amongst white Britons. *Anthropology and Medicine*, 14, 229–239.
James, O. (2007). *Affluenza*, Vermilion, London.
Kakar, S. (1994). *The Inner World of the Indian Child*, Oxford University Press, New Delhi.
Kakar, S. (1997). *The Inner World: A Psychoanalytic Study of Childhood and Society in India (Second Edition)*, Oxford University Press, New Delhi.
Kaplan, E. (1997). *Looking for the Other: Feminism, Film and Imperial Gaze*, Routledge, London.
Lari, A., Alaghehbandan, R., & Joghataei, M. (2005). Psychosocial and cultural motivations for self-inflicted burns among Iranian women. *International Psychiatry*, 9, 5-6.
LeFever, G.B., Dawson, K.V., & Morrow, A.D. (1999) The extent of drug therapy for attention deficit hyperactivity disorder among children in public schools. *American Journal of Public Health*, 89, 1359-1364.
LeVine, R.A., Dixon, S., LeVine, S., Richman, A., Leiderman, P.H., Keefer, C.H., & Brazelton, T.B. (1994) *Child Care and Culture: Lessons from Africa*, Cambridge University Press, Cambridge.
Maitra, B. (1996). Child abuse: A universal diagnostic category? *The International Journal of Social Psychiatry*, 42, 287-304.
Maitra, B. (2006). Culture and the mental health of children: The cutting edge of expertise. In: *Critical Voices in Child and Adolescent Mental Health,* S. Timimi & B. Maitra (Eds.), Free Association Books, London.
Manson, S. M., Bechtold, D. W., Novins, D. K., & Beals, J. (1997). Assessing psychopathology in American Indian and Alaska Native Children and Adolescents. *Applied Developmental Science*, l, 135-144.
Martin, J., & Sugarman, J., (2000). Between the modern and the postmodern: the possibility of self and progressive understanding in psychology. *American Psychologist*, 55, 397-406.
McMunn, A.N., Nazroo, J.Y., Marmot, M.G., Boreham, R., & Goodman, R. (2001) Children's emotional and behavioural well-being and the family environment: findings from the Health Survey for England. *Social Science and Medicine*, 53, 423-440.
Moncrieff, J. (2008) Neoliberalism and biopsychiatry: A marriage of convenience. In: *Libratory Psychiatry: Philosophy, Politics and Mental Health,* C. Cohen & S. Timimi (Eds.), Cambridge University Press, New York.
NHS Information Centre. (2010). *Prescription Cost Analysis, England – 2009*, available from: http://www.ic.nhs.uk/webfiles/publications/prescostanalysis2009/PCA_2009.pd f
National Institute of Drug Abuse. (2011). *Prescription Drug Abuse*, available from: http://www.nida.nih.gov/tib/prescription.html
Newman-Black, M. (1989). How can the convention be implemented in developing countries? In: *Making Reality of Children's Rights,* R. Barnen (Ed.), UNICEF, New York.
Obeyesekere, G. (1977). The theory and practice of psychological medicine in Ayurvedic tradition. *Culture, Medicine and Psychiatry*, 1, 155-181.

Olfson, M., Marcus, S.C., Weissman, M.M., & Jensen, P.S. (2002) National trends in the use of psychotropic medications by children. *Journal of the American Academy of Child and Adolescent Psychiatry*, 41, 514-21.

Organization of African Unity, (1990). *The African Charter on the Rights and Welfare of the Child Adopted by the 26th Ordinary Session of the Assembly of Heads of State and Government of the OAU*, OAU, Addis Ababa.

Petryna, A., Lakoff, A., & Kleinman, A. (2006) *Global Parmaceuticals: Ethics, Markets, Practices*, Duke University Press, Durham.

Pillai, A., Patel, V., Cardozo, P., Goodman, R., Weiss, H.A., & Andrew, G. (2008) Non-traditional lifestyles and prevalence of mental disorders in adolescents in Goa, India. *The British Journal of Psychiatry*, 192, 45–51.

Prout, A., & James, A. (1997). A new Paradigm for the sociology of childhood? Provenance, promise and problems. In: *Constructing And Re-Constructing Childhood: Contemporary Issues In The Sociological Study Of Childhood*, A. James, & A. Prout (Eds.), Falmer Press, London.

Read, J., Haslam, N., Sayce, L., & Davies, E. (2006). Prejudice and schizophrenia: A review of the 'Mental illness is an Illness like any other' approach. *Acta Psychiatrica Scandinavica*, 114, 303-318.

Richards, B. (1989). Visions of freedom. *Free associations*, 16, 31-42.

Robertson, M.M. (2000). No net loss: Wetland restoration and the incomplete capitalization of nature. *Antipode*, 32, 463-493.

Rose, N. (1999). *Powers of Freedom: Reframing Political Thought*, Cambridge University Press, New York.

Roland, A. (1980). Psychoanalytic perspectives on personality development in India. *International Review of Psychoanalysis*, 1, 73-87.

Segal, U. (1992). Child abuse in India: An empirical report on perceptions. *Child Abuse and Neglect*, 16, 887-908.

Sharav, V. (2006). *ADHD Drug Risks: Cardiovascular and Cerebrovascular Problems*. Available from: http://www.ahrp.org/cms/content/view/76/28/

Slater, D. (1997). *Consumer Culture and Modernity*, Polity, Cambridge.

Smith, R. (2003). An extreme failure of concordance. *British Medical Journal*, 327, 819.

Stephens, S. (1995) Children and the politics of culture in "Late Capitalism". In: *Children and The Politics Of Culture*, S. Stephens (Ed.) Princeton University, Press Princeton.

Summerfield, D. (2008). How scientifically valid is the knowledge base of global mental health? *British Medical Journal*, 336, 992-994.

Tait, G. (2006). A brief philosophical examination of ADHD. In: *Critical New Perspectives on ADHD*, G. Lloyd, J. Stead, & D. Cohen (Eds.), Routledge, Abingdon.

Timimi, S. (2002). *Pathological Child Psychiatry and the Medicalization of Childhood*, Brunner-Routledge, London.

Timimi, S. (2004). Rethinking childhood depression. *British Medical Journal*, 329, 1394-1396.

Timimi, S. (2005a). *Naughty Boys: Anti-Social Behaviour, ADHD, and the Role of Culture*, Palgrave Macmillan, Basingstoke.

Timimi, S. (2005b). Effect of globalisation on children's mental health. *British Medical Journal*, 331, 37-39.

Timimi, S. (2008a). Child psychiatry and its relationship to the pharmaceutical industry: Theoretical and practical issues. *Advances in Psychiatric Treatment*, 14, 3-9.

Timimi, S. (2008b). Children's mental health and the global market: an ecological analysis. In: *Libratory Psychiatry: Philosophy, Politics and Mental Health*, C. Cohen & S. Timimi (Eds.), Cambridge University Press, New York.

Timimi, S. (2009a). *A straight Talking Introduction to Children's Mental Health Problems*, PCCS Books, Ross-on-Wye.

Timimi, S. (2009b). The use of psycho-pharmaceuticals to control boys' behaviour: A tale of badly behaving drug companies and doctors. *Arab Journal of Psychiatry*, 20, 147 – 160.

Timimi, S. (2009c). The commercialization of children's mental health in the era of globalization. *International Journal of Mental Health*, 38, 5 – 27.

Timimi, S. (2010). The McDonaldization of childhood; Children's mental health in neo-liberal market cultures *Transcultural Psychiatry*, 47, 686-706.

Timimi, S., & Dwivedi, K. (2009) Child and adolescent psychiatry. In: *Psychiatry – An Evidence Based Text for the MRCPsych*, B. Puri & I. Treasaden (Eds.), Hodder-Arnold, London.

Timimi, S., & Maitra, B. (Eds.) (2006). *Critical Voices in Child and Adolescent Mental Health*, Free Association Books, London.

Timimi, S., & 33 co-endorsers. (2004). A critique of the international consensus statement on ADHD. *Clinical Child and Family Psychology Review*, 7, 59-63.

Timimi, S., Gardiner, N., & McCabe, B. (2010). *The Myth of Autism: Medicalising Men's and Boys' Social and Emotional Competence*, Palgrave MacMillan, Basingstoke.

Triandis, H.C. (1995). *Individualism and Collectivism*, Westview Press, Boulder.

Trommsdorff, G. (2002). An eco-cultural and interpersonal relations approach to development of the lifespan. In: *Online Readings in Psychology and Culture (Unit 12, Chapter 1)*, W.J. Lonner, D.L. Dinnel, S.A. Hayes, & D.N. Sattler (Eds.), Center for Cross-Cultural Research, Western Washington University, Washington DC.

UNICEF. (2001). *A League Table of Child Deaths by Injury in Rich Nations*. UNICEF Innocenti Research Centre, Florence.

UNICEF. (2007). *An Overview of Child Well-Being in Rich Countries*, UNICEF Innocenti Research Centre, Florence.

UNICEF. (2011). *Child Well-Being in the UK, Spain and Sweden: The Role of Inequality and Materialism*. Available from: http://www.unicef.org.uk/Documents/Publications/UNICEFIpsosMori_childwellbeing_reportsummary.pdf

United Nations General Assembly. (1989). *Adoption of a Convention on the Rights of the Child*, United Nations, New York.

University of Washington. (2011). Less depression for working moms who expect that they 'can't do it all'. *ScienceDaily*, August 25, 2011. Available from: http://www.sciencedaily.com/releases/2011/08/110820135309.htm

Warner, R. (2010) Does the scientific evidence support the recovery model? *The Psychiatrist*, 34, 3-5.

Watters, E. (2009). *Crazy like us: The Globalization of the American Psych*, Free Press, New York.

Whitaker, R. (2010). *Anatomy of an Epidemic*, Crown, New York.

Wolfenstein, M. (1955). Fun morality: An analysis of recent child-training literature. In: *Childhood in Contemporary Culture*, M. Mead & M. Wolfenstein (Eds.), The University of Chicago Press, Chicago.

Wong, I.C., Murray, M.L., Camilleri-Novak, D., & Stephens, P. (2004) Increased prescribing trends of paediatric psychotropic medications. *Archives of Disease in Childhood*, 89, 1131-2.

World Health Organisation. (2010). *mhGAP Intervention Guide*, WHO, Geneva.

Zito, J.M., Safer, D.J., Dosreis, S., Gardner, J.F., Boles, J., & Lynch, F. (2000) Trends in prescribing of psychotropic medication in pre-schoolers. *Journal of the American Medical Association*, 283, 1025-30.

22

Mental Health of Children from a Chronobiological and Epidemiological Point of View

Tetsuo Harada[1], Miyo Nakade[1,2], Kai Wada[1], Aska Kondo[1],
Mari Maeda[1], Teruki Noji[1] and Hitomi Takeuchi[1]
[1]*Kochi University,*
[2]*Tokai Gakuen University,*
Japan

1. Introduction

In 24-hour society seen especially in developed countries including Japan, fluctuations in the environmental conditions that act as zeitgebers for the circadian clock, such as light, meals and even social activities (e.g. "flextime") tend to become irregular and with decreasing amplitudes. Using mobile phones, playing video games, and frequenting 24-hour stores may accelerate this irregularity of environmental diurnal rhythms. These circumstances lead to weaker zeitgebers for entraining circadian clocks in children and promote a shift to the evening-typed diurnal rhythms in daily life. This evening-typed life style may potentially cause a decline in mental health in children via these three physiological mechanisms:

1. A tendency towards inner desynchronization of the two biological clocks (main clock and slave clock in the SCN, Honma & Honma, 1988) in evening-typed children
2. Lower serotonin levels in the daytime due to lower tryptophan consumption at breakfast (no breakfast or lower nutritional quality of breakfast)
3. Shortage of actual sleep duration

This chapter includes several sections in relation to mental health of children:

- Are Japanese children shifting towards evening-typed lifestyles?
- Are evening-typed children exhibiting poorer mental health?
- Environmental factors that promote evening-typed lifestyles 1 (Light environment)
- Environmental factors that promote evening-typed lifestyles 2 (Breakfast regularity and nutritional content)
- Environmental factors that promote evening-typed lifestyles 3 (24-hour commercialization of society: mobile phones, 24-hour convenience stores, video games, late night television)
- Intervention programs to promote morning-typed lifestyles and better mental health in kindergarten children.
- Intervention programs to promote morning-typed lifestyles and better mental health in elementary and junior high school students

- Conclusions: How can we change the environmental conditions surrounding children to promote better mental health?
- References

2. Are Japanese children shifting towards evening-typed lifestyles?

Due to the rapid advance of 24-hour society in Japan, Japanese children and students have been gradually shifting to evening-typed lifestyles, especially in the five year period from 1999-2004. Figure 1 shows an example of the rapid shift to evening-typed lifestyle in junior high school students, and especially girls. Scores improved between 2001 and 2006. Kochi is the most active place in Japan for the "Early to Bed, Early to Rise, and Don't Forget Your Breakfast" campaign being promoted throughout Japan since 2003. This campaign may have caused the improvement. However, girls are still more evening-typed than boys. A small chapter later on will discuss the reasons for girls being more evening-typed. From 8 years old (grade 1 of elementary school) to 13 years old (grade 1 of junior high school), morningness-eveningness (M-E) scores gradually decrease with age (Figure 2). Students aged 9-11 years (grade 3 to 5 of elementary school) showed significantly lower M-E scores (were more evening-typed) in 2003 and 2004 than in 1998 (Figure 2).

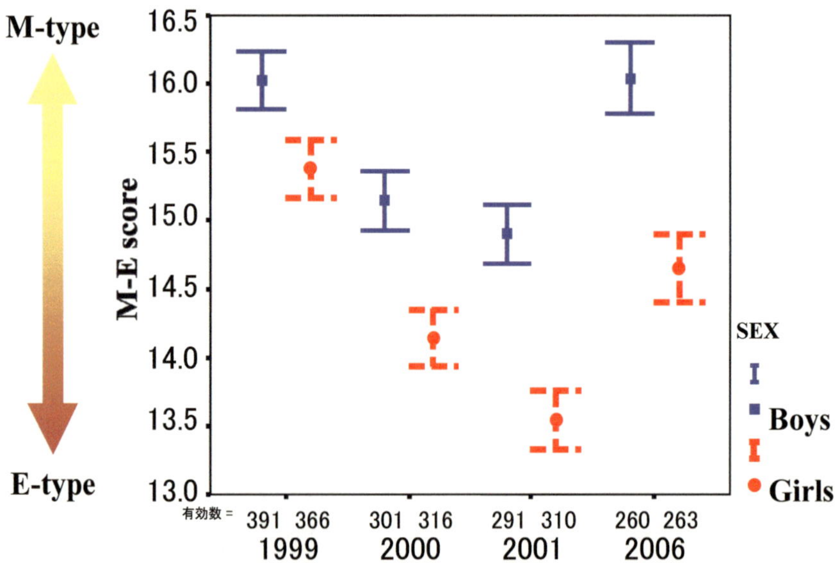

Fig. 1. Inter-annual variation in Morningness-Eveningness (M-E) scores of students attending a Japanese junior high school in Kochi (33°N).

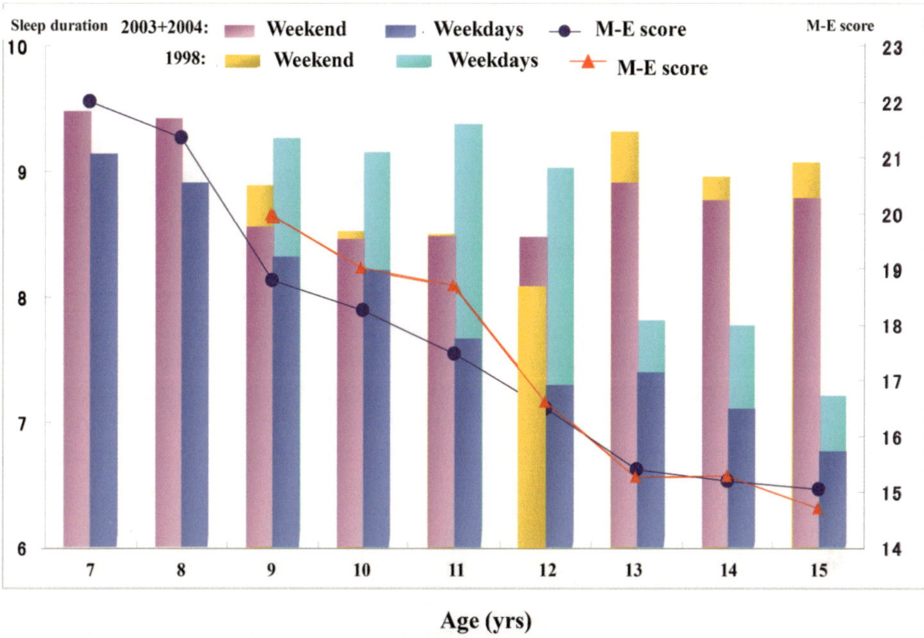

Fig. 2. Comparison between 1998 and 2003-2004 in variation of sleep duration and Morningness-Eveningness (M-E) scores by age in Japanese children attending elementary school (7-12 years) or junior high school (13-15 yrs) located in Kochi city (33°N).

Among older students aged 18-30 years, men were significantly or tended to be more evening-typed than women. However, this gender difference in M-E scores disappeared in 2009 (Table 1). This phenomenon can be explained by the recent rapid shifting to evening-type life observed only in women.

	2003	2004	2005	2006	2009
Females					
	15.89 ± 3.64 (220)	14.98 ± 4.47 (140)	15.30 ± 3.59 (353)	15.24 ± 3.54 (210)	15.15 ± 3.07 (198)
Males					
	14.66 ± 4.14 (236)	14.26 ± 3.3 (129)	14.15 ± 3.19 (211)	13.99 ± 3.311 (198)	14.73 ± 3.29 (198)
Mann-Whitney U-test: z , p					
	-3.391, 0.001	-1.700, 0.089	-3.679, <0.001	-3.904, <0.001	-1.067, 0.286
In total					
	15.25 ± 3.95 (457)	14.63 ± 4.901 (269)	14.89 ± 3.48 (574)	14.63 ± 3.49 (408)	14.97 ± 3.20(396)
Kruskal- Wallis test:	*χ2 value =9.952,*	*df=3,*	*p=0.019 (2003-2006)*		

Table 1. Inter-annual variation of M-E scores in Japanese university students and students of training schools for medical nurses and physical therapists aged 18-30 years in Kochi (30°N).

In conclusion of this section, females continue to be evening-typed through adolescence and adulthood. This evening-typed lifestyle for females is very dangerous in terms of mental and physical health, as extremely evening-typed lifestyle is associated with irregular menstrual cycles, severe symptoms of premenstrual syndrome, and more severe menstrual pain (Takeuchi et al., 2005). Especially for adolescent girls, a morning-typed lifestyle is critical for the development of a stable reproductive system including the regular menstrual cycle.

3. Are evening-typed children exhibiting poorer mental health?

Figures 3 & 4 show a significant relationship between chronotype of young Japanese children and mental health. Young children who became depressed frequently or frequently became angry due to a very small trigger are significantly more evening-typed than those who did not exhibit these symptoms. Figures 5 & 6 also indicate the relationship between chronotype of Japanese adolescents (junior high school students) and frequency to feel depression or irritation. Evening-typed adolescents felt more depressed and irritated more frequently than morning-typed adolescents.

In older Japanese students aged 18-30 years, students who lived in rooms with sufficient light exposure and had stable moods were significantly more morning-typed than those who did not (Figure 7). This phenomenon suggests that students who tried to expose themselves to sunlight even indoors shifted to morning-types with a more stable mood. Improvement of mood that accompanies greater morningness may be caused by better coupling of two internal oscillators (Honma & Honma, 1988) and by higher serotonin synthesis (Nakade et al., 2009).

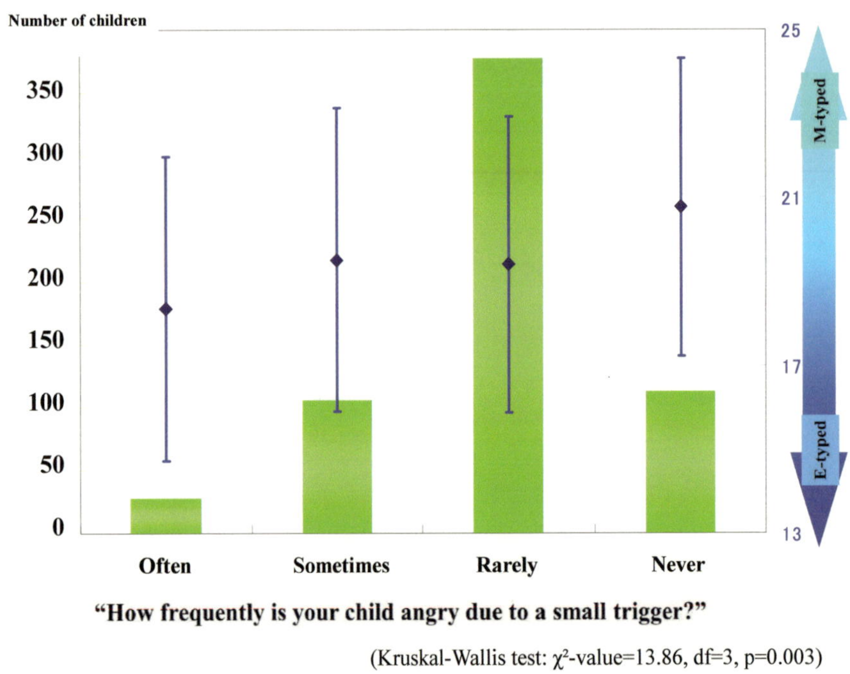

Fig. 3. Relationship between chronotype and frequency of becoming angry due to a small trigger in Japanese children aged 2-6years in 2003.

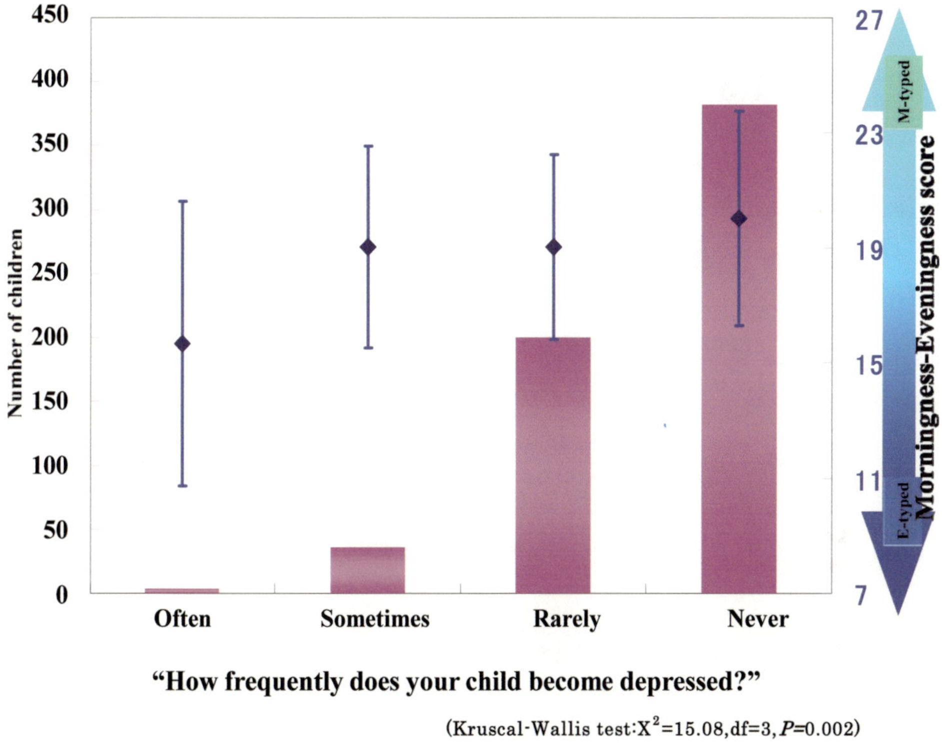

Fig. 4. Relationship between chronotype and frequency of becoming depressed in Japanese children aged 2-6years in 2003.

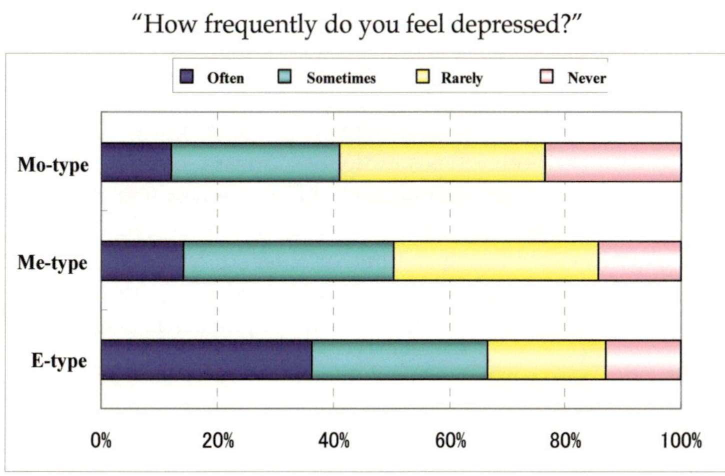

Fig. 5. Relationship between chronotype and frequency to feel depression in Japanese junior high school students in 2005. Mo-type =Morning-type: 25% of the distribution; Me-type=Medium-type: 50% of the distribution; E-type=Evening-type: 25% of the distribution.

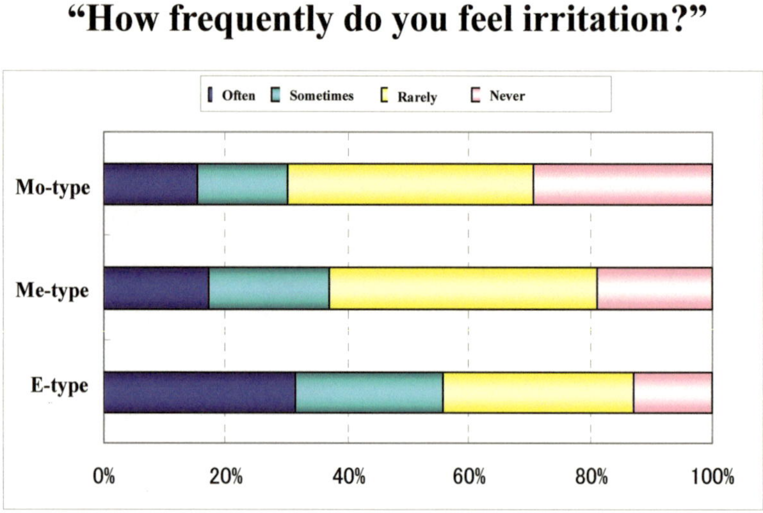

Fig. 6. Relationship between chronotype and frequency to feel irritation in Japanese junior high school students in 2005. Mo-type =Morning-type: 25% of the distribution; Me-type=Medium-type: 50% of the distribution; E-type=Evening-type: 25% of the distribution

4. Environmental factors that promote evening-typed lifestyles 1 (light environment)

Children aged 2-6 years who used black-out curtains or blinds (Mean ± SD, 20.27 ± 3.48, n=245) were more evening-typed than those who used cotton or lace curtains (21.09±3.39, 507) (Mann-Whitney U-test, z=-3.073, p=0.002), although no such differences were observed in older students (z=-1.449, p=0.147) (Figure 8). Children aged 2-6 years who used a fluorescent lamp as their evening lighting went to bed significantly later on nights before holidays than those who used other types of lighting (mostly orange color and other lower color temperature light bulbs), although no such difference was observed in older students aged 18-30 years (Figure 9). No significant differences due to evening lighting were seen in bed times on weekdays in either young children or older students (Figure 9). Actigraph data of a university student showed that use of blackout curtains in the summer (August) in Kochi (33°N) caused his bed times to become free running (Harada et al., 2003) (Figure 10).

Black-out curtains shut out early morning sunlight which has powerful potential for inducing a phase advance of human circadian oscillators, and use of such curtains induces a phase delay of the sleep-wake cycle. In the evening, blue light included in wave components emitted from fluorescent lamps may induce a phase delay of circadian rhythms. These results match those of light pulse experiments by Honma and Honma (1988).

Strong light from fluorescent lamps induces a phase advance of circadian rhythms in the early morning and a phase delay in the first half of subjective night. These phase altering effects may be observed even under weak 200-300 lux lighting.

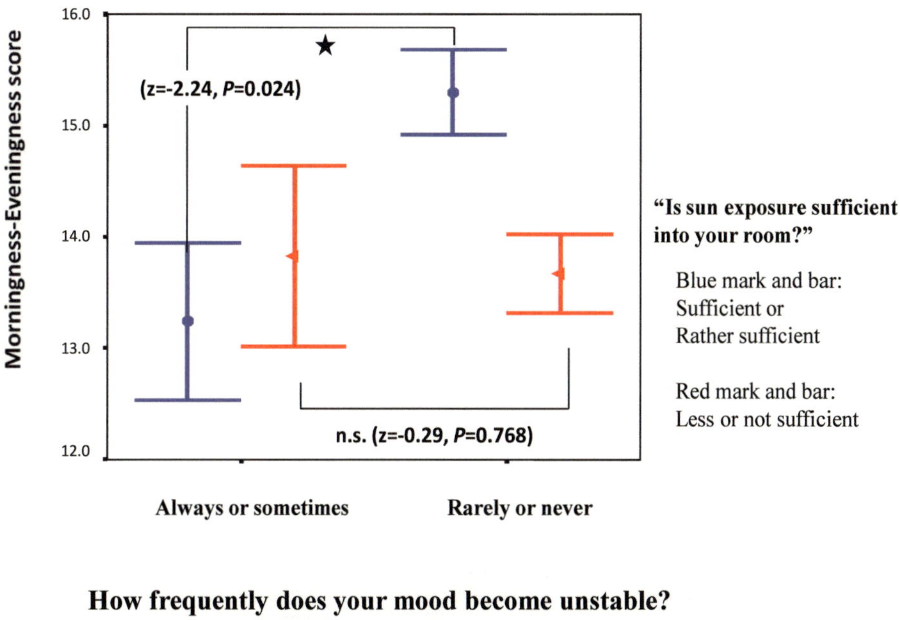

Fig. 7. Integrated relationship among circadian typology, sun-exposure extent and mood change in Japanese elder students aged 18-30 years in 2003.

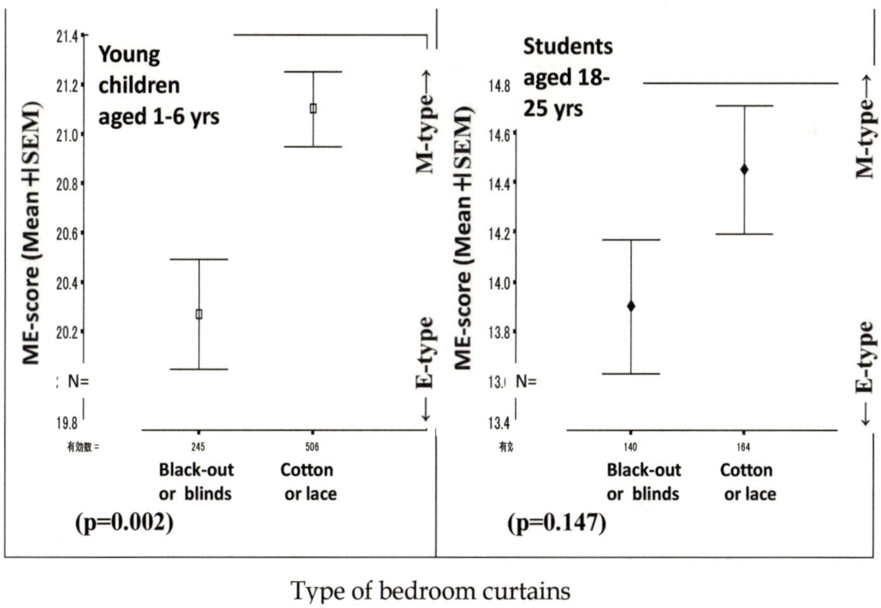

Fig. 8. Effects of type of bedroom curtain on circadian typology of young Japanese children and older students.

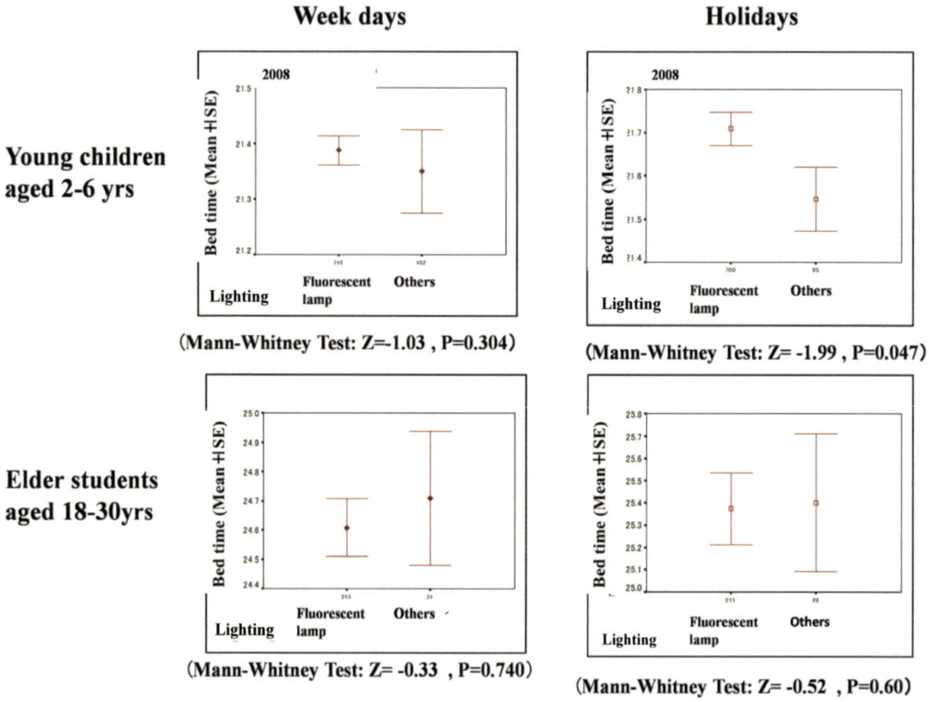

Fig. 9. Effects of evening lighting on circadian typology in young Japanese children and University students (2008).

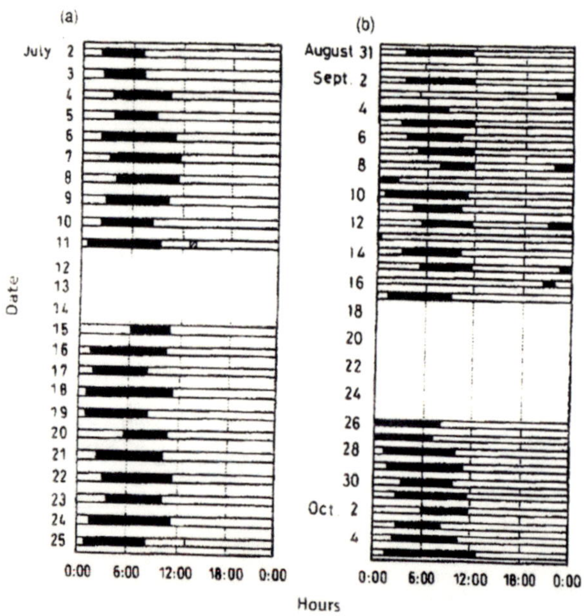

Fig. 10. Sleep-wake cycle of student A (a) before and (b) after changing to black-out curtains. Open bars: awakening, grey bars: nap and black bars: night sleep (Harada et al., 2003).

5. Environmental factors that promote evening-typed lifestyles 2 (Breakfast regularity and nutritional content)

Most young children eat breakfast at the same time everyday or almost every day. These children show significantly more morning-typed diurnal rhythms than children who frequently ate breakfast at irregular times. However, no clear relationship was observed between frequency of eating breakfast at a regular time and circadian typology in their parents (mostly mothers) (Figure 11).

Harada et al. (2007) calculated the amount of tryptophan consumed based on the tryptophan content of various food items and types of food eaten for breakfast, to create an index of estimated tryptophan intake. A significant positive correlation was seen between the tryptophan index and M-E scores (Figure 12 modified from Harada et al., 2007). Indices of tryptophan intake from supper did not differ among the three circadian types (morning type: 25% of the distribution, medium type: 50%, evening type: 25%), whereas the indices of tryptophan intake from breakfast were significantly higher in morning-type children than in medium- and evening-typed children (Figure 13).

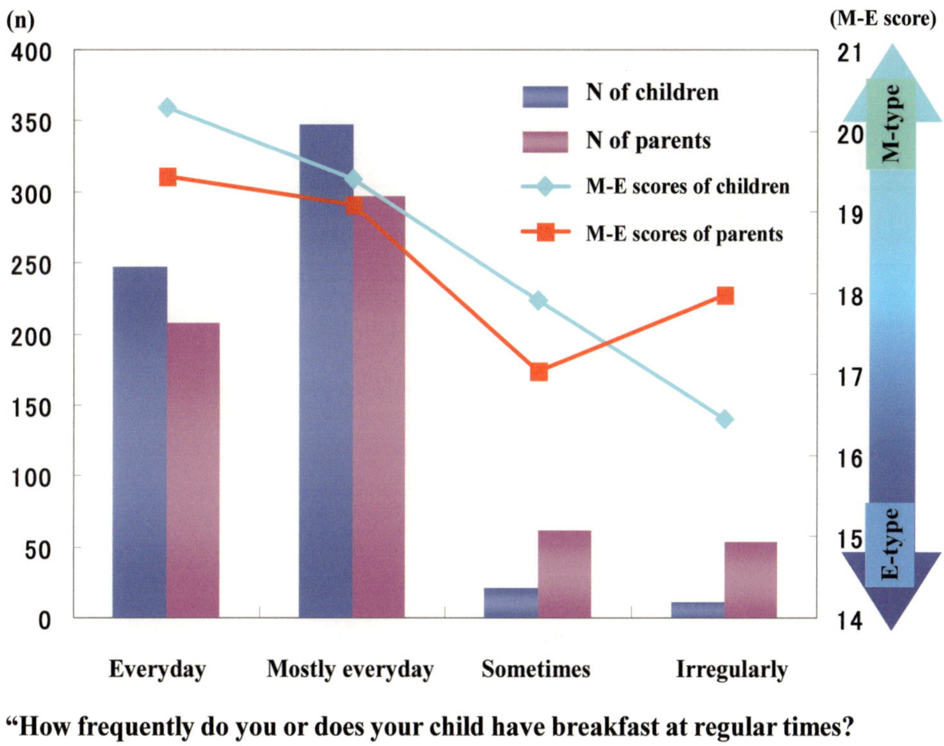

Fig. 11. Relationship between the frequency of having breakfast at regular times and circadian typology of Japanese children aged 2-6years and their mothers living in Kochi (33°N). Questionnaires were administered in June-July in 2004.

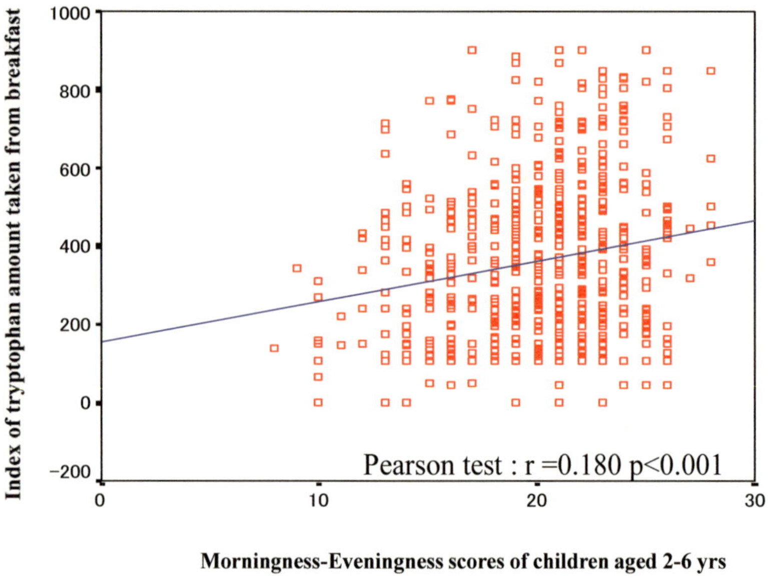

Fig. 12. Significant positive correlation between index of tryptophan intake from breakfast and circadian typology in young Japanese children living in Kochi (33°N). Questionnaires were administered in June-July, 2004. (Harada et al., 2007)

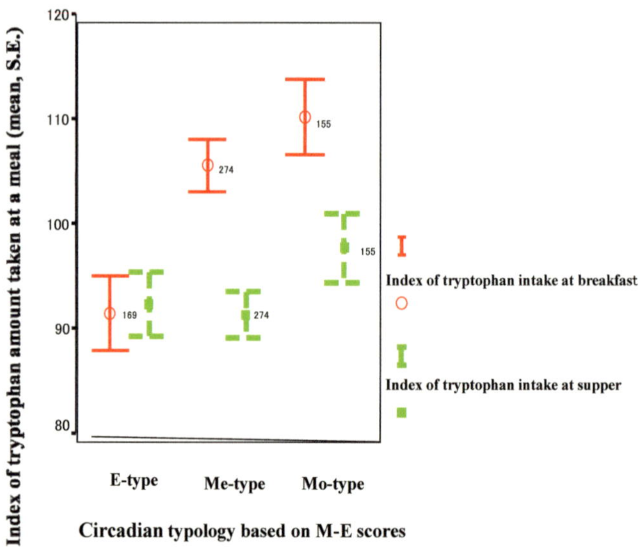

(Kruscal-Wallis U-test: Breakfast, χ^2=18.505, df=2, p<0.001,

Supper, χ^2=2.054, df=2, p=0.358)

Fig. 13. Relationship between circadian typology of Japanese children aged 2-6years and tryptophan intake at breakfast or supper. E-type, Me-type and Mo-type mean evening-type, medium type and morning-type, respectively. Morning-typed children show significantly higher tryptophan intake at breakfast but not at supper.

Nakade et al (2009) showed that children who ate one or more dishes including high amounts of protein were significantly more morning-typed than those who did not. Moreover, morning-type-promoting effects of sun exposure after the breakfast were shown only in children who ate high protein meals (Figure 14 from Nakade et al., 2009).

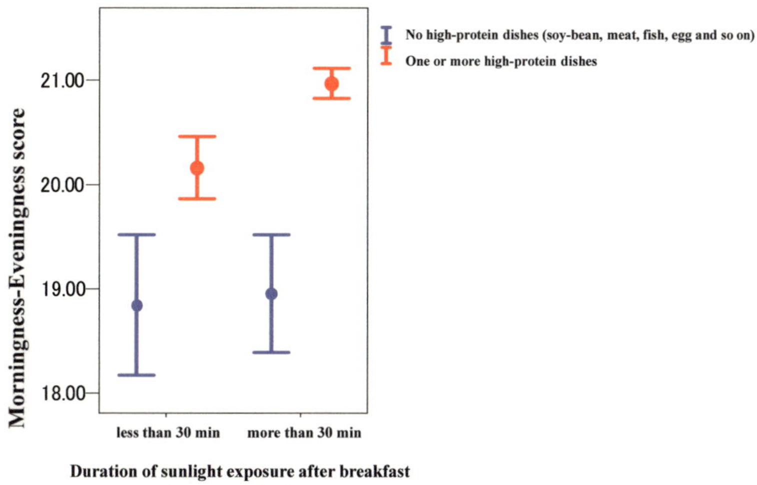

(**Mann-Whitneys U-test:** Effect of sunlight exposure on M-E scores, no high-protein dish(es) at breakfast, z=-0.098, p=0.922; high-protein dish(es), z=-2.293, p=0.022)

Fig. 14. Effect of sunlight exposure after breakfast on circadian typology depending on whether high-protein dish(es) is(are) included in children's dishes at breakfast. (Nakade et al., 2009).

Regular timing of breakfast could be an effective zeitgeber for circadian oscillators in preschool and kindergarten aged children. High intake of tryptophan at breakfast followed by exposure to sunlight may promote serotonin synthesis in the morning, and the accompanying high peak of extra-cellular brain concentration of serotonin may be a good internal zeitgeber for human circadian clocks.

6. Environmental factors that promote evening-typed lifestyles 3 (24-hour commercialization of society: mobile phones, 24-hour convenience stores, video games, late night television)

Partial results of an integrated analysis on the effects of using mobile phones, frequenting convenience stores and watching late night TV (starting at 11:00 p.m.) are shown in Figures 15, 16, and 17. Figure 15 shows that circadian typology in Junior high school students depends on the duration of each instance of mobile phone usage. This dependence is extreme in girls. Figure 16 demonstrates that a high frequency of visiting convenience stores leads to evening-typed diurnal rhythms in both girls and boys.

In contrast, boys who frequented convenience stores every day were significantly more morning-typed than those who did not. This result may seem odd, but can be explained as phase-advancing effect of bright light (1000-1500 lux) inside the store in the morning before school.

(Kruskal-Wallis test: boys, χ^2=5.040, df=3, p=0.167, girls, χ^2=16.838, df=3, p=0.001)

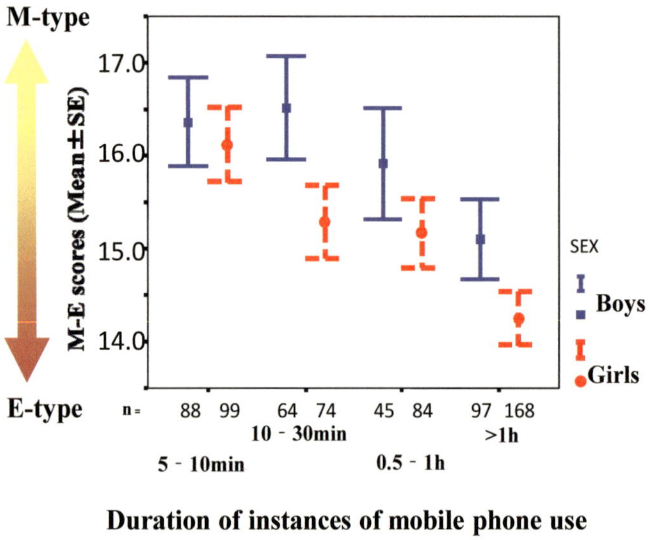

Fig. 15. Relationship between duration when mobile phone was once used and circadian typology in Japanese junior high school students living in Kochi (33°N). Questionnaires were administered in 2003-2006.

(Kruskal-Wallis test, boys, χ^2 =15.457, df=3, p=0.001, girls, χ^2=15.421, df=3, p=0.001)

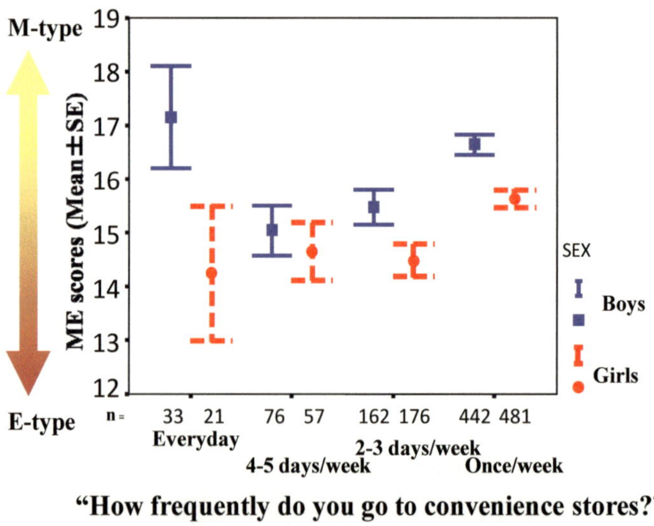

Fig. 16. Relationship between frequency of using convenience stores and circadian typology in Japanese junior high school students living in in Kochi (33°N). Questionnaires were administered in 2003-2006.

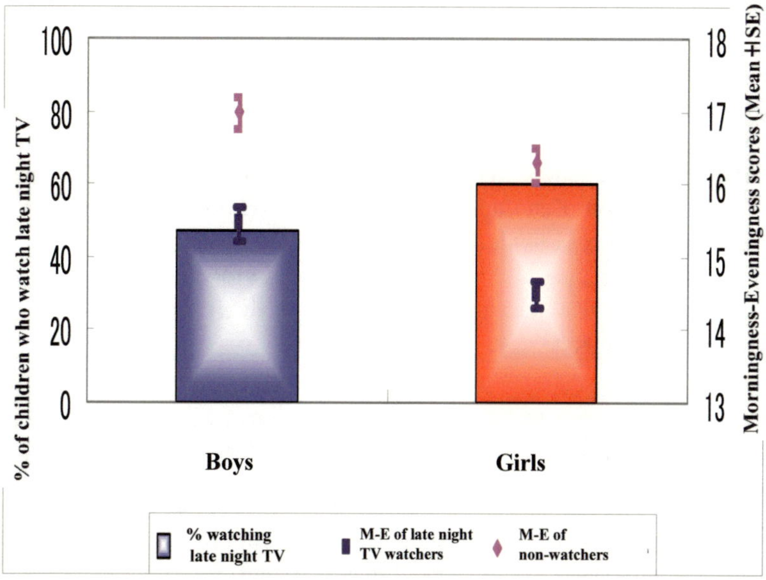

Fig. 17. Watchers of late night TV (from 11:00 p.m.) were much more evening-typed than non-watchers among both boys and girls attending a junior high school in Kochi (33°N). (Mann-Whitney U-test: boys, z=-4.92, p<0.001; girls, z=-6.14, p<0.001)

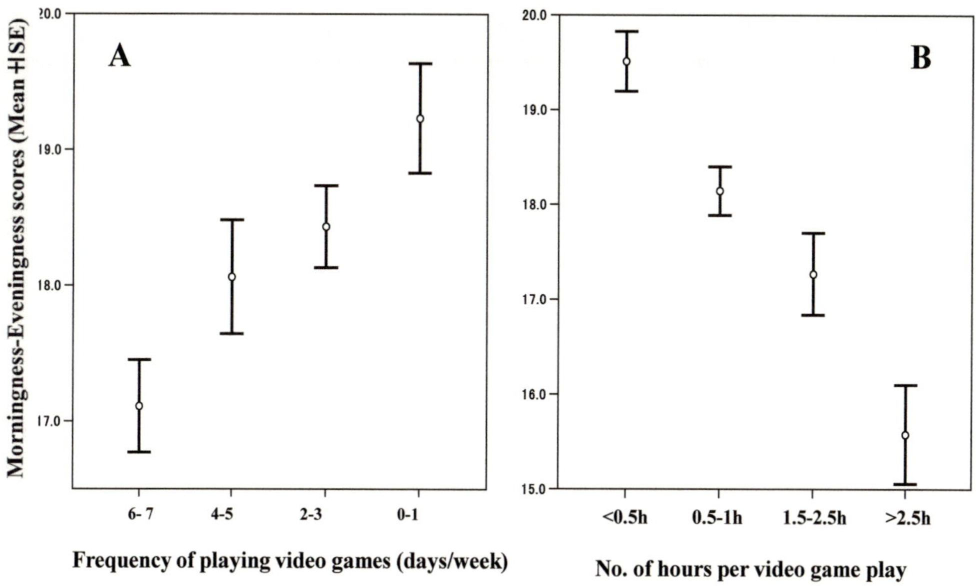

Fig. 18. Relationship between circadian typology and frequency of playing video games (A) and number of hours per instance of video game playing (B) in students attending an elementary school in Kochi (33°N).Questionnaires were administrated to all the students in 2007, and 560 students responded (response rate of about 70%).

Among Japanese adolescents, 60% of girls watch late night TV, while only 48% of boys do so (Figure 17). Junior high students who watch late night TV show much lower M-E scores (1.5-1.8 points lower) than those who do not, irrespective of gender (Figure 17). Figure 18 shows a clear negative correlation between circadian typology (M-E scores) and frequency of playing video games on a gaming device, and between typology and duration of each instance of playing video games, in elementary school students living in Kochi, Japan. These clear correlations suggest that Japanese elementary school students play video games mainly in the evening. Krejci et al. (2011) recently reported that Japanese children aged 2-6 years and Czech children aged 2-8 years mainly played video games from 6:00 to 9:00 p.m. in June, and from 3:00 to 6:00 p.m. in November, respectively, and usage shifted children in both countries to evening typology.

7. Intervention programs to promote morning-typed lifestyles and better mental health in kindergarten children (Kondo et al., unpublished)

The objective of this intervention program was to assess whether a newly produced month-long intervention program which consists of 9 intervention items is effective for shifting diurnal rhythms of Japanese children aged 2-6years to morning-type.

The first 2 items consisted of letting children affix stickers of "NO TV BOY"(Intervention-1) or "NO VIDEO GAME GIRL"(Intervention-2) to a mount if they did not watch TV or play videogames that day. A leaflet for changing to a morning-typed lifestyle was written by Harada et al (unpublished) and included 7 advices to parents:

1. Expose your child to early morning sunlight (Intervention-3)
2. Avoid using fluorescent lamps during the first half of subjective night (Intervention-4)
3. Give your child a nutritionally rich breakfast at the same time every day (Intervention-5)
4. Expose your child to sunlight after breakfast to increase efficiency of serotonin synthesis (Intervention-6)
5. Enforce bedtime discipline (Intervention-7)
6. Shift your own diurnal rhythms (as the parent) to morning-type (Intervention-8)
7. Avoid bringing your child to shops or restaurants after sunset (Intervention-9)

These 9 interventions were administered to 1367 children who attended one of 11 nursery schools or 1 kindergarten in Kochi for 1 month in June, 2008. Effects of the interventions were estimated using an integrated questionnaire on how many days in the 30-day period they could administer each of the 9 intervention items and an anonymous questionnaire on diurnal rhythms (including an M-E questionnaire that Torsvall and Åkerstedt (1980) constructed and questions on sleep habits, depression, anger, and other topics). The questionnaires were administered immediately preceding the start of the intervention period and 2 months after the end of the intervention period. Increasing number of items in which a child could participate for more than 20 days correlated to greater morningness ($p<0.01$) (Figure 19), higher quality sleep ($p<0.01$) and better mental health ($p=0.01$) (Figure 20).

	r	*P* (both)	N
Intervention3 (Morning light)	-0.30	0.00	460
Intervention4 (Fluorescent L	-0.13	0.00	463
Intervention5 (Breakfast)	-0.24	0.00	471
Intervention6 (Sunlight)	-0.16	0.00	459
Intervention7 (Descipline)	-0.29	0.00	468
Intervention8 (MtypeParents	-0.32	0.00	467
Intervention9 (No nightstore	0.03	0.47	471
Intervention1 (NoTV Boys)	-0.15	0.00	464
Intervention2 (No Game Girls)	-0.11	0.02	453

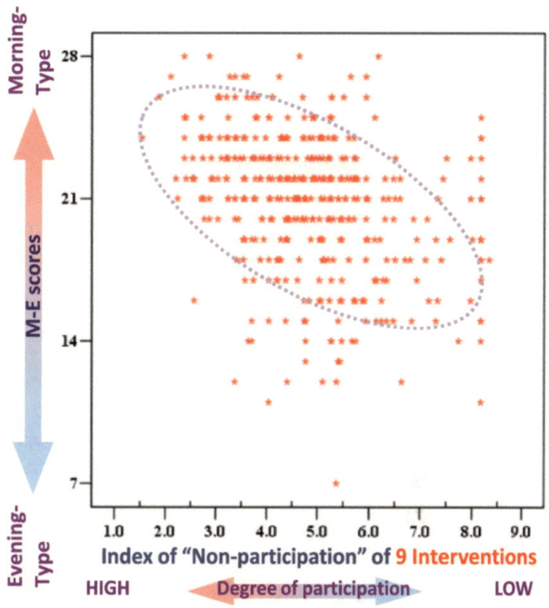

Fig. 19. Total scores of non-participation of Interventions 1-9 and M-E scores (Correlation analysis: r=0.348, p<0.01).

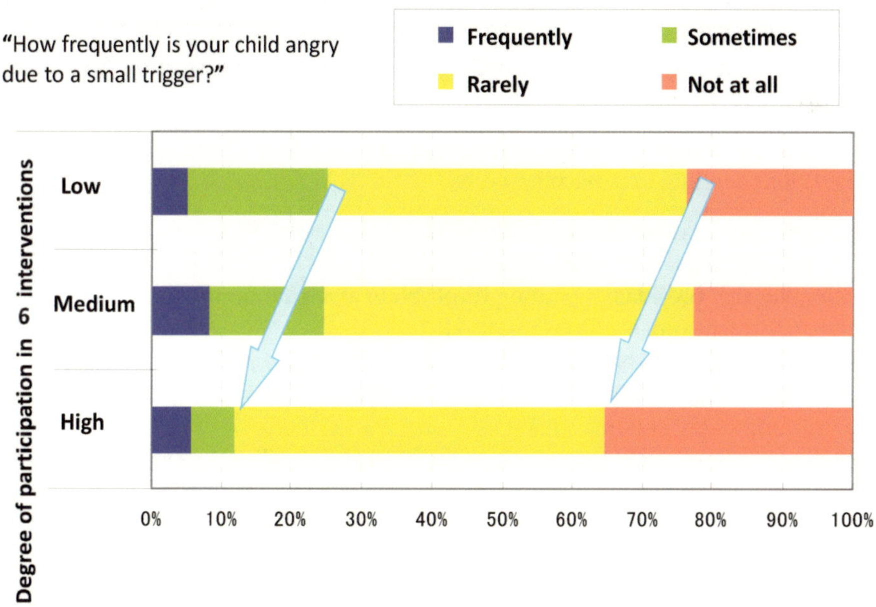

Fig. 20. High degree of participation of 9-Interventions leads to better mental health (frequency of anger triggered by something small) in Japanese children aged 1-6 years (p=0.012).

8. Intervention programs to promote morning-typed lifestyles and better mental health in elementary and junior high school students (Kondo et al., unpublished)

Girls are at a particular risk, as extremely evening-typed lifestyle leads to irregular menstruation cycle, severe pain accompanying menstruation and severe symptoms of premenstrual syndrome (PMS) (Takeuchi et al., 2005). Therefore, extremely evening-typed lifestyle in adolescent girls may impede normal development of the reproductive system and future reproductive function. In the current extreme situation, interventions are essential for maintaining better sleep, mental health and reproductive functioning in female junior high school students in Japan.

The type of intervention that is thought to be the most effective for maintaining their health is education in school classes that could help them control their own environmental factors by themselves to make their lifestyle more morning-typed. This intervention study attempted to evaluate the effectiveness of newly developed teaching materials and new lectures in class to promote better sleep and mental health by actual testing them and evaluating them from an epidemiological point of view.

The intervention project aimed to assess which of three following types of lectures is most effective for shifting adolescents to morning-type.

Type 1: Two back-to-back 50-minute lectures to explain the three following reasons why morning-type life styles lead to better grades:

1. Morning-types get adequate REM sleep which leads to the fixation of new memories,
2. Morning-types have better coupling of their two oscillators, which may promote better mental health, and
3. Tryptophan intake from a nutritionally rich breakfast is transformed into serotonin (that increases concentration).

Type 2: Two back-to-back 50-minute lectures to recommend 7 methods (Harada et al., unpublished) for changing to a morning-type:

1. Morning sunlight exposure before breakfast,
2. Avoidance of fluorescent lamps at night,
3. Nutritionally rich breakfast including tryptophan and vitamin B6,
4. Morning sunlight exposure after breakfast,
5. Avoidance of going to shops at night (convenience stores, video rental shops, 24-hour internet cafés, etc.),
6. Early morning study at home, and
7. Avoidance of using Visual Digital Terminals (video games) or watching TV at night

Type 3: One lecture to explain the three above reasons followed by one lecture to recommend the 7 above methods (combination lectures).

Type 4: Control group which received no lectures (no lectures).

Lectures were given by A. Kondo to 120 adolescents (60 girls, 60 boys) who attended a junior high school affiliated with the Faculty of Education of Kochi University, located at Kochi in June and July, 2009. Impact of the lessons was estimated using an integrated questionnaire on whether the adolescents could participate in the 7 methods after the lecture, a questionnaire on diurnal rhythms (including an M-E questionnaire that Torsvall and Åkerstedt (1980) constructed and questions on sleep habits, ID no., etc.) and a questionnaire about their understanding of "Morningness-Eveningness". Most questionnaires were administered immediately preceding the lectures and 1 month after the lectures. One-to-one comparisons of before-lecture data to after-lecture data were used for the statistical analysis.

Seven recommendations (Harada et al., unpublished) for changing to a morning-type included 10 detailed points:

1. Exposure to sunlight in the early morning.
2. Avoidance of light from fluorescent lamps in the evening.
3. Having breakfast at the same time each day.
4. Having a nutritionally rich breakfast including tryptophan and vitamin B6.
5. Exposure to sunlight after breakfast.
6. Avoidance of shops (convenience stores, rental video shops, internet cafés and so on) or restaurants open after sunset.
7. Home study early in the morning.
8. Avoidance of using mobile phones in the evening and at night.
9. Avoidance of playing video games in the evening and at night.
10. Avoidance of watching TV in the evening and at night.

In each detailed point, every 5 days of participation counts as 1 index for the participation score, so that the participation index distribution is from 0 to 50 (5 indices x 10 detailed items). The questionnaire data was statistically analyzed with SPSS 12.0 statistical software. The analysis of M-E scores, bedtimes, wake-up times, and sleep duration was standardized to non-parametric tests of Mann-Whitney U-test and Kruskal-Wallis-test, as such variables did not always show normal distribution. The other items of analysis which were measured along an ordinal scale were subject to chi-square tests and Fisher's test meta-analysis.

One-to-one individual comparisons of before-lecture data to after-lecture data showed a significantly higher increase in M-E scores and a significantly higher decrease in frequency of depression in Type 3 students compared to the other types ($p<0.05$ for both) (Table 2). Understanding of "Morningness-Eveningness" was gained in more students in the Type 2 and 3 groups than in the Type 1 and 4 groups (Table 2).

There were no significant differences in the participation index among students in Type 1-4 groups (Table 3). A negative correlation was seen between the participation index nd difference in bed times ($r=-0.161$, $p=0.086$) and sleep duration ($r=-0.238$, $p=0.011$, Figure 21) (value-before-lecture minus value-1month-after-lecture) between before and 1month after the lecture.

The improvements in Type 3 students suggest that a combination of classes on fundamental knowledge and detailed techniques to promote health including diurnal rhythms and sleep may be effective for preventing the shift of Japanese adolescents to evening-type and for promoting better sleep and mental health. However, no differences were seen in the participation index between Type 3 students and students in the other groups. While there was no difference in the "quantity" of participation, it is likely that psychological "quality" may have been higher in the Type 3 students compared to students in the other groups.

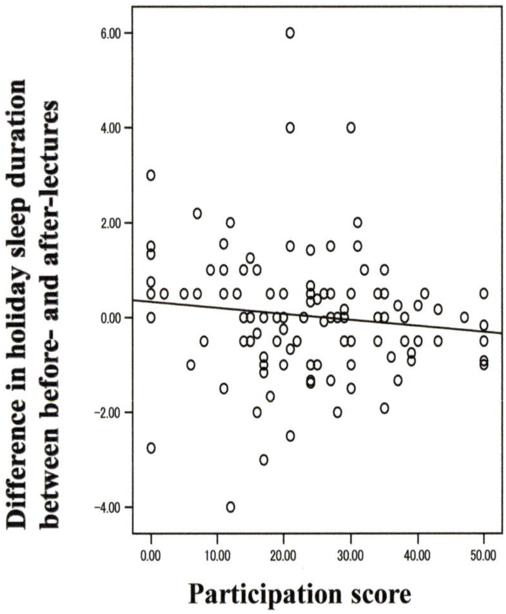

Fig. 21. Negative correlation between difference in sleep duration on holidays between before- and after-lectures (sleep-duration-before-lecture minus sleep-duration-1month-after-lecture) and participation score in the one-month period following the lecture (one-to-one analysis).

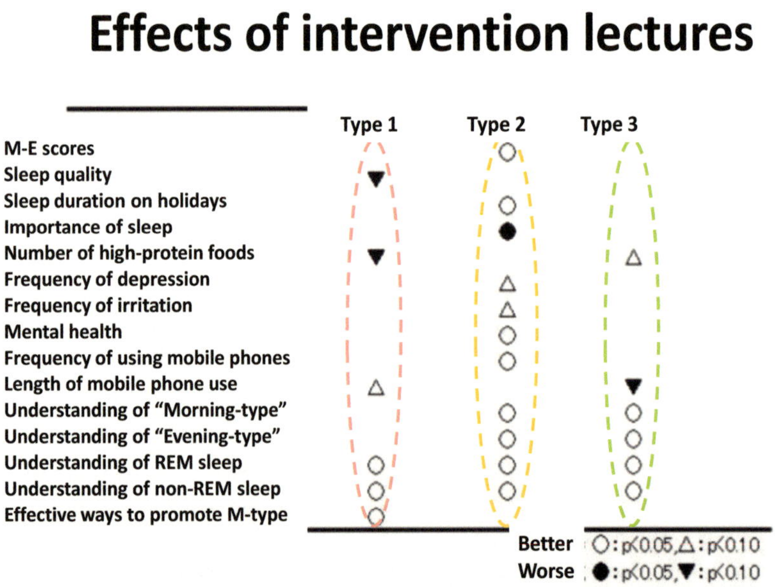

Fig. 22. Effects of intervention lectures consisting of Types 1-3.

A leaflet for changing to a morning-typed lifestyle produced by Harada et al (unpublished) and included 9 recommendations

1. Exposure to early morning sunlight **(Intervention-1)**
2. Avoidance of fluorescent lamps during the first half of subjective night **(Intervention-2)**
3. Having a nutritionally rich breakfast at the same time each day **(Intervention-3)**
4. Exposure to sunlight after having breakfast for efficient synthesis of serotonin **(Intervention-4)**
5. Bedtime discipline for young children aged 2-8 yrs **(Intervention-5)**
6. Diurnal rhythms of parents shifted to morning-type **(Intervention-6)**
7. Parents should not bring their children when they go to stores that are open after sunset **(Intervention-7)**
8. Making cram school classes earlier in the early evening and recommendation of studying at home early in the morning **(Intervention-8)**
9. Avoidance of watching TV, playing video games, working on computers and using mobile phones at night **(Intervention-9)**

Fig. 23. Nine recommendations to promote greater morningness in children which can promote better mental health.

Type	Change in M-E scores	Change in the knowledge on M-E	Change in depression
1	**0.45 (2.45)**	**0.21 (0.64)**	**-0.03 (0.91)**
2	**0.47 (2.35)**	**0.39 (0.50)**	**0.15 (0.71)**
3	**1.88 (3.38)**	**0.31 (0.67)**	**-0.32 (0.96)**
4	**-0.11 (2.56)**	**0.26 (0.44)**	**-0.26 (0.67)**
	Kruskal-Wallis test	***χ^2-test***	
χ^2-value	*8.934*	*15.352*	*24.663*
df	*3*	*6*	*15*
p-value	*0.03*	*0.018*	*0.055*

Table 2. Change in several parameters shown by students in three types of intervention lectures (Type 1-3) or in Type 4 with no intervention (Mean $\pm$ SD).

Participation score	*N in total (%)*	*Type 1(%)*	*Type 2(%)*	*Type 3(%)*	*Type 4(%)*
0	11(8.6)	1(3.0)	3(11.1)	6(20.7)	1(3.7)
1-10	19(16.2)	3(8.8)	1(3.7)	2(6.9)	2(7.4)
11-20	34(29.0)	10(29.4)	9(33.3)	6(20.7)	9(33.3)
21-30	34(29.0)	10(29.4)	9(33.3)	8(27.6)	7(25.9)
31-40	20(17.1)	7(20.6)	3(11.1)	4(13.8)	6(22.2)
41-50	10(8.5)	3(8.8)	2(7.5)	3(10.3)	2(7.4)

Kruskal-Wallis test

X^2-value= 2.497

df=3

p=0.476

Table 3. Distibution of scores for participation in the intervention program (Types 1-4).

9. Conclusions: How can we change the environmental conditions surrounding children to promote better mental health?

Figure 23 shows nine recommendations for promoting morning-typed lifestyles in children. The first recommendation is to induce a circadian phase advance by morning exposure to sunlight, while the second recommendation is to prevent the phase delaying effects of blue light emitted from fluorescent lamps in the first half of subjective night (Honma & Honma, 1988). The third and fourth recommendations are effective methods for inducing serotonin synthesis in the morning (Harada et al., 2007; Nakade et al., 2009). The fifth and sixth recommendations act as social zeitgebers for circadian clocks in children. The seventh to ninth recommendations help children avoid exposure to blue light emitted from strong fluorescent lamps in the evening on the roofs of cram schools for entrance examinations to high school and convenience stores, and the displays of mobile phones, televisions and computers in Japan.

10. References

Harada, T., Hirotani, A., Maeda, M., Nomura, H., & Takeuchi, H. (2007). Correlation between breakfast tryptophan content and Morningness-Eveningness in Japanese infants and students aged 0 - 15 years. *Journal of Physiological Anthropology,* 26, 201-207.

Honma, K., & Honma, S. (1998). A human phase-response curve for bright light pulses. *Japanese Journal of Psychiatry and Neurology,* 42, 167-168.

Krejci, M., Wada, K., Nakade, M., Takeuchi, H., Noji, T., &Harada, T. (2011) Effects of video game playing on the circadian typology and mental health of young Czech and Japanese children. *Psychology* 2, 674-680.

Nakade, M., Takeuchi, H., Taniwaki, N.,Noji, T., & Harada, T. (2009) An integrated effect of protein intake at breakfast and morning exposure to sunlight on the circadian typology in Japanese infants aged 2–6 years. *Journal of Physiological Anthropology,* 28,. 239–245.

Takeuchi, H., Oishi T., & Harada, T. (2005) Association between Morningness-Eveningness preference and mental/physical symptoms in Japanese femalses 12 to 31 years of age. *Chronobiology International,* 22, 1055-1068.

Torsvall, M. D., & Åkerstedt, T. A. (1980). Diurnal type scale construction, consistency and variation in shift work. *Scand Journal of Work Environment and Health,* 6, 283-290.

Section 5

Inter-Relationship Between Personality, Mental Health and Mental Disorders

23

Personality and Mental Health

Mohammad Ali Salehinezhad
University of Tehran, Tehran, Iran

1. Introduction

The importance of personality to mental health entails accurate definition of both personality and mental health. According to World Health Organization (WHO) health is defined as "a state of complete physical, mental and social well-being and not merely the absence of disease or infirmity (WHO, 2001b, p.1). Mental health and mental well-being are included in the foregoing definition of health which emphasizes on considering mental health as a construct interconnecting with other variables in a unified context. In addition of, this definition, psychologists deal with mental health in some terms. looking at the realm of mental health, we meet terms such as mental health (WHO, 2001), "psychological health" (Rosenthal & Hooley, 2010), well-being (Josefsson et al., 2011), "subjective well-being" or "happiness" (Lucas & Diener, 2008; Ryan and Deci, 2001), "Psychological well-being" or "eudaimonia" (Cloninger & Zohar 2011; Wood, Joseph, & Maltby, 2011) "mental hygiene" (Barenbaum & Winter, 2008) and "psychological wealth" (Diener & Biswas-Diener, 2008) that need to be explained in order to illustrate a correct definition and understanding of mental health. Thus, it is clear that, mental Health cannot be considered separately, and in order to have a better understanding of mental health, its major components such as physical, mental, and spiritual well-being should be considered together (Cloninger & Zohar, 2011).

Personality, which is the main concentration of this chapter, is defined as **an individual's characteristic style of behaving, thinking, and feeling**"(Schacter, Gilbert, & Wegner, 2009). Although there has been much debate about the definition of personality, two major themes have pervaded nearly all efforts at domain of personality theorizing: human nature and individual differences (Buss, 2008). The way we think, feel and behave and our unique individuality have significant contribution in our mental health as in our psychopathology. Some individuals are more prone to mental illness and psychopathology because of their characteristics and personality traits (Hampson & Friedman, 2008), whereas some others experience higher level of mental health because of their personality traits and characters (Cloninger, 1999, 2004; Seligman et al., 2005; Wood & Tarrier, 2010). Therefore, it seems that some individuals are more susceptible to mental illness, thereby threatening their mental health.

Another controversy in personality psychology addresses the nature and domain of personality. Do personality traits locate as some separate constructs that are either present or absent in individuals? Or they should be considered in a continuum? The answer to this question has grave theoretical and practical implications not only in personality psychology, but also in mental health. The purpose of this chapter is to explain and debate important role of personality in mental health in a comprehensive context and finally accentuate and propose prospective areas of personality regarding to both mental health and mental illness.

2. Domain of personality

Personality psychology seems to be the broadest and most integrative branch of the psychological sciences (Buss, 2008). The recent calls for integration in psychology, entails us to have a more unified and integrative approach toward behavior and psychological process of individuals. This integration has also addressed personality psychology (e.g., Mayer, 2005; Miscehl & Shoda, 2008). Integration in personality psychology is depicted in new frame work in personality suggested by Mayer (2005). In the field of personality, there used to be a perspective-by-perspective framework that causes personality psychology get fragmented by theories; however, Mayer (2005) suggests the systems framework for personality which leads to the integration of personality that can naturally promote integration as well as a vision of the whole person.

While, Mayer (2005) proposes integration of personality in a broad scale, encompassing all psychology, Miscel and Shoda (2008) on the other hand, argue about unification within personality theories and concepts. They point to the two main approaches in personality: dispositional approach and processing approach. Miscel and Shoda (2008), reconcile these two approaches within a unifying framework at least in the abstract. They analyze both the distinctive behavior patterns that characterize the exemplars of a disposition and the psychological processes and mediating units that underlie those.

On balance, Mayer's new frame work in personality (2005) seems more successful in regard to mental health because of its broad inclusion of biological, psychological, and social systems. Understanding that personality connects the biological and social helps identify its location. The biological, psychological, and social systems are connected, in part, along a continuum called the molecular–molar dimension (Mayer, 2005). In the figure 1 Mayer, illustrates the integration of personality psychology. The molecular end of the dimension refers to smaller systems of interest—at its extremes, subatomic particles. The molar end refers to larger systems—at its extremes, the entire universe as a system (Henriques, 2003; Levy-Bruhl, 1903). The middle range of this dimension separates psychology from its biological neighbors below and its larger sociological and ecological systems above.

Considering this approach to personality, the biological, psychological and social and cultural factors with regard to mental health are appreciated. Thus I believe that when we address mental health issues, personality as described above, can provide a broader as well as a more realistic view toward mental health. Each perspective may address mental health problems with more emphasize on a specific set of variables, rather than in a multivariable context. Thus, personality should be considered as an integral part whenever we tackle either mental health or mental illness. The role of personality in determining mental health and mental illness is quiet prominent and can lead to theoretical implications in the realm of research toward mental health and practical implications in community level.

2.1 Personality traits vs personality processes

I like to point briefly to a new developed approach in personality psychology that bring about new implications for issues in models of personality structure, methods of personality assessment, and identifying targets for personality interventions. As we know Reviews of studies documenting associations between personality traits and important life outcomes amply confirm the predictive power of personality. Personality traits predict consequential Outcomes for individuals (e.g., happiness, longevity), couples (e.g., relationship quality), groups, and society (e.g., volunteerism, criminality). These reviews provide an extensive catalogue of *what* personality predicts but do not examine *how* personality gives rise to these associations (Hampson, 2012). According to Hampson (2012) Understanding personality processes or "*how*" of personality, goes beyond describing individual differences by explaining the expression of Individual differences. Adopting this approach in personality researches allows us understanding the predictive power of personality in our life and how personality can mediate or moderate our mental states.

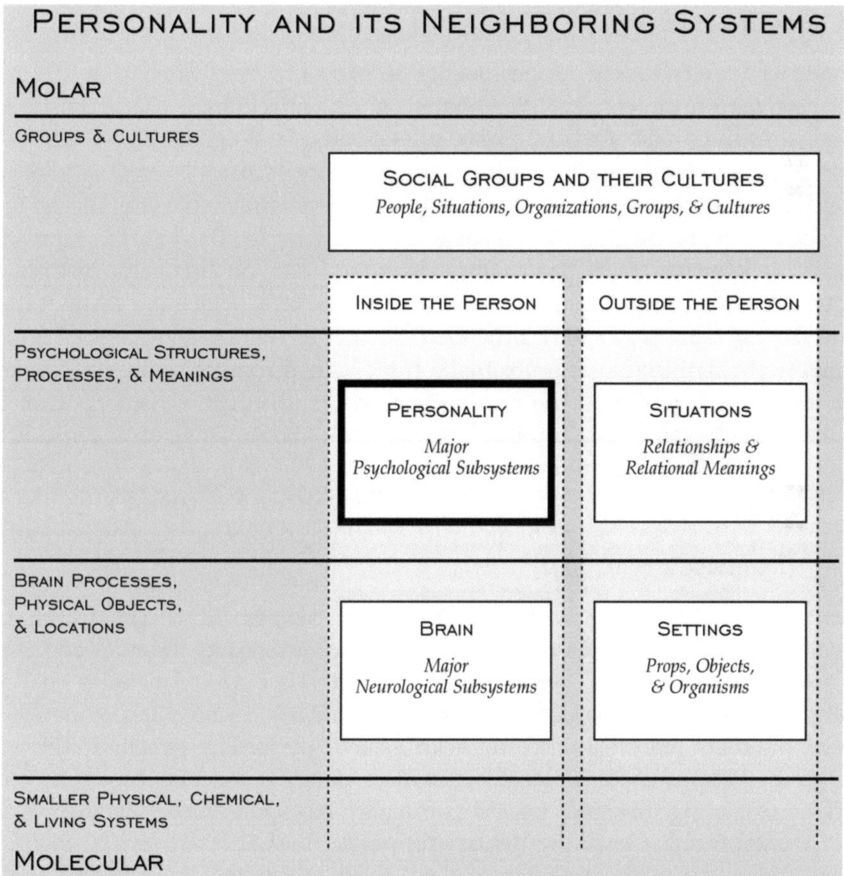

Note. The horizontal lines represent levels of the molecular-molar continuum. The "Inside the Person" box shows personality and its emergence from major psychological subsystems and from the brain. The "Outside the Person" box shows the psychological situation and the setting from which it emerges. Both personality and the situation are incorporated within larger social systems (shown above them). Adapted from Figure 1 in "Classifying Change Techniques According to the Areas of Personality They Influence: A Systems Framework Integration," by J. D. Mayer, 2004, *Journal of Clinical Psychology, 60,* p. 1296.

Fig. 1. Personality and its Neighboring Systems.

3. Relationship between personality and mental health: unidirectional or bidirectional?

What is the nature of relationship between personality and mental health? It is clear that personality traits and characters of individuals affect their mental health (Josefsson et al., 2011; Cloninger & Zohar, 2011). But the question is that how these personality traits and characters affect individuals in a way that promote mental health and wholesome behaviours. Is this relationship unidirectional, in a way that personality as an independent structure, determines mental states of individuals? Or personality can be affected by the presence or absence of mental health too? To answer this question we should primarily define both personality and mental health.

3.1 Definition of personality

Your intuitive understanding of personality is probably very similar to the way that psychologists define the concept. **Personality is an individual's characteristic style of behaving, thinking, and feeling** (Schacter, Gilbert, & Wegner, 2009). Consider this definition regarding the figure 1 in order to draw a more accurate concept of personality in your mind. Besidess of personality, personality disorders are notable with regard to mental illness. The conceptualization of personality disorders in DSM-IV-TR represents the categorical perspective that personality disorders are qualitatively distinct clinical syndromes (American Psychiatric Association, 2000, p. 689), which are distinct from each other and from general personality structures (Shedler & Westen, 2004; Skodol et al., 2006). This categorical classification is problematic from both theoretical and practical points of view. It has been argued that the current personality disorder classification in DSM is neither theoretically sound nor empirically validated (Aboaja, Duggan, & Park, 2011). The categorical model of classification has become so problematic that a Research Planning Work Group for DSM-V concluded that it will be "important that consideration be given to advantages and disadvantages of basing part or all of DSM-V on dimensions rather than categories" (Rounsaville et al., 2002).

In contrast to DSM-IV-TR, Psychodynamic Diagnostic Manual (PDM) and recent evidences (Rounsaville et al., 2002) suggest a dimensional model for personality disorders and personality traits. Dimensional model for personality suggest a spectrum relationship in regard to personality and personality disorders (Widiger & Smith, 2008). It would appear more likely that personality disorders are on a spectrum with general personality structure. This spectrum relationship may also exist for personality disorders and Axis I mental disorders. (Widiger & Smith, 2008). Adopting this view toward personality has some important implications with regard to mental health; Personality traits which affect mental health can be found in each individual. The intensity or weakness of these traits is different in individuals and these differences are responsible for mental states to be healthy or unhealthy. In what follows, I will discuss more about the consequences of spectrum relationship in mental health.

3.2 Definition of mental health

The term 'mental health literacy' was first coined by Jorm etal. (1997) meaning 'knowledge and beliefs about mental disorders which aid their recognition, management or prevention' (p.182). As it is said earlier, WHO has included mental well-being in the definition of health.

WHO famously defines health as: a state of complete physical, mental and social well-being and not merely the absence of disease or infirmity (WHO, 2001b, p.1). Three ideas central to the improvement of health follow from this definition: mental health is an integral part of health, mental health is more than the absence of mental illness, and mental health is intimately connected with physical health and behavior (WHO, 2001a). WHO has recently proposed that mental health is: a state of well-being in which the individual realizes his or her own abilities, can cope with the normal stresses of life, can work productively and fruitfully, and is able to make a contribution to his or her community (WHO, 2001b, p.1).

Realizing abilities, coping with stresses, and working productivity are some behaviors and according to definition of personality, these style of behaving are determined by personality. When we notice to definition of other related terms to mental health, we find the relationship between personality and mental health more vivid."Subjective well-being" has been defined as an individual's evaluation of his/her life as a whole (Diener, 1984;) this individual evaluation can be affected by the way of thinking or feeling in which personality account for this. Well-being is the other term in the realm of health and mental health. Well-being is a multidimensional concept that includes Various aspects of mental and physical health, supporting social relationships, and ability to cope with stressful situations (McDowell, 2010; Stokes, etal., 1982). Subjective well-being and subjective health are more highly correlated with each other than subjective health and objective physician assessed health (Jossefsson et al, 2011). Subjective well-being which is an integral component of well-being thus, is related with personality.

"Psychological health" (Rosenthal & Hooley, 2010), well-being (Josefsson et al., 2011), "subjective well-being" or "happiness" (Lucas & Diener, 2008; Ryan and Deci, 2001; Luhmann et al., 2012), "Psychological well-being" or "eudaimonia" (Cloninger & Zohar 2011; Wood, Joseph, & Maltby, 2011) "mental hygiene" (Barenbaum & Winter, 2008) and "psychological wealth" (Diener & Biswas-Diener, 2008) are terms and concepts in the realm of mental health each one points to psychological functioning and determines styles of behaving leading to healthy state. Therefore, personality which directs our ways of thinking, feeling and behaving is an undeniable construct in determining these healthy states. Finally we should appreciate the role of culture with its given values which can affect directly or indirectly health and mental health through beliefs, expectations, values and ingroup concepts (Bagherian, Rocca, Thorngate, & Salehinezhad, 2011)

3.3 Relationship between personality and mental health

We realized definition of personality and mental health. The question is that how their relationship is shaped? Many studies have shown the effect of personality, personality traits, and personality dimensions in mental health (e.g., Josefsson et al., 2011; Cloninger & Zohar, 2011; Cloninger, 1999; Cloninger, 2004; Cloninger, 2006; Diener & Biswas-Diener, 2008; Aboaja, Duggan, & Park, 2011; Chan & Joseph, 2000; Herero & Extremera, 2010; Wood & Tarrier, 2010; Joseph & Wood, 2010). A cumulating body of research suggests that there are variables such as personality traits that predispose individuals to experience specific life events (Luhmann et al., 2012). However, as we know, personality is conceptualised as an unchanging aspect of the person (Chan & Joseph, 2000) at least according to dispositional approach (Miscehl & Shoda, 2008). According to Widiger and Smith (2008) an Axis I disorder can alter the appearance or expression of premorbid personality traits. Persons who are very anxious, depressed, angry, or distraught will often fail to provide an accurate description of their general personality traits (i.e., their usual way of thinking, feeling, behaving, and relating to others). Presence of a mental disorder negatively affect individuals in realizing their abilities and coping with stress as well as making them dysfunctional in important areas of life and this is in opposition with mental health. Thus presence and absence of mental health can alter the appearance and expression of personality traits. Finally recent evidence even suggest that the relation between life events and subjective well-being may be bidirectional (Luhman et al., 2012)

4. Personality and mental illness

Mental illness or, in other word, "psychopathology" is a term that can facilitate our conceptualization of mental health. This is more intelligible when we consider that mental illness (MI) and mental health (MH) have been recently considered to be bipolar extremes of the same underlying dimension (Insel & Scolnick, 2006; Keyes, 2007; Pressman & Cohen, 2005). By measuring psychopathology symptoms in mental health studies, we can set the findings in a broader perspective of well-being and ill-health (Josefsson et al., 2011). The concept of mental health requires an understanding of abnormal behavior leading to mental illness. Normality and abnormality cannot be differentiated objectively. They reside on a continuum and slowly fade into the other (Millon et al. 2004). Mental health and mental illness are the same. They cannot be considered separately. An individual with mental illness does not experience the state of mental health. By recognizing and examining the personality factors related to psychopathology, the relationship between personality and mental health would be clear in turn.

It is notable that we consider, although mental illness (MI) and mental health (MH) have been considered to be bipolar extremes of the same underlying dimension, this viewpoint has begun to be questioned. There are now some indications that positive and negative aspects of psychological experience are mediated by different psychological systems (Keyes, 2007, 2009; MacLeod & Moore, 2000; Pressman & Cohen, 2005). Thus, low levels of a mental illness characteristic such as depression does not guarantee high levels of mental health characteristic such as optimism. What we can claim with more certainty is that various combinations of both MI and MH are possible (Keyes, 2007). Thus, with regard to psychological treatment of clients and considering researches in the realm of mental health we need to take into account the level and characteristics of MH as well as those of MI (Alterman et al., 2010).

Understanding the role of personality can help us understand mental health and that's why in this part, the relationship between personality and psychopathology is discussed. The importance of personality to psychopathology has been recognized since the beginnings of medicine (Widiger & Smith, 2008). Hippocrates (in the fourth century b.c.) distinguished between four fundamental dispositions (i.e., sanguine, melancholic, phlegmatic, and choleric) that were thought to provide a vulnerability to a variety of physical and psychological disorders (Maher & Maher, 1994). Moreover, in recent years personality and mental health have been studied in large amount of researches (e.g., Akiskal, Hirschfeld, & Yerevanian, 1983; Clark, Watson, & Mineka, 1994; Eysenck, 1987; Krueger, McGue, & Iacono, 2001). Contemporary theoretical models directly link personality with psychopathology (Pincus, Lukowitsky, & Wright, 2010; Widiger & Smith, 2008), and cross sectional research finds links between personality and psychopathology of most types and Personality disorders in particular (Wright, Pincus, & Lenzenweger, 2011).

Krueger, McGue, and Iacono (2001) provided interesting findings about relationship between personality and psychopathology. They found a connection between the higher-order structure of common DSM mental disorders and personality. This higher order structure includes internalization and externalization. These two fundamental dimensions of child psychopathology map well also onto the adult psychopathology and fundamental personality temperaments (Widiger & Smith, 2008). Krueger et al (2001) point to personality as a covariance, meaningfully account for comorbidity among mental disorders. They found that internalization was linked with higher negative emotionality and lower positive emotionality and externalization was linked with lower constraint. In general, they found that comorbidity could be modelled by hypothesizing the existence of broad, continuous variables underlying observed patterns of correlation among DSM constructs. These broad variables, in turn were linked to broad variables from the personality literature. This refers to a vulnerability model of the relationship between personality and mental disorder; a model in which personality contributes to the risk of experiencing mental disorder (Kruger et al, 2001).

It is notable that in relationship between personality and psychopathology, we should include both maladaptive personality functioning - as described within the American Psychiatric Association's (2000) Diagnostic and Statistical Manual of Mental Disorders (DSM-IV-TR) - as well as normal personality traits, as described within dimensional models of general personality structure such as Big Five theory. In respect to this relationship there are three important potential forms of interplay between personality and psychopathology: first, Personality and psychopathology can influence the presentation or appearance of one another (pathoplastic relationships); second, they can share a common, underlying etiology (spectrum relationships); and third, they can have a causal role in the development or etiology of one another (Widiger & Smith, 2008).

4.1 Pathoplastic relationship

The influence of personality and psychopathology on the presentation, appearance, or expression of each is typically characterized as a "pathoplastic relationship" (Widiger & Smith, 2008). As it was pointed earlier about bidirectional the relationship between personality and mental health, the relationship between personality and psychopathology is bidirectional too. Consequently, personality traits can affect on appearance of psychopathology and the appearance or presentation of personality can similarly be affected by the presence of a psychopathology.

4.1.1 Pathoplastic effects of personality on psychopathology

Mental disorders occur within the context of a premorbid personality structure that often has a profound effect on their presentation, course, or treatment (Millon et al., 1996). This is better intelligible when we know that mental disorders are clinically significant impairments in one or more areas of psychological functioning including one's thinking, feeling and behaving (American Psychiatric Association, 2000). Thus, a person's characteristic manner of thinking, feeling and behaving that we call it as personality, can affect these significant impairments.

As an example it can be refer to anorexia nervosa and bulimia nervosa (Widiger & Smith, 2008). The primary distinction between persons with anorexia nervosa and those with bulimia nervosa is perhaps simply that the former are pathologically successful in the effort to maintain a low body weight (i.e., are grossly underweight), whereas persons with bulimia nervosa are relatively unsuccessful, due partly to their binge eating and inadequate (but still excessive) compensatory behaviors. This fundamental distinction could be driven, in large part, by premorbid personality differences. It is possible that those who go on to develop anorexia are characterized in part by premorbid personality traits of very high conscientiousness (Widiger & Smith, 2008).

Another example in regard to this pathoplastic relationship of personality and psychopathology refers to depression. Studies about relationships between depression and Temperament and Character Inventory (TCI), usually show that depressed patients exhibit higher harm avoidance and self-transcendence scores as well as lower self-directedness and cooperativeness scores as compared to healthy controls (Hansenne et al, 1999; Marijnissen et al, 2002). Personality features may predispose an individual to depression; the personality can be modified after a depression; the personality can modify the clinical presentation of a depressive disorder; and finally the personality can be considered like a subclinical manifestation of a depressive disorder (e.g., Akiskal et al., 1983; Hirschfeld et al., 1997).

4.1.2 Pathoplastic effects of psychopathology on personality

Just as premorbid personality traits can alter the appearance or expression of an Axis I disorder, an Axis I disorder can alter the appearance or expression of premorbid personality traits (Widiger & Smith, 2008). Persons who are very anxious, depressed, angry, or distraught will often fail to provide an accurate description of their general personality traits (i.e., their usual way of thinking, feeling, behaving, and relating to others). Distortion in self-image is a well-established symptom of mood disorder (American Psychiatric Association, 2000), and it should not be surprising to find that persons who are depressed provide inaccurate descriptions of their usual way of thinking, feeling, and relating to others. Once their mood, anxiety, or other mental disorder is successfully treated, their self-description changes accordingly.

Some may argue that personality is a relatively stable structure and psychopathology cannot change or alter personality, however some well-documented studies reveal the existence of such a relationship (e.g., Clark & Harrison, 2001; Farmer, 2000; Vitousek & Stumpf, 2005; Widiger & Samuel, 2005). According to processing approach, personality is an organized system of mediating units (e.g., encodings, expectancies, goals, motives) and psychological processes or cognitive–affective dynamics, conscious and unconscious, that interact with the situation the individual experience (Mischel & Shoda, 2008). Personality in this approach is a dynamic construct which operates across social situations as well as it can be influence from social behaviour.

In sum, pathoplastic relationship between personality and psychopathology is a notion with practical implications, which should be considered in mental health research. An important theoretical and practical implication implies that psychological problems can predispose individuals to develop morbid personality traits which in turn can intensify the psychological problems. On the other hand there are some kinds of personality profiles which can promote mental health (e.g., Josefsson et al, 2011; Herero & Extremera, 2010; Chan & Joseph, 2000; Unterrainer et al, 2010) which will be discussed in this chapter.

4.2 Spectrum relationship

It used to be assumed that personality and psychopathology are distinct entities. Looking at Diagnostic and statistical manual of mental disorders, 4th edition (DSM-IV), show attempts in order to provide a more accurate diagnostic criteria in mental disorders, including personality disorders. The assumption of the diagnostic manual is that the categories refer to distinct clinical entities, each with its own distinguishable etiology, pathology, and treatment (Widiger & Mullins-Sweatt, 2007). However, personality and psychopathology may themselves fail, in some instances, to be distinct entities. They may instead exist along a common spectrum of functioning. For example, rather than contributing to the etiology of depression, neuroticism may itself be a form of a depression (Widiger & Smith, 2008). In contrast to DSM-IV-TR, Psychodynamic Diagnostic Manual (PDM) and recent evidences (Rounsaville et al., 2002) suggest a dimensional model for personality disorders and personality traits.

This spectrum relationship exists in some ways such as: Personality on a Spectrum with Personality Disorders, Personality Disorders on a Spectrum with Axis I Mental Disorders, and Axis I on a Spectrum with Personality (Widiger & Smith, 2008). This dimensional approach to personality, personality disorders and mental disorders accompanies with beneficial implication in the realm of mental health. The first and most important one involves our attitude toward mental health research; identification and differentiation of etiological relationships of personality and psychopathology cannot be considered with simplicity. Actually it is more complicated because of observable overlapping and comorbidity that exists among mental health problems specially. This approach affects the way clinicians meet mental disorders, as well as research guidelines we adopt toward psychopathology and mental illness problems. That is why the American Psychiatric Association (APA) subsequently cosponsored a series of international conferences devoted to further enriching the empirical database in preparation for the eventual development of DSM-V (Widiger & Smith, 2008).

The other important theoretical and practical implication refers to inclusion of mental health. Mental health is a pervasive issue which can be endangered and this can happen to everyone, rather than a specific group of afflicted people suffering from mental problems. In fact mental health issues can afflict each individual based on styles of thinking, feeling and behaving. By adopting this approach, community psychologist and researchers in the areas of mental health will have better conceptualization of mental health problems.

4.3 Causual relationship

The third form of interplay between personality and psychopathology refers that they can have a causal role in the development or etiology of one another. This causal relationship is again bidirectional: One's characteristic way of thinking, feeling, behaving, and relating to others can result in, or contribute to, the development of a mental disorder, just as a severe or chronic mental disorder can itself contribute to fundamental changes in personality (Widiger & Smith, 2008). Personality can change for the better or worse. The ICD-10 (World Health Organization, 1992) contains a number of mental disorder diagnoses that concern maladaptive changes to personality functioning occurring within adulthood; however, this is not noticeable in DSM-IV. As it is noted earlier personality is conceptualised as an unchanging aspect of the person (Chan & Joseph, 2000). This reluctance toward immutability of personality is because there is little empirical research to document the reliability or validity of such personality change (Chan & Joseph, 2000; Widiger & Smith, 2008).

The assertion that an individual's personality has changed or remained the same over time is ambiguous. It is conceivable that the experience of having suffered from a severe mental disorder, such as a psychosis or a major depression, might have a fundamental and lasting effect on one's characteristic manner of thinking, feeling, and relating to others (e.g., Caspi et al., 2005; Roberts & DelVecchio, 2000; Srivastava, John, Gosling, & Potter, 2003). Thus, severe mental problems and mental health problems can affect or even alter personality. Looking at other side of this relationship, the casual effects of personality on mental problems is well documented (e.g., Marijnissen. Et al., 2002; Furukawa et al., 1998; Krueger et al., 2001).

5. Personality and mental health

Much is known about the relationship of personality to psychopathology (Cloninger, 1999), but much less is known about the relationship of personality to health as a state of physical, mental, and social well-being (Cloninger, 2004). In recent decades, health-related researches and health care have focused on negative mental processes such as Psychological distress and dysfunction, while positive mental processes such as psychological well-being have been much less studied (Huber et al., 2008).Mental health professionals need to understand the relationship between personality, well-being and mental health in order to help motivate both the promotion of health and the reduction of distress and disability (Amering & Schmolke, 2009; Cloninger, 2006).

In contrast to previous studies of clinical psychologists who were interested in understanding distress (Wood & Tarrier, 2010) and alleviating human suffering (Joseph & Wood, 2010), positive psychology research can best impact on the scientific knowledge base of psychology, and be utilized to improve people's lives (Wood & Tarrier, 2010). Normal personality traits are described within the dimensional models of general personality structure. It has been proposed that most of the problems in treating personality disorders could be resolved based on normal personality (Aboaja, Duggan, & Park, 2011). By considering personality and personality disorders on a spectrum (Widiger & Smith, 2008), the contribution of personality in mental health and well-being would be more clear.

5.1 Models of personality

There are some prominent models of personality including: Eysenck's (1987) three dimensions of neuroticism, extraversion, and psychoticism; Harkness and McNulty's five factors of positive emotionality / extraversion, aggressiveness, constraint, negative emotionality / neuroticism, and psychoticism (Harkness, McNulty, & Ben-Porath, 1995); Tellegen's (1982) three dimensions of negative affectivity, positive affectivity, and constraint; Millon's six polarities of self, other, active, passive pleasure, and pain (Millon et al., 1996); the interpersonal circumplex dimensions of agency and communion (Pincus & Gurtman, 2006); Zuckerman's (2002) five dimensions of sociability, activity, aggression-hostility, impulsive sensation seeking, and neuroticism- anxiety; Cloninger's (2000) seven factors of novelty seeking, harm avoidance, reward dependence, persistence, self-directedness, cooperativeness, and self-transcendence; and the FFM dimensions of neuroticism, extraversion, openness, conscientiousness, and agreeableness (Costa & McCrae, 1990). However, according to Markon, Krueger, and Watson's (2005) meta-analysis which has been done in order to assemble a matrix of correlations among the 44 scales derived from all of these inventories obtained from 52 prior studies, no more than five major factors underlie variation in the 44 scales. These five factors strongly resembled the domains of the Five Factor Model (Widiger & Smith, 2008).

5.1.1 Five Factor Model of personality

Previous research mostly leaned on the Five Factor Model (FFM), as a dominant one in personality psychology (Aboaja, Duggan, & Park, 2011; Garcia, 2011; Jovanovic, 2011) And agree that individual differences in personality are captured by the dimensions of the five-factor model or Big Five taxonomy (Hapmson, 2012). Much of what psychologists mean by the term "personality" is summarized by the FFM, and the model has been of great utility to the field by integrating and systematizing diverse conceptions and measures (McCrae & Costa, 2008). Additionally, each of the DSM-IV-TR personality disorders can, in fact, be readily understood as a maladaptive or extreme variant of the domains and facets of the FFM (Widiger & Trull, 2007; Aboaja, Duggan, & Park, 2011). Therefore, an investigation of Big Five model scales and subscales would have useful outcomes in considering personality traits in mental health. FFM involves some assumptions about human nature and about what people are like. Noting these assumptions, illustrate the natural functioning of individuals and helps us discriminating how normal functioning is.

The five personality factors—Neuroticism, Extraversion, Openness, Agreeableness, and Conscientiousness— form the substantive nucleus of FFM. According to McCrae & Costa (2008) each of these factors are related to some Characteristic adaptations which can either promote or mar mental health. They are characteristic because they reflect the enduring psychological core of the individual, and they are adaptations because they help. Neuroticism (a tendency to experience dysphoric affect, sadness, hopelessness, guilt) is related to Low self-esteem, irrational perfectionistic beliefs, and pessimistic attitudes. Extraversion (a preference for companionship and social stimulation) is related to social skills, numerous friendships, enterprising vocational interests, participation in team sports, club memberships. Openness to experience (a need for variety, novelty, and change) is related to interest in travel, many different hobbies, knowledge of foreign cuisine, diverse vocational interests, friends who share tastes. Agreeableness (a willingness to defer to others during interpersonal conflict) is related to forgiving attitudes, belief in cooperation, inoffensive language, and reputation as a pushover. And Conscientiousness (strong sense of purpose and high aspiration levels) is related to leadership skills, long-term plans, organized support network, technical expertise.

Among the five factors neuroticism is shown to be related to psychopathology. For example neuroticism is shown to be significantly correlated with half of the personality disorder (e.g., Aboaja, Duggan, & Park, 2011; Blais, 1997; Costa & McCrae, 1990; Duggan, 2004; Egan et al., 2002). Both neuroticism and extroversion contribute in the conceptualization of personality disorder while openness was the least notable factor in the conceptualization of personality disorder. (Aboaja, Duggan, & Park, 2011). During recent decades, special interest has developed in the positive rather than the negative aspects of mental health (Seligman et al.,

2005) such as subjective well-being (Quevedo & Abella, 2011). In regard to mental health and well-being, well-being variables such as gratitude are positively correlated with extraversion, agreeableness, openness, and conscientiousness, and negatively correlated with neuroticism (e.g., McCullough et al., 2004, Wood, Joseph, et al., 2008; Wood, Maltby, Gillett et al., 2008; Wood, Maltby, Stewart et al., 2008). In regard to subjective well-being in which a broad range of studies has compellingly shown that personality is an important precursor of SWB (e.g., McCrae & Costa, 1991; Myers, 1992; Myers & Diener, 1995) it is notable that there is a robust negative relationship between neuroticism and SWB, and a robust positive relationship between extraversion and SWB. Moreover, the association has consistently been shown to be stronger for neuroticism than for extraversion (Gomez et al., 2009).

Recently, Steel, Schmidt, and Shultz (2008) conducted a comprehensive meta-analysis and evaluated the associations between each personality factor and SWB. Their findings support a strong relationship between neuroticism, extraversion, agreeableness, conscientiousness and all components of SWB, whereas openness to experience shows close associations with the SWB facets of happiness, positive affects, and quality of life. In another meta-analysis by DeNeve and Cooper (1998), Neuroticism was most closely related with happiness, life satisfaction and negative affect, and Extraversion with positive affect. Quevedo & Abella (2011) examined whether the facets of the Big Five Model and other personality characteristics not included in this model, such as optimism, self-esteem, and social support, are better predictors of SWB than Big Five broad dimensions. They found that Neuroticism was negatively correlated with positive affect and Extraversion inversely related with negative affect. Neuroticism and Extraversion were associated to happiness; individuals with low Neuroticism and high Extraversion showed increased happiness. The findings also showed that Facets accounted for double the variance of SWB than the Big Five, although only 7 of 30 facets were relevant. More importantly, optimism, self-esteem and social support better explained the relationship between personality and SWB.

In sum, the five personality factors—Neuroticism, Extraversion, Openness, Agreeableness, and Conscientiousness— form the substantive nucleus of the system; FFT traces their ramifications throughout the personality system. It also provides a framework in which to understand the development and operation of psychological mechanisms (such as need for closure) and the behavior and experience of individual men and women.

5.1.2 Temperament and Character Inventory (TCI)

Cloninger's theory of personality is based on a synthesis of information from family studies, studies of longitudinal development, and psychometric studies of personality structure, as well as neuropharmacologic and neuroanatomical studies of behavioral conditioning and learning in man and animals (Cloninger, 1987). His revised biosocial model of personality posits seven domains of personality as measured by the Temperament and Character Inventory (TCI) (Cloninger, 1994): four temperament (Harm Avoidance, Novelty Seeking, Reward Dependence and Persistence) and three character domains (Self-Directedness, Cooperativeness, and Self- Transcendence) (Cloninger, 1994). TCI has been extensively used in many studies in regard to health, mental health, mental illness, genetic and environmental relationship, mood states, brain regions, well-being and happiness (e.g.,

Cloninger, 1999; Cloninger, 2006; Gillespie, Cloninger, Heath, & Martin, 2003; Constantino et al., 2002; Svrakic, Przybeck, & Cloninger, 1992; Gardini, Cloninger, & Venneri, 2009; Josefsson et al., 2011; Cloninger & Zohar, 2011).

The TCI personality dimensions have been shown to be antecedent causes of individual differences in psychopathology and personality (Calvo et al., 2009; Ettelt et al., 2008; Smith et al., 2008; Zohar, Ebstein, & Pauls, 2005) showing a beneficial application of TCI in examining mental health and having predictive validity in prospective studies in the general population and with specific disorders that have extensive effects on all aspects of health (Cloninger & Zohar, 2011). Additionally, within the seven factor model of personality, by conceptualizing personality as a combination of several components rather than single dimensions examined separately, it is possible to understand processes within individuals and not just differences among individuals facing the biopsychosocial reality (Josefsson et al., 2011). In Temperament and Character Inventory (TCI), 8 different character profiles can be determined by combining only three character dimensions (Cloninger & Zohar, 2011; Josefsson et al., 2011); associations of these character profiles with well-being and mental health need to be explained. By characterizing temperament and character we can understand the natural course of personality development (Constantino, Cloninger, Clarke, Hashemi, & Przybeck, 2002). Character dimensions aim at depicting maturity and integration of personality (Josefsson et al., 2011); thus character traits have strong effects on the perception of well-being (Cloninger & Zohar, 2011). Regarding the dimensions of character such as Self-directedness, Cooperativeness and Self-transcendence (Cloninger, 1994) individuals with mature and immature, or normal and abnormal personalities are differentiable (Gillespie, Cloninger, Heath, & Martin, 2003).

In the Temperament and Character Inventory (TCI) character has been found to be strongly related to well-being whereas temperament traits are only weakly associated (Cloninger & Zohar, 2011; Cloninger, 2004; Ruini et al., 2003). Among the character dimensions, Self-directedness, Cooperativeness and Self-transcendence aim at depicting maturity and integration of personality and 8 character profiles are assumed base on these three character profiles (Josefsson et al., 2011; Cloninger & Zohar, 2011). Cloninger and zohar (2011) studied the relation between personality and health and happiness based on 8 character profiles including: creative (SCT), organized (SCt), fanatical (ScT), autocratic (Sct), moody (sCT), dependent (sCt), disorganized (scT) and depressive (Sct). They found that character has a strong impact on the perception of all aspects of health, including social, emotional, and physical well-being. Creative (SCT) profile was significantly higher than all others with the exception of organized (SCt) profile in positive affect while depressive (sct) profile was significantly lower than all 7others. Individuals who with creative (SCT) or organized (SCt) profiles are frequently in the best of health, whereas those who are depressive (sct) or disorganized (scT) are frequently in the worst of ill-health. Thus Character profiles have a strong association with individual differences in health, including both its non-affective aspect (i.e., "wellness") and its affective aspect (i.e., happiness).

Among the dimensions of character, three dimensions of character measured by the TCI contribute to individual differences in health. TCI Self-directedness clearly has the strongest impact as a foundation for the regulation of a person's hopes and desires, which influences all aspects of both wellness and happiness (Cloninger & Zohar, 2011), consistent with theories of self-efficacy and self-determination (Cervone, 2005; Ryan and Deci, 2000).

Cooperativeness has a strong impact on perceptions of social support, which also makes a substantial impact to increase wellness and reduce negative emotions, consistent with attachment and social engagement theories (Bowlby, 1983; Ryan and Deci, 2001). Self-transcendence has a strong impact on awareness of participation in what is beyond the individual self, which increases the experience of positive emotions, but has little or no impact on wellness or negative emotions, consistent with humanistic and existential theories (Cloninger, 2004; Jaspers, 1968; Rogers, 1995).

5.2 Personality and physical health

As we noticed, in the integrative definition of health and mental health, mental health is intimately connected with physical health and behavior (WHO, 2001a). One way personality can influence mental health is through physical health. In a broader view, mental health is a crucial component of health (Cloninger & Zohar, 2011); thus, considering the likelihood of disease regarding personality traits is notable. The effects of type A behavior pattern (e.g., Houston & Snyder, 1988;) and type D personality (Mols et al, 2010) in disease, and the influence of personality traits on other physical problems have been studied significantly (e.g., Olson & Dahli, 2009; Mols et al., 2010; Carver & Miller, 2006 & Goodwin & Friedman, 2006). These studies indicate the undeniable role of personality in determining mental health based on physical health. It is also notable that the relationship between physical and mental health is mutual according to the definition of health and mental health (WHO, 2001,a).

6. Personality related variables in mental health

The Broad literature in personality studies has demonstrated some particular variables contributing to mental health which might not be categorized in a personality model. In what follows I point to some of these variables based on previous studies.

6.1 Self-related variables

"Self-" related variables such as self-esteem (Rosenberg, 1979), self-monitoring (Snyder, 1987), and self- Regulation (Gailliot, Mead, & Baumeister, 2008) have strong effects on mental health. Self-esteem is shown to be associated with psychological health (e.g., Rosenthal & Hooley, 2010; Ni et al., 2010; Baumeister, Campbell, Krueger, & Vohs, 2003). Furthermore, self-regulation as an underlying structure of personality characterizes the structure and processes of everyday behavior especially the experience of stressor events (Carver, Scheier, & Fulford, 2008) and dependence on its level would be accounted for risky behaviors which are harmful for health (Arnaut, 2006). In what follows, I discuss about these variables in brief.

6.1.1 Self esteem

Self esteem is regarded as a positive personality feature, contribute in healthy functioning. High self esteem has elicited considerable interest in recent years (Zeigler-Hill, Chadha, & Osterman, 2008). Despite the association of high self esteem with markers of psychological adjustment such as subjective well-being (e.g., Baumeister, Campbell, Krueger, & Vohs,

2003; Diener, 1984; Robins, Hendin, & Trzesniewski, 2001; Tennen & Affleck, 1993), there also appears to be a dark side to high self-esteem. That is, high self-esteem has been linked to a variety of negative outcomes including prejudice, aggression and various strategies to maintain or enhance self-esteem (Zeigler-Hill, Chadha, & Osterman, 2008).

In an effort to better understand how high self-esteem can be associated with both positive and negative outcomes, contemporary theorists (e.g., Deci & Ryan, 1995; Kernis, 2003) have proposed that there are actually two forms of high self-esteem: secure high self-esteem and fragile high self-esteem. Secure high self-esteem reflects positive attitudes toward the self that are realistic, well-anchored, and resistant to threat. Individuals with secure high self esteem have a solid foundation for their feelings of self-worth that does not require constant validation. In contrast, fragile high self-esteem refers to feelings of self-worth that are vulnerable to challenge, require constant validation, and rely upon some degree of self-deception (Zeigler-Hill, Chadha, & Osterman, 2008). The model of self-esteem instability developed by Kernis and his colleagues (Kernis, 2005) is often used to distinguish between secure and fragile self-esteem. According to the model of self-esteem instability, individuals with stable high self-esteem are believed to possess a solid basis for their positive feelings of self worth. As a result, the self-esteem of these individuals is relatively unaffected by events that may have an evaluative component. That is, the solid foundation for their feelings of self-worth protects individuals with stable high self-esteem from the variety of adversities that individuals frequently encounter in their day-to-day lives. In contrast, individuals with unstable high self-esteem are thought to possess positive feelings about the self that are highly vulnerable to challenge which leads these individuals to behave as if their self esteem is constantly at stake (Greenier et al., 1999; Kernis, Brown, & Brody, 2000; Kernis et al., 1993; Kernis, Greenier, Herlocker,Whisenhunt, & Abend, 1997; Waschull & Kernis, 1996).

6.1.2 Self regulation

Self-regulation is a prominent component of personality. Early on, Freud (1962) theorized that personality consisted of three components: the id, ego, and superego (Gailliot, Mead, & Baumeister, 2008). Self-regulation allows the individual to resist behaviors such as engaging in unsafe or promiscuous sex, abusing drugs and alcohol, overeating, overspending, fighting or acting violently, procrastinating, and making lewd or negative remarks toward others. In one sense, self-regulation can be seen as a process that allows the influence of personality to outshine the influence of the situation and other factors Gailliot, Mead, & Baumeister, 2008).

Self-regulation influences many of the major problems faced by people individually and by society collectively and contribute in both negative and positive consequence based on its intensity. Poor self regulation can increase the spread of sexually transmitted diseases, contributes to crime and indeed is regarded as one of its most important causes (Gottfredson & Hirschi, 1990; Pratt & Cullen, 2000), undermines drinking restraint, thereby possibly contributing to alcoholism and other harmful effects, such as drunk driving. In contrast benefits of self-regulation include controlling monetary spending, performing well in school, and refraining from aggressive or violent behavior, preventing unhealthy or disordered eating. It is also beneficial to social interactions. Contextually appropriate self-regulation promotes harmonious interactions with others and the other important benefit of self regulation involves emotion regulation and control of emotions (Gailliot, Mead, & Baumeister, 2008). The latter one has o mutual relationship with self regulation in a way that controlling one's emotions can also deplete self-regulatory resources. With regard to mental health, we see that in most of mental disorders, there is problems with self regulation process such as substance use (Donohue, Farley, & French, 2006), borderline and antisocial personality disorder (Trull, Steep, & Solhan, 2006), eating disorders and sexual deviation (Murphy & Page, 2006), and externalizing problems (Whilmshurst, 2005).

6.2 Resilience, hardiness and mental toughness

The recent resurgence of an emphasis on positive psychology (e.g., Seligman & Csikszentmihalyi, 2000) is welcome and has spurred relevant theorizing and research (Maddi, 2006). During recent decades, special interest has developed in the positive rather than the negative aspects of mental health (Seligman et al., 2005). Resilience, hardiness and mental toughness are factors which act as protective ones and improve as well as promote well being and mental health. In contrast to pathological factors which their absence in beneficial, presence of these protective factors affect our mental state in healthy way and thus, must be considered in mental health issues.

6.2.1 Resilience

Resilience is a construct has flourished across many disciplines of psychology and health like positive psychology (Yi-Frazier, Smith, Vitalino, Yi, Mai, Hillman, & Weinger, 2009). Because of ambiguities of resilience in both definitions and terminology, it has often been criticized (Davydov et al., 2010). Resilience has had numerous meanings in prior research as a dynamic process of adaptation to adverse and unpleasant experiences (Luthar & Cicchetti, 2000; Masten, 2001) but generally refers to an individual capacity in the face of stressful events (Yi-Frazier et al., 2009) and a pattern of functioning indicative of positive adaptation in context of risk or adversity, underlying two conditions: (a) exposure to risk and (b) positive adaptation (Ong, Bergeman, & Boker, 2009). In other definitions it is called stress resistance (Garmzy, 1985) or post traumatic growth (Tedeschi, Park, & Calhoun, 1998). According to Bonanno (2004), resilience is more than surviving from life stresses and is not synonymous with invulnerability (Philippe, Lecours, & Beaulieu-Pelletier, 2009) but corresponds to successful adjustment (Donnellan, Conger, McAdams, & Neppl 2009), behavioral adjustment (Leve, Fisher, & Chamberlain, 2009) and hanging to balance after prior disequilibrium (Richardson, 2002).

Current theories of resilience regard it as a multidimensional construct including internal variables as temperament and personality and individual differences (Mancini & Bonanno, 2009; Campbell-sills, Cohan, & Stein, 2006) and external factors like social environment with a neurological functioning as mediating mechanism (Leve et al., 2009; Davis, Luecken, Lemery-Chalfant, 2009). Historically, resilience research has been largely the purview of developmental investigators dealing with early childhood and adulthood (Ong et al., 2009) and now has progressed to include early, middle, and late adulthood (Fava & Tomba, 2009). Clinical psychologists recently examined resilience in situations of economic hardship, social inequality and discrimination, psychological trauma, loss, bereavement, depression and pain (Davis et al., 2009; Donnellan et al., 2009; Keyes, 2009; Mancini & Bonanno, 2009; Southwick, Vythilingam, & Chamey, 2005; Zautra, Johnson, & Davis, 2005).

The consistent results approve positive and protective effects of resilience in stress resistance (Ong et al., 2009), successful adjustment (Donnellan et al., 2009), positive emotions (Philippe et al., 2009), better quality of relationships with others (Bonanno, Papa, Moskowitz, & Folkman, 2005), subjective well-being (Burns & Anstey, 2010), physical and psychological health and well-being (Davis et al., 2009; Fava & Tomba, 2009; Salehinezhad & Besharat, 2010), and even speedy recovery illness (Yi-Frazier et al., 2009). In opposite, low levels of resilience relates to vulnerability, low levels of well-being, psychological disorders , maladaptive coping behavior, and negative defenses (Campbell-sills et al., 2006; Fava & Tomba, 2009; Philippe et al., 2009; Yi-Frazier et al., 2009). Resilience has shown to be related not only to mental health but also to adapting performance and achievement in the field of sport, career and education (Salehinezhad & Besharat, 2010). This makes resilience not only a protective factor (Ong et al., 2009) but also an improving factor of emotions (Philippe et al., 2009), physical and psychological health and well-being (Davis et al., 2009; Fava & Tomba, 2009) and achievement (Salehinezhad & Besharat, 2010). Resilience has a particular feature in which turns it so applicable to mental health realm. This feature involves its extensive and broad application in different levels. People often show resilience in the face of adversity rather than ruminate over the bad things that happen in their lives (MacAdams, 2008). In a broader view, themes of resilience apply not only to individuals but to families and community (Zautra, 2009).

There is a significant theoretical and practical implication arising from resilience conceptualization which should be considered by researchers in the realm of mental health. Mono-causal models of psychopathology which is popular in clinical practice due to their simplicity in terms of theoretical, therapeutic and disorder prevention approaches, tends to ignore moderating, mediating and confounding effects of other biosocial variables, thereby undermining the multi-Causal nature of human health – from genes to cultures with developmental process mediating. However, construct of mental resilience can provide a means of integrating social and natural sciences taking into account both psychosocial and biological models of mental health pathways (Davydov et al., 2010). A guiding question in respect to resilience and mental health asks that while somatic disease, trauma and chronic stress are known to be common precedents of psychiatric disorder (Davydov et al., 2010) why majority of people who experience such stressful events do not develop psychopathology? And which resilience factors provide such mental 'immunity'? (Collishaw et al., 2007; Jin et al., 2009; Patel & Goodman, 2007). These kinds of questions address protective factors of mental health rather than preventing pathological factors. Concepts of 'mental immunity', 'mental hygiene' or 'mental resilience' have in common the aim of broadening research concepts in mental health beyond risk factors for pathology to include wellness enhancement and health promoting factors, in the same way that it has been important to identify the characteristics of infection-resistant groups during epidemics (Davydov et al., 2010). Thus the importance of mental health in terms of protective factor and good mental health rather than absence of unhealthy states should be more considered in further studies.

6.2.2 Hardiness

The other psychological construct, prominent in domain of mental health and positive psychology is hardiness (Salehinezhad & Besharat, 2010). Over the past 20 years, personality hardiness has emerged as a combination of attitudes that enhance performance, health, and mood despite stressful circumstances (e.g., Maddi, 1999, 2002; Maddi, Khoshaba, Harvey, Lu & Persico, 2001). It is also related to inspiring performance such as transformational leadership (Johnsen et al., 2009).

Hardiness is defined as the presence of three interrelated dispositions: commitment, control, and challenge (Kobasa, Maddi, & Kahn, 1982; Maddi et al., 2006). Control refers to the ability to feel and act as if one is in control of various life situations, commitment points, the tendency to involve rather than distance oneself from whatever one is doing; and challenge, addresses the ability to understand that change is normal (Horsburgh et al., 2009). Hardiness acts as a buffer to major life stressors (Maddi et al., 2006). High hardiness is associated with lower psychological distress, higher quality of life (Hoge, Austin, & Pollack, 2007) and high level of mental health (Salehinezhad & Besharat, 2010). The person high in hardiness is marked by increased commitment, sense of control, and challenge (Johnsen et al., 2009). Hardiness is a psychological style associated with resilience, good health, and good performance under a range of stressful conditions and is potentially a valuable personality style for highly demanding situations and occupations (Bartone, Roland, Picano, & Williams, 2008). Previous researches have established hardiness as a dispositional factor in preserving and enhancing performance and physical and mental health despite stressful circumstances (Maddi et al., 2006; Salehinezhad & Besharat, 2010).

In regard to mental health hardiness is indeed a measure of mental health and is not only negatively related to neuroticism, but also positively related to all four of the other factors in the Five Factor Model. Hardiness leads to beneficial health and performance effects by providing the courage and motivation needed to carry out coping, social support, and self-care efforts (Maddi et al., 2006 Maddi, 2002). Hardiness has emerged, over the years, as a positive dispositional force in encouraging an active, effective, healthy life (Maddi, 2002). A matter of interest, therefore, is its conceptual and empirical overlap with other proposed positive characteristics that also appear important in explaining effective functioning and health (Maddi et al., 2006)

6.2.3 Mental toughness

Mental toughness is newly defined construct (Horsburgh et al., 2009) and has recently been defined by Clough, Earl, and Sewell (2001). These researchers developed a definition of mental toughness based on the established psychological concept known as the 'hardy personality' that was first proposed by Kobasa (1979) (Horsburgh et al., 2009; Golby & Sheard, 2004) which consists of control, commitment and challenge. Mental toughness model requires a fourth category: confidence (Horsburgh et al., 2009). Thus Clough et al. (2001) created what they call the '4Cs model of mental toughness': control, commitment, challenge, and confidence and defined mental toughness as: Mentally tough individuals tend to be sociable and outgoing; as they are able to remain calm and relaxed, they are competitive in many situations and have lower anxiety levels than others. With a high sense of self-belief and an unshakeable faith that they control their own destiny, these individuals can remain relatively unaffected by competition or adversity (p. 38).

With regard to mental health, it is expected that mental toughness will be positively correlated with extraversion. Also from Clough et al's (2001) definition, it is expected that a positive correlation will be found between mental toughness and agreeableness and conscientiousness: people who are "relatively unaffected by competition or adversity" may also be viewed as being agreeable; and those who believe they "control their own destiny" or who score high on Commitment are likely to also be conscientious. Clough et al. (2001) also state that individuals high on mental toughness experience low anxiety and have a high sense of self-belief; from this, it is expected that a negative correlation will be found between mental toughness and neuroticism. An implications for potential therapeutic interventions designed to modify an individual's level of mental toughness is assumed. Mental toughness is influenced more by environmental factors and thus may be more malleable than those mainly influenced by genetic factors (Horsburgh et al., 2009)

6.3 Stress, coping and defense styles

Stress and mental health have been repeatedly found to vary inversely (e.g., DeLongis, Lazarus, & Folkman, 1988) and with likely reciprocal influence (Hammen, 2005). Defining stress as the organism's reaction to external survival-related demands (Lazarus & Folkman, 1984), and mental health as ". . . a state of well-being in which the individual . . . can cope with the normal stresses of life . . ." (World Health Organization, 2001), it is also clear that stress and mental health are linked by definition (Stead, Shanahan, & Neufeld, 2010). Within the Five Factor Model of personality, neuroticism is mostly strongly associated with poor stress regulation (Williams & Moroz, 2009; Lazarus & Folkman, 1984).

Stress and coping typically go hand in hand. When people find themselves hard-pressed to deal with some impediment or some looming threat, the experience is stressful (Carver, Scheier, & Fulford, 2008), and in these circumstances individuals use coping styles. Depending on what kind of coping people use, their well-being and psychological health could be better or worse because clearly, coping style is relevant to one's performance, conduct, and health under stress (Maddi, 2006). Most contemporary views of stress and coping can be traced, in one way or another, to the work of Lazarus and Folkman and their colleagues (e.g., Lazarus & Folkman, 1984). Lazarus and Folkman (1984) have defined coping as "the efforts to master, reduce, minimize or tolerate the negative consequences of internal or external demands." The importance of coping style in predicting scores across a number of mental health variables is well established (e.g., Maltby, Day, & Barber, 2004; Zeidner & Endler, 1996). Copings are different with different effects on health mental health. It is common to refer to three classes of responses: 1) Problem-focused coping consists of attempts to remove the obstacle or to minimize its impact 2) Emotion-focused coping consists of attempts to reduce the distress emotions caused by the obstacle 3) Avoidance coping is a class of responses that appear to be aimed either at avoiding any acknowledgment that the problem exists.

Difference in coping responses is considerable based on optimism and pessimism. Optimists tend to use more problem-focused coping strategies than pessimists. When problem-focused coping is not a possibility, optimists turn to adaptive emotion-focused coping strategies such as acceptance, use of humor, and positive reframing. These are strategies that keep them engaged with the effort to move forward with their lives. Pessimists tend to cope through overt denial and by disengaging from the goals with which the stressor is interfering. Moreover, these differences in coping responses appear to be at least partially responsible for differences between optimists and pessimists in the emotional well-being they experience (Carver, Scheier, & Fulford, 2008).

While coping strategies are aroused in stressful circumstances, the situations in which individuals feel anxious would evoke defense mechanisms. The role that defense mechanisms play in protecting against anxiety is integral to understanding many psychodynamic theories of personality and psychopathology (Freud, 1962). The function of the defense mechanism is to protect the individual from experiencing excessive anxiety (Cramer, 2009). Two theoretical models of defense use, based on the dimension of maturity, have been proposed by Vaillant (1971) and Cramer (2006). According to these models the 3 types of defenses people use reflect their level of personality maturity (Salehinezhad et al., 2011); therefore, defense styles also have contributions to mental health and well-being in term of personality.

6.4 Other related variables to mental health

Studies usually present many other factor related to mental health that are usually considered separately. Among these factors there are some interesting and relatively newly researched concepts in regard to mental health.

6.4.1 Religion and spirituality

Psychologists typically ignore religion. Religion is seen as an exotic specialty area, like sexual fetishes or the detection of random number sequences. Religion is like sex to a Victorian or dreams to a behaviorist—an awkward and embarrassing phenomenon best (Bloom, 2012). Religion has often been overlooked, neglected, minimized, and marginalized, despite the fact that religion was of great interest to the founding figures of the field, including Gordon Allport and Henry Murray. Across the lifespan, spirituality and religion are important, perhaps central, dimensions of human experience (Emmons, Barrett, & Schnitker, 2008) insofar as Piedmont (1999) proposed an extension of the Big Five dimensions of personality by considering a sixth factor named "Spiritual Transcendence". Thus, it should be considered more than before as we see this tendency in recent years specially, in the field of personality psychology. research in the context of mental health and quality of life has shown that Religious/Spiritual Well-Being is positively correlated with different parameters of psychological and physiological health (e.g., Koenig, McCullough, & Larson, 2001; Unterrainer et al., 2010; Dezutter, Soenens, & Hutsebaut, 2006; Maltby & Day, 2004). For example researches find that religious people, on average, report higher subjective well-being and also have fewer psychosocial pathologies such as domestic abuse (Diener & Tay, 2011)

Religious attitudes and orientations had a significant effect on psychological distress and/or psychological well-being whereas church attendance and belief salience showed no such effect (Dezutter, Soenens, & Hutsebaut, 2006). This is related to theoretical model of religious coping proposed by Maltby and Day (2003). They indicated that Intrinsic related positively with positive coping which, in turn, relates to higher levels of mental health. Extrinsic, on the other hand, tends to relate to maladaptive appraisals of stress and less positive coping, which serve to explain the negative association with mental health. Unterrainer et al. (2010) investigated the relationship between Religious/Spiritual Well-Being and indicators of Psychological Well-Being (including personality). They found that religiosity and spirituality could contribute to the genesis of mental health and disease (Unterrainer et al., 2010) with respect to sense of coherence, "positive" personality dimensions "Extraversion" and "Openness". To conclude, religiosity and spirituality may represent important aspects of human personality (Löckenhoff, Ironson, O'Cleirigh, & Costa, 2009). By introducing the concept of "religious/spiritual well- being", new studies are viable, concerning the consideration of religiosity/spirituality as an important personality trait in the context of Psychological Well-Being. Finally it is notable that although researches reveal the relation of religion with subjective well-being, however, Yet, people are rapidly leaving organized religion in economically developed nations where religious freedom is high. Thus, it appears that the benefits of religion for social relationships and SWB depend on the characteristics of the society (Diener & tay, 2011).

6.4.2 Sense of coherence

The other construct which is suggested to assist an individual to maintain physical and psychological well-being in the face of stressors is sense of coherence (SOC) (Antonovsky, 1987; Kobasa, 1979). Antonovsky (1993) proposed that with this global orientation, one has the feeling that life is comprehensible, manageable and meaningful. Sense of coherence is not a coping style, but has stress-buffering effects. It is the ability to perceive a stressor as comprehensible, manageable, and meaningful (Gauffin, Landtblom, & Räty, 2010). Individuals with a greater sense of coherence are more likely to respond to a stressor with adaptive and most suitable strategies which has a positive outcome for health and well-being (Modin, Ostberg, Toivanen, & Sundel, 2011; Pallant & Lae, 2002). This construct along with coping styles would highlight their effects not only on mental health and well-being (e.g., Modin et al., 2011) but also on physical well-being regarding to deseases (e.g., Gauffin, Landtblom, & Raty, 2010) in a mutual relationship (Bergman et al., 2011)

6.4.3 Emotional intelligence

Emotional intelligence consists of the interaction between emotion and cognition that leads to adaptive functioning (Salovey & Grewal, 2005). Mayer et al. (2004) argued that emotional intelligence is best conceived of as ability, similar to cognitive intelligence. However, emotional intelligence has also been conceptualized as a trait (Neubauer & Freudenthaler, 2005), similar to personality characteristics such as extraversion or conscientiousness. (Schutte et al., 2007). Better perception, understanding, and management of emotion of individuals with higher emotional intelligence make it less likely that they will experience mental health problems and emotional intelligence has useful additional predictive information over and above the Big Five Dimensions for mental health functioning (Schutte et al., 2007; Ciarrochi, Deane, & Anderson, 2002).

7. Conclusion

As Cloninger (2004) argued, much less is known about the relationship of personality to health as a state of physical, mental, and social well-being. Traditionally, the profession of clinical psychology has been interested in the alleviation of human suffering. Studies of positive psychological functioning have been far outweighed by those concerned with psychological distress and dysfunction (Joseph & Wood, 2010). It is time to pay more attention to healthy aspects of personality and mental process or in other words good mental health (Davydov et al., 2010) in order to find what kind of features are prominent in healthy individuals rather than what kind of features should not be seen in individuals and also in order to include wellness and mental health promoting factors. Considering the notion of clinicians who are really and actually engaged in psychopathology, and believe that general personality traits and personality disorders are placed in one spectrum, we can change our approach regarding mental health. Mental health and mental illness are not two distinct phenomena. They might have fluctuation in different situations and might appear in just some kind of situations considering psychological, social, cultural and situational factors. Even in defining abnormal traits there are divergence between social- personality perspectives and clinical perspectives (Rosenthal & Hooley, 2010). Is it really possible to draw a distinction border between health and illness? If yes, to what extent?

There has begun to be a profound shift in psychology's center of gravity– or its locus of control–from outside to inside the person (McCrae, 2002). We thought that psychopathology was the result of life stress, and those events such as marriage, retirement, and loss of spouse would surely bring about major transformations of intraspychic and interpersonal styles. We thought we would be happy if we won the lottery. We now know that these assumptions are naive, just to the extent that they leave out of account the contributions of the individual (Neyer & Asendorpf, 2001) and among many factors contributing in individuals, personality scores higher. Research among adults suggests that personality is a major determinant for adults 'well-being in recent 25 years ago (e.g., Grarcia, 2011; McCrae, 2002) and this is not limited to adulthood. The relationship of personality to well-being has been investigated among adolescents and shows similar results (e.g., Fogle, Huebner, & Laughlin, 2002; Garcia, 2011).

The same significant shift also involves researches about psychopathology, clinical psychology and mental health. And it is the increasing emphasis on the promotion of positive functioning in clinical psychology and mental health. This shift is important because of three main reasons: first of all clinical psychology has always been concerned with well-being but having adopted the language of psychiatry it has inadvertently restricted itself to a narrow definition of well-being which in practice is the absence of distress and dysfunction. The adoption of positive functioning serves to expand the remit of the field of clinical psychology and mental health realm. Secondly By adopting positive functioning as a goal there is the possibility that we are able to increase our ability to predict and treat distress and dysfunction (Jodeph & Wood, 2010; Wood & Tarrier, 2010). And finally, positive characteristics can buffer the impact of negative life events on distress, potentially preventing the development of disorder (Wood & Tarrier, 2010).

In respect to recent revolution in conceptualization of personality, personality disorders and mental disorders in a spectrum and recent tendency to put mental health research in the context of positive psychology (Seligman et al., 2005; Quevedo & Abella, 2011), prospective efforts ought to consider the ubiquitous shade of personality in mental health and psychological well being studies (Garcia, 2011; McCrae, 2002). Personality psychology has made striking advances in the past two decades, demonstrating the importance of individual differences in a wide variety of life domains (McCrae, 2002) insofar as Once again, personality psychology may become "the intellectual center of all the social sciences"(Baumeister,1999,p.371). This is enough to believe that researches, studies, policies and practical implication in respect to mental health and health can be better organized and conceptualized within the realm of personality psychology which incorporates not only all psychology within psychology, but also includes broad biological, psychological, and social systems within humans (Mayer, 2005)

8. References

Aboaja, A., Duggan, C., & Park., B. (2011). An exploratory analysis of the NEO-FFI and DSM personality disorders using multivariate canonical correlation. *Personality and Mental Health, 5,* 1-11.

Akiskal, H.S., Hirschfeld, R., Yerevanina, B. (1983). The relationship of personality to affective disorders. Archives ofGeneral Psychiatry 40, 801–810.

Alterman, A., Cacciola, J., Ivey, M., Coviello, D. M., Lynch, K., Dugosh, K., & Habing, B. (2010). Relationship of mental health and illness in substance abuse patients. *Personality and Individual Differences,* 49, 880-884.

American Psychiatric Association. (2000). Diagnostic and statistical manual of mental disorders, 4th edition Washington, DC: American Psychiatric Press text revision.

American Psychoanalytic Association. (2006). *Psychodynamic diagnostic manual (PDM).* Silver Spring, MD: Alliance of Psychoanalytic Organizations.

Amering, M., Schmolke, M. (2009). *Recovery in Mental Health*: World Psychiatric Association Evidence and Experience in Psychiatry. John Wiley & Sons, New York.

Antonovsky, A. (1987). *Unravelling the mystery of health.* San Francisco, California: Jossey-Bass.

Antonovsky, A. (1993). The structure and properties of the sense of coherence scale. *Social Science and Medicine, 36,* 725–733.

Arnaut, G. L. (2006). Sensation Seeking, Risk Taking, and Fearlessness. In J. C. Thomas, & D. L. Segal (Ed.), *Comprehensive handbook of personality and psychopathology* (pp. 322–341).Vol. 1. John Wiely & Sons, Inc.s

Bagherian, F., Rocca, C., Thorngate, W., & Salehinezhad, M. A. (2011). Beliefs and expectations about future among Iranian and Canadian studdents. *Procedia Social and Behavioral Sciences,* 30, 602-607.

Barenbaum, N. B., & Winter, D. G. (2008). History of Modern Personality theory and research. In O. P. John, & R. W. Robins, & L. A. Pervin (Eds.), Handbook of personality (pp. 3-28). New York: Guilford.

Bartone, P. T., Roland, R. R., Picano, J. J., & Williams, T. J. (2008). Psychological hardiness predicts success in US Army Special Forces Candidates. *International Journal of Selection and Assessment,* 16, 78-81.

Baumeister, R. F., Campbell, J. D., Krueger, J. I., & Vohs, K. D. (2003). Does high selfesteem cause better performance, interpersonal success, happiness, or healthier lifestyles? *Psychological Science in the Public Interest, 4,* 1–44.

Bergman, E., Malm, D., Ljungquist, B., Berterö, C., & Karlsson, J. (2011). Meaningfulness is not the most important component for changes in sense of coherence. European Journal of Cardiovascular Nursing. doi: 10.1016/j.ejcnurse.2011.05.005

Blais, M. (1997) Clinical ratings of the five factor model of personality and the DSM-IV personality disorders. Journal of Nervous and Mental Disease, 185/6, 338–394.

Bloom, P. (2012). Religion, morality, evolution. *Annual Review of Psychology,* 63, 179-199.

Bonanno, G. A. (2004). Loss, trauma, and human resilience: Have we underestimated the human capacity to thrive after extremely aversive events? *American Psychologist, 59,* 20–28.

Bonanno, G. A., Papa, A., Moskowitz, J. T., & Folkman, S. (2005). Resilience to loss in bereaved spouses, bereaved parents, and bereaved gay men. Journal of Personality and Social Psychology, 88, 827-843.

Bowlby, J., 1983. Attachment Second Edition: Attachment and Loss. Basic Books, New York.

Burns, R. A., & Anstey, J. K. (2010). The Connor-Davidson Resilience Scale (CD-RISC): Testing the invariance of a uni-dimensional resilience measure that is independent of positive and negative affect. Journal of Personality and Individual Differences, 48, 527-531.

Buss, D. M. (2008). Human Nature and Individual Differences. In O. P. John, & R. W. Robins, & L. A. Pervin (Eds.), *Handbook of personality* (pp. 29-60). New York: Guilford.

Calvo, R., Lazaro, L., Castro-Fornieles, J., et al., (2009). Obsessive-compulsive personality disorder traits and personality dimensions in parents of children with obsessive-compulsive disorder. *European Psychiatry, 24,* 201–206.

Campbell-Sills, L., Cohan, S. L., & Stein, M. B. (2006). Relationship of resilience to personality, coping, and psychiatric symptoms in young adults. Behaviour Research and Therapy, 44, 585-599.

Carver, C. S., & Miller, C. J. (2006). Relations of serotonin function to personality: Current views and a key methodological issue. *Psychiatry Research,* 144, 1–15.

Carver, C. S., Scheier, M. F., & Fulford, D. (2008). Self-regulatory processes, stress, and coping. In O. P. John, & R. W. Robins, & L. A. Pervin (Eds.), *Handbook of personality* (pp. 725-742). New York: Guilford.

Caspi, A., Roberts, B. W., & Shiner, R. L. (2005). Personality development: Stability and change. Annual Review of Psychology, 56, 453–484.

Cervone, D., 2005. Personality architecture: within-person structures and processes. *Annu. Rev. Psychol.* 56, 423–452.

Chan, R. & Joseph, S. (2000). Dimensions of personality, domains of aspiration, and subjective well-being. Personality and Individual Differences, 28, 347-354.

Ciarrochi, J., Deane, F., & Anderson S. (2002). Emotional intelligence moderates the relationship between stress and mental health. Pesronality and Individual Differences, 32, 197-209.

Clark, L. A., & Harrison, J. A. (2001). Assessment instruments. In W. J. Livesley (Ed.), Handbook of personality disorders: Theory, research, and treatment (pp. 277–306). New York: Guilford Press.

Clark, L. A., Watson, D., & Mineka, S. (1994) Temperament, personality, and the mood and anxiety disorders. *Journal of Abnormal Psychology,* 103, 103–116.

Cloninger, C. R. (1994). *The Temperament and Character Inventory (TCI): a guide to its development and use.* Washington University, St Louis, Missouri: Centre for Psychobiology of Personality.

Cloninger, C. R. (2000). A practical way to diagnosespersonality disorders: A proposal. *Journal of Personality Disorders, 14,* 99–108.

Cloninger, C. R., & Zohar, A. H. (2011). Personality and the perception of health and happiness. *Journal of Affective Disorders, 128,* 24-32.

Cloninger, C.R. (1999). *Personality and Psychopathology (American Psychopathological Association Series).* American Psychiatric Press, Washington, D.C.

Cloninger, C.R. (2004). *Feeling Good: the Science of Well-Being*. Oxford University Press, New York.

Cloninger, C.R. (2006). The science of well-being: an integrated approach to mental health and its disorders. *World Psychiatry, 5*, 71–76.

Cloninger, C.R., (1987). A systematic method for clinical description and classification of personality variants — a proposal. Arch. Gen. Psychiatry 44, 573–588.

Clough, P., Earl, K., & Sewell, D. (2001). Mental toughness: The concept and its measurement. In I.

Cockerill (Ed.), *Solutions in sport psychology* (pp. 32 42). London: Thomson.

Collishaw, S., Pickles, A., Messer, J., Rutter, M., Shearer, C., & Maughan, B. (2007). Resilience to adult psychopathology following childhood maltreatment: Evidence from a community sample. *Child Abuse & Neglect, 31*, 211–229.

Constantino, J. N., Cloninger, C. R., Clarke, A. R., Hashemi, B., & Przybeck, T. (2002). Application of the seven factor model of personality to early childhood. *Psychiatry Research*, 109, 229–243.

Costa, P. T., Jr., & McCrae, R. R. (1990). Personality disorders and the five-factor model of personality. *Journal of Personality Disorders, 4*, 362–371.

Cramer, P. (2006). Protecting the self: *Defense mechanisms in action*. New York : Guilford Press.

Cramer, P. (2009). The development of defense mechanisms from pre-adolescence to early adulthood: Do IQ and social class matter? A longitudinal study. *Journal of Research in Personality*, 43, 464–471.

Davis, M. C., Luecken, L., & Lemery-Chalfant, K. (2009). Resilience in common life: Introduction to the special issue. *Journal of Personality*, 77, 1637-1644.

Davydov, D. M., Stewart, R., Ritchie,. & Chaudieu, I. (2010). Resilience and mental health. Clinical Psychology Review, 30,479–495.

Deci, E. L., & Ryan, R. M. (1995). Human agency: The basis for true self-esteem. In M. H. Kernis (Ed.). *Efficacy, agency, and self-esteem* (pp. 31–50). New York: Plenum Press.

DeLongis, A., Lazarus, R., & Folkman, S. (1988). The impact of daily stress on health and mood: Psychological and social resources as mediators. *Journal of Personality and Social Psychology*, 54(3), 436–495.

DeNeve, K. M., & Cooper, H. (1998). The happy personality: A meta-analysis of 137 personality traits and subjective well-being. *Psychological Bulletin*, 124, 197–229.

Dezutter, J., Soenens, B., & Hutsebaut, D. (2006). Religiosity and mental health: A further exploration of the relative importance of religious behaviors vs. religious attitudes. *Personality and Individual Differences*, 40, 807–818.

Diener, E. (1984). Subjective well-being. *Psychological Bulletin*, 95(3),542–575.

Diener, E., & Tay, L. (2011). The religion paradox: If religion makes people happy, why are so many dropping out? *Journal of Personality and Social Psychology*, 101, 1278-1290.

Diener, E., Biswas-Diener, R. (2008). *Happiness: Unlocking the Secrets of Psychological Wealth*. Blackwell Publishing, Malden, MA.

Donnellan, M. B., Conger, K. J., McAdams, K. K., & Neppl, T. K. (2009). Personal characteristics and resilience to economic hardship and its consequences: Conceptual issues and empirical illustrations. *Journal of Personality*, 77, 1645-1676.

Donohue, B., Farley, A. M., & French, S. L. (2006). Drug abuse and dependence. In M. Hersen & J. C. (Eds.), *Comprehensive Handbook of personality and psychopathology* (pp. 354-369). Vol. 1. John Wiely & Sons, Inc.

Duggan, C. (2004). Does personality change and, if so, what changes? *Criminal Behaviour and Mental Health, 14/1*, 5–16.

Egan, V., Austin, E., Elliot, D., Patel, D., & Charlesworth, P. (2002). Personality traits, personality disorders and sensational interests in mentally disordered offenders. *Legal and Criminological Psychology*, 8, 51–62.

Emmons, R. A., Barrett, J. L., & Schnitker, S. A. (2008). Personality and the Capacity for religious and spiritual experience. In O. P. John, & R. W. Robins, & L. A. Pervin (Eds.), *Handbook of personality* (pp. 634-653). New York: Guilford.

Ettelt, S., Grabe, H.J., Ruhrmann, S., et al., (2008). Harm avoidance in subjects with obsessive-compulsive disorder and their families. *Journal of Affective Disorders, 107*, 265–269.

Eysenck, H. J. (1987). The definition of personality disorders and the criteria appropriate for their description. *Journal of Personality Disorders, 1*, 211–219.

Farmer, R. F. (2000). Issues in the assessment and conceptualization of personality disorders. *Clinical Psychology Review*, 20, 823–851.

Fava, G. A., & Tomba, E. (2009). Increasing psychological well-being and resilience by psychotherapeutic methods. *Journal of Personality*, 77, 1903-1934.

Fogle, L. M., Huebner, E. S., & Laughlin, J. E. (2002). The relationship between temperament and life satisfaction in early adolescence. Cognitive and behavioral mediation models. *Journal of Happiness Studies,* 3, 373–392.

Freud, S. (1962). The neuro-psychoses of defense. In J. Strachey (Ed., Trans.), *The standard edition of the complete psychological works of Sigmund Freud* (Vol. 3, pp. 43–68). London: Hogarth Press (Original work published 1894).

Furukawa, T., Hori, S., Yoshida, S., Tsuji, M., Nakanishi, M., & Hamanaka, T (1998). Premorbid personality traits of patients with organic, schizophrenic, mood and neurotic disorders according to five factor model of personality. *PsychiatryResearch,* 78, 179-187.

Gailliot, M. T., Mead, N. L., & Baumeister, R. F. (2008). Personality and Psychopathology. In O. P. John, & R. W. Robins, & L. A. Pervin (Eds.), *Handbook of personality* (pp. 472-491). New York: Guilford.

Garcia, D. (2011). Two models of personality and well-being among adolescents. *Personality and Individual Differences* , 50, 1208–1212.

Gardini, S., Cloninger, C. R., & Venneri, A. (2009). Individual differences in personality traits reflect structural varianceinspecific brain regions. *BrainResearchBulletin*, 79, 265–270.

Garmezy, N. (1985). Stress-resistant children: The search for protective factors. In J. E. Stevenson (Ed.), *Recent research in developmental psychopathology*. Journal of Child Psychology and Psychiatry Book Supplement No. 4. Oxford: Pergamon Press.

Gauffin, H., Landtblom, A., & Raty, L. (2010). Self-esteem and sense of coherence in young people with uncomplicated epilepsy:A 5-year follow-up. *Epilepsy & Behavior, 17*, 520–524.

Gillespi, N. A., Cloninger, C. R., Heath, A., & Martin, N. G. (2003). The genetic and environmental relationship between Cloninger's dimensions of temperament and character. *Personality and Individual Differences, 35,* 1931–1946.

Golby, J. & Sheard, M. (2004). Mental toughness and hardiness at different levels of rugby league. Personality and Individual Differences, 37, 933-942.

Gomez, V., Krings, F., Bangerter, A., & Grob, A. (2009). The influence of personality and life events on subjective well-being from a life span perspective. *Journal of Research in Personality,*43, 345–354.

Goodwin, R. G., & Friedman, H. S. (2006). Health status and the five factor personality traits in a nationally representative sample. *Journal of Health Psychology,* 11, 643–654.

Gottfredson, M. R., & Hirschi, T. (1990). A general theory of crime. Stanford, CA: Stanford University Press.

Hammen, C. (2005). Stress and depression. Annual Review of Clinical Psychology, 1(1), 293–319.

Hampson, S. E. (2012). Personality processes: mechanisms by which personality traits get outside the Skin. *Annual Review of Psychology,* 63, 315-339.

Hampson, S. E., & Friedman, H. S. (2008). Personality and Health. In O. P. John, & R. W. Robins, & L. A. Pervin (Eds.), *Handbook of personality* (pp. 770-794). New York: Guilford.

Hansenne, M., Reggers, J., Pinto, E., Karim, K., Ajamier, A., & Ansseau, M. (1999). Temperament and character inventory (TCI) and depression. *Journal of Psychiatric Research,* 33, 31-36.

Harkness, A. R., McNulty, J. L., & Ben-Porath, Y. S. (1995). The Personality Psychopathology Five (PSY 5): Constructs and MMPI-2 scales. *Psychological Assessment, 7,* 104–114.

Herero, V. G., & Extremera, N. (2010). Daily life activities as mediators of the relationship between personality variables and subjective well-being among older adults. *Personality and Individual Differences.* 49, 124-129.

Hirschfeld, R.M.A., Shea, M.T., Holzer, C.E., 1997. Personality dysfunction and depression. In: Honing, A., van Praag, H.M. (Eds.), *Depression: Neurobiological, Psychopathological and Therapeutic Advances.* John Wiley, New York, pp. 327–341.

Horsburgh,V. A., Aitken Schermer, J., Veselka, L., & Vernon, P. A.(2009). A behavioural genetic study of mental toughness and personality. *Personality and Individual Differences, 46,* 100–105.

Houston, B. K., & Snyder, C. R. (Eds.). (1988). *Type A behavior pattern: Research, theory, and intervention.* New York: Wiley.

Huber, A., Suman, A., Biasi., & Carli, G (2008). Predictors of psychological distress and well-being in women with chronic Musculoskeletal pain: Two sides of the same coin?. *Journal of Psychosomatic Research* ,64, 169–175.

Insel, T. R., & Scolnick, E. M. (2006). Cure therapeutics and strategic prevention: Raising the bar for mental health research. *Molecular Psychiatry,* 11, 11 17.

Jaspers, K., 1968. The phenomenological approach in psychopathology. *Br. J. Psychiatry* 114, 1313–1323.

Jin, J., Tang, Y. -Y., Ma, Y., Lv, S., Bai, Y., & Zhang, H. (2009). A structural equation model of depression and the defense system factors: A survey among Chinese college students. *Psychiatry Research, 165,* 288−296.

Johnsen, B. H., Eid, J., Pallesen, S., Bartone, P. T., & Nissestad, A. O. (2009). Predicting transformational in naval cadets: Effects of personality hardiness and training. *Journal of Applied Social Psychology*, 39, 2213-2235.

Jorm, A. F., Korten, A. E., Jacomb, P. A., Christensen, H., Rodgers, B., & Politt, P. (1997). 'Mental health literacy': a survey of the public's ability to recognize mental disorder and their beliefs about the effectiveness of treatment. *The Medical Journal of Australia*, 166,182–186.

Josefsson, K., Cloninger, C. R, Hintsanen, M., Jokela, M., Pulkki-Råback, L., & Keltikangas-Järvinen, L. (2011). Associations of personality profiles with various aspects of well-being: A population-based study. *Journal of Affective Disorders*, doi: 10.1016/j.jad.2011.03.023.

Joseph, S., & Wood, A. (2010). Assessment of positive functioning in clinical psychology: Theoretical and practical issues. *Clinical Psychology Review*, 30, 830–838.

Jovanovic,V. (2011). Personality and subjective well-being: One neglected model of personality and two forgotten aspects of subjective well-being. *Personality and Individual Differences*,50 ,631–635.

Kernis, M. H. (2003). Toward a conceptualization of optimal self-esteem. Psychological Inquiry, 14, 1–26.

Kernis, M. H. (2005). Measuring self-esteem in context: The importance of stability of self-esteem in psychological functioning. *Journal of Personality*, 73, 1–37.

Kernis, M. H., Brown, A. C., & Brody, G. H. (2000). Fragile self-esteem in children and its associations with perceived patterns of parent-child communication. *Journal of Personality*, 68, 225–252.

Kernis, M. H., Cornell, D. P., Sun, C. R., Berry, A. J., & Harlow, T. (1993). There's more to self-esteem than whether it is high or low: The importance of stability of self-esteem. *Journal of Personality and Social Psychology*, 65, 1190–1204.

Kernis, M. H., Greenier, K. D., Herlocker, C. E., Whisenhunt, C. R., & Abend, T. A. (1997). Self-perceptions of reactions to doing well or poorly: The roles of stability and level of self-esteem. *Personality and Individual Differences*, 22, 845–854.

Keyes, C. L. M. (2007). Promoting and protecting mental health as flourishing: A complementary strategy for improving national mental health. *American Psychologist*, 62(2), 95–108.

Keyes, C. L. M. (2009). The black-white paradox in health: Flourishing the face of social inequality and discrimination. *Journal of Personality*, 77, 1678-1705.

Kobasa, S. C. (1979). Personality and resistance to illness. *American Journal of Community Psychology, 7*, 413–423.

Kobasa, S. C. (1979). Stressful life events, personality, and health: An inquiry into hardiness. *Journal of Personality and Social Psychology*, 37(1), 1–11.

Kobasa, S. C., Maddi, S. R., & Kahn, S. (1982). Hardiness and health: A prospective study. *Journal of Peersonality and Social Psychology, 42*, 168-177.

Koenig, H. G., McCullough, M. E., & Larson, D. B. (2001). Handbook of religion and health. Oxford: Univ.Press

Krueger, R. F., Mc Gue, M., & Iacono, W. G. (2001). The higher-order structure of common DSM mental disorders: internalization, externalization and their connections to personality. *Personality and Individual Differences, 30*, 1245-1259.

Lazarus, R. S., & Folkman, S. (1984). *Stress, appraisal, and coping*. New York, NY: Springer.

Leve, L. D., Fisher, P. A., & Chamberlain, P. (2009). Multidimensional treatment foster care as a preventive intervention to promote resiliency among youth in the child welfare system. *Journal of Personality, 77*, 1870-1902.

Löckenhoff, C. E., Ironson, G. H., O'Cleirigh, C., & Costa, P. T. Jr., (2009). Five-factor model personality traits, spirituality/religiousness, and mental health among people living with HIV. *Journal of Personality, 77*, 1411–1436.

Lucas, R. E., & Diener, E. (2008). Personality and Subjective Well-Being. In O. P. John, & R. W. Robins, & L. A. Pervin (Eds.), *Handbook of personality* (pp. 795-814). New York: Guilford.

Luhmann, M., Hofmann, W., Eid, M., & Lucas, R. E. (2012). Subjective well-Being and adaptation to life events: A meta-analysis. *Journal of Personality and Social Psychology*, 102, 592-615.

Luthar, S. S., & Cicchetti, D. (2000). The construct of resilience: Implications for interventions and social policies. *Development and Psychopathology*, 12, 857-885.

MacAdams, D. P. (2008). Personal narratives and the life story. In O. P. John, & R. W. Robins, & L. A. Pervin (Eds.), *Handbook of personality* (pp. 243-262). New York: Guilford.

MacLeod, A. K., & Moore, R. (2000). Positive thinking revisited: Positive cognitions, well-being and mental health. *Clinical Psychology and Psychotherapy*, 7, 1–10.

Maddi, S. R. (1999). The personality construct of hardiness, I: Effects on experiencing, coping, and strain. *Consulting Psychology Journal*, 51, 83-94.

Maddi, S. R. (2002). The story of hardiness: Twenty years of theorizing, research, and Practice. *Consulting Psychology Journal*, 54, 173-185.

Maddi, S. R. (2006). Hardiness: The courage to be resilient. In J. C. Thomas, & D. L. Segal (Ed.), *Comprehensive handbook of personality and psychopathology* (pp. 306–321).Vol. 1. John Wiely & Sons, Inc.

Maddi, S. R., Harvey, R. H., Khoshaba, D. M., Lu, J. L., Persico, M., & Brow, M. (2006). The personality construct of hardiness, III: Relationships with repression, innovativeness, authoritarianism, and performance. *Journal of Personality*, 74, 575-598.

Maddi, S. R., Khoshaba, D. M., Harvey, R., Lu, J. & Persico, M. (2001). The personality construct of hardiness, II: Relationships with comprehensive tests of personality and psychopathology. *Journal of Research in Personality*, 36, 72-85.

Maher, B. A., & Maher, W. B. (1994). Personality and psychopathology: A historical perspective. *Journal of Abnormal Psychology*, 103, 72–77.

Maltby, J., & Day, L. (2003). Religious orientation, religious coping and appraisals of stress. *Personality and Individual Differences*, 34, 1209–1224.

Maltby, J., Day, L. (2004). Should never the twain meet? Integrating models of religious personality and religious mental health. *Personality and Individual Differences* ,36 ,1275–1290.

Maltby, J., Day, L., & Barber, L. (2004). Forgiveness and mental health variables: Interpreting the relationship using an adaptational-continuum model of personality and coping. *Personality and Individual Differences*, 37, 1629–1641.

Mancini, A. D., & Bonanno, G. A. (2009). Predictors and parameters of resilience to loss: Toward an individual differences model. *Journal of Personality*, 77, 1805-1832.

Marijnissen, G., TuinieR, S., Sijben, A., & Verhoeven, W. (2002). The temperament and character inventory in major depression. *Journal of Affective Disorders*,70, 219–223.

Markon, K. E., Krueger, R. F., & Watson, D. (2005). Delineating the structure of normal and abnormal personality: An integrative hierarchical approach. *Journal of Personality and Social Psychology*, 88, 139–157.

Masten, A. (2001). Ordinary magic: Resilience processes in development. American Psychologist, 56, 227-238.

Mayer, J. D., (2005). A Tale of Two Visions: Can a New View of Personality Help Integrate Psychology? *American Psychologist*, 60, 294–307.

Mayer, J. D., Salovey, P., & Caruso, D. (2004). Emotional intelligence: theory, findings, and implications. *Psychological Inquiry*, 15, 197–215.

McCrae, R. (2002). The maturation of personality psychology: Adult personality development and psychological well-being. *Journal of Research in Personality*, 36, 307–317.

McCrae, R. R., & Costa, P. T. (1991). Adding Liebe and Arbeit: The full five-factor model and well-being. *Personality and Social Psychology Bulletin*, 17, 227–232.

McCrae, R. R., & Costa, P. T. (2008). The five- factor theory of Personality. In O. P. John, & R. W. Robins, & L. A. Pervin (Eds.), *Handbook of personality* (pp. 159-181). New York: Guilford.

McCullough, M. E., Tsang, J.-A., & Emmons, R. A. (2004). Gratitude in intermediate affective terrain: Links of grateful moods to individual differences and daily emotional experience. *Journal of Personality and Social Psychology*, 86, 295–309.

McDowell, I., (2010).Measures of self-perceived well-being. *Journal of Psychosomatic Research*, 69,69–79.

Millon, T., Davis, R., Millon, C. M., Wenger, C. M., Van Zuilen, M. H., et al. (1996). *Disorders of personality: DSM-IV and beyond* (2nd ed.). New York: Wiley.

Millon, T., Grossman, S., Millon, C., Meagher, S., & Ramnath, R. (2004). *Personality Disorders in Modern Life*. (2nd ed.). John Wiley & Sons, New York.

Mischel, W., & Shoda, Y. (2008). Toward a unified theory of personality. In O. P. John, & R. W. Robins, & L. A. Pervin (Eds.), *Handbook of personality* (pp. 208-241). New York: Guilford.

Modin, B., Ostberg, V., Toivanen, S., & Sundell, K. (2011). Psychosocial working conditions, school sense of coherence and subjective health complaints. A multilevel analysis of ninth grade pupils in the Stockholm area. *Journal of Adolescence, 34*, 129–139.

Mols, F., Holterhues, C., Nijsten, T., & Poll-Franse, L. (2010). Personality is associated with health status and impact of cancer among melanoma survivors. *Europian Journal of Cancer*, 4 6, 5 7 3 –5 8 0.

Murphy, W. D. & Page, I. J. (2006). Sexual deviation. In M. Hersen & J. C. (Eds.), *Comprehensive Handbook of personality and psychopathology* (pp. 436-449). Vol. 1. John Wiely & Sons, Inc.

Myers, D. G. (1992). The pursuit of happiness: *Who is happy and why*. New York: William Morrow.

Myers, D. G., & Diener, E. (1995). Who is happy? *Psychological Science*, 6, 10–19.

Neubauer, A. C., & Freudenthaler, H. H. (2005). Models of emotional intelligence. In R. Schultz & R. D. Roberts (Eds.), *Emotional intelligence: an international handbook* (pp. 31–50). Cambridge, MA: Hogrefe.

Neyer, F. J., & Asendorpf, J. B. (2001). Personality-relationship transaction in young adulthood. *Journal of Personality and Social Psychology*, 81, 1190–1204.

Ni, C., Liu, X., Hua, Q., Lv, A., Wang, B., & Yan, Y. (2010). Relationship between coping, self-esteem, individual factors and mental health among Chinese nursing students: A matched case–control study. *Nurse Education Today, 30*, 338–343.

Olsson, I., & Dahl, A. (2009). Personality problems are considerably associated with somatic morbidity and health care utilization. *European Psychiatry*, 24, 442–449.

Ong, A. D., Bergeman, C. S., & Boker, S. M. (2009). Resilience comes of age: Defining features in later adulthood. *Journal of Personality*, 77, 1-28.

Pallant, J. F., & Lae, L. (2002). Sense of coherence, well-being, coping and personality factors: further evaluation of the sense of coherence scale. *Personality and Individual Differences*, 33, 39–48.

Patel, V., & Goodman, A. (2007). Researching protective and promotive factors in mental health. *International Journal of Epidemiology*, 36, 703−707.

Philippe, F. L., Lecours, S., & Beaulieu-Pelletier, G. (2009). Resilience and positive emotions: Examining the role of emotional memories. *Journal of Personality*, 77, 140-175.

Piedmont, R. L. (1999). Does spirituality represent the sixth factor of personality? Spiritual transcendence and the five-factor model. *Journal of Personality*, 67, 985–1013.

Pincus, A. L., & Gurtman, M. B. (2006). Interpersonal theory and the interpersonal circumplex: Evolving perspectives on normal and abnormal personality. In S. Strack (Ed.), *Differentiating normal and abnormal personality* (2nd ed., pp. 83–111). New York: Springer.

Pincus, A. L., Lukowitsky, M. R., & Wright, A. G. C. (2010). The interpersonal nexus of personality and psychopathology. In T. Millon, R. F. Kruger, & E. Simonsen (Eds.) *Contemporary directions in psychopathology: Scientific foundations for the DSM–V and ICD–11* (pp. 523–552). New York, NY: Guilford Press.

Pratt, T. C., & Cullen, F. T. (2000). The empirical status of Gottfredson and Hirschi's general theory of crime: A meta-analysis. *Criminology*, 38, 931–964.

Pressman, S. D., & Cohen, S. (2005). Does positive affect influence health? *Psychological Bulletin*, 131(6), 925–971.

Quevedo, R. ., & Abella, M. (2011). Well-being and personality: Facet-level analyses. *Personality and Individual Differences*, 50, 206–211.

Richardson, G. E. (2002). The metatheory of resilience and resiliency. Journal of Clinical Psychology, 58, 307-321.

Roberts, B. W., & DelVecchio, W. F. (2000). The rank-order consistency of personality traits from childhood to old age: A quantitative review of longitudinal studies. *Psychological Bulletin*, 126, 3–25.

Robins, R. W., Hendin, H. M., & Trzesniewski, K. H. (2001). Measuring global self-esteem: Construct validation of a single-item measure and the Rosenberg self-esteem scale. *Personality and Social Psychology Bulletin*, 27, 151–161.

Rogers, C.R., (1995). A Way of Being. Houghton Mifflin, Boston.

Rosenberg, M. (1979). Conceiving the self. New York: Basic Books.

Rosenthal, S. A., & Hooley, J. M. (2010). Narcissism assessment in social–personality research: Does the association between narcissism and psychological health result from a confound with self-esteem? *Journal of Research in Personality*, 44, 453–465.

Rounsaville, B. J., Alarcon, R. D., Andrews, G., Jackson, J. S., Kendell, R. E., & Kendler, K. (2002). Basic nomenclature issues for DSM-V. In D. J. Kupfer, M. B. First, & D. E. Regier (Eds.), *A research agenda for DSM-V* (pp. 1–29). Washington, DC: American Psychiatric Association.

Ruini, C., Ottolini, F., Rafanelli, C., et al., (2003). The relationship of psychological well-being to distress and personality.Psychother. *Psychosom.* 72, 268–275.

Ryan, R.M., Deci, E.L., (2000). Self-determination theory and the facilitation of intrinsic motivation, social development, and well-being. *Am. Psychol.* 55, 68–78.

Ryan, R.M., Deci, E.L., (2001). On happiness and human potentials: a review of research on hedonic and eudaimonic well-being. *Annu. Rev. Psychol.* 52, 141–166.

Salehinezhad, M. A., Besharat, M. A. (2010). Relations of resilience and hardiness with sport achievement and mental health in a sample of athletes. *Procedia social and behavioral science*, 5, 757–497.

Salehinezhad, M. A., Khodapanahi, M. K., Yekta, M., Mahmoodikahriz,. Ostadghafour, S. (2011). Defense styles in iternalizing and externalizing disorder. *Procedia Social and Behavioral Sciences*, 30, 236-241.

Salovey, P., & Grewal, D. (2005). The science of emotional intelligence. *Current Directions in Psychological Science*, 14, 281–285.

Schacter, D. L., Gilbert, D. T., & Wegner, D. M. (2009). *Psychology*. Worth Publishers: New York

Schutte, N. S., Malouff, J. F., & Thorsteinsson, E. B. (2007). A meta-analytic investigation of the relationship between emotional intelligence and health. *Personality and Individual Differences, 42*, 921–933.

Seligman, M. E. P., & Csikszentmihalyi, M. (2000). Positive psychology: An introduction. *American Psychologist*,55, 5–14.

Seligman, M. E. P., Steen, T. A., Park, N., & Peterson, C. (2005). Positive Psychology Progress. Empirical validation of interventions. *American Psychologist, 60*, 410–421.

Shedler, J., & Westen, D. (2004). Dimensions of personality pathology: An alternative to the five-factor model. *American Journal of Psychiatry, 161*, 1743–1754.

Skodol, A. E., Gunderson, J. G., Shea, M. T., Mc- Glashan, T. H., Morey, L. C., Sanislow, C. A., et al. (2006). The Collaborative Longitudinal Personality Disorders Study (CLPS): Overview and implications. *Journal of Personality Disorders, 20*, 487–504.

Smith, M.J., Cloninger, C.R., Harms, M.P., et al., (2008). Temperament and character as schizophrenia-related endophenotypes in non-psychotic siblings. *Schizophrenia. Research. 104*, 198–205.

Snyder, M. (1987). *Public appearances, private realities: The psychology of self-monitoring.* New York: Freeman.

Southwick, S. M., Vythilingam, M., & Charney, D. S. (2005). The psychobiology of depression and resilience to stress: Implications for prevention and treatment. *Annual Review of Clinical Psychology*, 1, 255-291.

Srivastava, S., John, O. P., Gosling, S. D., & Potter, J. (2003). Development of personality in early and middle adulthood: Set like plaster or persistent change? *Journal of Personality and Social Psychology,* 84, 1041–1053.

Stead, R., Shanahan,, M., & Neufeld, R. (2010). "I'll go to therapy, eventually": Procrastination, stress and mental health. *Personality and Individual Differences* ,49 ,175–180.

Steel, P., Schmidt, J., & Shultz, J. (2008). Refining the relationship between personality and subjective well-being. *Psychological Bulletin,* 134, 138–161.

Svrakic, D. M., Pryzbeck, T. R., & Cloninger, C. R., (1992). Mood states and personality traits. *Iournnl of Affectire Disorders,* 24, 217-226.

Tedeschi, R. G., Park, C. L., & Calhoun, L. F. (1998). Posttraumatic growth: positive changes in the aftermath of crisis. Mahwah, NJ: Lawrence Erlbaum Associates.

Tellegen, A. (1982). *Brief Manual for the Multidimensional Personality Questionnaire.* Unpublished manuscript, University of Minnesota, Minneapolis.

Tennen, H., & Affleck, G. (1993). The puzzles of self-esteem: A clinical perspective. In R. F. Baumeister (Ed.), Self-esteem: The puzzle of low self-regard (pp. 241–262). New York: Plenum Press.

Trull, T. J., Stepp, S. D., & Solhan, M. (2006). Borderline personality disorder. In M. Hersen & J. C. (Eds.), *Comprehensive Handbook of personality and psychopathology* (pp. 299-315). Vol. 1. John Wiely & Sons, Inc..

Unterrainer, H. F., Ladenhauf, K. H., Moazedi, M. L., Wallner-Liebmann, S. J., & Fink, A. (2010). Dimensions of Religious/Spiritual Well-Being and their relation to Personality and Psychological Well-Being. *Personality and Individual Differences, 49,* 192–197.

Vaillant,G.E.(1971).Theoretical hierarchy of adaptive ego mechanisms. *Archives of General Psychiatry,* 24, 107–118.

Vitousek, K. M., & Stumpf, R. E. (2005). Difficulties in the assessment of personality traits and disorders in eating-disordered individuals. *Eating Disorders,* 13(1), 37–60.

Waschull, S. B., & Kernis, M. H. (1996). Level and stability of self-esteem as predictors of children's intrinsic motivation and reasons for anger. *Personality and Social Psychology Bulletin,* 22, 4–13.

WHO (2001a). *Strengthening mental health promotion.* Geneva, World Health Organization.

WHO (2001b). *Mental Health: New Understanding, New Hope.* World Health Organization, Geneva

Widiger , T. A., & Smith , G. T.(2008). Personality and Psychopathology. In O. P. John, & R. W. Robins, & L. A. Pervin (Eds.), *Handbook of personality* (pp. 743-769). New York: Guilford.

Widiger, T. A., & Mullins-Sweatt, S. (2007). Mental disorders as discrete clinical conditions: Dimensional versus categorical classification. In M. Hersen, S. M. Turner, & D. Beidel (Eds.), *Adult psychopathology and diagnosis* (3rd ed., pp. 3–33). New York: Wiley.

Widiger, T. A., & Samuel, D. B. (2005). Evidence- based assessment of personality disorders. *Psychological Assessment,* 17, 278–287.

Widiger, T. A., & Trull, T. J. (2007). Plate tectonics in the classification of personality disorder: Shifting to a dimensional model. *American Psychologist, 62,* 71–83.

Williams, P., & Moroz, T. (2009) Personality vulnerability to stress-related sleep disruption: Pathways to adverse mental and physical health outcomes. *Personality and Individual Differences*, 46, 598–603.

Wilmshurst, L. (2005). Essentials of child psychopathology. New Jersey: John Wiely & Sons, Inc.

Wood, A. M., Joseph, S., & Maltby, J. (2011). Gratitude predicts psychological well-being above the Big Five facets. *Personality and Individual Differences*, 46, 443–447.

Wood, A. M., Maltby, J., Gillett, R., Linley, P. A., & Joseph, S. (2008). The role of gratitude in the development of social support, stress, and depression: Two longitudinal studies. *Journal of Research in Personality*, 42, 854–871.

Wood, A. M., Maltby, J., Stewart, N., Linley, P. A., & Joseph, S. (2008). A socialcognitive model of trait and state levels of gratitude. *Emotion*, 8, 281–290.

Wood, A. M., Tarrier, N. (2010). Positive Clinical Psychology: A new vision and strategy for integrated research and practice. *Clinical Psychology Review, 30,* 819–829.

World Health Organization. (1992). International classification of diseases (10th ed.). Geneva, Switzerland: Author.

Wright, A. G., Pincus, A. L., & Lenzenweger, M. F. (2011). Development of personality and the remission and onset of personality pathology. *Journal of Personality and Socail Psychology*, 101, 1351-1358.

Yi-Frazier, J. P., Smith, R. E., Vitalino, P. P., Yi, J. C., Mai, S., Hillman, M., & Weinger, K. (2009). A person-focused analysis of resilience resources and coping in patients with diabetes. *Stress and Health, 10,* 1-10.

Zautra, A. J. (2009). Resilience: One part recovery, two parts sustainability. Journal of Personality, 77, 1935-1943.

Zautra, A. J., Johnson, L. M., & Davis, M. C. (2005). Positive affect as a source of resilience for women in chronic pain. *Journal of Consulting and Clinical Psychology*, 73, 212-220.

Zeidner, M., & Endler, N. S. (1996). *Handbook of coping: Theory, research, applications*. London: John Wiley & Sons Inc.

Zeigler-Hill, V., Chadha, S., & Osterman, L. (2008). Psychological defense and self-esteem instability: Is defense style associated with unstable self-esteem*? Journal of Research in Personality* ,42, 348–364

Zohar, A.H., Ebstein, R.P., Pauls, D.L. (2005). TPQ profiles of patients with OCD and GTS and their first degree relatives. *World Journal of Biological Psychiatry, 6,* 151–152.

Zuckerman, M. (2002). Zuckerman–Kuhlman Personality Questionnaire (ZKPQ): An alternative five-factorial model. In B. de Raad & M. Perugini (Eds.), *Big five assessment* (pp. 377–396). Seattle, WA: Hogrefe & Huber.

24

Factors Associated with Positive Mental Health in a Portuguese Community Sample: A Look Through the Lens of Ryff's Psychological Well-Being Model

Helder Miguel Fernandes[1,2], José Vasconcelos-Raposo[1,2] and Robert Brustad[3]
[1]*Research Centre in Sport, Health and Human Development, Vila Real*
[2]*University of Trás-os-Montes and Alto Douro, Vila Real*
[3]*University of Northern Colorado, Colorado*
[1,2]*Portugal*
[3]*USA*

1. Introduction

Recent estimates of the extent of mental illness have revealed that about one in three individuals meet criteria for the diagnosis of at least one mental health disorder at some point of their lives (WHO International Consortium in Psychiatric Epidemiology, 2000). Studies have suggested that in any one-year time span at least one in five people is likely to be diagnosed with a mental disorder with anxiety and mood disorders (namely unipolar major depression) among the most commonly diagnosed disorders, with a lifetime prevalence of about 25% of the general population (Antony & Swinson, 1996). In Portugal, chronic anxiety and depression tend to represent about 17% of the reasons why citizens undergo a long-term medical treatment (DG SANCO, 2007). Additionally, the first Portuguese mental health epidemiological study revealed that almost 23% of the individuals in the study reported a diagnosable mental illness during the previous year (Caldas de Almeida, 2010).

Although much is known about the correlates, prevalence and treatment of psychological disorders, still more remains unknown about the "positive side" of mental health. Some authors have argued that explicit efforts should be made toward the establishment of criteria for positive psychological health given its significance (Keyes, 2005; Ryff & Singer, 1998; Seligman & Csikszentmihalyi, 2000). Several developments and models have been presented since the seminal work of Marie Jahoda. Such formulations have become directed toward defining the core features/indicators of well-being, which have originated a myriad of different terminologies and theoretical and conceptual boundaries (i.e., well-being, happiness, positive affect and emotions, life satisfaction, and quality of life).

For this reason, the study of well-being has proliferated during the last decades, predominantly under the umbrella of the positive psychology movement (Seligman &

Csikszentmihalyi, 2000). Ryan and Deci's (2001) prominent review article suggested that the extensive body of well-being research could be restricted to two distinct, but related models, rooted in two ancient traditions, namely the hedonic and eudaimonic perspectives. The subjective well-being (SWB) model consists of three components: positive and negative affect, and life satisfaction (Diener et al., 1999). The second model, psychological well-being (PWB), is arguably best represented by Ryff's multidimensional structure of positive psychological functioning. This dual perspective has received some empirical support through factor analytic studies (Compton et al., 1996; Linley et al., 2009). Therefore, a considerable overlap should be recognized between the hedonic and eudaimonic perspectives, both in terms of theoretical and empirical aspects. Nevertheless, Carol Ryff has contributed to the discussion by identifying points of convergence in several mental health, clinical, and life span developmental theories and translating them to an empirical form of assessment (Ryff, 1989). These points of convergence constitute the core dimensions of the model, namely the importance of autonomy, environmental mastery, personal growth, positive relations with others, purpose in life, and self-acceptance. Therefore, these theoretically and empirically founded set of indicators appear to represent the core components of human flourishing.

The three components of subjective well-being have been extensively related with different types of variables. Meta-analytic evidence indicates that sociodemographic variables (gender, age and education) have a small effect on subjective well-being (Diener et al., 2003). Other variables, including self-reported health, religion and marriage have also been positively associated with positive affect and life satisfaction, although such influence is weak and its causal direction is unclear (see Diener et al., 1999). It has also been suggested that wealth might contribute to happiness and life satisfaction by providing certain basic needs but this relationship is more relevant in low-income countries (Diener, 2000). This premise was later supported by the meta-analysis performed by Howell and Howell (2008), which concluded that the effect size between economic status and subjective well-being was higher among low-income developing nations and for least educated samples than for more developed and higher income nations. Additionally, several personality traits have been found to be moderately correlated to life satisfaction, positive affect and negative affect (DeNeve & Cooper, 1998). More recently, a study by Steel et al. (2008) indicated that the relationship between personality and SWB dimensions is higher (e.g., four times) than reported in previous meta-analyses. Other studies have also demonstrated that subjective well-being is positively related with self-esteem (especially in individualistic cultures), optimism and personal control (Diener & Diener, 1995; Scheier et al., 2001). Moreover, previous research has demonstrated that people who adopt a healthy lifestyle (e.g., exercising enough, non-smoking, drinking moderately) are happier and more satisfied with their life (Grant et al., 2009; Shahab & West, 2011), report lower levels of depression and anxiety (Mykletun et al., 2008; Rethorst et al., 2009; Wipfli et al., 2008), and have more favourable views about the self (Spence et al., 2005). These final psychosocial dimensions tend to be usually included under the umbrella of subjective well-being.

Compared with the hedonic perspective, the eudaimonic approach has been much less frequently studied, especially with large scale populations. Rare exceptions are the investigations directed by Carol Ryff, namely the MIDUS (Midlife in the United States)/MIDJA (Midlife in Japan), NSFH (National Survey of Families and Households), and WLS (Wisconsin Longitudinal Study). Previous empirical research has examined how eudaimonic well-being is influenced by sociodemographic factors, such as age, gender, socioeconomic status, race/ethnicity and culture. Aspects of well-being, such as positive relations and self-acceptance have consistently showed little age variation, while autonomy and environmental mastery have been found to be positively related to age. Moreover, cross-sectional data has shown evidence that purpose in life and personal growth decline across age periods (Ryff, 1989; Ryff & Keyes, 1995). However, Springer et al. (2011) have recently suggested that longitudinal age variations explain a very small proportion of the variance across the PWB dimensions. In addition, few gender differences have been identified, with women generally rating themselves higher on positive relations and personal growth than men (Ryff, 1989; Ryff & Keyes, 1995). With regard to socioeconomic status, available evidence has consistently demonstrated that educational attainment, occupational status and income are positive predictors of eudaimonic well-being (Keyes et al., 2002; Marmot et al., 1997; Ryff & Singer, 1996). A further line of inquiry has also investigated how well-being is affected by different challenges in life (e.g., parenthood, giving care to an ill or disabled significant other, experiencing relocation, health changes on later life) as well as by the individual's interpretations of these experiences (Heidrich & Ryff, 1993; Ryff & Heidrich, 1997). Previous correlational and factor-analytic studies have also demonstrated that self-esteem shows highest associations with self-acceptance, purpose in life and environmental mastery (Compton, 2001; Paradise & Kernis, 2002; Ryff, 1989). Eudaimonic well-being has also been linked with reduced biological risk, such as lower levels of daily salivary cortisol, pro-inflammatory cytokines, cardiovascular risk, and longer REM sleep duration (Lindfors & Lundberg, 2002; Ryff et al., 2004) and left prefrontal cortex activation (Urry et al., 2004), which is associated better emotional outcomes (Davidson, 2004). Furthermore, the relation between health-promoting behaviours and psychological well-being has been less explored. The scarce available evidence suggests that exercisers score significantly higher than non-exercisers on all PWB dimensions, with the highest effect sizes being reported for purpose in life, positive relations and self-acceptance (Edwards et al., 2005). Gunnell (2009) also observed a positive relationship (r= 0.22) between a measure of eudaimonic well-being (Subjective Vitality Scale) and leisure-time physical activity in individuals with osteoporosis. Additionally, Besenski (2009) suggested that the relationship between health-enhancing physical activity and psychological well-being is best explained by the *experience* during the activity, rather than the *level* (duration, frequency, intensity) of activity. Specifically with adolescent samples, Vleioras and Bosma (2005) found that avoiding facing identity issues is negatively related to all psychological well-being dimensions. Additionally, Fernandes and Vasconcelos-Raposo (2008) demonstrated that psychological well-being, as measured by an adaptation of Ryff's scales (Fernandes et al., 2010), is related to specific sociodemographic (gender and age), socio-cultural (parent-child relationship, family structure and place of residence), and psychological variables (self-esteem, school satisfaction and social anxiety) during adolescence.

According to Ryff and Singer (1998), positive human health should be conceptualized as a multidimensional dynamic process that includes physical, socio-cultural and mental components. Moreover, these authors suggested that future research should identify and understand the factors associated with positive psychological functioning and develop positive health interventions based upon this knowledge. To the best of our knowledge, few studies have analyzed the relation between health-promoting behaviours (exercise, non-smoking) and eudaimonic well-being (e.g., Besenski, 2009; Edwards et al., 2005; Kimiecik,

2011). As such, the present research makes an original contribution to the literature by identifying and evaluating some of the possible sociodemographic, lifestyle and psychosocial correlates of psychological well-being in a non-American sample (Portugal).

Therefore, the present empirical study aims to examine the influence of sociodemographic (gender, age, place of residence, educational attainment, and socioeconomic status), lifestyle (smoking and physical activity) and psychosocial (body satisfaction) factors on positive mental health in a large Portuguese community sample. Taking into account the above considerations, the six dimensions of Ryff's well-being model were designated as indicators of positive mental health (Keyes, 2005; Ryff & Singer, 1998), and were selected as the psychological outcomes to be studied.

2. Method

This study used a cross-sectional, descriptive, and correlational research design.

2.1 Participants

A sample of 783 individuals (355 men and 428 women) randomly recruited from the northern and central regions of Portugal participated in the study. The mean age of the sample was 34.45 (SD = 11.77) years, with an age range from 18 to 78 years. Age was divided into three age groups: young adults (≤ 29 yrs), midlife adults (30-54 yrs), and older adults (≥ 55 yrs). As a result, 339 individuals were referred to as young adults (43.3%), 403 were referred to as midlife adults (51.5%), and 41 were considered older adults (5.2%). A total of 358 (45.7%) individuals reported living a rural area, while 425 (54.3%) reported living in urban areas. Educational attainment was divided into three groups: 9 or fewer years of education (n= 324, 41.4%); 12 or fewer years of education (n= 253, 32.3%); and academic degree (n= 206, 26.3%). The mean for years of education was 9.25 (SD = 3.78). Regarding the sample's economic levels, 266 (34.0%) reported receiving one minimum monthly salary (MMS; nearly €485), 349 (44.6%) reported one to two MMS, 112 (14.3%) reported more than two and three MMS, while the remaining 56 (7.2%) individuals reported incomes higher than three MMS. The sample was divided in three socioeconomic status groups: low (1 MMS), moderate (1 to 2 MMS) and high (more than 2 MMS).

Data were collected using a street intercept survey method. All participants were informed of the study's goals and provided a signed informed consent.

2.2 Instruments

Initially, participants responded to a sociodemographic questionnaire. Educational attainment was assessed by the highest educational qualification achieved. The socioeconomic status (low, moderate or high) was measured by occupational level and monthly income. Body satisfaction was evaluated by one question ("How satisfied are you with your body/appearance?") using a 10-point response scale (1: very dissatisfied to 10: very satisfied). Smoking was assessed with a frequency item (number of cigarettes per day), while exercise measurement was based on a composite average of two single self-report items assessing the number of days individuals accumulated 30 or more minutes of moderate to vigorous physical activity during the past 7 days and for a typical week. Based on this form of screening measure, respondents were classified into one of three groups regarding levels of physical activity: inactive (< 1 day/week), insufficiently active (≥ 1 and < 5 days/week) and active (≥ 5 days/week). In relation to the recognized amount of physical activity needed to promote and maintain health, the American College of Sports Medicine (ACSM) and the American Heart Association (AHA) expert panel of scientists have recommended that "*...healthy adults aged 18–65 yr need moderate-intensity aerobic physical activity for a minimum of 30 min on five days each week*" (Haskell et al., 2007, p. 1083).

A Portuguese translation (Novo et al., 1997) of the 54-item version of the Scales of Psychological Well-being (Ryff, 1989) was used. Each dimension contains 9 items, positively or negatively worded with responses to a 5-point Likert scale (1: Strongly disagree to 5: Strongly agree). Negatively worded items were reversed before any subsequent analysis, allowing the calculation of a global score with possible scale values range from 9 to 45. Reliability coefficients (Cronbach's alpha) ranged between 0.68 (environmental mastery) and 0.77 (autonomy). The internal consistency value was 0.95 for the total psychological well-being score.

2.3 Statistical analysis

Descriptive statistics of data were presented as mean (M), standard deviation (SD), range and relative frequency (%), when appropriate. Skewness and kurtosis coefficients were computed for univariate normality analyses purposes, and all values were within ±1. Multivariate analysis of variance (MANOVA) followed by one-way analysis of variance (ANOVA) were used to investigate differences between gender, place of residence, educational attainment, socioeconomic status, smoking status and physical activity levels (inactive, insufficiently active and active) on the well-being dimensions. Partial eta-squared (η_p^2) was reported as a measure of the effect size between groups according to the following rule of thumb: small (> 0.01), medium (> 0.06) and large (> 0.14). Associations between variables were calculated using the Pearson product-moment coefficient. Additionally, hierarchical regression analysis was used to determine the influence of different blocks of variables (sociodemographic, lifestyle and psychosocial) on the dependent variables. All of these statistical analyses were conducted using SPSS (version 16.0).

3. Results

3.1 Descriptive and univariate normality analysis

Table 1 shows descriptive statistics (range, means and standard deviations) and univariate normality measures (skewness and kurtosis) for the measured variables.

Results indicate moderate to high values of smoking frequency and body satisfaction, and low levels of self-reported physical activity (about two days a week). Mean values of the PWB dimensions ranged between 32.48 (self-acceptance) and 34.69 (personal growth) on a possible scale range of 9 to 45. Absolute values of the univariate skewness and kurtosis were within the range of −1 to +1, and were interpreted as normally distributed. For study purposes, subjects were also divided according to their smoking and physical activity status. Frequency distribution analysis revealed a 36.3% prevalence rate of smoking and a 37.3% prevalence rate of physical inactivity. Only 11.0% of the total sample reported achieving recommended physical activity levels (minimum of 30 min on five or more days each week).

Variables	Range	M	SD	Skewness	Kurtosis
Smoking (cigarettes per day)	0–35	14.57	9.54	0.98	−0.77
Physical activity (days per week)	0–7	1.77	1.94	0.95	0.37
Body satisfaction	1–10	7.00	1.84	−0.40	0.09
Autonomy	15–45	33.63	4.94	−0.44	0.45
Environmental mastery	15–45	32.78	4.31	−0.31	0.81
Personal growth	21–45	34.69	4.54	−0.26	−0.14
Positive relations	16–45	33.45	4.78	−0.35	0.33
Purpose in life	12–45	34.12	4.80	−0.45	0.76
Self-acceptance	13–45	32.48	4.64	−0.52	0.96
Total PWB score	93–256	201.15	21.78	−0.43	0.91

Table 1. Descriptive and univariate normality analysis.

3.2 Comparative analysis

A MANOVA was conducted to compare the effect of gender on the six dimensions of psychological well-being. Results are summarized in Table 2.

Variables	Males M ± SD	Females M ± SD	*F*	*p*	η_p^2
Autonomy	33.64 ± 4.64	33.62 ± 5.18	0.01	0.943	0.00
Environmental mastery	33.35 ± 4.33	32.30 ± 4.23	11.60	0.001	0.02
Personal growth	34.57 ± 4.29	34.79 ± 4.75	0.46	0.500	0.00
Positive relations	33.49 ± 4.71	33.42 ± 4.84	0.05	0.822	0.00
Purpose in life	34.24 ± 4.70	34.01 ± 4.88	0.46	0.499	0.00
Self-acceptance	32.96 ± 4.10	32.09 ± 5.02	6.89	0.009	0.01
Total PWB score	202.26 ± 20.26	200.23 ± 22.94	1.69	0.194	0.00

Table 2. Means (M), standard deviations (SD) and univariate effects of the psychological well-being dimensions by gender.

A significant multivariate effect of gender was found ($F_{(6,776)}$= 3.93, p= 0.001, Wilk's λ= 0.97), although the eta value suggests a small effect (η_p^2 = 0.03). Simple main effects analysis showed that males reported higher levels of environmental mastery and self-acceptance ($p<$ 0.010). Moreover, a one-way ANOVA produced no significant differences in the total score (p= 0.194).

In order to identify possible gender differences by age groups, three independent MANOVAs were conducted for young, midlife and older adults. A significant effect was only found for young adults ($F_{(6,332)}$= 3.17, p= 0.005, Wilk's λ= 0.95, η_p^2= 0.06), indicating that the previous gender differences were only evident during this younger age period.

Table 3 presents the comparative analysis between age groups.

A one-way MANOVA was used to examine the association between age groups and well-being scores, revealing an overall main effect for age groups ($F_{(12,1550)}$= 4.54, p= 0.000, Wilk's λ= 0.93), but a small effect size (η_p^2= 0.04). Follow-up univariate analyses indicated significant differences in four of the six dependent variables. Post hoc comparisons using Scheffé's test indicated that young adults reported higher scores of personal growth (p=

Variables	Young adults M ± SD	Midlife adults M ± SD	Older adults M ± SD	*F*	*p*	η_p^2
Autonomy	34.09 ± 4.97	33.48 ± 4.77	31.22 ± 5.65	6.63	0.001	0.02
Environmental mastery	32.81 ± 4.38	32.67 ± 4.20	33.56 ± 4.71	0.82	0.440	0.00
Personal growth	35.48 ± 4.39	34.27 ± 4.49	32.34 ± 5.08	12.65	0.000	0.03
Positive relations	34.09 ± 4.61	32.94 ± 4.79	33.17 ± 5.46	5.48	0.004	0.01
Purpose in life	34.65 ± 4.89	32.94 ± 4.79	33.17 ± 5.45	3.91	0.021	0.01
Self-acceptance	32.88 ± 4.87	32.17 ± 4.41	32.29 ± 4.80	2.15	0.117	0.00
Total PWB score	204.00 ± 22.01	199.29 ± 20.93	195.83 ± 25.27	5.66	0.004	0.02

Table 3. Means (M), standard deviations (SD) and univariate effects of the psychological well-being dimensions by age groups.

0.001), positive relations (p= 0.005) and purpose in life (p= 0.042) than midlife adults, and higher levels of autonomy (p= 0.002) and personal growth (p= 0.000) than older adults. In addition, a decrement in autonomy scores was also observed between midlife and older adults (p= 0.019). A one-way ANOVA revealed a small detrimental effect as age groups increased on the total PWB score (p= 0.004).

The results of the psychological well-being scales comparison by place of residence are summarized in Table 4.

Variables	Rural M ± SD	Urban M ± SD	*F*	*p*	η_p^2
Autonomy	33.16 ± 4.98	34.03 ± 4.88	6.05	0.014	0.01
Environmental mastery	32.67 ± 4.20	32.87 ± 4.39	0.45	0.501	0.00
Personal growth	33.98 ± 4.68	35.29 ± 4.34	16.37	0.000	0.02
Positive relations	33.13 ± 4.71	33.73 ± 4.83	3.06	0.081	0.00
Purpose in life	33.86 ± 4.62	34.33 ± 4.94	1.82	0.178	0.00
Self-acceptance	32.22 ± 4.63	32.71 ± 4.64	2.13	0.145	0.00
Total PWB score	199.01 ± 21.70	202.95 ± 21.77	6.38	0.012	0.01

Table 4. Means (M), standard deviations (SD) and univariate effects of the psychological well-being dimensions by place of residence.

A significant multivariate effect of place of residence was found for the six dependent variables ($F_{(6,776)}$= 3.36, p= 0.003, Wilk's λ= 0.98), although the eta value was small (η_p^2= 0.03). Subsequent univariate analysis showed significant differences only in two dimensions, with urban residents reporting higher scores of autonomy and personal growth. A one-way ANOVA showed that rural residents revealed lower scores of the total PWB score (p= 0.012).

Next, a MANOVA was conducted to compare the effect of educational attainment on the six dimensions of psychological well-being. Results are summarized in Table 5.

A significant multivariate effect of educational attainment was found ($F_{(12,1550)}$= 11.24, p= 0.000, Wilk's λ= 0.85), with the eta value suggesting a moderate effect (η_p^2= 0.08). Simple main effects analysis showed that higher educational attainment (10 or more years of schooling completed) was associated with higher scores on all of the psychological well-being dimensions, when compared with the less educated group (≤ 9 years). A large effect

Variables	≤ 9 years M ± SD	≤ 12 years M ± SD	Academic M ± SD	F	p	η_p^2
Autonomy	32.51 ± 5.12	34.43 ± 4.82	34.41 ± 4.46	14.75	0.000	0.04
Environmental mastery	31.94 ± 4.53	33.26 ± 4.34	33.51 ± 3.64	10.89	0.000	0.03
Personal growth	32.61 ± 4.42	36.08 ± 4.19	36.27 ± 3.83	68.01	0.000	0.15
Positive relations	32.24 ± 4.64	34.32 ± 4.76	34.29 ± 4.62	18.61	0.000	0.05
Purpose in life	32.69 ± 4.55	34.99 ± 4.93	35.29 ± 4.44	26.26	0.000	0.06
Self-acceptance	31.43 ± 4.43	33.02 ± 5.06	33.50 ± 4.08	15.62	0.000	0.04
Total PWB score	193.41 ± 21.29	206.09 ± 21.54	207.25 ± 19.02	38.46	0.000	0.09

Table 5. Means (M), standard deviations (SD) and univariate effects of the psychological well-being dimensions by educational attainment.

size was found for personal growth (η_p^2= 0.15). As expected, a moderate incremental effect of educational attainment on the total PWB score was also observed (η_p^2= 0.09).

Table 6 presents the comparative analysis between socioeconomic status groups.

Variables	Low M ± SD	Moderate M ± SD	High M ± SD	F	p	η_p^2
Autonomy	32.97 ± 5.40	34.00 ± 4.65	33.91 ± 4.69	3.66	0.026	0.01
Environmental mastery	31.52 ± 4.67	33.12 ± 4.04	34.07 ± 3.71	21.00	0.000	0.05
Personal growth	33.97 ± 5.07	34.71 ± 4.24	35.82 ± 4.03	8.70	0.000	0.02
Positive relations	32.77 ± 4.93	33.70 ± 4.64	34.01 ± 4.73	4.30	0.014	0.01
Purpose in life	32.85 ± 5.26	34.44 ± 4.37	35.43 ± 4.42	17.11	0.000	0.04
Self-acceptance	31.37 ± 5.29	32.81 ± 4.16	33.58 ± 4.14	13.16	0.000	0.03
Total PWB score	195.44 ± 24.52	202.77 ± 19.75	206.80 ± 19.07	16.39	0.000	0.04

Table 6. Means (M), standard deviations (SD) and univariate effects of the psychological well-being dimensions by socioeconomic status.

A one-way MANOVA was used to examine the association between socioeconomic status and well-being scores, revealing a small effect ($F_{(12,1550)}$= 5.20, p= 0.000, Wilk's λ= 0.92, η_p^2= 0.04). Follow-up univariate analyses indicated significant differences in all dependent variables. Post hoc comparisons using Scheffé's test indicated that groups with higher levels of socioeconomic status reported higher scores of well-being, when compared with the lowest income group. A one-way ANOVA showed that the group with lower socioeconomic status revealed lower scores of the total PWB score (p= 0.000).

The results of the psychological well-being scales comparison by smoking status are summarized in Table 7. A one-way MANOVA was used to examine the association between smoking status and well-being scores, revealing an overall main effect for non-smoking/smoking groups ($F_{(6,776)}$= 7.44, p= 0.000, Wilk's λ= 0.95), but with a small to medium effect size (η_p^2= 0.06). Follow-up univariate analyses only indicated significant differences for two of the six dependent variables, with non-smokers reporting higher scores of environmental mastery and purpose in life (p< 0.001). Additionally, a one-way ANOVA by smoking status produced no significant differences in the total score (p= 0.143).

Lastly, a MANOVA was conducted to compare the effect of physical activity on the psychological well-being dimensions. Results are summarized in Table 8.

Variables	Non-smokers M ± SD	Smokers M ± SD	F	p	η_p^2
Autonomy	33.57 ± 4.74	33.74 ± 5.29	0.21	0.646	0.00
Environmental mastery	33.20 ± 3.92	32.03 ± 4.83	13.74	0.000	0.02
Personal growth	34.80 ± 4.43	34.50 ± 4.73	0.83	0.364	0.00
Positive relations	33.36 ± 4.63	33.61 ± 5.03	0.47	0.494	0.00
Purpose in life	34.57 ± 4.27	33.32 ± 5.52	12.29	0.000	0.02
Self-acceptance	32.51 ± 4.40	32.45 ± 5.05	0.03	0.867	0.00
Total PWB score	202.01 ± 19.91	199.64 ± 24.67	2.15	0.143	0.00

Table 7. Means (M), standard deviations (SD) and univariate effects of the psychological well-being dimensions by smoking status.

Variables	Inactive M ± SD	Insuf. active M ± SD	Active M ± SD	F	p	η_p^2
Autonomy	33.23 ± 4.92	33.76 ± 4.93	34.37 ± 4.99	2.05	0.130	0.01
Environmental mastery	32.19 ± 4.00	32.99 ± 4.37	33.78 ± 4.74	5.67	0.004	0.02
Personal growth	33.91 ± 4.78	35.06 ± 4.32	35.62 ± 4.41	7.60	0.001	0.02
Positive relations	32.78 ± 4.62	33.70 ± 4.76	34.58 ± 5.12	5.91	0.003	0.02
Purpose in life	33.81 ± 4.81	34.31 ± 4.73	34.22 ± 5.07	0.94	0.390	0.00
Self-acceptance	32.19 ± 4.51	32.58 ± 4.72	33.06 ± 4.70	1.33	0.265	0.00
Total PWB score	198.10 ± 21.30	202.39 ± 21.66	205.63 ± 22.74	5.40	0.005	0.02

Table 8. Means (M), standard deviations (SD) and univariate effects of the psychological well-being dimensions by physical activity status.

Results indicated a significant, albeit small (η_p^2= 0.02), multivariate effect of physical activity ($F_{(12,1550)}$= 2.67, p= 0.001, Wilk's λ= 0.96). Simple main effects analysis indicated significant differences in three of the six dependent variables. Post hoc comparisons using Scheffé's test indicated that active individuals reported higher scores of environmental mastery (p= 0.010) and positive relations (p= 0.009) than inactive adults. Moreover, physical activity groups (insufficiently active and active) reported higher personal growth scores than the inactive group (p< 0.01). A one-way ANOVA showed that the inactive group reported lower scores of the total PWB score (p< 0.01).

3.3 Correlation and regression analysis

Pearson correlation analysis were conducted to examine possible associations between sociodemographic (age, educational attainment, and socioeconomic status), lifestyle (smoking and physical activity), psychosocial (body satisfaction) factors and psychological well-being. Table 9 presents the bivariate correlations between these measures.

With regard to age, significant negative associations were found for autonomy, personal growth, positive relations with others and the total well-being score. Educational attainment and socioeconomic status were positively related with all well-being dimensions, with higher effects for personal growth. Body satisfaction was also positively correlated with all psychological well-being measures, with the highest association being with self-acceptance. Smoking frequency was negatively related with environmental mastery and purpose in life, while physical activity was positively correlated with environmental mastery, personal growth, positive relations with others, purpose in life and the total well-being score.

Variables	AUT	EM	PG	PR	PL	SA	PWB
Age	−0.11**	0.01	−0.23**	−0.12**	−0.11**	−0.06	−0.13**
Educational attainment (years)	0.21**	0.17**	0.39**	0.23**	0.24**	0.20**	0.31**
Socioeconomic status	0.16**	0.24**	0.32**	0.20**	0.27**	0.23**	0.30**
Smoking (cigarettes per day)	0.03	−0.15**	−0.03	0.01	−0.13**	0.02	−0.06
Physical activity (days per week)	0.04	0.15**	0.12**	0.15**	0.01	0.04	0.12**
Body satisfaction	0.15**	0.25**	0.14**	0.19**	0.16**	0.31**	0.25**

Note: AUT – Autonomy; EM - Environmental mastery; PG – Personal growth; PR – Positive relations; PL – Purpose in life; SA – Self-acceptance; PWB - Total PWB score. * $p< 0.05$; ** $p< 0.01$

Table 9. Correlations between sociodemographic, lifestyle and psychosocial factors, and measures of psychological well-being.

Additionally, significant negative associations were found between age and educational attainment ($r= -0.29$, $p< 0.001$), and between smoking and physical activity ($r= -0.12$, $p< 0.01$). As expected, a high correlation was observed between educational attainment and socioeconomic status ($r= 0.81$, $p< 0.001$). Body satisfaction was equally related with educational attainment and socioeconomic status ($r_s= 0.11$, $p< 0.01$), and a positive relationship was also observed with physical activity ($r= 0.15$, $p< 0.001$).

In order to determine the proportion of variance explained by each variable/factor (predictor), independent hierarchical regressions were conducted on each psychological well-being dimension (criterion). The first block of variables included the sociodemographic factors (gender: 1= male, 2= female; age; place of residence: 1= rural, 2= urban; educational attainment; and socioeconomic status). The second block included the two measured lifestyle factors (smoking and physical activity). Lastly, the third block was constituted by the only psychosocial variable (body satisfaction). The results of the sequential analyses are summarized in Table 10. For clarity purposes only the significant relationships are reported.

Criterion and predictor	β	R^2	ΔR^2
Autonomy			
Block 1		0.05	–
Educational attainment	0.15*		
Block 2		0.05	0.00
Block 3		0.07	0.02
Body satisfaction	0.13**		
Environmental mastery			
Block 1		0.07	–
Gender	−0.07*		
Socioeconomic status	0.27**		
Block 2		0.10	0.03
Smoking	−0.14**		
Physical activity	0.07*		
Block 3		0.14	0.04
Body satisfaction	0.21**		

Table 10. Summary of hierarchical regression analysis for predictors of psychological well-being dimensions.

Criterion and predictor	β	R^2	ΔR^2
Personal growth			
Block 1		0.18	–
Age	−0.17**		
Place of residence	0.08*		
Educational attainment	0.22**		
Socioeconomic status	0.13*		
Block 2		0.19	0.01
Physical activity	0.08*		
Block 3		0.20	0.01
Body satisfaction	0.09*		
Positive relations			
Block 1		0.06	–
Age	−0.09*		
Educational attainment	0.12*		
Block 2		0.08	0.02
Physical activity	0.11**		
Block 3		0.10	0.02
Body satisfaction	0.15**		
Purpose in life			
Block 1		0.08	–
Age	−0.12**		
Socioeconomic status	0.26**		
Block 2		0.10	0.02
Smoking	−0.14**		
Block 3		0.12	0.02
Body satisfaction	0.13**		
Self-acceptance			
Block 1		0.07	–
Socioeconomic status	0.21**		
Block 2		0.07	0.00
Block 3		0.14	0.07
Body satisfaction	0.28**		
Total PWB score			
Block 1		0.12	–
Age	−0.11**		
Socioeconomic status	0.21**		
Block 2		0.14	0.02
Physical activity	0.10*		
Block 3		0.18	0.04
Body satisfaction	0.21**		

Note: * $p< 0.05$; ** $p< 0.01$

Table 10. Summary of hierarchical regression analysis for predictors of psychological well-being dimensions (*continued*).

Results of the regression analyses demonstrated that sociodemographic variables explained 5% (autonomy) to 18% (personal growth) of the variance in the well-being dimensions. Within these block of variables, socioeconomic status followed by age and educational attainment were the most important predictors of the psychological well-being measures. The inclusion of lifestyle factors explained a small additional amount of variance (between 0% and 3%) in the outcome dimensions. After controlling for the effects of the two first blocks, body satisfaction predicted 1% (personal growth) to 7% (self-acceptance) of additional variance in the criterion variables.

4. Discussion

The present cross-sectional research study aimed to extend knowledge on the positive mental health of Portuguese people by (1) using a multidimensional model of psychological well-being (Ryff, 1989), (2) studying a large non-American community sample and therefore extending previous findings, and (3) identifying the influence of specific sociodemographic, lifestyle and psychosocial factors on various well-being dimensions.

4.1 The effects of sociodemographic factors

By examining comparative and correlational analyses, it was possible to identify the multivariate and univariate effects of sociodemographic data (gender, age, place of residence, educational attainment, and socioeconomic status) on the explained well-being variance.

Previous empirical evidence has shown that women rate themselves higher on positive relations and personal growth than men (Ryff, 1989; Ryff & Keyes, 1995). However, in the present study, males reported higher levels of environmental mastery and self-acceptance, but these differences were only observed during the young adulthood age range. A possible explanation for our findings might rely on the extensive body of research that has repeatedly found a higher incidence of certain psychological problems among women, such as depression and anxiety (WHO, 2004). Several explanations have been suggested in order to elucidate such sex differences, namely: the typical roles that women assume in the family, at home and in work settings (Almeida & Kessler, 1998); the greater frequency of childhood and adulthood trauma reported by females (Nurullah, 2010); the differentiated manner of responding to stressful situations (Hankin & Abramson, 2001); and potential biological determinants (Fitzgerald & Dinan, 2010) among others. On one hand, our results suggest that, during this life transition between adolescence and midlife adulthood, males report a stronger sense of mastery, control and competence in managing the surrounding context and possess a more positive attitude towards the past and present self, including favourable and unfavourable qualities. On the other hand, there is also evidence to suggest that women are able to overcome responsibilities and adversities of emerging adulthood, since no other gender differences were observed in the following age periods.

The analysis of age effects on eudaimonic well-being showed a declining pattern in strength of autonomy, personal growth, positive relations, purpose in life and total well-being score across groups. Compared with previous cross-sectional data, our results provide mixed conclusions regarding meaningful trajectories of eudaimonic well-being across the life course. Findings from Carol Ryff's initial studies (Ryff, 1989; Ryff & Keyes, 1995) suggested age increments for environmental mastery and autonomy, and a declining pattern for purpose in life and personal growth. More recently, Springer et al. (2011) investigated longitudinal age variations in the six well-being dimensions. Although age trends were not consistent between samples (WLS and MIDUS) and small proportions of variance were explained by age, it was possible to examine declining scores for autonomy (in WLS waves), personal growth, purpose in life and self-acceptance (in WLS waves). Thus, our findings support the assumption that experiences/opportunities for autonomy, personal growth, positive relations and purpose in life may be limited for cohorts of older persons or that these age groups place less value to these psychosocial dimensions when compared with the younger cohorts (or their past life). Obviously, future longitudinal research with population-based surveys is needed in order to better understand how the aging process affects the positive mental health of the Portuguese people.

Regarding the effects of the place of residence, differences were found for autonomy, personal growth and total well-being scores across rural and urban groups. Given the scarce body of literature on this subject, such results need to be interpreted with caution, without neglecting the possible indirect effects of variables such as educational attainment, occupational status, income, access to health services, among others. Several studies have identified rural-urban disparities in psychiatric disorders and quality of life (Peen et al., 2007, 2010). Among a Portuguese adolescent sample, Fernandes and Vasconcelos-Raposo (2008) found that urban residents reported higher scores for personal growth, purpose in life, self-acceptance and total well-being. In a more general sense, it is possible to suggest that this results from the discrepancy between the aspirations and expectations of the individual and their ability to satisfy them within his environment/place of residence (Wilkening & McGranahan, 1978). As such, our results suggest that urban residents are more self-determining and independent, more able to regulate social pressures to think and act in certain ways, less concerned with the evaluations and expectations of (significant) others, more open to new experiences and have a higher sense of continued development (realizing his/her potential). A possible explanation for this assumption is the higher levels of educational attainment ($F_{(1,781)}$= 40.50, p= 0.000, η_p^2= 0.05) and socioeconomic status ($F_{(1,781)}$= 48.47, p= 0.000, η_p^2= 0.06) reported by our urban sample group, which we analyse next.

Educational attainment and socioeconomic status were positively associated with all the psychological well-being dimensions, and were the sociodemographic variables that explained the greatest proportion of variance. These findings are consistent with previous cross-sectional empirical research (Keyes et al., 2002; Marmot et al., 1997; Ryff & Singer, 1996), which has identified these factors as positive predictors of eudaimonic well-being. For example, Ryff (1989) revealed that self-rated finances was a leading predictor variable, especially for self-acceptance, environmental mastery, purpose in life and personal growth ($R^2 \geq$ 13%). Therefore, this correlational evidence supports the assumption that a lower position in the social order not only increases the likelihood of negative health outcomes but that it also decreases the chances of psychological well-being (Ryff et al., 1999). Furthermore, Kaplan et al. (2008) examined the cumulative impact of different income measures in five of the six scales of psychological well-being. A longitudinal analysis showed a consistent increase of purpose in life, self-acceptance, personal growth and environmental mastery as mean income increased over the last three decades. These results emphasize the primary influence of economic well-being on psychological well-being and reflect the accumulation of socioeconomic advantage/disadvantage on eudaimonic well-being, throughout the adult life course. Therefore, if adults face significant challenges in their efforts and abilities to maintain a sense of purpose, self-realization and personal development, it is not surprising that a better socioeconomic condition affords important mediated or direct preventive and protective mechanisms in the face of stress, challenge, adversity and risk of disease. Thus, our results suggest that social class inequalities in education and income should represent important issues for public policies and intervention programs that aim to develop the positive mental health of the Portuguese population.

4.2 The effects of lifestyle factors

When testing the effects of lifestyle factors (smoking and exercising) on eudaimonic well-being, results from the comparative and correlational analyses indicated that these variables had a small effect (0% to 3% of the explained variance). Cigarette smoking was negatively associated with environmental mastery and purpose in life, while physical activity was positively correlated with environmental mastery, personal growth, positive relations and total well-being score.

Available empirical evidence has demonstrated that smoking affects not only a person's physical health (USDHHS, 2004), but also his mental health and well-being (Lawrence et al., 2009). In addition, review articles have indicated that smoking is more prevalent in people with mental health problems (e.g., Campion et al., 2008; Scott & Happell, 2011). Physical activity, in turn, has been also associated with higher levels of happiness, life satisfaction and self-esteem (Grant et al., 2009; Shahab & West, 2011; Spence et al., 2005), and with lower levels of depression and anxiety (Mykletun et al., 2008; Rethorst et al., 2009; Wipfli et al., 2008). The literature linking physical (in)activity and mental health is extensive, but for some reason, researchers have neglected the study of eudaimonic well-being. The effects of physical activity on one's mental well-being have been mainly interpreted by reducing anxiety, stress and depression, or through mood, self-esteem and quality of life enhancement. However, leading a life of purpose, having quality connections to others and experiencing continued growth are unique facets of eudaimonic well-being and distinct from indicators of subjective well-being (Ryff & Singer, 1998). Such a premise is supported by our results, in which, higher levels of environmental mastery, personal growth and positive relations were reported by physically active individuals, especially those who met the ACSM/AHA recommendations. Previous research with a sample of Portuguese older adults (60-95 years) also found a positive association between physical activity levels and positive mental health, with a stronger effect for the more active group who met the ACSM/AHA guidelines (Fernandes et al., 2009). Nevertheless, the low effect sizes obtained in the present study require some caution regarding the interpretation of a direct/unidirectional effect of physical activity on eudaimonic well-being. First, Besenski (2009) suggested that psychological well-being is best explained by the experience during health-enhancing physical activity, rather than its level (duration, frequency, intensity). Thus, experiencing eudaimonia during a physical activity (e.g., doing something you believe in, developing your potential, pursuing excellence, developing trusting interpersonal relations) is expected to be more strongly related with psychological well-being (Huta & Ryan, 2010; Kimiecik, 2011), although hedonia might also be experienced (Waterman et al.,

2008). Second, our cross-sectional results cannot establish causality. Explicitly, physical activity may promote increments of some well-being dimensions, but individuals with higher well-being levels may also easily adopt health-promoting practices. Third, the low effect sizes and percentage of explained variance after adjusting for the sociodemographic variables, may also suggest that this association is mediated by other variables (e.g., fitness levels, self-efficacy, body satisfaction, self-esteem).

Within the positive health agenda, Ryff and Singer (1998, 2000) have suggested that people who fail to adhere to health behavioural practices may have a lack of meaningful life/work opportunities, personal development experiences, consistent relationships and social support, and feelings of meaningful life pursuits and environmental mastery. As such, individuals with a positive, purposive and meaningful life are likely to adopt or sustain practices of positive psychological functioning, such as taking care of one's physical, social and mental health. On the whole, our results provide preliminary empirical support for these assumptions, with differential patterns of associations between smoking, exercising and well-being measures. Therefore, the need for integrating key behavioural factors on positive health promotion policies and programs is of maximal importance. Thus, approaches to health promotion should not only emphasize the prevention and treatment of problem behaviours, but also the inclusion of the promotion of optimal health behaviours and sustaining supportive environments (Ryff & Singer, 2000; Singer & Ryff, 2001). However, future research should also clarify the nature of the relationship between health-promoting behaviours and eudaimonic well-being.

4.3 The effects of psychosocial factors

Psychosocial factors were only measured by a single-item of body satisfaction. Despite this limitation, positive associations were found between this measure and all well-being dimensions, explaining 1% to 7% of additional variance after adjusting for socio-demographic and lifestyle factors. The highest correlations were obtained for self-acceptance, environmental mastery, positive relations with others and purpose in life. This evidence is in accordance with previous research that revealed stronger associations of global self-esteem with self-acceptance, purpose in life and environmental mastery (Compton, 2001; Paradise & Kernis, 2002; Ryff, 1989).

Body satisfaction can be defined in terms of the thoughts and feelings about one's body image/appearance. It can be assessed as the difference between the perceived (current) and the ideal physical appearance (Damasceno et al., 2011), as the evaluation of one's body size, shape, muscularity, muscle tone and weight (Grogan, 2008), or as a specific domain of evaluation within a hierarchical multidimensional model of self-perceptions (e.g., Fox & Corbin, 1989). Our results extend previous empirical evidence by showing that a specific domain of self-perceptions provides a basis for positive psychological functioning, even after controlling for sociodemographic and lifestyle factors.

Another associated point of extreme importance is the consistent relationship between physical activity and body satisfaction reported in the literature (Hausenblas & Fallon, 2006) and also found in the present study ($r = 0.15$, $p < 0.001$). Thus, body satisfaction may be a mediator variable between exercise and eudaimonic well-being, which is particularly important for women. Firstly, this mediation argument has been confirmed for the relationship between physical activity and subjective well-being (Rejeski et al., 2001). Secondly, a recent meta-analysis indicated that gender differences in self-esteem vary depending on the specific domain (Gentile et al., 2009). Results showed a male advantage in physical appearance self-esteem through all age periods which was most pronounced during adulthood. Therefore, we suggest that the environmental mastery and self-acceptance scores of women could be increased trough physical activity participation mediated by body satisfaction changes. Nevertheless, future research should focus on this type of interaction processes and related outcomes.

4.4 Study limitations

Some limitations should be considered regarding the obtained results. Firstly, although this community sample was randomly recruited from the northern and central regions of Portugal, it is not necessarily representative of the entire population, so additional caution is needed when generalizing from this data. Secondly, this is a cross-sectional study and, therefore, causal inferences should not be made.

5. Conclusion

In conclusion, the results of the present study allowed for the identification of factors associated with eudaimonic well-being. Sociodemographic (gender, age, place of residence, educational attainment and socioeconomic status), lifestyle (smoking and physical activity) and psychosocial (body satisfaction) variables exhibited different patterns of associations with positive mental health, as measured through Ryff's scales. Males, younger adults, urban residents and higher socioeconomic groups reported higher levels of well-being scores. Additionally, health behaviour practices (non-smoking and exercising) presented significant relations with some psychological well-being dimensions, underscoring the importance of the inclusion of key behavioural factors on positive health promotion policies and programs. Finally, body satisfaction exerted significant influences on all well-being scales and both direct and indirect effects on eudaimonic well-being were explored.

Overall, these results demonstrate that multiple factors (sociodemographic, lifestyle and psychosocial) are associated with positive mental health in a Portuguese community sample. Moreover, we expect that this evidence provides guidance to health sector reforms and other health policies focused on the creation and sustainment of supportive environments designed to promote positive mental health and well-being.

6. References

Almeida, D. & Kessler, R. (1998). Everyday stressors and gender differences in daily distress. *Journal of Personality and Social Psychology*, Vol.75, pp. 670-680, ISSN 0022-3514

Antony, M. & Swinson, R. (1996). *Anxiety disorders: Future directions for research and treatment: A discussion paper*. Health Canada/Minister of Supply and Services, ISBN 0-662-24980-1 Ottawa, Ontario, Canada

Besenski, L. (2009). *Health-enhancing physical activity and eudaimonic well-being*. Master's thesis, University of Saskatchewan, Saskatoon, Canada

Caldas de Almeida, J. (2010). *Estudo epidemiológico nacional de saúde mental*. Faculdade de Ciências Médicas, Lisboa

Campion, J.; Checinski, K.; Nurse, J. & McNeill, A. (2008). Smoking by people with mental illness and benefits of smoke-free mental health services. *Advances in Psychiatric Treatment*, Vol.14, pp. 217-228, ISSN 1472-1481

Compton, W. (2001). Toward a tripartite factor structure of mental health: Subjective well-being, personal growth, and religiosity. *The Journal of Psychology*, Vol.135, No.5, pp. 486-500, ISSN 0022-3980

Compton, W.; Smith, M.; Cornish, K. & Qualls, D. (1996). Factor structure of mental health measures. *Journal of Personality and Social Psychology*, Vol.71, No.2, pp. 406-413, ISSN 0022-3514

Damasceno, V.; Vianna, J.; Novaes, J.; Lima, J.; Fernandes, H. & Reis, V. (2011). Relationship between anthropometric variables and body image dissatisfaction among fitness center users. *Revista de Psicología del Deporte*, Vol.20, No.2, pp. 367-382, ISSN 1988-5636

Davidson, R. (2004). Well-being and affective style: Neural substrates and biobehavioral correlates. *Philosophical Transactions of the Royal Society of London B*, Vol.359, pp. 1395-1411, ISSN 0080-4622

DeNeve, K. & Cooper, H. (1998). The happy personality: A meta-analysis of 137 personality traits and subjective well-being. *Psychological Bulletin*, Vol.124, No.2, pp. 197-229, ISSN 0033-2909

DG SANCO (2007). *Health in the European Union. Special Eurobarometer 272e/ Wave 66.2-TNS Opinion & Social*. Office for Official Publications of the European Communities, Luxembourg

Diener, E. & Diener, M. (1995). Cross-cultural correlates of life satisfaction and self-esteem. *Journal of Personality and Social Psychology*, Vol.69, No.1, pp. 120–129, ISSN 0022-3514

Diener, E. (2000). Subjective well-being: The science of happiness and a proposal for a national index. *American Psychologist*, Vol.55, No.1, pp. 34-43, ISSN 0003-066X

Diener, E.; Oishi, S. & Lucas, R. (2003). Personality, culture, and subjective well-being: Emotional and cognitive evaluations of life. *Annual Review of Psychology*, Vol.54, pp. 403-425, ISSN 0066-4308

Diener, E.; Suh, E.; Lucas, R. & Smith, H. (1999). Subjective well-being: Three decades of progress. *Psychological Bulletin*, Vol.125, No.2, pp. 276-302, ISSN 0033-2909

Edwards, S.; Ngcobo, H.; Edwards, D. & Palavar, K. (2005). Exploring the relationship between physical activity, psychological well-being and physical self-perception in different exercise groups. *South African Journal for Research in Sport, Physical Education & Recreation*, Vol.27, pp. 75-90, ISSN 0379-9069

Fernandes, H. & Vasconcelos-Raposo, J. (2008). *O bem-estar psicológico em adolescentes: Uma abordagem centrada no florescimento humano*. CEDAFES-UTAD, ISBN 978-972-6698-42-5, Vila Real, Portugal

Fernandes, H.; Vasconcelos-Raposo, J. & Teixeira, C. (2010). Preliminary analysis of the psychometric properties of Ryff's Scales of Psychological Well-Being in Portuguese adolescents. *The Spanish Journal of Psychology*, Vol.13, No.2, pp. 1032-1043, ISSN 1138-7416

Fernandes, H.; Vasconcelos-Raposo, J.; Pereira, E.; Ramalho, J. & Oliveira, S. (2009). A influência da actividade física na saúde mental positiva de idosos. *Motricidade*, Vol.5, No.1, pp. 33-50, ISSN 1646-107X

Fitzgerald, P. & Dinan T. (2010). Biological sex differences relevant to mental health, In: *Oxford textbook of women and mental health*, D. Kohen, (Ed.), 30-41, Oxford University Press, ISBN 978-0199214365, Oxford, Great Britan

Fox, K. & Corbin, C. (1989). The physical self-perception profile: Development and preliminary validation. *Journal of Sport and Exercise Psychology*, Vol.11, pp. 408-430, ISSN 0895-2779

Gentile, B.; Grabe, S.; Dolan-Pascoe, B.; Twenge, J.; Wells, B. & Maitino, A. (2009). Gender differences in domain-specific self-esteem: A meta-analysis. *Review of General Psychology*, Vol.13, No.1, pp. 34-45, ISSN 1089-2680

Grant, N.; Wardle, J. & Steptoe, A. (2009). The relationship between life satisfaction and health behavior: A cross-cultural analysis of young adults. *International Journal of Behavioral Medicine*, Vol.16, pp. 259-268, ISSN 1070-5503

Grogan, S. (2008). *Body image: Understanding body dissatisfaction in men, women, and children* (2nd ed.). Routledge, ISBN 978-041-5147-85-9, East Sussex, Great Britain

Gunnell, K. (2009). *Leisure-time physical activity in individuals with osteoporosis: Associations with psychological well-being*. Master's thesis, Brock University, Ontario, Canada

Hankin, B. & Abramson, L. (2001). Development of gender differences in depression: An elaborated cognitive vulnerability-transactional stress theory. *Psychological Bulletin*, Vol.127, pp. 773-796, ISSN 0033-2909

Haskell, W.; Lee, I.; Pate, R.; Powell, K.; Blair, S.; Franklin, B.; Macera, C.; Heath, G.; Thompson, P. & Bauman, A. (2007). Physical activity and public health: Updated recommendations for adults from the American College of Sports Medicine and the American Heart Association. *Circulation*, Vol.116, pp. 1081-1093, ISSN 0009-7322

Hausenblas, H. & Fallon, E. (2006). Exercise and body image: A meta-analysis. *Psychology and Health*, Vol.21, pp. 33-47, ISSN 0887-0446

Heidrich, S. & Ryff, C. (1993). Physical and mental health in later life: The self-system as mediator. *Psychology and Aging*, Vol.8, No.3, pp. 327-338, ISSN 0882-7974

Howell, R. & Howell, C. (2008). The relation of economic status to subjective well-being in developing countries: A meta-analysis. *Psychological Bulletin*, Vol.134, No.4, pp. 536-560, ISSN 0033-2909

Huta, V. & Ryan, R. M. (2010). Pursuing pleasure or virtue: The differential and overlapping well-being benefits of hedonic and eudaimonic motives. *Journal of Happiness Studies*, Vol.11, pp. 735-762, ISSN 1389-4978

Kaplan, G.; Shema, S. & Leite, C. (2008). Socioeconomic determinants of psychological well-being: The role of income, income change, and income sources during the course of 29 years. *Annals of Epidemiology*, Vol.18, No.7, pp. 531-537, ISSN 1047-2797

Keyes, C. (2005). Mental illness and/or mental health? Investigating axioms of the complete state model health. *Journal of Consulting and Clinical Psychology*, Vol.73, No.3, pp. 539-548, ISSN 0022-006X

Keyes, C.; Shmotkin, D. & Ryff, C. (2002). Optimizing well-being: The empirical encounter of two traditions. *Journal of Personality and Social Psychology*, Vol.82, No.6, pp. 1007-1022, ISSN 0022-3514

Kimiecik, J. (2011). Exploring the promise of eudaimonic well-being within the practice of health promotion: The how is as important as the what. *Journal of Happiness Studies*, Vol.12, pp. 769-792, ISSN 1389-4978

Lawrence, D.; Mitrou, F. & Zubrick, S. (2009). Smoking and mental illness: Results from population surveys in Australia and the United States. *BMC Public Health*, Vol.9, doi: 10.1186/1471-2458-9-285, ISSN 1471-2458

Lindfors, P. & Lundberg, U. (2002). Is low cortisol release an indicator of positive health? *Stress and Health*, Vol.18, pp. 153-160, ISSN 1532-3005

Linley, P.; Maltby, J.; Wood, A.; Osborne, G. & Hurling, R. (2009). Measuring happiness: The higher order factor structure of subjective and psychological well-being measures. *Personality and Individual Differences*, Vol.47, pp. 878-884, ISSN 0191-8869

Marmot, M.; Ryff, C.; Bumpass, L.; Shipley, M. & Marks, N. (1997). Social inequalities in health: next questions and converging evidence. *Social Science and Medicine*, Vol.44, No.6, pp. 901-910, ISSN 0277-9536

Mykletun, A.; Overland, S.; Aarø, L.; Liabø, H. & Stewart, R. (2008). Smoking in relation to anxiety and depression: Evidence from a large population survey - the HUNT study. *European Psychiatry*, Vol.23, No.2, pp. 77-84, ISSN 0924-9338

Novo, R.; Duarte-Silva, E. & Peralta, E. (1997). O bem-estar psicológico em adultos: Estudo das características psicométricas da versão portuguesa das escalas de C. Ryff. In: *Avaliação psicológica: Formas e contextos*, M. Gonçalves; I. Ribeiro; S. Araújo; C. Machado; L.S. Almeida & M. Simões, (Ed.), vol. V, 313-324, APPORT/SHO, Braga, Portugal

Nurullah, A. (2010). Gender differences in distress: The mediating influence of life stressors and psychological resources. *Asian Social Science*, Vol.6, No.5, pp. 27-35, ISSN 1911-2017

Paradise, A. & Kernis, M. (2002). Self-esteem and psychological well-being: Implications of fragile self-esteem. *Journal of Social and Clinical Psychology*, Vol.21, No.4, pp. 345-361, ISSN 0736-7236

Peen, J.; Dekker, J.; Schoevers, R.; Have, M.; de Graaf, R. & Beekman, A. (2007). Is the prevalence of psychiatric disorders associated with urbanization? *Social Psychiatry and Psychiatric Epidemiology*, Vol.42, No.12, pp. 984-989, ISSN 0933-7954

Peen, J.; Schoevers, R.; Beekman, A. & Dekker, J. (2010). The current status of urban-rural differences in psychiatric disorders. *Acta Psychiatrica Scandinavica*, Vol.121, No.2, pp. 84-93, ISSN 0001-690X

Rejeski, W.; Shelton, B.; Miller, M.; Dunn, A.; King, A. & Sallis, J. (2001). Mediators of increased physical activity and change in subjective well-being: Results from the Activity Counseling Trial (ACT). *Journal of Health Psychology*, Vol.6, No.2, pp. 159-168, ISSN 1359-1053

Rethorst, C.; Wipfli, B. & Landers, D. (2009). The antidepressive effects of exercise: A meta-analysis of randomized trials. *Sport Medicine*, Vol.39, pp. 491-511, ISSN 0112-1642

Ryan, R. & Deci, E. (2001). On happiness and human potentials: A review of research on hedonic and eudaimonic well-being. *Annual Review of Psychology*, Vol.52, pp. 141-166, ISSN 0066-4308

Ryff, C. & Heidrich, S. (1997). Experience and well-being: Explorations on domains of life and how they matter. *International Journal of Behavioral Development*, Vol.20, No.2, pp. 193-206, ISSN 0165-0254

Ryff, C. & Singer, B. (1996). Psychological well-being: Meaning, measurement, and implications for psychotherapy research. *Psychotherapy and Psychosomatics*, Vol.65, pp. 14-23, ISSN 0033-3190

Ryff, C. & Singer, B. (1998). The contours of positive human health. *Psychological Inquiry*, Vol.9, No.1, pp. 1-28, ISSN 1047-840X

Ryff, C. & Singer, B. (2000). Interpersonal flourishing: A positive health agenda for the new millennium. *Personality and Social Psychology Review*, Vol.4, No.1, pp. 30-44, ISSN 1088-8683

Ryff, C. (1989). Happiness is everything, or is it? Explorations on the meaning of psychological well-being. *Journal of Personality and Social Psychology*, Vol.57, No.6, pp. 1069-1081, ISSN 0022-3514

Ryff, C.; Magee, W.; Kling, K. & Wing, E. (1999). Forging macro-micro linkages in the study of psychological well-being. In: *The self and society in aging processes*, C.

Ryff & V. Marshall, (Ed.), 247-278, Springer, ISBN 978-0826112675, New York, USA

Ryff, C.; Singer, B. & Love, G. (2004). Positive health: Connecting well-being with biology. *Philosophical Transactions of the Royal Society B: Biological Sciences*, Vol.359, pp. 1383-1394, ISSN 0962-8436

Scheier, M.; Carver, C. & Bridges, M. (2001). Optimism, pessimism, and psychological well-being. In: *Optimism and pessimism: Implications for theory, research, and practice*, E. C. Chang, (Ed.), pp. 189–216, American Psychological Association, ISBN 978-1557986917, Washington, DC, USA

Scott, D. & Happell, B. (2011). The high prevalence of poor physical health and unhealthy lifestyle behaviours in individuals with severe mental illness. *Issues in Mental Health Nursing*, Vol.32, No.9, pp. 589-597, ISSN 0161-2840

Seligman, M. & Csikszentmihalyi, M. (2000). Positive psychology: An introduction. *American Psychologist*, Vol.55, No.1, pp. 5-14, ISSN 0003-066X

Shahab, L., & West, R. (2011). Differences in happiness between smokers, ex-smokers and never smokers: Cross-sectional findings from a national household survey. *Drug and Alcohol Dependence*, doi: 10.1016/j.drugalcdep.2011.08.011, ISSN 0376-8716

Singer, B. & Ryff, C. (Eds.) (2001). *New horizons in health: An integrative approach*. National Academy Press, ISBN 978-0-309-07296-0, Washington, DC, USA

Spence, J.; McGannon, K. & Poon, P. (2005). The effect of exercise on global self-esteem: A quantitative review. *Journal of Sport & Exercise Psychology*, Vol.27, No.3, pp. 311-334, ISSN 0895-2779

Springer, K.; Pudrovska, T. & Hauser, R. (2011). Does psychological well- being change with age? Longitudinal tests of age variations and further exploration of the multidimensionality of Ryff's model of psychological well-being. *Social Science Research*, Vol.40, pp. 392-398, ISSN 0049-089X

Steel, P.; Schmidt, J. & Shultz, J. (2008). Refining the relationship between personality and subjective well-being. *Psychological Bulletin*, Vol.134, No.1, pp. 138-161, ISSN 0033-2909

U.S. Department of Health and Human Services – USDHHS (2004). *The health consequences of smoking: A report of the Surgeon General*. USDHHS, CDCP, NCCDPHP, OSH, ISBN 0-16-051576-2, Atlanta, USA

Urry, H.; Nitschke, J.; Dolski, I.; Jackson, D.; Dalton, K.; Mueller, C.; Rosenkranz, M.; Ryff, C.; Singer, B. & Davidson, R. (2004). Making a life worth living: Neural correlates of well-being. *Psychological Science*, Vol.15, No.6, pp. 367-372, ISSN 0956-7976

Vleioras, G. & Bosma, H. A. (2005). Are identity styles important for psychological well-being? *Journal of Adolescence*, Vol.28, No.3, pp. 397-409, ISSN 0140-1971

Waterman, A., Schwartz, S. & Conti, R. (2008). The implications of two conceptions of happiness (hedonic enjoyment and eudaimonia) for the understanding of intrinsic motivation. *Journal of Happiness Studies*, Vol.9, pp. 41-79, ISSN 1389-4978

WHO (2004). *Gender in mental health research*. World Health Organisation, ISBN 92-4-159253-2, Geneva, Switzerland

WHO International Consortium in Psychiatric Epidemiology (2000). Cross-national comparisons of the prevalences and correlates of mental disorders. *Bulletin of the World Health Organization*, Vol.78, No.4, pp. 413-426, ISSN 0042-9686

Wilkening, E. & McGranahan, D. (1978). Correlates of subjective well-being in Northern Wisconsin. *Social Indicators Research*, Vol.5, pp. 211-234, ISSN 0303-8300

Wipfli, B.; Rethorst, C. & Landers, D. (2008). The anxiolytic effects of exercise: A meta-analysis of randomized trials and dose-response analysis. *Journal of Sport & Exercise Psychology*, Vol.30, pp. 392-410, ISSN 0895-2779

25

Towards a Paradigmatic Shift in Mental Health Care?

Ragnfrid E. Kogstad
Hedmark University College
Norway

1. Introduction

Mental health care has its professional and theoretical foundation in-between medicine and the social sciences. Its history is marked by tensions between humanism, recovery orientation, client-centred approaches and "being with" as principles on the one hand, and custodialism, instrumentalism, manualized therapy, diagnostic cultures, medical care delivery and biogenetic understanding on the other. In recent years, spokesmen in the field have promoted a so-called integrated biopsychosocial model, saying there are some genetic dispositions, along with individual psychology and social factors that together predict the development of mental disabilities. In this chapter, the content of and evidence behind such an integrated model will be discussed, with reference to the possibility of combining such varied approaches as biogenetic and humanistic understandings, the status of genetic research, new findings when it comes to the causes behind mental suffering and the historical and recent consequences of a mental health care, in which the etiology and understanding of the phenomena have been limited and unsure. As we know, these methods have historically often had fatal consequences. But also today, the reports about degrading, humiliating and painful experiences are numerous. Reactions to this reality differ between strong efforts to improve existing services and campaigns to change attitudes and a contrasting fundamental criticism towards the laws that govern mental health care and the paradigm on which the laws are built.

2. An integrated biopsychosocial model?

Several researchers operate with two main approaches in psychiatry or mental health care, e.g. medical or contextual understandings (Wampold, 2001), or psychosocial or biogenetic explanations (Walker & Read, 2002). These approaches do not represent distinct, exclusive perspectives, but instead they borrow from each other. Nevertheless, it is still possible to distinguish between views based on a fundamental belief which say that mental suffering should be understood and treated as relational/psychosocial problems, the results of trauma, anxiety or existential suffering related to loneliness and the loss of meaning on the one hand, and beliefs which say that we are approaching the discovery of a biogenetic foundation for illnesses with emotional or behavioural expressions on the other. Until now, the conclusions have been unsure. Researchers talk about "genetic predispositions" and an interaction between "genes and environment" (Andreassen, 2005; Caspi et al., 2003; Surtees et al., 2007; Nesvåg, 2008), but cannot document the existence of biological or genetic markers.

Recently, the field of epigenetics has shed some new light on the antagonism between the biogenetic and humanistic-contextual approaches, as epigentic studies have revealed that conditions outside the gene can change its genetic expression (Fosse, 2009; Getz et al., 2011). With both animals and human beings, relational stress and assaults seem to influence behaviour and brain development by changing epigenetic control mechanisms, which can be interpreted as support for a stronger relational and contextual orientation.

Philosophers have pointed to the search for meaning as being genuinely imbedded in human nature (Bachtin, 1997; Vetlesen & Nordtvedt, 1994; Wifstad 1997). For example, within a bio-genetic perspective, medicalization may gain priority at the cost of helping to focus on existential dilemmas and search for meaning. As emphasized by Stenfeldt-Foss (1997), "The uncritical use of neuroleptic drugs and minor tranquilizers, instead of proper psychosocial and psychotherapeutic procedures, is an increasing danger in services for weaker groups lacking professional resources, thus threatening the patient-doctor relationship" (Medical Ethics and Medical Conduct, 1997, p. 14).

As Bentall (2003) points out, it is logically possible to both believe in genetic causes and be human, but at the same time, it is the heritage from Kraeplin, with his hypothesis about clearly distinguishable groups of illnesses with their respective biogenetic reference points, which made possible several of the cruelties found in the history of psychiatry. The biogenetic reference points legitimated a strong division between "us" and "them".

Still, we have yet to find a tenable rationale behind this division between "us" and "them". The question about what constitutes serious mental illness has no simple answer, while shifting trends also govern how diagnoses are developed and described. In 2011, two former editors of DSM (III & IV), Robert Spitzer and Allan Frances, warned against a development in which psychiatric diagnoses fit almost everybody, and young people can be recruited into the psychiatric system based on indicators that pathologize "normal" adolescent reactions (Angell, 2011). They referred to the National Institute of Mental Health in the US, which says that one-fourth of all Americans receive one psychiatric diagnosis every year. At the age of 32, 50% have suffered from some type of anxiety syndrome and 40% from depression. The former editors ask: Which numbers will we then see when these people get to the ages of 50, 65 or 80? This increase in diagnoses is seemingly at odds with findings from the comprehensive, longitudinal WHO's multi-centre study (see among others Hopper et al., 2007). The study started in 1966 as a large-scale, cross-cultural study conducted simultaneously in Columbia, Czechoslovakia, Denmark, India, Nigeria, China, the Soviet Union, Great Britain and the US. Summing up after 25 years, the authors could state that people with schizophrenia recover in spite of the methodological challenges. Globally, 60% had recovered when the study was finished. A striking finding was that the rate of recovery largely varied between industrialized and developing countries, though in favour of the latter. The recovery rate in developing countries approached 70%, whereas it was only 20% in the industrialized countries. Because of these findings, it becomes urgent to understand mental illnesses in contexts, not only for professional and scientific reasons, but also ethical ones. Since the neuro concepts have become metaphors for what is human and what happens in our consciousness, we have some special ethical challenges (Kollek, 2004).When psychological and cognitive phenomena are explained as causal effects of brain chemistry, human dignity, liberty and autonomy are affected. Metaphors can help facilitate communication, but may also carry with them some potentially dangerous conceptual baggage. Explaining biology (for example, somatic disease) with biology is unproblematic, but to explain consciousness with biology may have consequences for social interaction and stigma. As one example, it may now seem more opportune and legitimate to talk about bad genes than bad parents (Joseph, 2004), which has comprehensive consequences for stigma, as a biogenetic etiology has been shown to increase stigma, while a psychosocial etiology reduces it (Walker & Read, 2002).

What is often called a biopsychosocial model may in practice resemble a primarily biological model. The implementation of psychosocial therapeutic models easily lose terrain related to more instrumental means. The paradox in this field lies in the lack of evidence of an etiology which could legitimate those instrumental means. The Office of the United Nations High Commissioner for Human Rights says that: "The medical and charity model is completely abandoned in favor of a human rights and social model" (OHCHR, 2007). As a result of this, mental disabilities should be met with good relations, dialogues and the satisfaction of universal human, material and psychosocial needs.

3. Definitions of otherness

To make a division between "us" and "them" seems to be a phenomenon deeply imbedded in our culture. As we will also see, this division is sustained in several ways . Definitions of otherness are often based on special individual- and group properties, but also exist without such distinguishing properties. Medical, juridical, sociological and philosophical perspectives can be helpful in order to understand the reasons behind the definitions of otherness, in this case related to persons with mental disabilities.

As previously mentioned, there has been a long-lasting belief that mental illnesses can be explained by some organic failure/damage. As early as the 19th century, psychiatrists campaigned for adding some kind of hard science to the humanistic orientation in moral treatment institutions and to define mental illnesses as neurological, located in the brain (Withaker, 2004). But still, in 2011 no biological markers can tell when mental health has changed into mental illness. In spite of this weak ability to distinguish different psychiatric diagnoses from each other and tell when illnesses arise, new diagnoses have been developed for the next DSM version, and new groups will be included in existing diagnoses. Diagnoses are also closely associated with medication, with 500,000 children in the US now taking some type of anti-psychotic medicines (Angell, 2011), which must necessarily be based on some biological/genetic explanations. Ideas about biological changes and inherited vulnerability still exist and contribute to the justification of special approaches to persons diagnosed with serious mental illnesses, as will be elaborated on in the next paragraph.

According to Norwegian legislation, serious mental illness is a basic condition for involuntary confinement and treatment, and an additional condition is that the treatment is needed for health reasons, *or* that the person represents a danger to his/her own or other persons' lives or physical health (Norwegian Mental Health Act 1999, § 3-3- and 4-4). These paragraphs invite judicial assessment, as there are large variations in both involuntary confinement and treatment among different geographical regions in Norway. Some regions have 10 times as much forced treatment than others in relation to the population (Bremnes et al. 2008a+b), which in a clear way illustrates the arbitrariness in coercive treatment and the effects of a law that says: Forced treatment may be effectuated when it is obviously no use in attempting voluntary treatment, when benefits from the treatment clearly outweigh the disadvantages, and when the treatment is in accordance with acknowledged professional psychiatric methods and justified clinical practice (Norwegian Mental Health Act §3-3,1 and §4-4,1).

As early as 1994, the European Council expressed concerns over the high number of complaints related to bad treatment, which were just within the limits of mistreatment, such as over-medication and the devaluation of the client's needs (Council of Europe, 1994). The available knowledge about alternative approaches and treatments is highly relevant when it comes to a client's legal status. The European Convention on Human Rights states that the "least encroaching treatment" should always be used (Palm & Ericsson, 2005; Bartlett et al., 2007; Thune, 2008).

Knowledge about non-infringing or less infringing treatments has existed for a long time, for example with the Soteria House model, with the "being with" principle as opposed to long-term medication (Soerensen, 1982; Bola & Mosher, 2003; Bola et al., 2006). But as long as concepts about otherness, as expressed in the concept of "serious mental illness", exist in the law and imply a comprehensive professional power (the right to receive treatment based on a free and informed consent can be set aside), it has been difficult to protect mental health clients against degrading and infringing treatment, though now there are signs of a change to come. The disproportion between the arbitrariness in labelling people as seriously mentally ill on the one hand, and the huge consequences such diagnoses cause on the other has become more visible, not least with the United Nations (UN) and survivors organizations around the world having made a common effort to abolish discriminatory settlements for *all* disabled people (mental disabilities included), which has resulted in the Convention on the Rights of Peoples with Disabilities (CRPD). The convention legally took effect in 2008, and is an important step towards the abolition of forced institutionalization and treatment on the basis of disability. Its purpose is to "protect and ensure the full and equal enjoyment of all human rights and fundamental freedom by all persons with disabilities, and to promote respect for their inherent dignity" (Art. 1). The convention further states that "persons with disabilities include those who have long-term physical, mental, intellectual or sensory impairments" and that "persons with disabilities enjoy equal capacity on an equal basis with others in all aspects of life" (Art. 12). If they require support in order to exercise their legal capacity, this shall be provided. Regarding health care, this shall be of the same quality for persons with disabilities as it is for others, "including on the basis of free and informed consent" (Art. 25). The convention is a sign of changes in a more humanistic direction, which will be further elaborated on later in the chapter. The European Court of Human Rights may take the lead in the process towards a more humanistic direction and affirm that serious infringements are not redefined as necessary treatment.

Concepts about "otherness" related to mental health clients, in medical as well as legal contexts, are changing. Definitions of otherness are culturally bound, which may indicate that societies need a division between "us" and "them" for the sake of social integration, at least that is what social scientists say. With reference to Foucault (1973), Thomas Scheff (1999) describes how societies need excluded and stigmatized groups in order to secure the identity of the people inside the society. One example of this is how the big institutions in

France were filled with new groups in the 17th century as leprosy disappeared. Scheff's analysis is important in order to understand social mechanisms on the macro level, thereby creating change. His deviation theories should not be seen as fatalistic statements, saying that there must always be excluded groups. Maybe there will, but with the help of ethics theory, other perspectives can also be outlined. The philosopher Emanuelle Levinas (1993) challenged our concepts about otherness by saying that there will always be people we cannot understand, and that we should accept that we cannot fully understand another human being. Instead of defining and categorizing (and deciding whether people belong "inside" or "outside"), we should accept that it is not about understanding and control, but about love, respect and feeling responsible. We may not be able to avoid notions about otherness, but it should be possible to counteract social exclusion of groups based on their disabilities.

4. Degrading and painful experiences

Even if the history of psychiatry for the most part is seen from a professional perspective, patients have also told and published their stories. Larsen and Andersen (2011) have studied psychiatric patients' autobiographies from 1918 to 2008, and some of them talk about "a holy duty" when they explain their reasons for writing down and publishing their experiences from psychiatric care; they want to inform the community about conditions in the treatment system that ought to be changed. In 1925, one of the authors wrote from his heart that he wanted to prevent others from experiencing the same horrors and monstrosities he himself had endured. In the last period studied by Larsen and Andersen (1980-2008), there had been comprehensive reforms in the mental health service systems, as user involvement had become a central objective. Even so, no fundamental changes seem to have taken place from the patients' points of view, although it is possible that patients' experiences are not seen as being valid sources of knowledge. It could also be that patients' experiences indicate that more fundamental changes in understanding and basic values are needed, as Larsen and Andersen ask. Ekeland (2011) has elaborated on this point of view, and says that the darker sides of the history of psychiatry can be understood as a result of an epistemological mistake; instead of acknowledging human beings' subjectivity, objectification has taken place. This occurs when phenomena are created, communicated and interpreted by human beings (subject ontological phenomena) and treated as phenomena that exist independent of human beings. The phenomena studied in psychiatry and mental health care can hardly be counted as object ontological. In this field, we have to relate to cultural products and experiences picked up during dialogical processes such as emotions, behaviour, expectancies, hope, trust, etc. The phenomena should be acknowledged as human, individual and context-dependant. In order for health policy to take a more recovery-oriented and user-involved stance, a new foundation for research is needed that is based on the insight that interpretations and normative evaluations determine what we see and find. In this field, we cannot catch the ontology independently of those interpretations and evaluations.

When human subjectivity is wrongly exposed to objectification, ethical values are also at risk: When the suffering person and his/her relation with him/herself or the world is studied by an objectifying look, there is danger afoot because we all need to support the Other as a subject in order to protect ourselves against our own inhuman tendencies (Ekeland, 2011).

For more than 150 years, psychiatric and mental health care has been mainly based on a medical epistemology in which human beings are exposed to the medical glance, searching for medical symptoms rather than human, individual, context-related and interpreted phenomena. This is also mirrored in narratives about users' experiences from psychiatric and mental health care over the latest 10 years (Kogstad, 2009), from which I will give some examples.

The data was collected in cooperation with the national user organization in Norway, Mental Health Norway (MHN), which was chosen because it is the largest user organization in Norway. The organization has a good relationship with the government, as well as a well-developed administrative system that was able to facilitate the collection of data. During the period of data collection, there were approximately 5,000 members throughout the entire country, and about 4,000 of them were chosen randomly and invited to take part in the study, with a response rate of nearly 20%. Out of these, 492 (151 men and 341 women, aged 19– 90 years) also answered one or both of the open questions at the end of the questionnaire. These respondents have experience from all parts of the mental health care system, including traditional psychiatric institutions, outpatient clinics, day centres and individual therapy. Sixty-seven percent received a disability pension, 13% had a job and 20% a combined disability pension with a job or studies.

The material presented here consists of stories written in response to the question: If you have had a strong negative experience, would you like to describe such an event?

Although several informants said it was too difficult to write about negative and humiliating experiences, 335 nevertheless wrote about such episodes. A statistical representation related to user organization, or mental health clients in general, cannot be claimed, though distribution by gender, age, disability pension, education, job, in addition to the fact that the informants have experience from all parts of the health care system, suggests that the experiences and chosen categories are applicable across many user categories. The narratives vary in length from one line to several pages, and the longer stories often give in-depth information concerning background, causes, experiences, feelings and concrete elements in the recovery process or the traumatic experience, although quite brief reports also sometime contain important information such as: "Strong, painful effects of Trilafon." Out of the 335 negative stories, 267 were seen as being informative enough to be included in the analysis. The material is still rich and, most importantly, it is written by people who have first-hand knowledge of the experiences they describe.

The 267 stories about negative experiences were divided into three main categories: Experienced miscommunication, rejection and humiliation, with some of the narratives from the categories of rejection and humiliation shown below.

Subcategories under "rejection" were: "no treatment in institution apart from medicinal treatment", "no access to treatment or institution/no follow-up after discharge", "negative experiences at state welfare institutions", "social dilemma and religious needs rejected", "confidence lost because of deception", "childhood traumas and war experiences rejected" and "children/family not cared about when person is committed". All subcategories are illustrated in the stories:

I was forcibly sent to the hospital because I said I felt like committing suicide. I was heavily medicated and had only one talk with the doctor during my entire stay. I felt I was left totally on my own, together with other patients who screamed and smashed furniture. I shared a room with people who scared me. It was a painful experience. (*woman, age 45*)

I attempted suicide in the early 1980s. I was taken to the hospital by ambulance, my stomach was pumped and then I was sent home by taxi, dirty and wearing only my pants. I worried a lot about meeting my mother and my employer. I had no one to talk to after this incident. (*man, age 57*)

My GP would not accommodate my wishes when I asked for sick leave. The result was that I lost my job and just wanted to commit suicide. (*woman, age 55*)

I got the clear feeling that the psychiatric ward did what they could to help me when I was an inpatient. But when problems that had been brewing underneath came to the surface and childhood traumas emerged, I was once again alone with no help available. (*man, age 50*)

Once when I was in my thirties, I was in the hospital. The anxiety came back and I asked if I could talk to a psychiatrist. I thought that at last I would be able to open up and talk about the incest I had experienced as a child. His answer was: It was such a long time ago and should just be forgotten. (*woman, age 53*)

I was committed and had to leave my children, aged 2–19 years. No help was offered. I was neither listened to nor taken seriously, and did not get any help from the community health services. I was just given medicines with painful side effects. (*woman, age 60*)

Subcategories under "humiliation" were: "accused and made a fool of", "negative experiences with medication", "commitment", "forced medication", "punishment", "forced removal of medicines", "incorrect diagnoses" and "forced sterilization":

I was filled with anxiety the whole night when I was put in a room on my own with a night duty employee who didn't talk to me, but threatened to give me an injection if I didn't calm down. (*woman, age 44*)

I was not believed when I told them I had an adverse reaction to that special medicine. I had convulsions for a long period before I was given the proper antidote. (*woman, age 45*)

After less than half an hour, this strange doctor concluded that I should be sent to the hospital. I objected and said: "It will not help." But a person in my situation suddenly has no right to express herself. The doctor said: "Then it is a compulsory admission!" I objected and objected, but my voice did not count any longer. My husband signed the paper (after the doctor threatened that if he didn't, the police would do so). I don't think I have ever felt so deceived before. I was angry, sad and empty (…), and overwhelmed by the feeling of being totally turned down. I had lost everything. It felt like mental rape. This happened four to five years ago, though I can still feel it all today. The emotions have become embedded inside me and will always remain with me. (*woman, age 38*)

I was medicated by depot injection, but the way they did it was wrong. I didn't want the medicine. Four-five people were in the room. One gave the injection, while the others held me. I resisted. I was afraid. After this, they all left. I was alone. Later, I didn't want contact with the staff at all. I hid under the bedspread. Medication was the only physical contact I experienced during the stay. I think I needed the medicines. That was not the problem. After having been medicated several times, one person sat down at the bedside. This was a help of course, but all my bad feelings were still there. (*woman, age 32*)

I was confined and did not want to get out of bed. I was punished with no more cigarettes. They took away all I had and locked me into a room for three days. That weekend it was my birthday. (*man, age 37*)

Several times they have given or taken away medicines without telling me what was going on. (*man, age 37*)

I was given a wrong diagnosis. I wasn't believed when I told about my problem and was "stored away" in a nursing home in the countryside. The doctor told me that I would never recover and that this would be my home forever. But I met one person who understood that something was wrong. She was unskilled at that time, but she listened to me, encouraged and supported me, and helped me get away from that place. Today I have been taken off the sick list; I no longer take any medicines, live in my own house, work as a volunteer and study at the university. (*woman, age 64*)

It is difficult to talk about what I have experienced. When my third child was born, my husband was a psychiatric patient and sterilization was forced on me. The child died after five weeks. I didn't get help, but I became ill because of the bereavement and was sent to the hospital. The hospital contributed to furthering my mental problems. I have struggled a lot with this, and feel that the system does not believe in me. (*woman, age 67*)

Even if these stories represent only a small part of the narratives pertaining to humiliating experiences that infringe on clients' rights, the documentation is dramatic. The informants talk about situations in which the service system contributes further harm and trauma to the clients. Many stories are marked by an instrumental attitude to the service users and describe actions that can hardly be understood if they are not motivated by outdated views and the stigmatization of mental health clients, who tell about how their voices, feelings and opinions are of minor importance. Some of the episodes happened years ago, while others are quite new. But even if some experiences may belong to the past, the "victims" still fight with the aftermath of stigmatizing attitudes. Lawyers have underscored that encroachment in a person's private life demands treatment and recovery programmes of the highest quality (Syse & Nilstun, 1997). As long as this quality does not exist, then the right to intervene dramatically into people's lives must be questioned. Commitment and forced medication are often described by clients as being an extreme and often disabling experience. When we read clients' stories, we also get the impression that such actions are directed towards the stereotype of a mentally ill person and not at one who tells a detailed, thoughtful and emotional story. Several studies carried out in recent years show that there is little difference between the attitudes of the general public and psychiatrists towards people with mental health problems (Lauber et al., 2006). The studies even indicate that psychiatrists have more of a negative stereotypical view than the general public or other mental health professionals. The lack of responsiveness to clients' voices emerges as a major problem, thus causing reasons for concern regarding the protection of human rights for mental health clients.

5. Humanistic and contextual approaches

A humanistic perspective has both an ethical and scientific basis. Human beings live in a dimension of meaning that can primarily be experienced through dialogic relations. Dialogic relations are also fundamental for our existence and for a feeling of control and dignity, and because dialogic relations are fundamental, they cannot be rejected (Bachtin, 1997; Kirmayer, 1993; Sampson, 1993; Vetlesen & Nordtvedt, 1994; Wifstad, 1997). A humanistic perspective involves understanding emotional pain within both an existential and contextual perspective, a perspective in which the picture of human experiences and relations are sustained in its social complexity, without being reduced to biological or intrapsychic mechanisms. Still, with a contextual perspective, one cannot claim a meta-perspective. Whatever the position, efforts are needed to get into a dialogue with other positions, e.g. positions which are closer to the clinical field, with its more practical orientation and often acute problems that must be solved immediately. Of special interest here is how the positions of service users can be made more visible. Can researchers help? Maybe not, if we operate with absolute divisions between positions and only acknowledge knowledge obtained by personal experiences, although by such divisions, neither the users nor the professional's position makes sense. No single person can cover the experiences of an entire group, as some ability to generalize from one's own experiences must be taken for granted. We all have some kind of user experiences and a genuine, humanistic engagement can also help in understanding users' experiences. At the same time, it is important to bear in mind that some experiences are so traumatic that it is difficult or impossible to believe in dialogue and constructive solutions.

For ages, philosophers have discussed human beings' abilities to handle existential fragility, loss and anxiety. Being a human being means to be exposed to uncontrollable and unforeseen events which necessarily disturb our souls and make anxiety an existential modus (Yalom, 1980; Nussbaum, 1994; Hall, 2000). Platonic and Aristotelian philosophers had different solutions to these dilemmas. Platonic philosophers recommended transcendence and withdrawal, while the Aristotelians emphasized that love and relations is what give meaning and happiness and that the challenge is "a robust embrace of the human" (Hall, 2000:179) which included love and close relations, as well as the natural anxiety about death and separation. After having reflected upon fundamental, universal existential questions, Martha Nussbaum points to the ability to reflect over these questions as therapy for anxiety and fragility that is naturally embedded in our human existence. With this reflection, she says that the fundamental choice between rejection or the embracing of our living conditions becomes clearer.

Rollo May (1971) was one of the founders of humanistic psychology, and also focused on the ability to make fundamental choices based on a person's own values. Humanistic psychology has its roots in existentialism and Rollo May stressed that human conditions such as loneliness and a feeling of lost meaning could only be handled if the person discovered his/her own values and became responsible for his/her own choices.

Based on this way of thinking about emotional suffering, Hummelvoll (1997) has outlined the following principles for meetings with persons in crisis situations: Equality, mutuality, presence and acceptance, so that the person's self respect is strengthened and his/her own solutions acknowledged, support in making responsible choices and in the search for meaning, coherence and hope, an openness in dealing with moral conflicts and feelings of guilt, and help in the process of gaining independence, freedom, honesty and a life based on one's own values. These principles can also be seen as therapeutic guidelines.

6. A real biopsycho-social model

Through comprehensive review studies, Read et al. (2008) have provided a considerable contribution to the understanding of contextual factors, as well as illustrating that what is often seen as a genetically inherited vulnerability to stress can be acquired via adverse life events. As stated earlier by Zubin and Spring (1977), vulnerability can be acquired by trauma experiences, specific diseases, perinatal complications, family experiences, adolescent peer interactions and other life events, although their description of a biopsychosocial model was either misunderstood or misused. According to Read et al. (2008), asking about one's childhood and trying to understand the contextual meaning of symptoms has been outweighed by an approach that merely counts symptoms, gives the person a diagnosis and medication. This trend is clearly mirrored in research in which the focus on biological causes is on the rise. Out of 1,284 publications about childhood schizophrenia between 2000 and 2008, only five were related to child abuse and eight to poverty. The authors document how crucial factors such as child abuse and poverty really are, while revealing that poverty is even more strongly related to schizophrenia and psychosis than to other disorders. Based on the weighted average in 59 studies, the authors found that 64.5% of the women and 55% of the men had been subjected to either child sexual abuse or child physical abuse, with the combined rate at 60.02%. But estimating the prevalence of childhood maltreatment by using only child sexual or physical abuse as indicators leads to underestimation, as studies among first-episode schizophrenia spectrum inpatients also found that childhood emotional abuse mounted to 94 %, childhood emotional neglect to 89% and childhood physical neglect to 89%. Furthermore, studies of psychosis and schizophrenia have consistently found high rates of affectionless control parenting. There is also a pattern emerging in which the strongest relationships with abuse and neglect appear to be for hallucinations and the relationship between child abuse and hallucinations also exists across diagnostic boundaries.

In 2005, a review based on four population studies and a myriad of other studies (Read et al., 2005) concluded that child abuse is a causal factor for psychosis and schizophrenia. In the media, the research was presented as something that could cause the psychiatric establishment to "experience an earthquake that will shake its intellectual foundations" (James, 2005).

Since the 2005 review, seven more population-based studies have been published. The 2008 review (Read et al., 2008) then built on 11 population-based studies by seven independent research teams, using nine different samples drawn from six countries. In all of the studies, higher levels of child maltreatment or neglect were found in the psychosis groups.

The probability of a causal effect between child maltreatment or neglect and psychosis is increased if we find that the first not only predicts the second, but that more of the first – greater severity or frequency of abuse – is more related to the second, i.e. that there is a dose-response. The eight studies that investigated this dose-response hypothesis confirmed the hypothesis. According to the authors, it seems that the hypothesis that there is a specific genetic disposition for schizophrenia is turning out to be one of the costliest blind alleys in the history of medical research. This statement is supported by other researchers, e.g. example Hamilton (2008), who by then had conducted the most comprehensive genetic association study of genes. Hamilton wrote that "none of the polymorphisms were associated with the schizophrenia phenotype at a reasonable threshold for statistical significance" (Hamilton, 2008, p. 420) and that "The distribution of test statistics suggests nothing outside of what would be expected by chance" (Hamilton, 2008, p. 421). None of the researchers referred to by Read et al. (2008) argued that biological processes are irrelevant. There are biological processes underlying the mechanisms by which trauma leads to psychosis, and all mental processes have neurological and biochemical correlates, but even if these correlates can be identified, we have not discovered a *cause*. Read et al. (2008) compare such an argument with assuming that because grief also causes reactions in the brain, it is the brain that causes the grief and sadness. In contrast to this, the Trauma Neurodevelopmental Model (TN) of psychosis says that changes in the brain such as overactivity of the HPA axis, dopamine, norephinephrine and serotonin abnormalities, ventricular enlargement, etc. happen because of the brain's reaction to the environment. Biological differences found in the brains of persons with psychosis are also found in the brains of abused children, which is a finding that supports the theory that a heightened sensitivity to stress as traced in the brain's stress regulation mechanisms can be caused by childhood trauma.

This documentation implies that psychosis can be prevented. If child abuse is a causal factor for psychosis to the same extent as with other psychological problems, the authors then argue that the same primary prevention programmes that work for other problems will also work for psychosis. It is about keeping children safe and supporting families.

Another gain from accepting this well documented theory is that persons with diagnoses that say they have schizophrenia or psychosis are not seen as being genuinely different from "us", which is essential when it comes to a discussion about human rights for persons under mental health care. An important question is whether their disabilities qualify for treatment according to a special law and exemptions from the European Convention on Human Rights - indicating reduced decision capacity - or should they enjoy the same rights and freedoms as other groups in society when they need assistance from the health service systems?

The UN Convention on the Rights of Persons with Disabilities (CRPD), which was signed in 2006, builds on a social model which says that disabilities are the result of an interaction between an individual and barriers in a society. Therefore, the convention also adopts a human rights and social model for disabilities, including mental disabilities, as underscored by the UN High Commissioner on Human Rights. This new model also means a new legal position for mental health clients. As we shall see in the next paragraph, the CRPD states that all health care must be based on a free and informed consent.

7. Signs of a paradigmatic shift

After the CRPD was signed, 20 countries soon ratified the convention so that it could also be ratified as an international convention. As of 2011, approximately 100 countries had ratified, thus allowing mental disabilities to be included on equal basis with other disabilities. The convention states that *"persons with disabilities enjoy equal capacity on an equal basis with others in all aspects of life"* (Art. 12). It further states that health care shall be of the same quality for persons with disabilities as it is for others, *"including on the basis of free and informed consent"* (Art. 25).

The CRPD takes the legal protection of mental health clients a step further in relation to the European Convention on Human Rights (ECHR) from 1950, in which exceptions could be made for mental health clients, depending on medical judgments. It seems as if the time is now ripe for the European Court to take a more independent attitude towards medical judgments in the mental health care system, which is supported by the CRPD.

As stated by the UN Special Rapporteur on the right of everyone to enjoy the highest attainable standard of physical and mental health (Report of the UN Special Rapporteur on the right of everyone.. 2005): *"The Mental Illness Principles recognize that no treatment shall be given without informed consent. This is consistent with fundamental tenets of international human rights law, such as the autonomy of the individual. But this core provision in the Principles is subject to extensive exceptions and qualifications. (…) in practice their combined effect tends to render the right of informed consent almost meaningless."*

The CRPD was developed from the insight that the human rights of people with disabilities in many areas still have a weaker protection then the rights of other groups. The main objective of the convention is to prevent discrimination against people with disabilities, while also moving away from a model in which disabilities are seen as something individual - and people with disabilities as objects for medical and other interventions - to a model and practice in which all people have dignity and human rights on equal basis with other human beings. The CRPD substitutes the medical model with a social and human rights model (Orefellen, 2011). The Office of the United Nations High Commissioner for Human Rights (OHCHR) supports this point of view: *"First the Convention recognizes that disabilities are the result of interaction between an individual with impairment and the physical, attitudinal and other barriers in society. The medical and charity model is completely abandoned in favour of a human rights and social model"* (OHCHR, 2007).

The OHCHR also emphasizes the legal capacity of persons with disabilities: *"Article 12 of the Convention requires States parties to recognize persons with disabilities as individuals before the law, possessing legal capacity, including the capacity to act, on an equal basis with others" (OHCHR, 2009),* and further says: *"The Convention on the Rights of Persons with Disabilities (CRPD) states clearly that deprivation of liberty based on the existence of a disability is contrary to international human rights law, is intrinsically discriminatory, and is therefore unlawful. Such unlawfulness also extends to situations where additional grounds – such as the need for care, treatment and the safety of the person or the community – are used to justify deprivation of liberty.*

Under international human rights law, persons with disabilities are entitled to enjoy their rights to liberty and security on an equal basis with others, and can be lawfully deprived of their liberty only for the reasons, and in accordance with the procedures, that are applicable to other persons in the same jurisdiction" (OHCHR, 2008a). This citation also implies that crime is crime irrespective of diagnoses and disabilities, and that the judicial system and the health care system should not be mixed. The point is made clear in the following paragraphs:

"(…)Where additional grounds such as dangerousness, (…) are put forward to justify the restriction of liberty of a person with a mental and intellectual disability, such a person shall be subjected to detention on such grounds only in as much and on the same grounds as any other person, with no reference to his or her mental or intellectual condition" (OHCHR, 2008b).

"Laws contemplating dangerousness as a ground for deprivation of liberty should be equally applied to all" (OHCHR, 2007).

Article 12 seems to not open up for a reduced legal capacity or exemptions in any case, whether serious disabilities or comprehensive needs for help. (Orefellen, 2011). Instead, the CRPD builds on a model in which persons with disabilities should be ensured of getting the needed support in order to make decisions: *"This year as we focus on the right to act, let us recognize all people's right to make their own choices, and take their own actions as they see fit.*

Whenever people with disabilities need assistance they should be supported by people of their own free choice in making decisions, but never replaced in their legal capacity to act under no circumstance" (CRPD –committee, 2009c).

To ensure full inclusion and equal rights, it is necessary to tear down physical, judicial and other barriers that particularly affect people with disabilities, and to offer assistance in such a way that fundamental rights can be enjoyed on an equal basis with other groups. This implies a rethinking of both practice and legislation, which also demands comprehensive processes of increasing awareness (Orefellen, 2011).

The fundamental principles in the CRPD convention are dignity, autonomy, the freedom to make one's own choices, equality and non-discrimination, which also implies that institutionalization without a person's free and informed consent must be abolished:

"Legislation authorizing the institutionalization of persons with disabilities on the grounds of their disability without their free and informed consent must be abolished. This must include the repeal of provisions authorizing institutionalization of persons with disabilities for their care and treatment without their free and informed consent, as well as provisions authorizing the preventive detention of persons with disabilities on grounds such as the likelihood of them posing a danger to themselves or others, in all cases in which such grounds of care, treatment and public security are linked in legislation to an apparent or diagnosed mental illness" (OHCHR, 2009).

Additionally, Article 17 of the CRPD, which is about the right to respect in relation to physical and mental integrity for all peoples, including persons with disabilities, seems to be important in regard to coercive treatment in psychiatric and mental health care. When the CRPD committee examined Tunisia in April of 2011, Article 17's "Protecting the integrity of persons" was included in the "List of issues", and Tunisia was asked to document legislation that protects persons with disabilities from medical experiments and treatment without their free and informed consent, as well as outlining arrangements which will ensure that persons are not exposed to mechanically coercive means and coercive treatment in mental health care (CRPD, 2010b; Orefellen, 2011).

Serious infringements that would normally be classified as mistreatment in mental health care could be redefined as "necessary" health care, which is seen as a problem under the new paradigm that the CRPD represents:

"Medical treatments of an intrusive and irreversible nature, when they (...) aim at correcting or alleviating a disability, may constitute torture and ill-treatment if enforced or administered without the free and informed consent of the person concerned."

"The administration in detention and psychiatric institutions of drugs, including neuroleptics that cause trembling, shivering and contractions and make the subject apathetic and dull his or her intelligence, has been recognized as a form of torture."

"The Special Rapporteur notes that forced and non-consensual administration of psychiatric drugs, and in particular of neuroleptics, for the treatment of a mental condition needs to be closely scrutinized. Depending on the circumstances of the case, the suffering inflicted and the effects upon the individual's health may constitute a form of torture or ill-treatment" (SRT, UN special Rapporteur on Torture, 2008).

The Human Rights Council (2009) has underscored that there are *no* exemptions from the articles that protect people against the deprivation of liberty:

"Prior to the entrance into force of the Convention, the existence of a mental disability represented a lawful ground for deprivation of liberty and detention under international human rights law. The Convention radically departs from this approach by forbidding deprivation of liberty based on the existence of any disability, including mental or intellectual, as discriminatory."

8. The possibility of change

According to Kuhn (1970), Paradigmatic shifts take place when scientific discipline is thrown into a crisis. There have been several discussions over both the concept paradigm and paradigm shifts. New theories and ideas should be very comprehensive in order to qualify for the term, paradigm shift. Kuhn wrote that paradigm shifts usually happen via revolution and that the language and theories of various paradigms are incommensurable, though of course it can be doubted as to whether languages or theories *can* be incommensurable with one another.

In relation to psychiatric and mental health care, it is difficult to estimate as to what degree fundamental changes will take place and if so, whether the changes qualify for a paradigm shift, i.e. if there really is a scientific revolution taking place. Arguments in favour of the position that fundamental changes will come are the long-lasting tensions between a medical and psychosocial discourse, the unsuccessful attempts at documenting the existence of genetic and biological markers, the dark side of history as represented by very negative and painful user experiences over the centuries, the humanistic and successful alternatives outlined, and not least, the international ratification of the Convention on the Rights of Peoples with Disabilities, which is based on an international consensus about the need for substituting the medical and charity model with a human rights and social model.

What we are also seeing now is an intellectual battle between the followers of the different "paradigms". It seems as if this will not result in any reconciliation between the two main approaches. Arguments and documentation in favour of an approach at odds with mainstream professional thinking are not easily integrated into existing models. The documentation can be registered, but neglected when it comes to policymaking, which is what seems to have occurred in the Norwegian, government-appointed group, whose mandate it was to give a report on legislation related to coercive treatment in mental health care (NOU, 2011:9); acknowledging the weak, and at the same time often harmful effects of psychotropic drugs, but still allowing forced medication.

That there may be sudden changes instead of a rational and controlled process based on evidence and scientific documentation is indicated by the former lead editor of DSM-IV, Allan Frances. Frances, who earlier did not want to be "a crusader of the world", said in an interview in 2010 that ,"The idea of more kids getting unneeded antipsychotics that would make them gain 12 pounds in 12 weeks hit me in the gut. It was uniquely my job and my duty to protect them. If not me to correct it, who? I was stuck without an excuse to convince myself" (Interviewed by Gary Greenberg for Wired, December 27, 2010; published January 2011). Frances fears that by use of the proposed diagnostic category, "psychosis risk syndrome", as well as other newly constructed diagnoses, "DSM-5 will take psychiatry off a cliff".

There is no doubt that the mainstream thinking in psychiatric and mental health care is challenged from different sides and that changes will come, though in what way and how comprehensive are not easy to predict. Thus, we are facing exciting times.

9. Acknowledgement

This chapter is dedicated to Hege Orefellen for her groundbreaking work with human rights for mental health clients.

10. References

Andreassen, O. (2005) Har arv noen betydning for utvikling av relasjoner? I: Opjordsmoen, S., Vaglum, P., Block-Thoresen, G.R. (red.) Oss imellom. S 23-32. Stavanger: Hertvig forlag

Angell, M. (2011) The illusion of psychiatry. Book reviews: Kirsch, Whitaker, Charlat and DSM IV. The New York Review of books, 14. July

Bachtin, M (1997) Det dialogiska ordet. Gråbo: Bokförlaget Anthropos

Bartlett, P., Lewis, O., Thorold, O. (2007) Mental Disability and the European Convention on Human Rights. The Netherlands: Martinus Nijhoff Publishers Leiden/Boston

Bentall, Richard P. (2003): Madness explained. Psychosis and human nature. London: Penguin Books

Bola J, Lehtinen K, Aaltonen J, Rakkolainen V, Syvalahti E, Lehtinen V. Predicting medication-free treatment response in acute psychosis: cross-validation from the Finnish Need-Adapted Project. J Nerv Ment Dis 2006;194(10):732-739

Bremnes, R., Hatling, T., Bjørngaard, J.H. (2008) Tvungent psykisk helsevern med døgnopphold i perioden 2001-2006. Sluttrapport A4319. SINTEF Helse, Avd. Psykisk helse

Bremnes, R., Hatling, T., Bjørngaard, J.H. (2008) Bruk av tvangsmidler i psykisk helsevern i 2001, 2003, 2005 og 2007. SINTEF Helse A8231

Caspi, A., Sugden, K., Moffit, T.E., Taylor, A., Craig, I.W., Harrington, H.L., McClay, J., Mill, J., Martin, J., Braitwaite, A., Poulton, R. (2003) Influence of like stress on depression: Moderation by a polymorphism in the 5-HTT gene. *Science*, 301: 201-293

Council of Europe's Report on Psychiatry and Human Rights (1994). Parliamentary Assembly.

CRPD - Convention on the Rights of Persons With Disabilities (2006) Adopted by the UN general Assembly on Dec. 13th

CRPD-komitèen (2009c). *Committee on the Rights of Persons with Disabilities. Week long program of celebrations of the International Day of Persons with Disabilities, 3 – 9 December 2009. A World Appeal forAction! "Let us empower people with disabilities with the right to act!" Mohammed Al-Tarawneh, Chairperson, UN Committee on the rights of persons with disabilities, 3. December 2009: http://www.ohchr.org/EN/HRBodies/CRPD/Pages/InternationalDay122009.aspx*

CRPD-committee (2010b). List of issues to be taken up in connection with the consideration of the initial report of Tunisia (CRPD/C/TUN/1): http://www2.ohchr.org/SPdocs/CRPD/4thsession/CRPD.C.TUN.Q.1_en.doc

Ekeland, TJ (2011) Ny kunnskap – Ny praksis. Et nytt psykisk helsevern. Nasjonalt senter for erfaringskompetanse innen psykisk helse, rapp 1/2011

Fosse, R. (2009) Arv og miljø. Ingen gener for psykiske lidelser. *Tidsskrift for norsk psykologforening*. Vol 46, nummer 6: 596-600

Foucault, M. (1973). Galskapens historie: Oslo: Gyldendal kjempefakkel

Getz, L., Kirkengen, A.L., Ulvestad, E. (2011) Menneskets biologi - mettet med erfaring. Tidsskr Nor Legeforen nr. 7, 2011; 131: 683-7

Hamilton, S. (2008) Schizophrenia candidate genes: are we really coming up blank. Am J Psychiatry: 165 (4): 420-423

Hopper, K., Harrison, G., Janca, A & Satorius, N (eds) (2007) Recovery from Schizophrenia: An International Perspective, Oxford University Press.

Human Rights Council, tenth session. A/HCR/10/48, 26 January 2009. Thematic Study by the Office of the United Nations High Commissioner for Human Rights on enhancing awareness and understanding of the Convention on the Rights of Persons with Disabilities. Advance edited version.

Hummelvoll, J.K. (1997) psykiatrisk sykepleie - en holistisk-eksistensiell tilnærming. I: Hummelvoll, J.K. og Lindström, U.Å. (red.): Nordiska perspektiv på psykiatrisk omvårdnad. Lund: Studentlitteratur

James, O. (2005) Think again: new research on schizophrenia suggests that the drugs won't always work. The Guardian (UK) October 22.

Joseph, J. (2004). The Gene Illusion. Genetic Research in Psychiatry and Psychology Under the Microscope. New York: Algora Publishing

Kirmayer, L (1993) "Healing and the intervention of metaphor. The effectiveness of symbols revisited". *Culture, Medicine and Psychiatry.* 17: 161-195, Kluver, Academic Publisher.

Kogstad, R. (2009) Protecting Mental Health Clients' Dignity - the Importance of Legal Control. *International Journal of Law and Psychiatry, Vol 6, number 32: 383-391*

Kollek, Regine (2004) Mind, metaphors, neurosciences and ethics. I: D. Rees & S. Rose: The new brain sciences. Perils and Prospects. Cambridge: University press

Kuhn, T. (1970) The structure of scientific revolutions. 2nd. ed., Chicago: Univ. of Chicago Press

Larsen, IB & Andersen, AJW (2011) A Holy Duty - How do users of the mental health care system describe themselves, and what are their reasons for turning their experiences into written texts? *Klinisk Sygepleie*, 25, nr.1

Lauber, C., Nordt, C., Braunschweig, C., Rössler, W. (2006) Do mental health professionals stigmatise their patients? *Acta Psychiatr Scandinavia, 113 (Suppl 429):* pp. 51-59.

Levinas, E. (1993) Den annens humanisme. Thorleif Dahls kulturbibliotek. Oslo: Aschehoug

May, R. (1971) Menneskets dilemma i vår tid. Oslo: Aschehoug

Nesvåg, R. (2008). Characterization of brain morphology in patients with schizophrenia. Oslo: Faculty of medicine, University of Oslo

Norwegian Mental Health Act, Ot. Prp 11, 1998–99 (1999) Om lov om etablering og gjennomføring av psykisk helsevern.

NOU 2011:9, Økt selvbestemmelse og rettssikkerhet

Nussbaum, Martha (1994) The therapy of Desire: Theory and Practice in Hellenistic Ethics. Princeton: Princeton University Press

Orefellen, H. (2011) Selvbestemmelse og frihet på lik linje med andre. Lovutvalg for vurdering av regler om tvang mv. i psykisk helsevern. Dissens

Ot.prp 3, 1998–99: Om lov om styrking av menneskerettighetenes stilling i norsk rett (menneskerettighetsloven).

OHCHR (2007) Final Report of OHCHR Expert Seminar on Torture and Persons with Disabilities: http://www2.ohchr.org/english/issues/disability/documents.htm

OHCHR. (2008a). Office of the High Commissioner for Human Rights. Information Note No. 4. Persons with Disabilities.Dignity and Justice for Detainees Week: http://www.ohchr.org/EN/UDHR/Documents/60UDHR/detention_infonote_4.pdf

OHCHR (2008b). Office of the High Commissioner for Human Rights , August 2008 A review of the Ugandan Legal Framework Relevant to Persons With Disabilities. Comparative Analysis to the Convention on the Rights of Persons with Disabilities.

OHCHR (2009). Human Rights Council, tenth session. A/HCR/10/48, 26 January 2009. Thematic Study by the Office of the United Nations High Commissioner for Human Rights on enhancing awareness and understanding of the Convention on the Rights of Persons with Disabilities. Advance edited version: http://www2.ohchr.org/english/bodies/hrcouncil/docs/10session/A.HRC.10.48.pdf

Palm, E. & Ericsson, M. (2005). Att klaga til Europadomstolen. Stockholm: Jure.

Read, J. van Os, J., Morrison, A, Ross, C. (2005) Childhood trauma, psychosis and schizophrenia: a literature review with theoretical and clinical implications. Acta Psychiatr Scand: 112 (5): 330-350

Read, J., Fink, PJ; Rudegeair, T, Felitti, V, Whitfield, CL (2008) Child Maltreatment and Psychosis: A Return to a Genuinely Integrated Bio-Psycho-Social Model. Clinical Schizophrenia & Related Psychoses, Comprehensive Review, October

Report of the UN Special Rapporteur on the right of everyone to the enjoyment of the highest attainable standard of physical and mental health, Paul Hunt.(2005). E/CN.4/2005/51.

Sampson, E.E. (1993) Celebraiting the Other. A dialogic account of Human Nature. New York, London, Toronto, Sidney, Tokyo, Singapore: Harvester Wheatsheaf

Scheff, T.J. (1966) Being mentally Ill: A Sociological Theory. Chicago: Aldine

SRT (2008) UN Special Rapporteur on Torture. Interim report A/63/150. 28. July 2008. http://www2.ohchr.org/english/issues/disability/docs/torture/A_63_175_en.doc.

Steenfeldt- Foss, OW (1997), p. 14 in: Medical Ethics and Medical Conduct. Proceedings of the Conference on Human Rights. Ohrid. The former Yugoslav republic of Macedonia, 23-24. May. Oslo: The Norwegian Medical Association

Surtees, P.G., Wainwright, N.W., Willis-Owen, S.A., Sandhu, M.S., Luben, R., Day, N.E. (2007) The brain-derived neurotrophic factor Val66Met polymorphism is associated with sense of coherence in a non-clinical community sample of 7335 adults. *J Psychiatric Res,* 41: 707-710

Syse, A., & Nilstun, T. (1997). Ulike regler — lik lovforståelse? Om tvangsregulering og verdikonflikter i nordisk psykiatri. Tidsskrift for Rettsvitenskap, 5, 837–918.

Sørensen, T. (1982) Trenger vi det psykiatriske sykehuset? I: Norsk psykiatri i 80-årene. En innstilling om vitenskapelige og samfunnsmessige forhold som er av betydning for utviklingen av det psykiske helsevern. Oslo: Universitetsforlaget

Thune, G.H. (2008) Overgrep. Søkelys på psykiatrien. Oslo: Abstrakt Forlag

Vetlesen, A.J. & Nortvedt, P. (1994) Følelser og moral. Oslo: Ad Notam, Gyldendal

Walker, I., & Read, J. (2002). The differential effectiveness of psychosocial and biogenetic causal explanations in reducing negative attitudes toward "mental illness". Psychiatry, 65(4), 313–326.

Wampold, B. E. (2001). The Great Psychotherapy Debate. Models, Methods and Findings. Mahwa, N.J., Lawrence Erlbaum Associates

Wifstad, Å (1997). Vilkår for begrepsdannelser og praksis i psykiatri. Oslo: Tano-Aschehoug.

Whitaker, R. (2002). Mad in America, Bad Science, Bad Medicine and the Enduring Mistreatment of the Mentally Ill. NY Basic Books.

Zubin, J., Spring, B. (1977) Vulnerability: a new view of schizophrenia. J Abnorm Psychol, 86 (2):103-126

Yalom, I. (1980) Existential Psychotherapy. New York: Basic Books.

Section 6

Mental Health and Medicine

26

Depression in the Context of Chronic and Multiple Chronic Illnesses

Melinda Stanners and Christopher Barton
Discipline of Psychiatry, University of Adelaide, South Australia
Social Health Sciences, Flinders University, South Australia
Australia

1. Introduction

As an individual ages, the likelihood of living with a chronic illness increases. So too does the likelihood of a person living with multiple chronic illnesses. Current projections for ageing suggest that 25% of the populations of developed countries will be aged 65 years and over by the year 2050. Epidemiological research has identified that individuals living with chronic physical illnesses, such as heart disease, diabetes and respiratory diseases, are more likely to experience depression than those without chronic illness. These individuals experience worse quality of life, are more likely to be non-compliant with treatment regimens and more likely to suffer additional morbidity and premature mortality.

The impact of the interaction between chronic disease, disability and depression, therefore, is of increasing relevance in the pursuit of healthy ageing. In this chapter we will report findings from a review of the literature together with emerging findings from our own research program to highlight the epidemiology of depression and multi-morbidity, innovations in the management of persons living with multiple chronic illnesses and opportunities for improving the quality of mental health care for these people.

2. Epidemiology of chronic illness and depression

Chronic illnesses are the leading source of morbidity and mortality in developed nations. In the United States for example, nearly half of the US population experiences one or more chronic illnesses (Adams, Barnes et al. 2009) and chronic illnesses are among the leading causes of death (Kung, Hoyert et al. 2008). Likewise, mental health problems are common in the community and pose a significant burden of disease (Murthy, Bertolote et al. 2001). Of the mental health problems, depression is one of the most common mental health conditions experienced amongst populations, and is found in people of all regions, all countries and all societies (Murthy, Bertolote et al. 2001). The global burden of disease study estimated the 12 month prevalence of uni-polar depressive episodes to be between 5.8% and 9.5% (Murthy, Bertolote et al. 2001).

The incidence, prevalence and persistence of depression is not evenly distributed in the community. Depression is more common amongst those who are younger, female (Murthy, Bertolote et al. 2001), who have lower income or education (Lorant, Delliege et al. 2003;

Muntaner, Eaton et al. 2004; Melchior, Chastang et al. 2011), live in poverty or who live in poorer neighbourhoods (Murthy, Bertolote et al. 2001; Mair, Diez-Roux et al. 2008; Paczkowski and Galea 2010).

Another group that is particularly vulnerable to depression is those with chronic illness. There is now an extensive body of research documenting the epidemiology of chronic illness and depression. This is seen most clearly when comparing prevalence of depression in community settings where the prevalence is typically low (3%-5%) compared with primary care and inpatient settings where the prevalence is higher (5%-10% to 10%-14% respectively) (Katon 2003). Principally however, studies have reported increased prevalence of major depression in individuals diagnosed with specific medical illnesses such as cardiovascular disease (including myocardial infarct, stroke and cerebrovascular disease), type II diabetes, chronic obstructive pulmonary disease, arthritis and chronic pain, asthma and cancer (Lett, Blumenthal et al. 2004; Iosifescu 2007; Mezuk, Eaton et al. 2008; Patten, Williams et al. 2008; van der Feltz-Cornelis, Nuyen et al. 2010; Renn, Feliciano et al. 2011; Dong, Zhang et al. 2012).

The impact of co-occurring depression with chronic medical illness is significant. Once people develop chronic medical illness, depression is associated with increased symptom burden (perhaps arising from poorer adherence to treatment regimens and poorer perception of medical symptoms), additive functional impairment, greater medical utilisation costs and worse quality of life (Katon and Chiechanowski 2002; Katon 2011). Depressive disorders can adversely impact the course of medical illnesses (Benton, Staab et al. 2007) and recent evidence suggests that patients with depression die 5 to 10 years earlier than patients without depression (Chang, Hayes et al. 2010).

In the past decade, studies have identified depression as a risk factor for future chronic illness and not just arising from illness (Katon 2011). For example, Patten reported hazard ratios associated with major depression for several long term medical conditions identified as part of the Canadian National Public Health Survey(Patten, Williams et al. 2008). The age and sex adjusted risk of developing heart disease (1.6), arthritis/rheumatism (1.9), asthma (2.0) back pain (1.4), chronic obstructive pulmonary disease (2.4) and hypertension (1.7) were all statistically significantly raised for individuals with major depression at baseline, during the 8 year follow up period of the study.

It is increasingly clear that the relationship between chronic illness and depression is most likely bidirectional, whereby having depression increases risk of chronic illness, and conversely, having chronic illness increases risk of depression (Benton, Staab et al. 2007; Iosifescu 2007; Katon 2011; Renn, Feliciano et al. 2011). Conceptual models highlight the complex interactions between risk factors for major depression and chronic medical illness such as genetic and biological vulnerability, childhood adversity, stressful life events, and health risk behaviours such as smoking, sedentary lifestyle and over eating (Katon 2003; Katon 2011). While the mechanisms by which disease and depression interact are still to be resolved, it is clear that patients with chronic disease and comorbid anxiety or depression experience greater disease burden (Katon, Lin et al. 2007; Findley, Shen et al. 2011) and disability (Arnow, Hunkeler et al. 2006; Scott, Von Korff et al. 2009).

Most research investigating relationships between depression and chronic illness have focused on individual conditions and either exclude those patients with multiple chronic illnesses or do not consider conditions together. However, as the population ages, there are increasing numbers of individuals living with more than one chronic illness, and studies are only now beginning to investigate the prevalence and impact of depression in patients with multimorbidity.

3. Definition and epidemiology of multimorbidity

The term 'multimorbidity' is often used to describe the presence of two or more chronic conditions in an individual (Batstra, Bos et al. 2002), in contrast to the term 'comorbidity', which is defined as the presence of any disease in addition to an 'index' disease under study (Feinstein, 1967, quoted in (de Groot, Beckerman et al. 2003)).

Practical application of the term 'multimorbidity' differs across the literature. In Marengoni et. al.'s (Marengoni, Angleman et al. 2011) thorough systematic review of the literature to date, three major operational definitions are described:

- Number of concurrent diseases in an individual – the definition most frequently used in epidemiological research, but which does not differentiate between patients living symptom-free and patients experiencing severe functional loss.
- Cumulative indices measuring both number and severity of conditions – used in clinical studies for identifying patients at risk of negative health outcomes.
- Cumulative effect of conditions, symptom burden, and cognitive and physical dysfunction – used where care needs and use of services are addressed.

Attempts to estimate the prevalence and patterns of multimorbidity have provided inconsistent results. Studies investigating multimorbidity have been conducted worldwide, including the Netherlands (van den Akker, Buntinx et al. 1998) Canada (Fortin, Bravo et al. 2005), Sweden (Marengoni, Winblad et al. 2008), Australia (Britt, Harrison et al. 2008), United States (Wolff, Starfield et al. 2002), and Ireland (Glynn, Valderas et al. 2011), producing prevalence estimates ranging from 64.7% to 98.7% of patients over 65, although prevalence tends to be lower amongst persons aged less than 65 (Taylor, Price et al. 2010). Differences in data collection methods, defining and scoring multimorbidity, categorising ages, and modelling of prevalence data, limit the extent to which these studies can be compared. Data drawn from administrative databases and surveys (van den Akker, Buntinx et al. 1998) presented a much lower prevalence of multimorbidity than data drawn from medical records (2005). Recent studies propose patient record review as the most accurate method of multimorbidity data collection (Glynn, Valderas et al. 2011), as databases and surveys may provide incomplete information. As yet no resolution to these confounding factors has been reached.

Most studies published to date tend to define and measure multimorbidity as a simple disease count, which does not reflect disease burden. However, scales such as the Charlson Comorbidity index (Charlson, Pompei et al. 1987), the Index of Co-Existent Diseases (ICED) (Greenfield, Apolone et al. 1993) and the Cumulative Illness Rating Scale (CIRS) (Linn, Linn et al. 1968) have been developed to provide a measure of severity in multimorbidity research. The Charlson index provides a weighted score on the basis of disease count and severity, the ICED includes disease count, severity and physical impairment, and the CIRS classifies diseases by organ domains and attributes a severity score to each. Where the CIRS has been used in the literature, multimorbidity is defined as ...'the presence of illness in two or more morbidity domains' (pp73) (Britt, Harrison et al. 2008).

A systematic review of multimorbidity studies identified an inverse relationship between disease count and health-related quality of life (HRQOL), but the studies reviewed were limited by inconsistency of measures and definitions, and the absence of disease burden measures (Fortin, Lapointe et al. 2004). A recent study looking at multi-morbidity and self-rated health found that the effect of having a single chronic disease on perception of health was larger than the cumulative effect of chronic conditions, but that from the first disease onwards, multi-morbidity is associated with a smaller cumulative decline, suggesting that some form of adaptation occurs (Galenkamp and Braam et al. 2011). Whilst disease count has been associated with decline of physical functioning in both cross-sectional (Verbrugge, Lepkowski et al. 1989) and longitudinal (Kriegsman, Deeg et al. 2004) studies, disability has been found to be more predictive of mortality than disease count (Marengoni, von Strauss et al. 2009).

Disability has also been found to be more predictive of depression than age (Roberts, Kaplan et al. 1997). Roberts, Kaplan and Shema et al.' s (1997) analysis of the prevalence of major depressive episodes from the 1994 cohort of the Alameda County Study found that, when all risk factors were accounted for, age-related increases in depression were attributable to declines in physical health, physical function and perceptions of well-being. This finding, supported by subsequent research (Luszcz 2007), contradicts the assumption that depression is an inevitable effect of ageing, and highlights the impact of disease and disability on mental wellbeing.

While the relationship between disability and depression has been known for some time, few studies have investigated the occurrence of depression in people living with multimorbidy. An Australian study involving more than 7500 patients recruited from 30 General Practices found the prevalence of probable depression increased with increasing number of chronic physical conditions (Gunn, Ayton et al. 2010). For 2 conditions the age, sex and location adjusted odds of depression was 2.4 and for 5 or more conditions it was 3.45.

Another study of primary care patients reported increased psychological distress amongst 238 patients in Quebec, Canada. Multivariate analyses showed that psychological distress was increased when multimorbidity was measured by a simple illness count, but was significantly greater when measured using the CIRS. The risk of psychological distress was almost 5 times in the group with the highest burden of disease.

4. Challenges in management of the patient with multimorbidity and depression

A number of challenges have been identified in the treatment of the patient with co-morbid depression and chronic illness (Cimpean and RE. 2011; Katon 2011), however, while high quality trials of antidepressant treatments and psychotherapies demonstrate the effectiveness of these treatments in depressed medically ill patients, the efficacy of these treatments is lower in this population than in depressed individuals who are not medically ill (Iosifescu 2007). More intensive collaborative treatments that include antidepressants, psychotherapy, education and case management can be effective in this patient group (Iosifescu 2007).

But what of the patient with multimorbidity? Although the effect of depression on patterns of treatment, expenditures and outcomes for chronic medical conditions has received significant attention, the impact of multimorbidity on the treatment of depression is only now being investigated. It might be expected that additional challenges will present themselves in the identification of the depression, particularly in elderly patients, and the treatment of the depression in multimorbid patients. These challenges are outlined in further detail below.

4.1 Identification of depression in the elderly, multimorbid patient

A worldwide study conducted by the World Health Organisation (WHO) found that depression occurs more frequently in people with a chronic condition (Moussavi, Chatterji et al. 2007). Depression is also associated with increased risk of the development of other health conditions and increased symptom burden (Katon, Lin et al. 2007); therefore, timely detection and management of depression should be a priority where chronic illness is present.

At the frontline of mental health medicine, GPs struggle to detect and diagnose clinical depression in older patients. Depressive symptom presentation differs in older adults as compared with younger adults. Older patients suffering from depression will complain of irritability or feeling down, or admit to having lost interest in previously pleasurable activities (Mulsant and Ganguli 1999), but more often experience depression in a somatic form. The denial of psychological symptoms whilst emphasising physical symptoms is referred to as 'somatisation' (Lipowski 1988). A study of Canadian GPs found that the style of clinical presentation strongly affected clinician detection of depression in patients presenting with physical symptoms of depression (Kirmayer, Robbins et al. 1993). Complicating the presentation of depressive illness is the higher likelihood of older patients experiencing chronic disease, loss of function, and pain, where symptoms such as low energy, poor appetite, weight loss or cognitive decline may be related to depression, or disease, or both (Mulsant and Ganguli 1999). Chronically ill patients may also complain of medically unexplained symptoms or higher levels of pain (Katon, Lin et al. 2007). Consequently, where a chronic disease is present, depression is at risk of being undiagnosed or untreated (Redelmeier, Tan et al. 1998).

Differentiating between depression and other psychological and social problems continues to pose a challenge even after GP education has occurred. After ten years of education and guidelines, GPs in the Netherlands still struggled to differentiate depression from social problems in patients over 55 (Volkers, Nuyen et. al. 2004). Justification of the presence of depression further complicates diagnosis, as identified by a recent meta-synthesis of papers addressing GP depression diagnosis in the United Kingdom (Barley, Murray et al. 2011). Where social or physical circumstances were viewed as justifying the presence of depression, some clinicians were found to take a 'normalising' approach to the patient's depressive symptoms. Reluctant to medicalise social problems, these clinicians struggled to differentiate between distress and clinical depression (Barley, Murray et al. 2011). This poses a risk for clinicians who view depression in multimorbid patients as a natural response to illness and disability, as they may fail to recognise clinical depression and consequently withhold treatment by normalising and justifying patient depression.

Grief further complicates depression diagnosis. Older patients face the loss of spouses and peers, and although a grief reaction may take the appearance of a depressive episode (1994), in a healthy grief process the bereaved moves from acute grief to a state of integration and recovery of pleasure in life (Zisook and Shear 2009). Where acute grief lingers and becomes pathological, however, clinicians may misattribute and normalise symptoms of depression in bereaved patients, and inadvertently deprive patients of treatment (Zisook and Shear 2009). Pathological grief and bereavement-related depression have been identified as unique conditions separate from major depression (Prigerson, Bierhals et al. 1996), and have also been differentiated from major depressive disorder in the elderly (Kim and Jacobs 1991; Prigerson, Bierhals et al. 1996).

Scales like the Geriatric Depression Scale (Yesavage, Brink et al. 1983), the Beck Depression Inventory (Beck, Steer et al. 1996), and the Hospital Anxiety and Depression Scale (Zigmond and Snaith 1983), have been developed using criteria drawn from the DSM-IV to assist with the identification and diagnosis of depression. As yet, no validation of any of these scales has been attempted in multimorbid patient groups; this raises concerns about their reliability where depressive symptoms overlap with symptoms of disease (McFarlane, Ellis et al. 2008), particularly where somatic symptoms are addressed in the scale questionnaire. Geriatric Depression Scale item #13 (Sheikh and Yesavage 1986), for example, asks, 'Do you feel full of energy?'. A negative answer to this question is attributed to depression, but in a patient experiencing one or more chronic conditions, a lack of energy could equally be a vicissitude of their illnesses or medications as a symptom of depression. In a recent study by the authors of this chapter, 77.8% of multimorbid participants interviewed using the GDS endorsed a lack of energy, with the high endorsement rate suggesting that this question may not be appropriate as a depression screening criterion in this population. Item #2 of the GDS may be similarly inappropriate for patients with multiple chronic conditions, as an endorsement of the question 'Have you dropped many activities or interests?' could also be attributable to disability due to disease. The Beck Depression Inventory (Beck, Steer et al. 1996) also relies on somatic symptoms to detect depression. Additionally, emotionally-dependent questions relating to feelings of sadness, worthlessness or suicidality may not be useful where patients deny psychological symptoms. The Hospital Anxiety and Depression Score's exclusion of somatic symptoms gives it a higher degree of face validity, but no validation of the Hospital Anxiety and Depression Score in the multimorbid population has yet been published.

5. Treatment of depression

Once diagnosed with depression, depression can remain untreated for a variety of reasons such as competing demands on the time spent in consultation, patient resistance to discussing the depression or accepting treatment, polypharmacy, fear of antidepressant side effects, and limited access to treatment and services.

Due to increasingly tight time limitations in general practice, when depression presents alongside multiple physical conditions, the treatment of physical conditions often takes precedence (Ford 2008). Where patients prioritise symptoms to maximise their limited time with GPs, they may be unwilling to take time away from higher priority concerns to discuss their mental health; consequently, where physical symptoms are the patient's primary cause for concern, GPs may be unwilling to raise the issue of treatment for depression when patients have not complained about psychological suffering (Kendrick, Dowrick et al. 2009).

Patient acceptance of the diagnosis is a critical hurdle for general practitioners in providing depression treatment for older chronically ill patients, as many older patients deny or normalise depressive symptoms or attribute them to physical illness (Lipowski 1988; Mulsant and Ganguli 1999). Patient engagement is necessary for successful depression treatment (Zivin and Kales 2008), with general practitioners providing education and encouragement for patients to accept the need for some form of intervention.

5.1 Treatment: pharmacotherapy

Antidepressant treatment is the recommended first course of action in depression treatment (Montano 1999) and has good evidence of success in older patients (Frazer, Christensen et al. 2005). Antidepressant treatment remains the leading treatment mode in multimorbid patients, with one study in the United States identifying that amongst multimorbid adults with a diagnosis of depression, twice as many patients (56.2%) were prescribed antidepressants compared with those who received psychotherapy (21.4%). The remaining 22.5% received no treatment for depression (Vyas and Sambamoorthi 2011).

In patients with multiple chronic conditions, and particularly in elderly multimorbid patients, polypharmacy and medication side effects are salient concerns. Whilst software programs are available that support general practitioners attempting to navigate the minefield of multiple medication management, both patients and GPs are wary of disrupting a successful medication combination that may have taken some trial and error to reach. Even where GPs may be confident in their choice of antidepressant, patient anxiety around disrupting their medication plan may result in continued resistance to treatment.

Additionally, potential side effects of medications may exacerbate particular vulnerabilities in the elderly, such as dizziness increasing the risk of falls, and result in GP reluctance to prescribe and patient reluctance to trial them.

5.2 Non-compliance with medication

Even where GPs have prescribed an antidepressant, patient non-compliance presents a barrier to depression treatment. Zivin and Kales (Zivin and Kales 2008) observed that antidepressant medication non-adherence ranges from 40-75% in depressed elderly patients, identifying treatment preferences, resistance regarding depression's status as a medical illness, social support, cost of treatment and stigma as variables that effect non-adherence. Prior negative experiences, fear of adverse reactions, fear of antidepressant addiction, and polypharmacy also impacted negatively on medication adherence, as well as fear that the antidepressant would prevent the occurrence of natural sadness (Zivin and Kales 2008). Other studies have identified that expectation of positive benefits from taking medication, social support, and cognitive function are critical factors for antidepressant adherence, but that the same factors are also negatively impacted on by depression (DiMatteo, Lepper et al. 2000).

5.3 Treatment: psychotherapy

There is a noticeable gap in the literature on the subject of multimorbidity and psychotherapy. Psychotherapy is often used in the management of pain (Turk, Wilson et al. 2011), and has been observed to occur in multimorbid patients (Vyas and Sambamoorthi 2011), but no research to date has examined psychotherapy techniques or efficacy in this population.

5.4 Other strategies: exercise

Exercise has been found to alleviate depressive symptoms and improve mood as well as physical health in depressed adults with and without a range of chronic diseases (Dinas, Koutedakis et al. 2011). No studies have yet addressed the efficacy of exercise in patients with multiple chronic conditions, but exercise appropriate to the patient's capability may alleviate depressive symptoms in this population.

5.5 Other strategies: socialisation strategies

Whilst a gap remains in the literature examining loneliness and depression in patients with multiple chronic conditions, physical incapacity to engage in previously enjoyed activities, tiredness resulting from illness, medication side effects or depression, and the deaths of peers or spouse, foster an environment in which loneliness can develop. Loneliness has been found to be associated with depression in a range of studies worldwide (Kara and Mirici 2004); consequently, interventions that encourage or facilitate social engagement are often recommended for depressed chronically ill patients.

6. Innovations in the treatment of multimorbidity and implications for mental health

As we have described in the previous section, there are a number of challenges in the treatment of the patient with multimorbidity. While Western medical systems and health care professionals struggled to adapt to the shift in disease burden from acute, primarily infectious disease to chronic illness through the second half of the 20th Century, now these systems of care need to adapt again to support the treatment of increasingly older patients with multiple chronic illness.

There is momentum now in the move away from traditional medical care models, where patients see specialists for care of individual conditions with limited or no interaction between care providers, towards a more collaborative, integrated model of care, where patients play a central role in decision making about their treatment.

To help improve chronic care, there is a need to strengthen the primary care system, encourage care coordination, and promote care management of high cost patients with complex conditions (Shea, Shih et al. 2008; Boult, Green et al. 2009).

Multidisciplinary approaches have been trialled and discussed in a range of health care settings, including maternity and child health services (Schmied, Mills et al. 2010), chronic headache care (Gaul, Bromstrup et al. 2011), community-dwelling elders (Vedel, De Stampa et al. 2009), eczema sufferers (van Gils, van der Valk et al. 2009) and has been found to optimise patient outcomes in palliative care for lung cancer (Borneman, Koczywas et al. 2008) and short bowel syndrome (Modi, Langer et al. 2008). The dynamics of multidisciplinary teams have been studied in post-cancer follow-up care (Leib, Cieza et al. 2011) and maternity care (McIntyre, Francis et al. 2011), as well as in a hospital setting (Hogan, Barry et al. 2011). A 2004 systematic review of systematic reviews of integrated care programs found that despite considerable heterogeneity of care models, integrated care programs improved fragmentation, continuity and coordination of care, and provided an overall improvement in patient care (Ouwens, Wollersheim et al. 2005).

Several successful models of care for older persons with chronic conditions have been evaluated, and a recent systematic review of models of comprehensive care for older adults with chronic conditions describes 15 of these (Boult, Green et al. 2009). The models primarily involved interdisciplinary primary care, or services that enhance traditional primary care (Boult, Green et al. 2009). However, community based approaches, such as chronic disease self-management, have also been found to be effective, including for patients with multimorbidity and depression (Harrison, Reeves et al. 2011)

As the first line of medical care, the role of coordinator of care often falls to primary care providers. This may prove problematic in complex patients, as complex patients frequently accessing specialty care have been found to experience less continuity of care with their primary care provider, suggesting that high use of specialist services may compromise the primary care provider's ability to provide adequate coordination of care (Liss, Chubak et al. 2011). Where complex patients receive large amounts of specialty care, it may be more effective to share coordination of care with other care providers; this could be achieved where the specialist is part of a multidisciplinary team.

Other solutions continue to emerge. For example, dedicated multidisciplinary clinics with the express goal of providing coordinated care to multimorbid patients are a fairly recent phenomenon that have been successful in improving coordination of care and patients outcomes in Ireland (Hogan, Barry et al. 2011), and such clinics have been implemented elsewhere.

The Multidisciplinary Ambulatory Consulting Service (MACS) clinic, operated out of the clinical pharmacology unit at the Royal Adelaide Hospital, South Australia, provides a useful model for multidisciplinary care for multimorbid patients with complex care needs. The MACS clinic team is comprised of several specialists, including a pharmacologist, cardiologist, and complex disease management specialists; registrars on rotation; pharmacists; and nurses. Patients are referred to a specific specialist in the clinic. Patients attending the clinic see first the nurse, who takes their weight and blood pressure measurements and discusses contextual stressors and potential support needs such as community services or domiciliary care. Patients then meet with the pharmacist, and bring all medications and other vitamins and supplements for the pharmacist to review. Patients then meet with the specialist to whom they have been referred. After the clinic, the members of the team meet together to discuss patient needs, and collaborate on patient care plans. A detailed report is sent to the patient's primary care provider after each clinic visit.

An acknowledged limitation of the clinic in its current form is the absence of psychological or psychiatric care – a challenge that is frequently faced in primary care. Whilst many patients are burdened with comorbid mental health problems, recent research in the USA identified that the segregation of physical and mental health administration in Medicare is the greatest barrier to providing mental health care in a primary care setting (Kathol, Butler et al. 2010). This segregation is also present in health systems with Universal health care, such as Australia, which includes psychological therapy as an 'allied health' service as opposed to a general medical service, and limits the number of Medicare-subsidised psychological service visits to twelve. The administrative and ideological segregation between 'medical' care providers and 'allied health' providers presents a substantial barrier to integration of care (Kathol, Butler et al. 2010), particularly where multidisciplinary teams are in place to manage complex patients. As depression and anxiety increase with symptom burden (Katon, Lin et al. 2007; Findley, Shen et al. 2011), incorporation of mental health care into multidisciplinary models seems a logical step in the development of coordinated and integrated care. It is clear, however, that some ideological shifts may be required before such integration is possible.

7. Conclusion

A large body of research, spanning several decades, confirms that individuals with chronic illness are more likely to have depression than those without chronic illness. Research published in the past decade indicate that the relationship between chronic illness and depression is most likely bi-directional, and conceptual models are now emerging that help to explain the mechanisms underlying this bi-directional relationship.

As populations age, the number of people living with chronic illness, and increasingly, multiple chronic illness increases. Prevalence of depression is higher amongst patients with more functional disability and those with multiple chronic illness. There are additional challenges to treating depression amongst this group compared to those without chronic illness, or those with a single chronic illness, but systems and processes, such as coordinated care and multi-disciplinary clinics, are emerging to support health care providers to meet these challenges.

Few studies to date have investigated depression treatment in a specifically multimorbid patient population. A clearer understanding of the concerns and motivations of the patient with multiple chronic conditions will aid in developing treatment approaches appropriate for this population. Furthermore, many studies have maintained a pharmacological focus, leaving issues relating to nonpharmacological treatment and the patient's broader context largely unexplored. With the expanding multimorbid patient population and increased risk of depression in these groups, future high quality trials are needed to establish the most effective approaches to identification and treatment of depression in multimorbid populations.

8. References

-. "Better access to mental health care." Retrieved 25th October, 2011, from http://www.health.gov.au/internet/main/publishing.nsf/Content/mental-pubs-b-better.

(1994). American Psychiatric Association. Diagnostic and Statistical Manual of Mental Disorders. Washington DC, American Psychiatric Association.

Adams, P., Barnes PM, et al. (2009). Summary health statistics for the US Population: National Health Interview survey, 2008. Hyattsville, MD., US Department of Health and Human Services, Centres for Disease Control and Prevention, National Center for Health Statistics.

Arnow, B. A., E. M. Hunkeler, et al. (2006). "Comorbid depression, chronic pain, and disability in primary care." Psychosom Med 68(2): 262-268.

Barley, E., J. Murray, et al. (2011). "Managing depression in primary care: A meta-synthesis of qualitative and quantitative research from the UK to identify barriers and facilitators." BMC Family Practice 12(1): 47.

Batstra, L., E. H. Bos, et al. (2002). "Quantifying psychiatric comorbidity--lessions from chronic disease epidemiology." Soc Psychiatry Psychiatr Epidemiol 37(3): 105-111.

Beck, A. T., R. A. Steer, et al. (1996). Manual for the Beck Depression Inventory-II. San Antonio, TX, Psychological Corporation.

Benton, T., Staab J, et al. (2007). "Medical co-morbidity in depressive disorders." Annals of Clinical Psychiatry 19(4): 289-303.

Borneman, T., M. Koczywas, et al. (2008). "An interdisciplinary care approach for integration of palliative care in lung cancer." Clin Lung Cancer 9(6): 352-360.

Boult, C., Green AF, et al. (2009). "Successful models of comprehensive care for older adults with chronic conditions: Evidence for the Institute of Medicines “Retooling for an Aging America” Report." Journal of the American Geriatric Society 57: 2328-2337.

Britt, H. C., C. M. Harrison, et al. (2008). "Prevalence and patterns of multimorbidity in Australia." Med J Aust 189(2): 72-77.

Chang, C.-K., Hayes RD, et al. (2010). "All-cause mortality among people with serious mental illness (SMI), substance abuse disorders, and depressive disorders in southeast London: a cohort study. ." BMC Psychiatry 10(77).

Charlson, M. E., P. Pompei, et al. (1987). "A new method of classifying prognostic comorbidity in longitudinal studies: Development and validation." Journal of Chronic Diseases 40(5): 373-383.

Cimpean, D. and D. RE. (2011). "Treating co-morbid chronic medical conditions and anxiety/depression." Epidemiology and Psychiatric Sciences. 20: 141-150.

de Groot, V., H. Beckerman, et al. (2003). "How to measure comorbidity. a critical review of available methods." J Clin Epidemiol 56(3): 221-229.

DiMatteo, M. R., H. S. Lepper, et al. (2000). "Depression is a risk factor for noncompliance with medical treatment: meta-analysis of the effects of anxiety and depression on patient adherence." Arch Intern Med 160(14): 2101-2107.

Dinas, P. C., Y. Koutedakis, et al. (2011). "Effects of exercise and physical activity on depression." Ir J Med Sci 180(2): 319-325.

Dong, J.-Y., Zhang Y-H, et al. (2012). "Depression and risk of stroke: A meta-analysis." Stroke 43: In Press.

Findley, P., C. Shen, et al. (2011). "Multimorbidity and persistent depression among veterans with diabetes, heart disease, and hypertension." Health Soc Work 36(2): 109-119.

Ford, D. E. (2008). "Optimizing outcomes for patients with depression and chronic medical illnesses." Am J Med 121(11 Suppl 2): S38-44.

Fortin, M., G. Bravo, et al. (2005). "Prevalence of multimorbidity among adults seen in family practice." Ann Fam Med 3(3): 223-228.

Fortin, M., L. Lapointe, et al. (2004). "Multimorbidity and quality of life in primary care: a systematic review." Health Qual Life Outcomes 2: 51.

Frazer, C. J., H. Christensen, et al. (2005). "Effectiveness of treatments for depression in older people." Med J Aust 182(12): 627-632.

Galenkamp, H., A.W. Braam, et al. (2011). "Somatic multimorbidity and self-rated health in the older population." J Gerontol B Psychol Sci Soc Sci 66B(3):380-386

Gaul, C., J. Bromstrup, et al. (2011). "Evaluating integrated headache care: a one-year follow-up observational study in patients treated at the Essen headache centre." BMC Neurol 11(1): 124.

Glynn, L. G., J. M. Valderas, et al. (2011). "The prevalence of multimorbidity in primary care and its effect on health care utilization and cost." Fam Pract 28(5): 516-523.

Glynn, L. G., J. M. Valderas, et al. (2011). "The prevalence of multimorbidity in primary care and its effect on health care utilization and cost." (1460-2229 (Electronic)).

Greenfield, S., G. Apolone, et al. (1993). "The importance of co-existent disease in the occurrence of postoperative complications and one-year recovery in patients undergoing total hip replacement. Comorbidity and outcomes after hip replacement." Med Care 31(2): 141-154.

Gunn, J., Ayton DR, et al. (2010). "The association between chronic illness, multimorbidity and depressive symptoms in an Australian primary care cohort." Social Psychiatry Epidemiology EPub ahead of print.

Harrison, M., Reeves D, et al. (2011). "A secondary analysis of the moderating effects of depression and multimorbidity on the effectiveness of a chronic disease self-management programme." Patient Education and Counselling In Press.

Hogan, C., M. Barry, et al. (2011). "Healthcare professionals' experiences of the implementation of integrated care pathways." Int J Health Care Qual Assur 24(5): 334-347.

Iosifescu, D. (2007). "Treating depression in the medically ill." Psychiatry Clinics of North America 30: 77-90.

Kara, M. and A. Mirici (2004). "Loneliness, depression, and social support of Turkish patients with chronic obstructive pulmonary disease and their spouses." J Nurs Scholarsh 36(4): 331-336.

Kathol, R. G., M. Butler, et al. (2010). "Barriers to physical and mental condition integrated service delivery." Psychosom Med 72(6): 511-518.

Katon, W. (2003). "Clinical and health service relationships between major depression, depressive symptoms and general medical illness." Biological Psychiatry 54: 216-226.

Katon, W. (2011). "Epidemiology and treatment of depression in patients with chronic medical illness." Dialogues in Clinical Neuroscience 13(1): 7-23.

Katon, W. and P. Chiechanowski (2002). "Impact of major depression on chronic medical illness." Journal of Psychosomatic Research 53: 859-863.

Katon, W., E. H. Lin, et al. (2007). "The association of depression and anxiety with medical symptom burden in patients with chronic medical illness." Gen Hosp Psychiatry 29(2): 147-155.

Kendrick, T., C. Dowrick, et al. (2009) "Management of depression in UK general practice in relation to scores on depression severity questionnaires: analysis of medical record data." British Medical Journal 338: b750 DOI: 10.1136/bmj.b750.

Kim, K. and S. Jacobs (1991). "Pathologic grief and its relationship to other psychiatric disorders." J Affect Disord 21(4): 257-263.

Kirmayer, L. J., J. M. Robbins, et al. (1993). "Somatization and the recognition of depression and anxiety in primary care." Am J Psychiatry 150(5): 734-741.

Kriegsman, D. M., D. J. Deeg, et al. (2004). "Comorbidity of somatic chronic diseases and decline in physical functioning:; the Longitudinal Aging Study Amsterdam." J Clin Epidemiol 57(1): 55-65.

Kung, H., D. Hoyert, et al. (2008). Deaths: final data for 2005. National Vital Statistics Reports Available from: http://www.cdc.gov/nchs/data/nvsr/nvsr56/nvsr56_10.pdf.

Leib, A., A. Cieza, et al. (2011). "Perspective of physicians within a multidisciplinary team: Content validation of the comprehensive ICF core set for head and neck cancer." Head Neck.

Lett, H., Blumenthal JA, et al. (2004). "Depression as a risk factor for coronary artery disease: Evidence, mechanisms and treatment." Psychosomatic Medicine 66: 305-315.

Linn, B. S., M. W. Linn, et al. (1968). "Cumulative illness rating scale." J Am Geriatr Soc 16(5): 622-626.

Lipowski, Z. J. (1988). "Somatization: the concept and its clinical application." Am J Psychiatry 145(11): 1358-1368.

Liss, D. T., J. Chubak, et al. (2011). "Patient-reported care coordination: associations with primary care continuity and specialty care use." Ann Fam Med 9(4): 323-329.

Lorant, V., Delliege D, et al. (2003). "Socioeconomic inequalities in depression: A meta-analysis." American Journal of Epidemiology 157(2): 98-112.

Luszcz, M., L. Giles, et al. (2007). The Australian Longitudinal Study of Ageing: 15 years of ageing in South Australia: Adelaide: South Australian Department of Families and Communities.

Mair, C., Diez-Roux AV, et al. (2008). "Are neighbourhood characteristics associated with depressive symptoms? A review of evidence." Journal of Epidemiology and Community Health 62: 940-946.

Marengoni, A., S. Angleman, et al. (2011). "Aging with multimorbidity: A systematic review of the literature." (1872-9649 (Electronic)).

Marengoni, A., E. von Strauss, et al. (2009). "The impact of chronic multimorbidity and disability on functional decline and survival in elderly persons. A community-based, longitudinal study." J Intern Med 265(2): 288-295.

Marengoni, A., B. Winblad, et al. (2008). "Prevalence of chronic diseases and multimorbidity among the elderly population in Sweden." Am J Public Health 98(7): 1198-1200.

McFarlane, A. C., N. Ellis, et al. (2008). "The conundrum of medically unexplained symptoms: questions to consider." Psychosomatics 49(5): 369-377.

McIntyre, M., K. Francis, et al. (2011). "The struggle for contested boundaries in the move to collaborative care teams in Australian maternity care." Midwifery.

Melchior, M., Chastang JF, et al. (2011). "Socioeconcomic position predicts long-term depression trajectory: a 13 year follow up of the GAZEL cohort study." Molecular Psychiatry: 1-10.

Mezuk, B., Eaton W, et al. (2008). "Depression and type 2 diabetes over the lifespan: a meta analysis. ." Diabetes Care 31: 2383-2390.

Modi, B. P., M. Langer, et al. (2008). "Improved survival in a multidisciplinary short bowel syndrome program." J Pediatr Surg 43(1): 20-24.

Montano, C. B. (1999). "Primary care issues related to the treatment of depression in elderly patients." J Clin Psychiatry 60 Suppl 20: 45-51.

Moussavi, S., S. Chatterji, et al. (2007). "Depression, chronic diseases, and decrements in health: results from the World Health Surveys." Lancet 370(9590): 851-858.

Mulsant, B. H. and M. Ganguli (1999). "Epidemiology and diagnosis of depression in late life." J Clin Psychiatry 60 Suppl 20: 9-15.

Muntaner, C., Eaton W, et al. (2004). "Socioeconomic position and major mental disorders." Epidemiologic Reviews 26: 53-62.

Murthy, R., Bertolote JM, et al. (2001). The World health report 2001: Mental health - new understanding, new hope.

Ouwens, M., H. Wollersheim, et al. (2005). "Integrated care programmes for chronically ill patients: a review of systematic reviews." Int J Qual Health Care 17(2): 141-146.

Paczkowski, M. and S. Galea (2010). "Sociodemographic characteristics of the neighbourhood and depressive symptoms. ." Current Opinion in Psychiatry 23: 337-341.

Patten, S., Williams J, et al. (2008). "Major depression as a risk factor for chronic disease incidence: longitudinal analyses in a general population cohort." General Hospital Psychiatry 30: 407-413.

Prigerson, H. G., A. J. Bierhals, et al. (1996). "Complicated grief as a disorder distinct from bereavement-related depression and anxiety: a replication study." Am J Psychiatry 153(11): 1484-1486.

Redelmeier, D. A., S. H. Tan, et al. (1998). "The treatment of unrelated disorders in patients with chronic medical diseases." N Engl J Med 338(21): 1516-1520.

Renn, B., Feliciano L, et al. (2011). "The bi-directional relationship of depression and diabetes: A systematic review." Clinical Psychology Review 31: 1239-1246.

Roberts, R. E., G. A. Kaplan, et al. (1997). "Prevalence and correlates of depression in an aging cohort: the Alameda County Study." J Gerontol B Psychol Sci Soc Sci 52(5): S252-258.

Schmied, V., A. Mills, et al. (2010). "The nature and impact of collaboration and integrated service delivery for pregnant women, children and families." J Clin Nurs 19(23-24): 3516-3526.

Scott, K. M., M. Von Korff, et al. (2009). "Mental-physical co-morbidity and its relationship with disability: results from the World Mental Health Surveys." Psychol Med 39(1): 33-43.

Shea, K., Shih A, et al. (2008). Health care opinion leaders' views on health care delivery system reform. Commonwealth Fund Commission on a High Performance Health System Data Brief. New York, NY.

Sheikh, J. I. and J. A. Yesavage (1986). "Geriatric Depression Scale (GDS): Recent evidence and development of a shorter version." Clinical Gerontologist 5(1-2): 165-173.

Taylor AW, Price K, et al. (2010). "Multi-morbidity - not just an older person's issue. Results from an Australian biomedical study." BMC Public Health 10: 718.

Turk, D. C., H. D. Wilson, et al. (2011). "Treatment of chronic non-cancer pain." Lancet 377(9784): 2226-2235.

van den Akker, M., F. Buntinx, et al. (1998). "Multimorbidity in general practice: prevalence, incidence, and determinants of co-occurring chronic and recurrent diseases." J Clin Epidemiol 51(5): 367-375.

van der Feltz-Cornelis, C., Nuyen J, et al. (2010). "Effect of interventions for major depressive disorder and significant depressive symptoms in patients with diabetes mellitus: a systematic review and meta analysis. ." General Hospital Psychiatry 32: 380-395.

van Gils, R. F., P. G. van der Valk, et al. (2009). "Integrated, multidisciplinary care for hand eczema: design of a randomized controlled trial and cost-effectiveness study." BMC Public Health 9: 438.

Vedel, I., M. De Stampa, et al. (2009). "A novel model of integrated care for the elderly: COPA, Coordination of Professional Care for the Elderly." Aging Clin Exp Res 21(6): 414-423.

Verbrugge, L. M., J. M. Lepkowski, et al. (1989). "Comorbidity and its impact on disability." Milbank Q 67(3-4): 450-484.

Volkers, A. C., J. Nuyen, et al. (2004). "The problem of diagnosing major depression in elderly primary care patients." Journal of Affective Disorders 82: 259-263.

Vyas, A. and U. Sambamoorthi (2011). "Multimorbidity and depression treatment." Gen Hosp Psychiatry 33(3): 238-245.

Wolff, J. L., B. Starfield, et al. (2002). "Prevalence, expenditures, and complications of multiple chronic conditions in the elderly." Arch Intern Med 162(20): 2269-2276.

Yesavage, J. A., T. L. Brink, et al. (1983). "Development and validation of a geriatric depression screening scale: A preliminary report." Journal of Psychiatric Research 17(1): 37-49.

Zigmond, A. S. and R. P. Snaith (1983). "The hospital anxiety and depression scale." Acta Psychiatr Scand 67(6): 361-370.

Zisook, S. and K. Shear (2009). "Grief and bereavement: what psychiatrists need to know." World Psychiatry 8(2): 67-74.

Zivin, K. and H. C. Kales (2008). "Adherence to depression treatment in older adults: a narrative review." Drugs Aging 25(7): 559-571.

27

Long-Lasting Mental Fatigue After Recovery from Meningitis or Encephalitis – A Disabling Disorder Hypothetically Related to Dysfunction in the Supporting Systems of the Brain

Lars Rönnbäck and Birgitta Johansson
Institute of Neuroscience and Physiology, Sahlgrenska Academy, University of Gothenburg and Sahlgrenska University Hospital, Gothenburg, Sweden

1. Introduction

Fatigue may originate from peripheral or central causes, thus being "physical" or "cognitive" (mental) in nature. Some authors also put forward the concepts "primary" or "secondary" fatigue (DeLuca, 2005). It may be that the different dimensions of fatigue have different neurobiological and neurophysiological correlates (see also Chaudhuri and Behan, 2000; 2004). The big problem, however, is that in-depth analyses of different types of fatigue have yet to be performed.

In this paper we focus on cognitive, or mental, fatigue (Johansson & Rönnbäck, 2012; Rönnbäck & Hansson, 2004), which in some cases can be long-lasting after meningitis or encephalitis. According to the International Classification of Diseases, 10th revision (ICD-10), the cognitive symptoms are covered by the diagnoses "mild cognitive disorder" or "neurasthenia" and according to the *Diagnostic and Statistical Manual of Mental Disorders*, 4th edition (DSM-IV) (American Psychiatric Association, 1994) they are included in the group of "mild neurocognitive disorders". According to the diagnostic classification by Lindqvist and Malmgren (1993), the symptoms belong to the "astheno-emotional syndrome".

The fatigue that we describe is characterized by a pronounced fatigability that may appear even after moderate mental activity. Characteristically the recovery time after being exhausted is long. We discuss diagnostics and we extend our previously proposed cellular mechanisms underlying this mental fatigue in brain disorders (Rönnbäck & Hansson, 2004) and suggest that functions of the supporting systems, namely the glial cells, in the brain are out of balance. Thus, dysfunction in the blood-brain barrier (BBB) permeability (see Abbott et al, 2006) due to inflammatory activity with microglial activation and the production of cytokines might be responsible for an attenuated astroglial fine-tuning and support of the neuronal glutamate signalling, which is of utmost importance for information processing in the brain.

2. Symptoms associated with the mental fatigue

A number of symptoms often appear in relation to the mental fatigue. These are noise- and light sensitivity, irritability, affect-lability, stress-intolerance and headache (table 1).

- DECREASED CONCENTRATION CAPACITY
- SUBJECTIVE MEMORY DISTURBANCE
- NOISE SENSITIVITY
- LIGHT SENSITIVITY
- AFFECT LABILITY
- IRRITABILITY
- STRESS SENSITIVITY
- SLEEP DISTURBANCE
- HEAD ACHE

Table 1. Symptoms often accompanying the mental fatigue in CNS infections/ inflammations or brain disorders.

3. Mental fatigue and depression

Fatigue and depression are important topics, to some degree overlapping as fatigue is on one hand a dominant symptom of and on the other hand, has been considered a risk factor for depression (Johnson et al., 1996). There is evidence supporting the idea that states of fatigue present variations of depression, while other studies argue for a more pure fatigue state, with little overlap with depression. Many studies on brain injury report increased susceptibility to depression after the injury, even if fatigue is also very common (Ashman et al., 2004; Silver et al., 2009; Whelan-Goodinson et al., 2009). Depression and mental fatigue can occur alone, but they sometimes occur simultaneously in states of CNS inflammation, infection or degeneration. The two states may overlap in symptomatology, but the core symptoms included in depression and mental fatigue, respectively, are different. Mental fatigue is mostly related to concentration and attention, especially over time, and is dependent on the degree of mental load. The fatigue fluctuates over the day, and the recovery period after mental exhaustion is mostly un-proportionally long. Persons suffering from depression, on the other hand, present low-spiritedness and a decreased interest in their surroundings. Many also find it difficult to feel pleasure. These persons may even experience fatigue but mostly throughout the day (see also Lerdal et al., 2011). The long-term mental problems after a well rehabilitated infection or inflammation in the CNS may relate to mental fatigue, as depression, if present, usually alleviates after some period while the mental fatigue persists.

Our hypothesis includes a tentative explanation on the basis of transmitter pathophysiology that persons suffering from long-lasting mental fatigue may be more vulnerable to depression (see below and figure 3).

4. On the diagnostics of mental fatigue

4.1 Assessment of mental fatigue: In clinical practice, fatigue is often noticed, but not always as important and central as it could be. This may be due to that it is subjective and there are limited possibilities to assess it objectively. Therefore, the problems caused by mental fatigue have not until now generated any extensive research. Mental fatigue is treated by many professionals as an issue of secondary importance.

As mental fatigue has such a great impact on many functions, it is important to consider the problem from a wide perspective and to look at the issue with an open mind, in order to develop an understanding of the cause of the problem. Mental fatigue is something specific, but it is easy to misunderstand this symptom. It could be mistaken for apathy if the person has difficulties with getting things done during the day, is not interested in learning new things and is not doing things that interest him or her. However, these problems, instead, could be the result of low energy levels, as is typical for mental fatigue. In this state it might be too exhaustive to carry out activities that demand a high degree of concentration, as talking to friends, reading and learning new things.

4.1.1 Self-assessment of mental fatigue

Fatigue is usually assessed as a subjective problem with self-report questionnaires, and there are many self-assessment scales trying to catch different forms of fatigue in various states or diseases. As life-prolonging therapy exists for persons with HIV/AIDS, chronic fatigue is one disabling symptom among these persons. A 56-item self-report instrument was developed by Pence and co-workers (2008) to specifically describe HIV-related fatigue with the aim to measure the intensity and consequences of fatigue as well as the circumstances surrounding fatigue in people living with HIV.

We focused on the mental fatigue which we consider as the limitation for work and social activities in different infectious and inflammatory CNS diseases and we constructed a self-assessment scale partly adapted from Rödholm et al (2001). This self-reported questionnaire contains 15 questions which cover the most common symptoms occurring after brain injury (TBI) (King et al., 1995). The selection of items is based on many years of clinical experience and reports (Lindqvist & Malmgren, 1993). The questions include symptoms reported early on, as well as a long time after a brain injury or neurological diseases. The questions relate to fatigue in general, lack of initiative, mental fatigue, mental recovery, concentration difficulties, memory problems, slowness of thinking, sensitivity to stress, increased tendency to become emotional, irritability, sensitivity to light and noise, decreased or increased sleep as well as 24-hour variations.

The items are based on common activities and the estimation relates to intensity, frequency and duration with exemplified alternatives. The intention was to make the scale more consistent between individuals and also between ratings for the same individual. Each item comprises examples of common activities to be related to four response alternatives. A higher score reflects more severe symptoms. A rating of 0 corresponds to normal function, 1 indicates a problem, 2 a pronounced symptom and 3 a maximal symptom. It is also possible to provide an answer which falls in between two scores (see example below).

Example of a question from the self-assessment scale of mental fatigue.

Mental fatigue

Does your brain become fatigued quickly when you have to think hard? Do you become mentally fatigued from things such as reading, watching TV or taking part in a conversation with several people? Do you have to take breaks or change to another activity?

0 I can manage in the same way as usual. My ability for sustained mental effort is not reduced.

0.5

1 I become fatigued quickly but am still able to make the same mental effort as before.

1.5

2 I become fatigued quickly and have to take a break or do something else more often than before.

2.5

3 I become fatigued so quickly that I can do nothing or have to abandon everything after a short period (approx. five minutes).

The self-assessment scale for mental fatigue and related items was evaluated. Significant correlations were found between all the 14 questions (24-hour variation was not included as only 'yes' and 'no' responses were measured). The 14 questions had adequate internal consistency. The Cronbach's alpha scale was used, giving a reliability coefficient of 0.944 (Johansson, et al., 2009). This indicates that the core problem with mental fatigue comprises a broader spectrum of relevant items with either primary or secondary symptoms. The response alternatives are refined in such a way as to make the self reports more consistent. This might have resulted in a more definite deviation from the healthy controls (the scale can be downloaded at www.mf.gu.se).

Many participants gave spontaneous comments on the scale as it includes important, key items which had previously been confusing for them. From a clinical viewpoint, the self-assessment scale can be a valuable therapeutic tool for the patient as it can clearly describe mental fatigue and common symptoms which co-occur. A better understanding of the problem is a very good starting point for further treatment (see also below). The self assessment scale may be valuable even for people with infectious or inflammatory CNS diseases and we hope that this scale will facilitate research on the prevalence, etiology and consequences of mental fatigue among persons suffering from diseases or disorders in the CNS.

4.1.2 Cognitive tests

With the intention of finding sensitive neuropsychological tests to assess mental fatigue, we chose tests measuring information processing speed (the time required to execute a cognitive task within a finite time period) (DeLuca & Kalmar, 2007), attention, working memory, verbal fluency and reading speed. The tests were digit symbol-coding from the WAIS-III NI (Wechsler, 2004), measuring information processing speed. Attention and working memory, both auditory and visual, were measured by means of the digit span and spatial span (Wechsler, 2004). Both tests included repetition of forward series of random numbers or blocks in order as well as in reverse. The verbal fluency test (FAS) measures the ability to generate as many words as possible beginning with a specific letter within one minute (Ellis et al., 2001). Parts A and B of the Trail Making Test (TMT), (Reitan & Wolfson, 1985) were used to measure visual scanning, divided attention and motor speed (Lezak et al., 2004). The test consists of a series of connect-the-circle tasks. The tasks in part A is to connect the circles in a sequence with a numerical order of 1 to 25. Part B comprise letters and digits in alternating numerical and alphabetical order, which have to be completed as quickly as possible. In order to evaluate higher demands such as dual tasks, a series of new tests was constructed with three and four factors, respectively. The same number of circles (25) was used in all parts. The alternation between factors was similar to part B but months was added in part C and both months and days of the week in chronological order in part D. In the latter, the order of letters and digits was changed. The reading speed was measured using the DLS reading speed test used for the screening of dyslexia (Madison, 2003).

After TBI information processing speed and attention tasks were found to be most sensitive and were significantly decreased compared to healthy control, while no such effect was found for both visual and auditory working memory. The subjective rating of mental fatigue and related symptoms was primarily linked to processing speed and attention and processing speed was found to be the primary predictor for mental fatigue. The total sum of scores also correlated significantly with percentages for sick leave (Johansson, et al., 2009). Information processing speed is also the cognitive function most likely to be affected after a brain injury (Frencham et al., 2005; Madigan et al., 2000; Martin et al., 2000).

The self-assessment scale in combination with tests that primarily measure information processing speed and a high cognitive load on attention might make it possible to evaluate problems described by patients with mental fatigue, as subjective mental fatigue at least after mild TBI and TBI are suggested to primarily correlate with objectively measured information processing speed. If cognitive decline within these neuropsychological regions are evident, the mental loading can be even higher.

We now turn to the cellular level to visualise what happens during a mental process. We focus on the glutamate signalling under normal conditions and in disorders, preferentially infections or inflammations within the CNS, when the astroglial support is attenuated.

5. Astroglial support of neuronal glutamate signaling (figures 1 and 2)

It is estimated that the human brain consists of 10^{11} neurons and 3-5 times as many glial cells. One single neuron may have contacts with many thousand other neurons. Thus it is easy to understand that the human brain has the prerequisites for extensive communication with both the surrounding milieu and with other neurons within the brain. Glutamate is the most frequent excitatory transmitter, which is also involved in mental activities including learning and memory formation. When the transmitter has fulfilled its functions at the post-synaptic neuron, it must be removed to allow new impulse traffic. The astrocytes, the prominent supporting cell type in the CNS, regulate the extracellular glutamate levels ($[Glu]_{ec}$) and are thus responsible for clearing the extracellular space from excessive glutamate. It is generally considered that the $[Glu]_{ec}$ has to be maintained at approximately 1–3 μM in order to avoid excitotoxic actions of glutamate on neurons (Choi, 1992), and also to assure a high signal-to-noise ratio (high precision) in normal glutamate neurotransmission (Yudkoff et al., 1993). The astrocytes express high-affinity Na^+-dependent electrogenic transporters: the glutamate aspartate transporter (GLAST) and glutamate transporter 1 (GLT-1) which are most abundantly located on astrocyte processes surrounding synapses of glutamatergic neurons (Danbolt, 2001). GLT-1 is today considered as the most important transporter for removal and regulation of $[Glu]_{ec}$ at synaptic transmission. GLT-1 is expressed on astrocytes only in the presence of glutamatergic neurons (Björklund et al., 2010), and the amount and efficiency increase when there is a high neuronal activity (Perego et al., 2000) (figure 1).

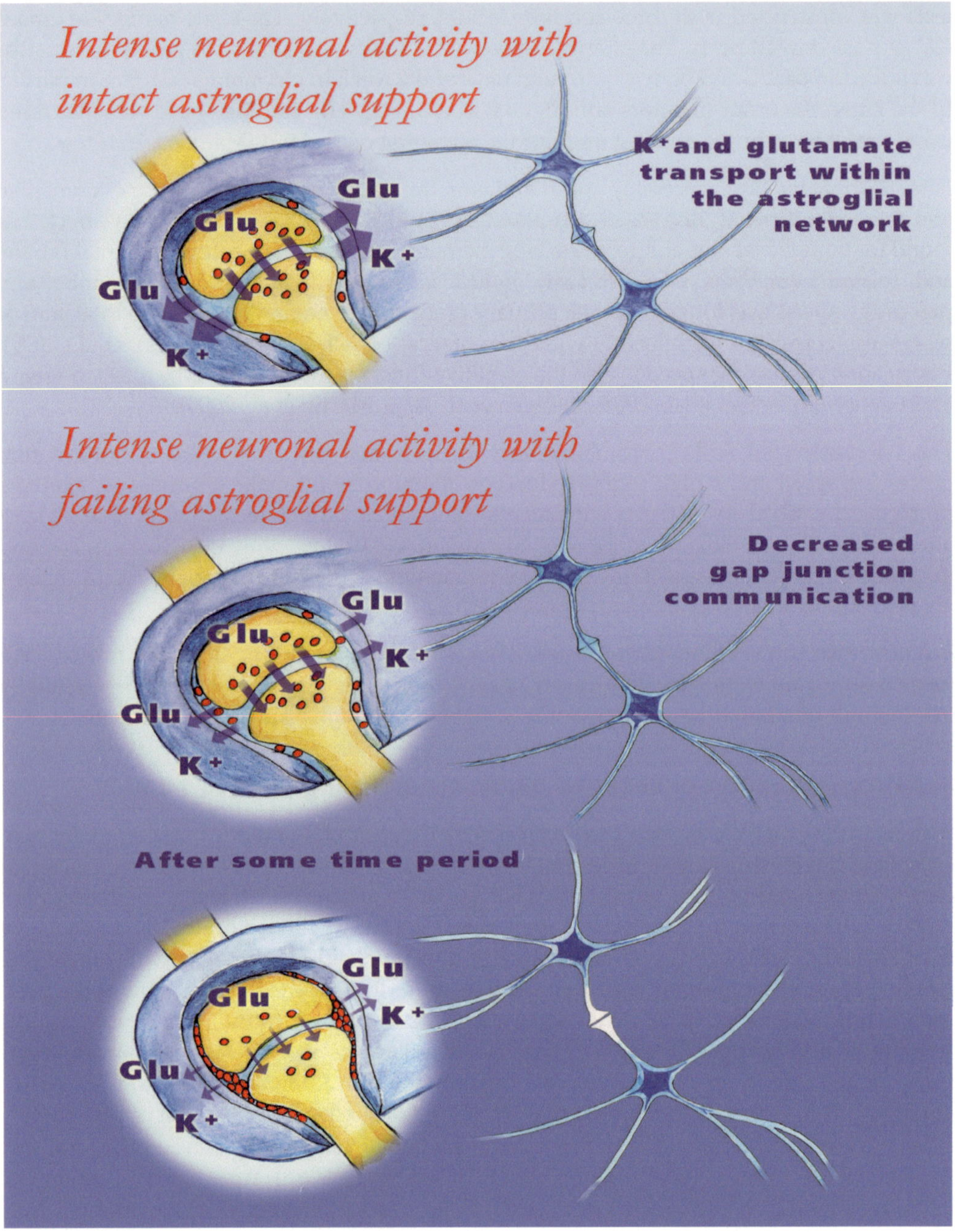

Fig. 1. Glutamate is released from the presynaptic terminal and affects postsynaptic glutamate receptors (left; upper figure). Thereafter glutamate is rapidly removed from the synaptic region by surrounding astroglial cells. A diminished astroglial glutamate uptake capacity leads to a decreased precision (signal-to-noise ratio) in the glutamatergic transmission (left; middle and lower figure). Astroglial networks that support neuronal glutamate signaling are shown to the right in the figures. (modified from Hansson & Rönnbäck, 2004 and drawn by Eva Kraft, Gothenburg, Sweden)

Let us make a simplified description of the situation around a neuron that is active in a mental process. This neuron is connected to other neurons in a network and signals are propagated from and to other neurons (figure 2). The propagation depends on the state of a number of synapses on the cell body and on the processes so that the neuron is polarized in a suitable way.

A great number of synapses could be activated in this process. Astroglial processes reach every synapse, and the astroglial cells regulate glutamate and ion levels in the synaptic cleft to set the proper sensitivity for an action potential (Hansson & Rönnbäck, 1995; 2003; Hertz & Zielke, 2004). When the astroglial cells take up glutamate their cell volume will increase somewhat, primarily due to osmosis, and normally this limited swelling is restored when the glutamate is transformed within the astroglial cell. If we perform intense mental activity, the neuron is reactivated frequently and the restoration done by the astrocytes will be delayed. In this situation the astrocytes can recruit help from other, nearby situated, astrocytes. The number of adjacent, activated neurons may also increase prominently. This may limit the support that can be provided from nearby astrocytes. If there is an intense neuronal activity for a longer period of time, the astroglial support can reach a state of saturation in which the transport capacity of extracellular substances is limited due to e.g. decreased extracellular space. As a consequence the neuronal polarization level will be continuously high, action potentials will be spontaneously triggered, and the mental precision will probably decrease - we experience fatigue. After a short break, however, we are mentally ready for new activities, or ready to continue the previously performed mental work.

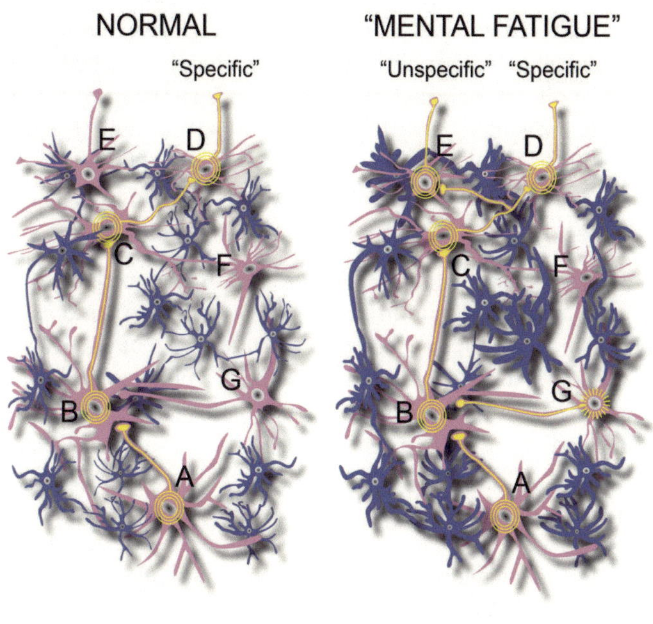

Fig. 2. Illustration of neuronal networks consisting of the nerve cells A-G (red) under physiological conditions (left figure). Cell A activates (yellow) B synaptically whereafter C, and later D is activated. Surrounding astroglial cells (blue) recognize the neuronal activity and interact with the neurons. The result will be that the "specific" response is carried forwards.

After a brain injury or other brain disorder (right figure) there could be a sprouting, which results in the activation of both neurons D and E by neuron C. Through the mechanism of glutamate "spill-over", and also due to the slightly increased level of extracellular glutamate, neuron G will be activated, which in turn lead to the activation of neuron B. The overall result will be activation of larger neuronal circuits, astroglial swelling, and "unspecific" signalling in addition to the "specific" one. Thus, the "noise" in the signaling is somewhat increased. The increased swelling of the glial cells further strengthens and reinforces these processes due to the decreased extracellular space.

6. Impaired astroglial glutamate uptake capacity in neuroinflammation

After brain injury the GLT-1 expression is down-regulated and the glutamate uptake impaired (Torp et al., 1995; Rao et al., 1998; Szymocha et al., 2000; Legay et al., 2003; Yi et al., 2004; Persson & Rönnbäck, 2012). The mechanisms underlying this down-regulation are not fully understood. The GLT-1 protein is sensitive for oxidative stress due to its content of cysteins that are sensitive to oxidative formation of cystein bridges. Furthermore, GLT-1 is sensitive to the acidic milieu and the pro-inflammatory cytokines TNF-alpha and IL-1beta (for ref, see Rönnbäck & Hansson, 2004).

7. Cellular mechanisms underlying mental fatigue – a hypothesis (figure 3)

If the astroglial fine-tuning of $[Glu]_{ec}$ is impaired, there would be decreased precision in the glutamate signalling. This is, according to our hypothesis, the basic cellular disturbance underlying the impaired concentration and memory capacity, which we experience as cognitive or mental fatigue (see Rönnbäck & Hansson, 2004). As a consequence, the signals taken into the brain will be handled in a less distinct way, resulting in ambiguous information. Due to its indistinct character, more information will be recognized as "new" by sensory brain centers, and will therefore be allowed to travel to the cerebral cortex and be processed there. The overall result may be that more, and larger, neuronal circuits would be activated over time (figure 2). With impaired GLT-1 function, local $[Glu]_{ec}$ could increase.

In CNS infections or inflammations, meningitis or encephalitis, pro-inflammatory cytokines are produced due to microglial activation (Andersson et al., 2005), and as GLT-1 is sensitive to TNF-alpha and also IL-1beta, the astroglial glutamate uptake capacity is impaired. Locally increased $[Glu]_{ec}$ could give rise to astroglial swelling, whereby the extracellular space shrinks (Sykova, 2001). The result would be disturbed fine-tuning of the glutamate signaling, and impaired transport of substances in the extracellular space (volume transmission). Astroglial swelling would give rise to relative depolarization of the astroglial cell membrane, with a further decreased astroglial glutamate uptake capacity, and in addition, a decreased capacity of the astrocytes to remove $[K^+]_{ec}$. Even moderately increased (up to 8–10 mM) $[K^+]_{ec}$ levels have been shown in experimental systems to inhibit glutamate release (Meeks & Mennerick, 2004). It should be noted that in states of decreased astroglial glutamate uptake capacity, even astroglial glucose uptake, and consequently the supply of metabolic substrates to the neurons, has been reported to decrease (see Hertz & Zielke, 2004). In addition, glutamate release from the presynaptic terminals could decrease due to impaired glutamine supply of the neurons. The result will be metabolic exhaustion and thereby decreased transmission.

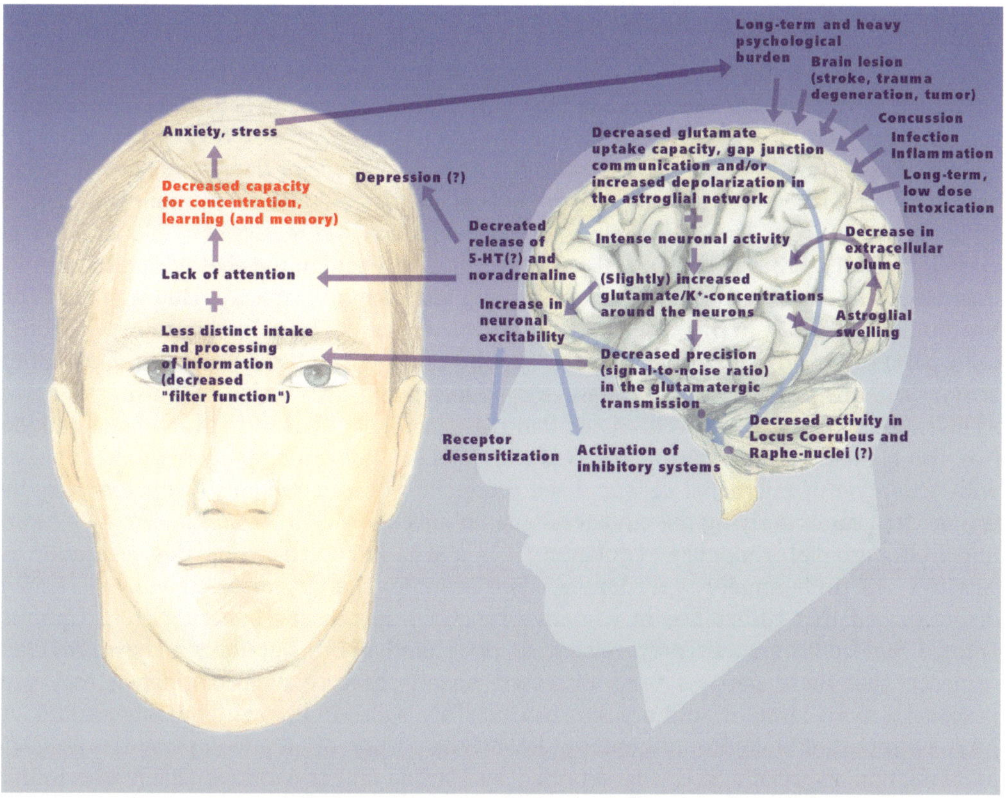

Fig. 3. A model for the development of mental fatigue due to brain disorder. Astroglial glutamate uptake capacity is impaired due to infection/inflammation, stroke or brain trauma (upper right in the figure). When there is an intense neuronal activity, this decreased capacity by the astroglial cells to clear extracellular glutamate levels could lead to impaired fine-tuning of glutamate and K^+ levels around the neurons. The result might be impaired precision (signal-to-noise ratio) in the glutamatergic transmission. Astroglial swelling will further impair the regulation of neuroactive substances in the extracellular space due to decreased extracellular space volume. Furthermore, it is known from animal experiments that increased neuronal excitability in the frontal lobe impair the activities in the Locus Coeruleus and the Raphe nuclei (Sara & Hervé-Minvielle, 1995). If this is the case even in humans, we could have a neurobiological basis for decreased attention, which is commonly experienced by the patient, due to decreased dopamine, 5-HT and noradrenaline levels. The person (left in the figure) might experience information intake and processing to be less distinct and in combination with the impaired attention, experience mental fatigue upon mental activity. Secondary anxiety and stress could aggravate the symptoms by interaction with the glucocorticoid system, which is also known to interact with astroglial glutamate regulation (Zschocke et al. 2005; Persson & Rönnbäck, 2012; drawn by Eva Kraft, Gothenburg, Sweden)

Our hypothesis, presented schematically in figure 3, can thus explain why persons with these mental fatigue symptoms could perform cognitive tasks well for short periods, but in situations with increased sensory stimulation, they become completely exhausted, and it takes a long time for them to recover their cognitive capacity.

8. Support for our hypothesis

It is well accepted today that, in addition to meningitis or encephalitis, ischemia, TBI as well as degenerative disorders are associated to neuroinflammation with activation of microglial cells and the production of cytokines within the CNS (see e.g. Persson & Rönnbäck, 2012 for review). Even in states of no obvious neuronal damage, like major depression, lack of sleep, and so called sickness-behavior, where the mental fatigue could be very prominent, there is an inflammatory reaction in the brain with the production and release of cytokines (see e.g. Hashioka, 2011). From experimental systems it is also well-known that administration of interleukin (IL)-1 can result in decreased learning and memory capacity (Huang et al., 2010; Imamura et al., 2011). In this respect it is of utmost interest to note that in states with long-term pain, in which the permeability of the BBB is shown to be increased, inflammatory activity with the production and release of cytokines in the CNS is also demonstrated. From a clinical point of view it is well known that these patients often suffer from mental fatigue (see also Hansson & Rönnbäck, 2004; Nijs et al., 2012). Thus, inflammation within the CNS with activation of microglial cells and the production of inflammatory mediators may be one mechanism underlying the mental fatigue, in which one cellular mechanism may be an impaired astroglial glutamate regulation. It is a well-known fact that this regulation is sensitive to inflammatory mediators. Furthermore, Lange and co-workers (2005) demonstrated that difficulties in cognitive functions in persons suffering from Chronic Fatigue Syndrome are not only related to poor motivation, but indeed they provided evidence that these persons used increased neural resource allocation when they are processing more complex auditory information. This is also in line with our suggestions. A further support of biological origin for at least some portion of fatigue in persons with CNS inflammation, especially SLE, was reported by Harboe and co-workers (2008) who found fatigue associated with cerebral white matter hyperintensities.

9. Can mental fatigue be treated?

Pathologic mental fatigue can be induced by CNS infections, inflammations or irreparable neuronal injuries. This is the case in MS, stroke and TBI, as well as in degenerative disorders. In these states it is of utmost importance to start treatment early, before new neural inter-connections are established (see Dancause et al., 2005; Hansson & Rönnbäck, 2003). It is important to diminish the risk for secondary anxiety. After infections or mild TBI, the mental fatigue can be prominent even in the absence of significant neuronal injury. Early information about the often good prognosis of the disorder is therefore important. In addition, it is important for the person to learn about the symptoms and his/her own possibilities to limit the symptoms for instance by avoiding stress, and thereby avoid getting into mental exhaustion. Drugs which inhibit inflammation and cell swelling might be of value if our hypothesis turns out to be correct. Furthermore, inhibition of pro-inflammatory cytokines is probably of value in order to strengthen the glutamate uptake capacity by the astroglial cells. Such drugs do not exist in the market today and it is interesting to note that late results have shown that local glutamate levels dictates adenosine receptor regulation of neuroinflammation (Dai et al., 2010) suggesting the requirement of a fine-tuning of drugs being effective in the treatment of mental fatigue. However, promising results at least concerning the wakefulness were reported by Rabkin and co-workers (2011) using Armodafinil. We have tested a mindfulness-based stress reduction (MBSR) program on stroke or TBI victims with promising results (Johansson et al., in preparation). It has to be investigated whether such therapy is valuable even for persons suffering from long-lasting mental fatigue after a meningitis or encephalitis.

10. Conclusion

Fatigue, especially mental fatigue, is common in states with infection or inflammation in the central nervous system (CNS) (Schmidt et al., 2006; Berg et al., 2010) as well as after a stroke (Choi-Kwon & Kim, 2011) or in degenerative diseases as Parkinson´s disease (Friedman et al., 2011). For most persons the fatigue attenuates timely in parallel with the alleviation of the infection, but in a number of persons the mental fatigue may remain over months or years, even after recovery from the infection. Characteristic for this mental fatigue is that the person is able to be mentally active just for short periods, and a prominent fatigability may arise upon even moderate mental activity. Typically the recovery time, i.e. the time to get the mental energy back, is long. It may be difficult for the person to go back to work, as our high-technology society with its increasing demands on peoples´ mental capacity does not accept anything but full engagement, even over time.

From a neurobiological point of view, the mental fatigue could be due to impairment of information processing capacity in the brain. Information processing is energy consuming and requires wide-spread and specific neural signaling. In states of brain dysfunction the information processing capacity is reduced.

In meningitis or encephalitis there is a neuro-inflammation with production of cytokines and other inflammatory compounds. It is well known that several of these substances impair the astroglial capacity to remove glutamate from the extracellular space. Glutamate signaling is essential for information processing in the brain, including learning and memory formation. Astroglial cells are responsible for the fine-tuning of extracellular glutamate which is considered necessary to keep a high efficiency in the information handling within the CNS.

We here extend our previously presented hypothesis on probable cellular mechanisms underlying mental fatigue after brain trauma and suggest that a remaining slightly impaired astroglial glutamate handling may at least partly explain long-lasting mental fatigue after recovery from a meningitis or encephalitis. The reason that the mental fatigue may be long-lasting in a number of such victims, but far from all, is not known (see Wait & Schoeman, 2010). Genetic or pre-morbid factors or states could be of importance (see also Lundin et al., 2006; Loeb et al., 2008).

11. Acknowledgements

The work performed in the authors´ laboratory was supported by the Swedish Research Council and by LUA/ALF from the Sahlgrenska University Hospital and Edit Jacobson's Foundation.

12. References

Abbott, N.J., Rönnbäck, L. & Hansson, E. (2006). Astrocyte-endothelial interactions at the blood-brain barrier. *Nature Rev Neurosci,* 7,41-53.

American Psychiatric Association, *Diagnostic and statistical menual of mental disorders,* 4th ed. Washington DC: American Psychiatric Association, 1994.

Andersson, A.K., Rönnbäck, L. & Hansson, E. (2005). Lactate induces tumour necrosis factor-alpha, interleukin-6 and interleukin-1beta release in microglial- and astroglial-enriched primary cultures. *J Neurochem,* 93, 1327-1333.

Ashman, T. A., Spielman, L. A., Hibbard, M. R., Silver, M. J., Chandna, T., & Gordon, W. A. (2004). Psychiatric challenges in the first 6 years after traumatic brain injury: Cross-sequential analyses of axis I disorder. *Arch Phys Med Rehabil, 85*(Suppl 2), S36-S42.

Berg, P.J., Smallfield, S. & Svien, L. (2010). An investigation of depression and fatigue post West Nile virus infection. *S D Med,* 63, 127-129.

Björklund, U., Persson, M., Rönnbäck, L. & Hansson, E. (2010). Primary cultures from cerebral cortex and hippocampus enriched in glutamatergic and GABAergic neurons. *Neurochem Res,* 35, 1733-1742.

Chaudhuri, A. & Behan, P.O. (2000). Fatigue and basal ganglia. *J Neurol Sci,*179,34-42.

Chaudhuri, A., & Behan, P. O. (2004). Fatigue in neurological disorders. *Lancet 363,* 978-988.

Choi, D.W. (1992). Excitotoxic cell death. *J Neurobiol,* 23,1261-1276.

Choi-Kwon, S. & Kim, J.S. (2011). Poststroke fatigue: an emerging, critical issue in stroke medicine. *Int J Stroke,* 6, 328-336.

Dai, S.S., Zhou, Y.G., Li, W., An, J.H., Yang, N., Chen, X.Y., Xiong, R.P., Liu, P., Zhao, Y., Shen, H.Y., Zhu, P.F. & Chen J.F. (2010) Local glutamate level dictates adenosine A2A receptor regulation of neuroinflammation and traumatic brain injury. *J Neurosci,* 30, 5802-5810.

Danbolt, N.C. (2001). Glutamate uptake. *Prog Neurobiol,* 65,1-105.

Dancause, N., Barbay, S., Frost, S.B., Plautz, E.J., Chen, D., Zoubina, E.V., Stowe, A.M. & Nudo, R.J. (2005). Extensive cortical rewiring after brain injury. *J Neurosci,* 25:10167-10179.

DeLuca, J. (ed.) (2005). Fatigue as a Window to the Brain. A Bradford Book, The MIT Press, Cambridge, Massachusetts, London, England, 336pp.

DeLuca, J., & Kalmar, J. H. (Eds.). (2007). *Information processing speed: How fast, how slow, and how come? In: Information processing speed in clinical population*: Taylor and Francis group, New York.

Ellis, D. C., Kaplan, E., & Kramer, J. H. (Eds.). (2001). *Delis-Kaplan Executive Function System – D-KEFS.* San Antonio, TX: The Psychological Corporation.

Frencham, K. A. R., Fox, A. M., & Maybery, M. T. (2005). Neuropsychological studies of mild traumatic brain injury: a meta-analytical review of research since 1995. *J Clin Exp Neuropsychol, 27*(3), 334-351.

Friedman, J.H., Abrantes, A. & Sweet, L.H. (2011). Fatigue in Parkinson´s disease. *Expert Opin Pharmacother* 12, 1999-2007

Hansson, E. & Rönnbäck, L. (1995). Astrocytes in glutamate neurotransmission. *FASEB J,* 9,343-50.

Hansson, E. & Rönnbäck, L. (2003). Glial neuronal signaling in the central nervous system. *FASEB J,* 17,341-348.

Hansson, E. & Rönnbäck, L. (2004). Altered neuronal-glial signaling in glutamatergic transmission as a unifying mechanism in chronic pain and mental fatigue. *Neurochem Res,* 29,989-996.

Harboe, E., Greve, O.J., Beyer, M., Goransson, L.G., Tjensvoll, A.B., Maroni, S. & Omdal, R. (2008). Fatigue is associated with cerebral white matter hyperintensities in patients with systemic lupus erythematosus. *J Neurol Neurosurg Psychiatry,* 79, 199-201.

Hashioka, S. (2011). Antidepressants and neuroinflammation: can antidepressants calm glial rage down? *Mini Rev Med Chem,* 11, 555-564.

Hertz, L. & Zielke, H.R. (2004). Astrocytic control of glutamatergic activity: astrocytes as stars of the show. *TRENDS in Neurosci,* 27,735-43.

Huang, Z.B. & Sheng, G.Q. (2010). Interleukin-1β with learning and memory. *Neurosci Bull,* 26, 455-468.

Imamura, Y., Wang, H., Matsumoto, N., Muroya, T., Shimazaki, J., Ogura, H. & Shimazu, T. (2011). Interleukin-1β causes long-term potentiation deficiency in a mouse model of septic encephalopathy. *Neuroscience,* 187,63-69

Johansson, B., Berglund, P., & Rönnbäck, L. (2009). Mental fatigue and impaired information processing after mild and moderate traumatic brain injury. *Brain Injury, 23*(13-14), 1027-1040.

Johansson, B. & Rönnbäck, L. (2012). Mental fatigue; a common long term consequence after a brain injury. InTech, ISBN Brain Injury - Functional Aspects, Rehabilitation and Prevention (ISBN 979-953-307-025-3), Vienna, Austria.

Johnson, S.K., DeLuca, J. & Natelson, B.H. (1996). Depression in fatiguing illness: comparing patients with chronic fatigue syndrome, multiple sclerosis and depression. *J Affect Disord,* 39, 21-30.

King, N. S., Crawford, S., Wenden, F. J., Moss, N. E. G., & Wade, D. T. (1995). The Rivermead post concussion symptoms questionnaire: a measure of symptoms commonly experienced after head injury and its reliability. *J Neurol Neurosurg Psychiatr, 24,* 587-592.

Lange, G., Steffener, J., Cook, D.B., Bly, B.M., Christodoulou, C., Liu, W.C., Deluca, J. & Natelson, B.H. (2005). Objective evidence of cognitive complaints in Chronic Fatigue Syndrome: a BOLD fMRI study of verbal working memory. *Neuroimage,* 26, 513-524.

Legay, V., Deleage, C., Beaulieux, F., Giraudon, P., Aymard, M. & Lina, B. (2003). Impaired glutamate uptake and EAAT2 downregulation in an enterovirus chronically infected human glial cell line. *Eur J Neurosci,* 17,1820-1828.

Lerdal, A., Gay, C.L., Aoulzerat, B.E., Portillo, C.J. & Lee, K.A. (2011). Patterns of morning and evening fatigue among adults with HIV/AIDS. *J Clin Nurs,* 20, 2204-2216.

Lezak, M. D., Howieson, D. B., & Loring, D. W. (Eds.). (2004). *Neuropsychological assessment* (4th ed.). New York:: Oxford University Press.

Lindqvist, G., & Malmgren, H. (1993). Organic mental disorders as hypothetical pathogenetic processes. *Acta Psychiatr Scand, 88*(suppl 373), 5-17.

Loeb, M., Hanna, S., Nicolle, L., Eyles, J., Elliott, S., Rathbone, M., Drebot, M., Neupane, B., Fearon, M., & Mahony, J. (2008). Prognosis after West Nile virus infection. *Ann Intern Med,* 149, 232-241.

Lundin, A., de Boussard, C., Edman, G., & Borg, J. (2006). Symptoms and disability until 3 months after mild TBI. *Brain Injury 20*(8), 799-806.

Madigan, N. K., DeLuca, J., Diamond, B. J., Tramontano, G., & Averill, A. (2000). Speed of information processing in traumatic brain injury: modality-specific factors. *J Head Trauma Rehabil 15*(3), 943-956.

Madison, S. (2003). *Läsdiagnos.* Lund: Läs och skrivcentrum.

Martin, T. A., Donders, J., & Thompson, E. (2000). Potential of and problems with new measures of psychometric intelligence after traumatic brain injury. *Rehabil Psychol, 45*(4), 402-408.

Meeks, J.P. & Mennerick, S. (2004). Selective effects of potassium elevations on glutamate signaling and action potential conduction in hippocampus. *J Neurosci,* 24,197-206.

Nijs, J., Meeus, M., Van Oosterwijck, J., Ickmans, K., Moorkens, G., Hans, G. & De Clerck, L.S. (2012). In the mind or in the brain? Scientific evidence for central sensitisation in chronic fatigue syndrome. *Eur J Clin Invest,* 42, 203-212.

Pence, B.W., Barroso, J., Leserman, J., Harmon, J.L., & Salahuddin, N. (2008). Measuring fatigue in people living with HIV/AIDS: psychometric characteristics of the HIV-related fatigue scale. *AIDS Care,* 20, 829-837.

Perego, C., Vanoni, C., Bossi, M., Massari, S., Basudev, H., Longhi, R. & Pietrini, G. (2000). The GLT-1 and GLAST glutamate transporters are expressed on morphologically distinct astrocytes and regulated by neuronal activity in primary hippocampal cocultures. *J Neurochem,* 75,1076-1084.

Persson, M. & Rönnbäck, L. (2012). Microglial self-defence mediated through GLT-1 and glutathione. *Amino Acids,* 42, 207-219

Rabkin, J.G., McElhiney, M.C. & Rabkin, R. (2011). Treatment of HIV-related fatigue with Armodafinil: a placebo-controlled randomized trial. *Psychosomatics,* 52, 328-336.

Rao, V.L., Baskaya, M.K., Dogan, A., Rothstein, J.D. & Dempsey, R.J. (1998). Traumatic brain injury down-regulates glial glutamate transporter (GLT-1 and GLAST) proteins in rat brain. *J Neurochem,* 70,2020-2027.

Reitan, R. M., & Wolfson, D. (Eds.). (1985). *The Halstead-Reitan neuropsychological Test Battery. Theory and clinical interpretation*. Tucson. AZ: Neuropsychology Press.

Rödholm, M., Starmark, J.-E., Svensson, E., & von Essen, C. (2001). Asteno-emotional disorder after aneurysmal SAH: reliability, symptomatology and relation to outcome. *Acta Neurol Scand, 103,* 379-385.

Rönnbäck, L. & Hansson, E. (2004). On the potential role of glutamate transport in mental fatigue. *J Neuroinflammation,* 1, 22.

Sara, S.J. & Hervé-Minvielle, A. (1995). Inhibitory influence of frontal cortex on locus coeruleus neurons. *Proc Natl Acad Sci U S A,* 92, 6032-6036.

Schmidt, H., Heimann, B., Djukic, M., Mazurek, C., Fels, C., Wallesch, C.W. & Nau, R. (2006). Neuropsychological sequelae of bacterial and viral meningitis. *Brain* 129, 333-345.

Silver, J. M., Mc Allister, J. W., & Arciniegas, D. B. (2009). Depression and cognitive complaints following mild traumatic brain injury. *Am J Psychiatry, 166*(6), 653-661.

Syková, E. (2001). Glial diffusion barriers during aging and pathological states. *Prog Brain Res,* 132, 339-363.

Szymocha, R., Akaoka, H., Dutuit, M., Malcus, C., Didier-Bazes, M., Belin, M.F. & Giraudon, P. (2000). Human T-cell lymphotropic virus type 1-infected T lymphocytes impair catabolism and uptake of glutamate by astrocytes via Tax-1 and tumor necrosis factor alpha. *J Virol,* 74,6433-6441.

Torp, R., Lekieffre, D., Levy, L.M., Haug, F.M., Danbolt, N.C., Meldrum, B.S. & Ottersen, O.P. (1995). Reduced postischemic expression of a glial glutamate transporter, GLT-1, in the rat hippocampus. *Exp Brain Res,* 103,51-58

Wait, J.W. & Schoeman, J.F. (2010). Behaviour profiles after tuberculous meningitis. *J Trop Pediatr,* 56, 166-171.

Wechsler, D. (Ed.). (2004). *Wechsler Adult Intelligence Scale – third edition, WAIS-III NI, Swedish version.* Stockholm: Pearson Assessment.

Whelan-Goodinson, R., Ponsford, J., & Schönberger, M. (2009). Validity of the hospital anxiety and depression scale to assess depression and anxiety following traumatic brain injury as compared with the structured clinical inteview for DSM-IV. *J Affect Disorder.* 114, 94-102

Yi, J.H., Pow, D.V. & Hazell, A.S. (2005). Early loss of the glutamate transporter splice-variant GLT-1v in rat cerebral cortex following lateral fluid-percussion injury. *Glia,* 49,121-133.

Yudkoff, M., Nissim, I., Daikhin, Y., Lin, Z.P., Nelson, D., Pleasure, D. & Erecinska, M. (1993). Brain glutamate metabolism: neuronal-astroglial relationships. *Dev Neurosci,* 15,343-350.

Zschocke, J., Bayatti, N., Clement, A.M., Witan, H., Figiel, M., Engele, J. & Behl, C. (2005). Differential promotion of glutamate transporter expression and function by glucocorticoids in astrocytes from various brain regions. *J Biol Chem,* 280,34924-34932.

28

Physiological Response as Biomarkers of Adverse Effects of the Psychosocial Work Environment

Åse Marie Hansen[1,2], Annie Hogh[2] and Eva Gemzøe Mikkelsen[3]
[1]*The National Research Centre for the Working Environment, Copenhagen,*
[2]*University of Copenhagen, Copenhagen*
[3]*CRECEA A/S,*
Denmark

1. Introduction

Throughout medical history, measurement of hormones and other physiological parameters have been used in clinical settings with the purpose of detecting and monitoring progress of disease. During the past three or four decades, however, hormones and other physiological effect markers have been increasingly used in occupational settings for purposes of assessing the effects of psychosocial circumstances and of occupational stress. Accordingly, the focus has partly drifted from detecting and monitoring disease to including the detection and monitoring of precursors of disease and risk factors for poor health in otherwise healthy subjects before medical manifests. Because the majority of the workforce is in good health, differences in hormonal and other physiological parameters are often expected to be less pronounced than the differences that typically render clinical interest. Salivary cortisol has increasingly been used in the study of the responsiveness of the hypothalamic pituitary adrenal (HPA) axis in occupational stress studies and employed in both field studies and experimental studies (for review see (Chida & Steptoe, 2009)). The reason for the increasing use of salivary cortisol in occupational settings is that it is a simple, non-invasive, harm-free and pain-free measure that allows the longitudinal study of HPA-axis activity without substantial interference with the subject's normal habits and environment. Since cortisol in saliva is stable for at least two week, it provides the possibility of self-sampling and mailing the samples by post (Garde & Hansen, 2005b). This chapter will use salivary cortisol as an example of a biomarker of adverse effects of work stress.

The biological pathways linking stress and health need to be better investigated (Kudielka & Wüst, 2010). In the understanding of the adaptation processes and in the pathogenesis of chronic diseases and adverse psychosocial working environment endocrine factors have become increasingly relevant. Exposure to adverse psychosocial working environment initiates a number of physiological reactions, regulated by hormones (Henry, 1992). The locus coeruleus-noradrenaline/autonomic (sympathetic) nervous system (Chrousos & Gold, 1992) and the hypothalamus-pituitary-adrenal (HPA) axis are the major physiological stress response systems in the body (Chrousos & Gold, 1992; Gold et al., 1995; Heim et al., 2000;

McEwen, 1998; McEwen & Seeman, 1999; Raison & Miller, 2003; Tsigos & Chrousos, 2002). The characterization of an individual's HPA axis activity, reactivity pattern to psychosocial stress and inter- and intra-individual variability appear to be of major interest (Hellhammer et al., 2009; Mason, 1968). Measurement of hormones and other physiological parameters have been used in clinical settings with the purpose of detecting and monitoring progress of disease. During the past three or four decades, however, hormones and other physiological effect markers have been increasingly used in occupational settings for purposes of assessing the effects of psychosocial circumstances and of occupational stress. According to Selye *"stress is the nonspecific response of the body to any demand"* (Selye, 1975). The stress response may be identified as changes in physiological indicators, e.g. endogenous substances measurable in blood, urine or saliva. Physiological indicators are therefore potential intermediate biomarkers of effect as defined by the World Health Organization (WHO) (1993): *'Biomarker for effect: a measurable biochemical, physiological, behavioural or other alteration within an organism, that depending upon the magnitude, can be recognized as associated with an established or possible health impairment or disease'.* However, the majority of the workforce is in good health, and differences in hormonal and other physiological parameters are often expected to be less pronounced than the differences that typically render clinical interest, such as manifestation of disease.

The aim of the present chapter is twofold: One is to provide the reader with insight into the present evidence for how different physiological responses may be used as potential biomarkers of the psychosocial working environment and health. The other aim is to address and thereby bring to awareness to potential sources of variations and confounders.

2. Job stress theories

The Job Demand–Control model identifies two crucial job aspects: job demand and job control (Karasek & Theorell, 1990). Job demand refers to the workload, and has been operationalized mainly in terms of time pressure and role conflicts. Job control refers to the person's ability to control his or her work activities. The job content questionnaire (JCQ) has been used to characterize the psychosocial working environment according to the Job Demand-Control model (Karasek et al., 1998). The underlying theoretical explanation may be that low control causes chronic disease through chronic de-regulation of our highly integrated physiological systems (Karasek, 2006). The Effort-Reward Imbalance (ERI) model is a model of occupational stress, focusing on a negative trade-off between experienced 'costs' and 'gains' at work. In this model, high ratio of effort spent relative to rewards received in terms of money, esteem, job security, and career opportunities, elicits sustained stress responses and ill health (Siegrist et al., 2004).

The cognitive theory of stress (CATS) offers a psychobiological explanation for the assumed relationship between stressful events and health (Reme et al., 2008; Ursin & Eriksen, 2004). CATS incorporate the cognitive evaluation of the situation and a core element in CATS is expectancy outcome. It is the person's experience and evaluation of demands and expectancies of outcomes that determine whether the demands cause a stress response which may affect the health. In CATS, coping with stressors is defined as positive outcome expectancy and is related to psycho-physiology. In a stressful situation, it is not enough with control. People must expect that this control leads to a good result. If this is not the case they may develop hopelessness (Reme et al., 2008).

According to the CATS a stress response is a general alarm in a homeostatic system, producing general and unspecific neurophysiological activation from one level of arousal to more arousal (Ursin & Eriksen, 2004). The stress response occurs whenever there is something missing, for instance a homeostatic imbalance, or a threat to homeostasis and life of the organism. The stress response, therefore, is an essential and necessary physiological response. The unpleasantness of the alarm is no health threat. However, if sustained, the response may lead to illness and disease through established pathophysiological processes ('allostatic load') (McEwen & Wingfield, 2003). It is the person's experience and evaluation of demands and expectancies of outcomes that determine whether the demands cause a stress response which may affect the health.

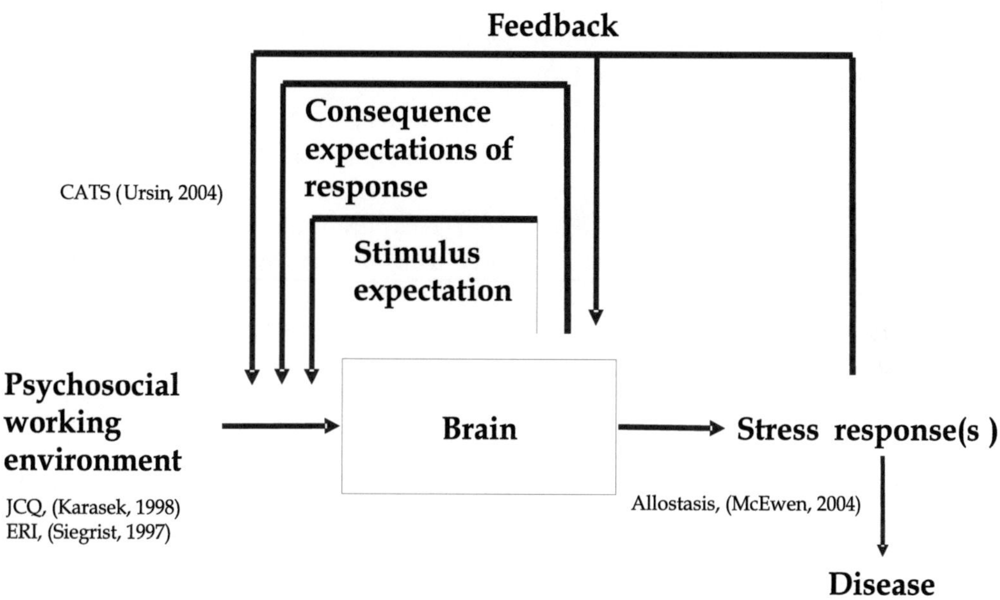

Fig. 1. A model of the association between the psychosocial working environment and disease.

Figure 1 presents a model of how the psychosocial working environment in theory may lead to disease. Theoretically, stress reactions may affect health either by a direct biological, prolonged physiological activation and lack of restitution, or by affecting health through lifestyle and health behaviours. The stress response occurs when homeostasis is threatened or perceived to be threatened and is mediated by the stress system. Cortisol is an indicator of the responsiveness of the HPA axis. Cortisol is a natural energy-releasing hormone with a distinct diurnal rhythm being highest in the morning and decreasing to the lowest in the evening. The acute stress response is in that sense a healthy response that adapts the organism to handle a challenge. However, prolonged stress leads over time to wear-and-tear on the body (allostatic load) (McEwen, 2004). Hormones and other mediators, such as neurotransmitters, cytokines, and other hormones are essential for adaption to challenges of daily life as well a major life stressors. One potential pathway to disease is when hormones and other mediators are not turned off when the stress is over. (McEwen, 2004). Frankenhaueser and Johansson (1986) studied excretion of adrenaline in urine during the day and in the evening among office workers before during and after a period of overtime work. Urinary adrenaline was consistently elevated during the overtime period and 4 weeks after the overtime period ended (Frankenhaeuser & Johansson, 1986). Increased risk of cardiovascular diseases has been found among employees performing mentally straining work (Karasek et al., 1981; LaCroix & Haynes, 1984; Pieper et al., 1989), monotonous work (Christensen, 1986; Kristensen, 1989; Putz-Anderson et al., 1992), as well as a high pace and shiftwork (Kristensen, 1989). Debilitated immune defence system may lead to cancer, infections and allergy. Long-term stress has been shown to influence the immune system and susceptibility to infection (Cohen & Williamson, 1991).

3. Early indicators of psychosocial work environment and health – exposure to workplace bullying as an example

Stressful and poorly organized work environments as well as deficiencies in leadership may facilitate work-related bullying and negative behaviour either directly or by creating a work climate in which bullying can flourish. In Denmark, it has been estimated that 8.3% of the working population between 20 and 59 years of age has been subjected to bullying within the past year. Of these, 1.6% reported frequent bullying, that is, weekly or daily (Ortega et al., 2008). Similar results have been reported in other countries (Lallukka et al., 2011; Matthiesen & Einarsen, 2007; Niedhammer et al., 2009). The most studied health outcomes of bullying are psychological symptoms and emotional reactions such as depression, burnout, anxiety, and aggression. However, psychosomatic and musculoskeletal health complaints have also been in focus (Hogh et al., 2010).

Systematic negative behaviour at work such as bullying or mobbing may have devastating effects on the health and well-being of the exposed individuals. Previous research covers cross-sectional studies, a few case-control studies and clinical interviews, as well as recent longitudinal studies. The early cross-sectional studies found correlations between exposure to bullying and chronic fatigue, psychosomatic, psychological and physical symptoms, general stress, insomnia, and mental stress reactions etc. (for reviews see e.g., (Dofradottir & Høgh, 2002; Einarsen & Mikkelsen, 2003; Moayed et al., 2006)). Common symptoms such as musculo-skeletal complaints, anxiety, irritability and depression were reported by targets in different European countries (Einarsen et al., 1996; Niedl, 1996; O'Moore et al., 1998; Zapf et al., 1996). Some victims displayed a pattern of symptoms indicative of Posttraumatic Stress Disorder (PTSD) (Björkqvist et al., 1994; Einarsen et al., 1999; Leymann & Gustafsson, 1996; Mikkelsen & Einarsen, 2002). Self-hatred and suicidal thoughts have also reported (Einarsen et al., 1994; Thylefors, 1987). Qualitative studies (Kile, 1990; Mikkelsen & Iversen, 2002; O'Moore et al., 1998; Price Spratlen, 1995; Thylefors, 1987) have demonstrated consequences such as reduced self-confidence, low self-worth, shyness, an increased sense of vulnerability as well as feelings of guilt and self-contempt. Moreover, some targets reported that their physical health and mental well-being had been permanently damaged (Mikkelsen, 2001). Longitudinal studies offer the possibility of measuring exposure and effects at different time points thus making it easier to conclude on the direction of the association from exposure to effect. Two recent Norwegian longitudinal studies have found that bullying predicts mental distress two years later (Finne et al., 2011; Nielsen et al., 2011). A longitudinal Finnish hospital study of primarily female employees showed a much higher risk of cardiovascular disease for targets of prolonged bullying as well as a four times higher risk of developing depressive symptoms. The longer time the bullying had taken place the higher risk of depression. (Kivimäki et al, 2003). Two Danish studies showed long-term health effects of exposure to bullying. For instance that exposure to bullying behaviour such as nasty teasing may generate both early and long-term stress reaction as shown in a 5-year follow-up study of the Danish working population; and that being bullied during your education may have health effects one year later as demonstrated by a prospective study of health care workers in care of the elderly (Høgh et al., 2007). Finally, longitudinal studies have also shown an increase in sickness absence among bullied targets (Clausen et al., 2011; Kivimäki et al., 2000; Ortega et al., 2011), as well as a risk of ending up on early retirement pension (Dellve et al., 2003)

According to transactional stress models, the nature and severity of emotional reactions following exposure to bullying may be a function of a dynamic interplay between event characteristics and individual appraisal- and coping processes. Definitions of bullying at work commonly entail descriptions that emphasize prolonged exposure to interpersonal acts of a negative nature, with which the target is unable to cope. These negative acts may be person related and/or work related. Together, these factors are likely to make up a highly stressful situation characterized by lack of control. Attributions of control and predictability are salient features of the individual's appraisal processes (Joseph, 1999; Lazarus, 1999). In transactional models such as the cognitive activation theory of stress (CATS) (Ursin & Eriksen, 2004) and the allostasis model (McEwen, 2004) the link between cognitive processes and physiology is emphasized. Yet, until now only few studies have studied the physiological consequences of bullying.

The stress response is the activation of the autonomic nervous system and hypothalamo-pituitary-adrenal (HPA) axis. Activation is a normal response and as such not unhealthy. However, inadequate or excessive adrenocortical and autonomic function is deleterious for health and survival. It is when the "fight/flight" response occurs too frequently or is greatly prolonged that we begin to experience the negative effects of stress. This prolonged elevation may be due to anxiety, to constant exposure to adverse environments involving interpersonal conflict, and to changes in life-style and health-related behaviours that result from being under chronic stress (McEwen, 2007). Recent research has pointed to a functional link between stress, disturbed sleep, psychiatric disorders, ageing, and neuroendocrine dysfunctions. In particular, elevated plasma cortisol levels have been shown in physiological ageing and patients with psychiatric disorders. Salivary cortisol has increasingly been used to study occupational stress and the responsiveness of the HPA-axis in both field studies and experimental studies (Aardal-Eriksson et al., 1999; Evans & Steptoe, 2001; Kirschbaum et al., 1989; van Eck et al., 1996; Zeier, 1994).

A few studies have addressed the physiological consequence of workplace bullying with biological measurements among targets who were still working (Hansen et al., 2006; Hansen et al., 2011; Kudielka & Kern, 2004). Kudielka and Kern presented tentative evidence of an altered circadian cycle of cortisol secretion among targets. Likewise, Hansen and colleagues observed signs of an altered HPA-axis activity among 22 targets manifested as a lower excreted amount of salivary cortisol in the morning (Hansen et al., 2006) and in among 161 frequently and occasionally occupationally active bullied persons (Hansen et al., 2011). Recently results pointing in the same direction were reported among young adults in as much as salivary cortisol levels and systolic blood pressure were lower in male targets who reported having no feelings of anger about their experience compared to controls and those who did report anger (Hamilton et al., 2008). While these observations are interesting and potentially clarifying as regards to how bullying might get "under the skin", it is equally clear that the study designs and methods used have limitations. In the Hansen et al (2006) study the definition of bullying did not account for frequency or duration, which are often considered important aspects despite controversies as to how they should be incorporated in a definition (Leymann, 1996; Zapf & Einarsen, 2005). A recent study of a large number of occupationally active persons was designed to counter methodological weaknesses inherent in previous studies involving salivary cortisol (Hansen et al., 2011). Results showed that frequently bullied employees, irrespective of gender had poorer psychological health and a lower level of salivary cortisol compared to a non-bullied reference group. Occasionally bullied employees only had a poorer psychological health compared to a reference group. These findings underline results reported among young adults (Hamilton et al., 2008) where the most affected individuals showed long-term effects on salivary cortisol.

4. The physiological response and the psychosocial working environment

Exposure to psychosocial stressors initiates a number of physiological reactions, regulated by hormones. Endocrine factors have become increasingly relevant for the understanding of the adaptation processes and in the pathogenesis of chronic diseases caused by occupational stressors. An intricate network of hormones and hormone-like activities is implicated in the stress response. Until now, neuro-endocrinological parameters have been widely used to estimate the biological effects of stress in field research.

A recent review compiled the literature on the psychosocial working environment and biological measures in blood and urine (Hansen et al., 2009). Job demands and job control were the most intensely studied factors of the psychosocial work environment. The result was clearest on HbA_{1c}, where all studies reported positive associations to both job demands (Cesana et al., 1985; Grossi et al., 2003; Hansen et al., 2003a; Kawakami et al., 2000) and job control (Grossi et al., 2003; Hansen et al., 2003a; Kawakami et al., 2000; Riese et al., 2000). Concentrations of testosterone were negatively associated with job demands (Hansen et al., 2003b) and job control (Berg et al., 1992; Hansen et al., 2003a; Theorell et al., 1990), whereas concentrations of fibrinogen were positively associated with job demands in all population based studies (Clays et al., 2005; Kittel et al., 2002; Steptoe et al., 2003; Tsutsumi et al., 1999), but not in workplace studies (Ishizaki et al., 2001; Riese et al., 2000). The result were mixed when evaluating prolactin in blood where both negative associations to job demands (Hansen et al., 2003b; Ohlson et al., 2001; Su, 2001), and positive associations between prolactin and job control were found (Berg et al., 1992; Hansen et al., 2003a; Ohlson et al., 2001; Su, 2001; Theorell et al., 1990; Theorell et al., 1993).

Only few studies were included on the effort reward model with mixed effect. One of two studies found cholesterol to be positively associated with effort reward (Kobayashi et al., 2005; Vrijkotte et al., 1999). No association between cortisol, fibrinogen and effort reward were found (Irie et al., 2004; Vrijkotte et al., 1999).

Concerning leadership five studies found a positive association with cortisol, one study when reporting poor leadership (Härenstam & Theorell, 1990), three when lacking of social support (Härenstam & Theorell, 1990; Payne et al., 1984; Schnorpfeil et al., 2003) and a single study on low job satisfaction (Payne et al., 1984). A positive association with concentrations of HbA_{1c} was found in three studies of poor social support (Grossi et al., 2003; Hansen et al., 2003a; Kawakami et al., 2000) and one of low job satisfaction (Kawakami et al., 1989).

Six studies found a positive association of catecholamines with organisational factors; two associated monotony and high work pace to catecholamines (Lundberg et al., 1989; Timio et al., 1979) where four studies found a positive association between catecholamines and having shift work (Fujiwara et al., 2004; Fujiwara et al., 1992; Levitt & Derrick, 1991; Mulders et al., 1982). Positive associations with HbA_{1C} were found for both having shift work (Cesana et al., 1985) and organizational changes where the participants rated their psychosocial working environment poorer at follow-up (Netterstrøm & Hansen, 2000). Low testosterone was found among employees having shift work (Axelsson et al., 2003; Touitou et al., 1990).

In summary the above mentioned studies point in the direction of adverse psychosocial working environment being associated with increased HbA_{1c} and fibrinogen in blood and decreased serum testosterone indicating an increased catabolic activity and decreased anabolic activity.

5. Potential variation and confounders in physiological response to adverse psychosocial working environment – cortisol used as an example

Biological measures will also reflect normal cyclic biological variations (e.g. diurnal and seasonal variations), effects of lifestyle factors, as well as the performance of the selected analytical methods and errors (Hansen et al., 2008). The magnitude of variations can, however, be estimated, statistically modelled and attributed to variations within the individual (intra-individual variation) as well as variations between individuals (inter-individual variation) (Costongs et al., 1985; Fraser et al., 1989; Garde et al., 2000; Hansen et al., 2001; Maes et al., 1997; Nicolau et al., 1984).

Measurement of saliva cortisol has been found to be an excellent indicator of unbound concentrations of cortisol in serum (Ahn et al., 2007; Neary et al., 2002; Putignano et al., 2001). The studies find a good correlation between mean saliva cortisol and mean serum cortisol (approx. $r = 0.6$) and that concentration of cortisol in serum was 10-20 times higher than measured in saliva. Also similar circadian fluctuations has been reported for cortisol in saliva and plasma (Umeda et al., 1981). It is however not only the total concentrations of cortisol that have rendered interest. A number of derived measures that are thought to better describe the dynamics of the stress response have been invented and put into common use. The two most common examples are the awakening response (ACR) and recovery (Kudielka et al., 2007). The ACR is sometimes called reactivity and recovery is sometimes referred to as "fall-during-the-day". The ACR is typically defined as the difference between concentrations of cortisol in the first saliva sample in the morning and the second sample. Recovery is typically defined as the difference between the highest concentration of cortisol in morning samples and the evening sample. Another derivate measure is the area under the curve, which is used as a proxy for the total concentrations during a pre-defined time period.

An important factor of compliance is the time of sampling. Some studies have used electronic devices to track when participants actually accessed the cotton swab, or tampon. In one study it was observed that 74% of the participants accessed the tampon according to the study protocol, whereas 26% failed to access the tampon on the proper time at least with one out of six samples. Of this latter group of non-compliants, 55% failed to take the second morning sampling correctly after 30 minutes. Participants, who were not informed that their sampling was being tracked, were significantly less compliant than informed participants (Kudielka et al., 2003). In another study that examined participant adherence found that 71% of participants, which were unaware they were being monitored, correctly followed the protocol. Their self-reported compliance was however 93%. Among the persons who were aware of being monitored, the objective compliance was 90%, consistent with the self-reported compliance of 93% (Wright & Steptoe, 2005). In both studies, the non-adherent participants had significantly lower morning cortisol values than the adherent participants.

In research projects, samples are often required to be stored for longer periods of time either because of the protocol of the project or because of lack of funding for analysis. A study on long-term storage found no effects on cortisol concentrations after storage of saliva at 5 degrees C for up to 3 months or at -20 degrees C and -80 degrees C for up to one year. In contrast, concentrations of cortisol were found to decrease by 9.2% (95% confidence interval (CI): 3.8%; 14.3%) per month in samples stored at room temperature. Repeated freezing and thawing of samples up to four times before analysis did not affect the measured concentrations of cortisol. Centrifuged saliva samples for analysis of cortisol may be stored at 5 °C for up to 3 months or at -20 °C or -80 °C for at least one year. However, long-term storage at room temperature cannot be recommended. Repeated cycles of freezing and thawing did not appear to affect the concentrations of cortisol (Garde & Hansen, 2005a; Hansen et al., 2005).

In summary it is important to reduce unnecessary variability in the study design (diurnal and seasonal variation), and to provide suggestions for dealing with variability in cases where such influences are unavoidable. Some examples are given for using salivary cortisol, which may not be relevant for other biomarkers.

6. Conclusion

The present chapter provides the reader with insight into the existing evidence on how different physiological responses may be used as potential biomarkers of the adverse effects of the psychosocial working environment. Adverse psychosocial working environment was found to be associated with increased HbA_{1c} and fibrinogen in blood and decreased serum testosterone indicating an increased catabolic activity and decreased anabolic activity. Further when using and interpreting the measured physiological response it is important to be aware of potential confounders directly addressed to the selected biological measure. In this context it is also important to reduce unnecessary variability in the study design (diurnal and seasonal variation), and to provide suggestions for dealing with variability in cases where such influences are unavoidable.

7. References

Biomarkers - Biomarkers and Risk Assessment: Concepts and principles. (1993). WHO. [155]. Geneva, WHO. Environmental Health Criteria. ISBN: 92-4-157155-1; ISSN: 0250-863x

Aardal-Eriksson, E., Eriksson, T. E., Holm, A.-C., & Lundin, T. (1999). Salivary cortisol and serum prolactin in relation to stress rating scales in a group of rescue workers. *Biological Psychiatry, 46,* 850-855.

Ahn, R. S., Lee, Y. J., Choi, J. Y., Kwon, H. B., & Chun, S. I. (2007). Salivary cortisol and DHEA levels in the Korean population: age-related differences, diurnal rhythm, and correlations with serum levels. *Yonsei.Med J, 48,* 379-388.

Axelsson, J., Åkerstedt, T., Kecklund, G., Lindqvist, A., & Attefors, R. (2003). Hormonal changes in satisfied and dissatisfied shift workers across a shift cycle. *Journal of Applied Physiology, 95,* 2099-2105.

Berg, M., Arnetz, B. B., Lidén, S., Eneroth, P., & Kallner, A. (1992). Techno-stress. A psychophysiological study of employees with VDU- associated skin complaints. *Journal of Occupational Medicine, 34,* 698-701.

Björkqvist, K., Österman, K., & Hjelt-Bäck, M. (1994). Aggression among university employees. *Aggressive Behavior, 20,* 173-184.

Cesana, G., Panza, G., Ferrario, M., Zanettini, R., Arnoldi, M., & Grieco, A. (1985). Can glucosylated hemoglobin be a job stress parameter. *Journal of Occupational Medicine, 27(5),* 357-360.

Chida, Y. & Steptoe, A. (2009). Cortisol awakening response and psychosocial factors: a systematic review and meta-analysis. *Biological Psychology, 80,* 265-278.

Christensen, N. J. (1986). Katekolaminer og psykisk stress. *Ugeskrift for Læger, 148,* 233-237.

Chrousos, G. P. & Gold, P. W. (1992). The concepts of stress and stress system disorders. Overview of physical and behavioral homeostasis. *Journal Of the American Medical Association, 267,* 1244-1252.

Clausen, T., Hogh, A., Borg, V., & Ortega, A. (2011). Acts of offensive behaviour and risk of long-term sickness absence in the Danish elder-care services: a prospective analysis of register-based outcomes. *International Archives Of Occupational And Environmental Health, e-pub-a-head-of-print.*

Clays, E., De, B. D., Delanghe, J., Kittel, F., Van, R. L., & De, B. G. (2005). Associations between dimensions of job stress and biomarkers of inflammation and infection. *Journal of Occupational and Environmental Medicine, 47,* 878-883.

Cohen, S. & Williamson, G. M. (1991). Stress and infectious disease in humans. *Psychological Bulletin, 109(1),* 5-24.

Costongs, G. M. P. J., Janson, P. C. W., Bas, B. M., Hermans, J., van Wersch, J. W. J., & Brombacher, P. J. (1985). Short-term and long-term intraindividual variations and critical differences of clinical chemical laboratory parameters. *Journal of Clinical Chemistry and Clinical Biochemistry, 23,* 7-16.

Dellve, L., Lagerström, M., & Hagberg, M. (2003). Work-system risk factors for permanent work disability among home-care workers: a case-control study. *International Archives Of Occupational And Environmental Health, 76,* 216-224.

Dofradottir, A. & Høgh, A. (2002). *Mobning på arbejdspladsen. En kritisk gennemgang af dansk og international forskningslitteratur (Bullying at work. A critical review of Danish and international research)* (Rep. No. 10). København: Arbejdsmiljøinstituttet.

Einarsen, S., Matthiesen, S. B., & Mikkelsen, E. G. (1999). *Tiden leger alle sår? Senvirkninger av mobbing i arbetslivet / Time heals? Late effects of bullying at work* Bergen: Institutt for Samfunnspsykologi - Universitetet i Bergen.

Einarsen, S. & Mikkelsen, E. G. (2003). Individual effects of exposure to bullying at work. In S.Einarsen, H. Hoel, D. Zapf, & C. L. Cooper (Eds.), *Bullying and Emotional Abuse in the Workplace. International perspectives in research and practice* (1 ed., pp. 127-144). London and New York: Taylor and Francis.

Einarsen, S., Raknes, B. I., Matthiesen, S. B., & Hellesøy, O. (1994). *Mobbing og harde personkonflikter. Helsefarlig samspill på arbeidsplassen (Bullying and serious interpersonal conflicts. Unhealthy interactions at the workplace).* Bergen: Sigma Forlag A.S.

Einarsen, S., Raknes, B. I., Matthiesen, S. B., & Hellesøy, O. H. (1996). Helsemessige aspekter ved mobbing i arbeidslivet. Modererende effekter av sosial stotte og personlighet. / The health-related aspects of bullying in the workplace: The moderating effects of social support and personality. *Nordisk Psykologi, 48,* 116-137.

Eller, N. H. (2007). Total power and high frequency components of heart rate variability and risk factors for atherosclerosis. *Auton.Neurosci., 131,* 123-130.

Evans, O. & Steptoe, A. (2001). Social support at work, heart rate, and cortisol: a self-monitoring study. *Journal of Occupational Health Psychology, 6,* 361-370.

Finne, L. B., Knardahl, S., & Lau, B. (2011). Workplace bullying and mental distress - a prospective study of Norwegian employees. *Scandinavian Journal of Work Environment & Health, 37,* 276-286.

Frankenhaeuser, M. & Johansson, G. (1986). Stress at work: psychobiological and psychosocial aspects. *International Reviews of Applied Psychology, 35,* 287-299.

Fraser, C. G., Cummings, S. T., Wilkinson, S. P., Neville, R. G., Knox, J. D. E., Ho, O. et al. (1989). Biological variability of 26 clinical chemistry analytes in elderly people. *Clinical Chemistry, 35,* 783-786.

Fujiwara, K., Tsukishima, E., Kasai, S., Masuchi, A., Tsutsumi, A., Kawakami, N. et al. (2004). Urinary catecholamines and salivary cortisol on workdays and days off in relation to job strain among female health care providers. *Scand J Work Environ Health, 30,* 129-138.

Fujiwara, S., Shinkai, S., Kurokawa, Y., & Watanabe, T. (1992). The acute effects of experimental short-term evening and night shifts on human circadian rhythm: the oral temperature, heart rate, serum cortisol and urinary catecholamines levels. *International Archives Of Occupational And Environmental Health, 63,* 409-418.

Garde, A. H. & Hansen, A. M. (2005a). Long-term stability of salivary cortisol. *Scand J Clin Lab Invest, 65,* 433-436.

Garde, A. H. & Hansen, Å. M. (2005b). Long-term stability of salivary cortisol. *Scand J Clin Lab Invest, 65,* 433-436.

Garde, A. H., Hansen, A. M., Skovgaard, L. T., & Christensen, J. M. (2000). Seasonal and biological variation of blood concentrations of total cholesterol, dehydroepiandrosterone sulfate, hemoglobin A(1c), IgA, prolactin, and free testosterone in healthy women. *Clinical Chemistry, 46,* 551-559.

Gold, P. W., Licinio, J., Wong, M. L., & Chrousos, G. P. (1995). Corticotropin relasing homone in the pathophysiology of melancholic and atypical depression and in the

mechanim of action of antidepressant drugs. *Annals of the New York Academy of Science, 771,* 716-729.
Grossi, G., Perski, A., Evengard, B., Blomkvist, V., & Orth-Gomer, K. (2003). Physiological correlates of burnout among women. *Journal of Psychosomatic Research, 55,* 309-316.
Hamilton, L. D., Newman, M. L., Delville, C. L., & Delville, Y. (2008). Physiological stress response of young adults exposed to bullying during adolescence. *Physiol Behav., 95,* 617-624.
Hansen, Å. M., Garde, A. H., Arnetz, B., Knardahl, S., Kristenson, M., Lundberg, U. et al. (2005). *A model database for salivary cortisol in occupational studies* (Rep. No. 2005:533). Copenhagen: Nordic Council of Ministers.
Hansen, Å. M., Garde, A. H., & Persson, R. (2008). Sources of biological and methodological variation in salivary cortisol and their impact on measurement among healthy adults: a review. *Scand J Clin.Lab Invest, 68,* 448-458.
Hansen, Å. M., Garde, A. H., Skovgaard, L. T., & Christensen, J. M. (2001). Seasonal and biological variation of urinary epinephrine, norepinephrine, and cortisol in healthy women. *Clinica Chimica Acta, 309,* 25-35.
Hansen, Å. M., Hogh, A., & Persson, R. (2011). Frequency of bullying at work, physiological response, and mental health. *Journal of Psychosomatic Research, 70,* 19-27.
Hansen, Å. M., Høgh, A., Persson, R., Karlson, B., Garde, A. H., & Ørbæk, P. (2006). Bullying at work, health outcomes, and physiological stress response. *Journal of Psychosomatic Research, 60,* 63-72.
Hansen, Å. M., Kaergaard, A., Andersen, J. H., & Netterstrøm, B. (2003a). Associations between repetitive work and endocrinological indicators of stress. *Work & Stress, 17,* 264-276.
Hansen, Å. M., Larsen, A. D., Rugulies, R., Garde, A. H., & Knudsen, L. E. (2009). A Review of the Effect of the Psychosocial Working Environment on Physiological Changes in Blood and Urine. *Basic and Clinical Pharmacology and Toxicology, 105,* 73-83.
Hansen, Å. M., Kaergaard, A., Andersen, J. H., & Netterstrøm, B. (2003b). Associations between repetitive work and endocrinological indicators of stress. *Work & Stress, 17,* 264-276.
Härenstam, A. & Theorell, T. (1990). Cortisol elevation and serum gamma-glutamyl transpeptidase in response to adverse job conditions: how are they interrelated? *Biological Psychology, 31,* 157-171.
Heim, C., Ehlert, U., & Hellhammer, D. H. (2000). The potential role of hypocortisolism in the pathophysiology of stress-related bodily disorders. *Psychoneuroendocrinology, 25,* 1-35.
Hellhammer, D. H., Wüst, S., & Kudielka, B. M. (2009). Salivary cortisol as a biomarker in stress research. *Psychoneuroendocrinology, 34,* 163-171.
Henry, J. P. (1992). Biological basis of the stress response. *Integr.Physiol.Behav.Sci., 27,* 66-83.
Hogh, A., Mikkelsen, E. G., & Hansen, Å. M. (2010). Individual Consequences of Workplace Bullying/Mobbing. In S.Einarsen, H. Hoel, D. Zapf, & C. L. Cooper (Eds.), *Bullying and Harassment in the Workplace: Developments in Theory, Research, and Practice* (Second ed., pp. 107-128). CRC Press.
Høgh, A., Ortega, A., Giver, H., & Borg, V. (2007). *Mobning af personale i ældreplejen* (Rep. No. 17). København: Det Nationale Forskningscenter for Arbejdsmiljø.

Hubl, W., Taubert, H., Freymann, E., Meissner, D., Stahl, F., & Dörner, G. (1984). A sensitive direct enzyme immunoassay for cortisol in plasma and saliva. *Experimental Clinical Endocrinology, 84,* 63-70.

Irie, M., Tsutsumi, A., Shioji, I., & Kobayashi, F. (2004). Effort-reward imbalance and physical health among Japanese workers in a recently downsized corporation. *International Archives Of Occupational And Environmental Health, 77,* 409-417.

Ishizaki, M., Martikainen, P., Nakagawa, H., Marmot, M., & The Japan work stress and health cohort-study group (2001). Socioeconomic status, workplace characteristics and plasma fibrinogen level of Japanese male employees. *Scand J Work Environ Health, 27,* 287-291.

Joseph, S. (1999). Attributional processes, coping and post-traumatic stress disorders. In W.Yule (Ed.), *Post-traumatic stress disorders. Concepts and therapy* (pp. 52-70). Chichester: John Wiley & Sons.

Karasek, R. (2006). The stress-disequilibrium theory: chronic disease development, low social control, and physiological de-regulation. *Med Lav., 97,* 258-271.

Karasek, R., Brisson, C., Kawakami, N., Houtman, I., Bongers, P., & Amick, B. (1998). The Job Content Questionnaire (JCQ): an instrument for internationally comparative assessments of psychosocial job characteristics. *Journal of Occupational Health Psychology, 3,* 322-355.

Karasek, R. & Theorell, T. (1990). Job structure and physiological response. In R.Karasek & T. Theorell (Eds.), *Healthy work. Stress, productivity, and the reconstruction of working life* (pp. 103-109). New York: Basic Books, Inc.

Karasek, R. A., Baker, D., Marxer, F., Ahlbom, A., & Theorell, T. (1981). Job decision latitude, job demands, and cardiovascular disease: A prospective study of swedish men. *American Journal of Public Health, 71(7),* 694-705.

Kawakami, N., Akachi, K., Shimizu, H., Haratani, T., Kobayashi, F., Ishizaki, M. et al. (2000). Job strain, social support in the workplace, and haemoglobin A1c in Japanese men. *Occup Environ Med, 57,* 805-809.

Kawakami, N., Araki, S., Hayashi, T., & Masumoto, T. (1989). Relationship between perceived job-stress and glycosylated hemoglobin in white-collar workers. *Industrial Health, 27,* 149-154.

Kile, S. M. (1990). *Helsefarlig lederskab. Ein eksplorerande studie (Health endangering leadership. An exploratory study)* Bergen: University of Bergen: department of Psychosocial Science.

Kirschbaum, C., Strasburger, C. J., Jammers, W., & Hellhammer, D. (1989). Cortisol and behavior: 1. adaptation of a radioimmunoassay kit for reliable and inexpensive salivary cortisol dertermination. *Pharmacology, Biochemistry and Behavior, 34,* 747-751.

Kittel, F., Leynen, F., Stam, M., Dramaix, M., de, S. P., Mak, R. et al. (2002). Job conditions and fibrinogen in 14226 Belgian workers: the Belstress study. *European Heart Journal, 23,* 1841-1848.

Kivimäki, M., Elovainio, M., & Vahtera, J. (2000). Workplace bullying and sickness absence in hospital staff. *Occupational Environmental Medicine, 57,* 656-660.

Kobayashi, Y., Hirose, T., Tada, Y., Tsutsumi, A., & Kawakami, N. (2005). Relationship between two job stress models and coronary risk factors among Japanese part-time female employees of a retail company. *Journal of Occupational Health, 47,* 201-210.

Kristensen, T. S. (1989). Cardiovascular diseases and the work environment. A critical review of the epidemiologic literature on nonchemical factors. *Scandinavian Journal of Work Environment & Health, 15,* 165-179.

Kudielka, B. M., Broderick, J. E., & Kirschbaum, C. (2003). Compliance with saliva sampling protocols: electronic monitoring reveals invalid cortisol daytime profiles in noncompliant subjects. *Psychosom.Med, 65,* 313-319.

Kudielka, B. M., Buchtal, J., Uhde, A., & Wüst, S. (2007). Circadian cortisol profiles and psychological self-reports in shift workers with and without recent change in the shift rotation system. *Biological Psychology, 74,* 92-103.

Kudielka, B. M. & Kern, S. (2004). Cortisol day profiles in victims of mobbing (bullying at the work place): preliminary results of a first psychobiological field study. *Journal of Psychosomatic Research, 56,* 149-150.

Kudielka, B. M. & Wüst, S. (2010). Human models in acute and chronic stress: assessing determinants of individual hypothalamus-pituitary-adrenal axis activity and reactivity. *Stress, 13,* 1-14.

LaCroix, A. & Haynes, S. (1984). Occupational exposure to high demand/low control work and coronary heart disease incidence in the Framingham cohort. *American Journal of Epidemiology, 120,* 481.

Lallukka, T., Rahkonen, O., & Lahelma, E. (2011). Workplace bullying and subsequent sleep problems - the Helsinki Health Study. *Scand J Work Environ Health, 37,* 204-212.

Lazarus, R. S. (1999). *Stress and emotion - a new synthesis*. London: Free Associations Books.

Levitt, M. A. & Derrick, G. R. (1991). An evaluation of physiological parameters of stress in the emergency department. *American Journal of Emergency Medicine, 9,* 217-219.

Leymann, H. (1996). The content and development of mobbing at work. *European Journal of Work and Organizational Psychology, 5,* 165-184.

Leymann, H. & Gustafsson, A. (1996). Mobbing at work and the development of post-traumatic stress disorder. *European Journal of Work and Organizational Psychology, 5,* 251-275.

Lundberg, U., Granqvist, M., Hansson, T., Magnusson, M., & Wallin, L. (1989). Psychological and physiological stress responses during repetitive work at an assembly line. *Work and Stress, 3(2),* 143-153.

Maes, M., Mommen, K., Hendricks, D., Peeters, D., D´Hondt, P., Ranjan, R. et al. (1997). Components of biological variation, including seasonality, in blood concentrations of TSH, TT3, FT4, PRL, cortisol and testosterone in healthy volunteers. *Clinical Endocrinology, 46,* 587-598.

Mason, J. W. (1968). A review of psychoendocrine research on the pituitary-thyroid system. *Psychosomatic Medicine, 30,* 666-681.

Matsukawa, T., Gotoh, E., Uneda, S., Miyajima, E., Shionoiri, H., Tochikubo, O. et al. (1991). Augmented sympathetic nerve activity in response to stressors in young borderline hypertensive men. *Acta Physiologica Scandinavica, 141,* 157-165.

Matthiesen, S. B. & Einarsen, S. (2007). Perpetrators and targets of bullying at work: Role stress and individual differences. *violence and victims, 22,* 735-753.

McEwen, B. S. (1998). Protective and damaging effects of stress mediators. *New England Journal of Medicine, 338,* 171-179.

McEwen, B. S. (2004). Protection and damage from acute and chronic stress. Allostasis and allostatic overload and relevance to the pathophysiology of psychiatric disorders. *Annals of the New York Academy of Science, 1032,* 1-7.

McEwen, B. S. (2007). Physiology and neurobiology of stress and adaptation: central role of the brain. *Physiol Rev., 87,* 873-904.

McEwen, B. S. & Seeman, T. (1999). Protective and damaging effects of mediators of stress. Elaborating and testing the concepts of allostasis and allostatic load. *Annals of the New York Academy of Science, 896,* 30-47.

McEwen, B. S. & Wingfield, J. C. (2003). The concept of allostasis in biology and biomedicine. *Hormones and Behavior, 43,* 2-15.

Mikkelsen, E. G. (2001). *Workplace bullying: Its incidence, aetiology and health correlates.* University of Århus. Department of Psychology.

Mikkelsen, E. G. & Einarsen, S. (2002). Basic assumptions and symptoms of post-traumatic stress among victims of bullying at work. *European Journal of Work and Organizational Psychology, 11,* 87-111.

Mikkelsen, E. G. & Iversen, G. F. (2002). Bullying at work: Perceived effects on health, well-being and present job situation. In A. P. D. Liefooghe & H. Hoel (Eds.), (pp. 31). London: Birkbeck, University of London.

Moayed, F. A., Daraiseh, N., Shell, R., & Salem, S. (2006). Workplace bullying: a systematic review of risk factors and outcomes. *Theoretical Issues in Ergonomics Science, 7,* 311-327.

Mulders, H. P. G., Mejman, T. F., O'Hanlon, J. F., & Mulder, G. (1982). Differential psychophysiological reactivity of city bus drivers. *Ergonomics, 25(11),* 1003-1011.

Neary, J. P., Malbon, L., & McKenzie, D. C. (2002). Relationship between serum, saliva and urinary cortisol and its implication during recovery from training. *Journal of Science and Medicine in Sport, 5,* 108-114.

Netterstrøm, B. & Hansen, Å. M. (2000). Outsourcing and stress: Physiological effects on bus drivers. *Stress Medicine, 16,* 149-160.

Nicolau, G. Y., Lakatua, D., Sackett-Lundeen, L., & Haus, E. (1984). Circadian and circannual rhythms of hormonal variables in elderly men and women. *Chronobiology International, 1,* 301-319.

Niedhammer, I., David, S., Degioanni, S., Drummond, A., Philip, P., Acquarone, D. et al. (2009). Workplace Bullying and Sleep Disturbances: Findings from a Large Scale Cross-Sectional Survey in the French Working Population. *Sleep, 32,* 1211-1219.

Niedl, K. (1996). Mobbing and well-being: Economic and personnel development implications. *European Journal of Work and Organizational Psychology, 5,* 239-249.

Nielsen, M. B., Hetland, J., Matthiesen, S. B., & Einarsen, S. (2011). Longitudinal relationships between workplace bullying and psychological distress. *SJWEH, online first: doi:10.5271/sjweh.3178.*

O'Moore, M., Seigne, E., McGuire, L., & Smith, M. (1998). Victims of bullying at work in Ireland. *The Journal of Occupational Health and Safety - Australia and New Zealand, 14,* 569-574.

Ohlson, C. G., Söderfeldt, M., Söderfeldt, B., Jones, I., & Theorell, T. (2001). Stress markers in relation to job strain in human service organizations. *Psychother.Psychosom, 70,* 268-275.

Ortega, A., Christensen, K. B., Hogh, A., Rugulies, R., & Borg, V. (2011). One year prospective study on the effect of workplace bullying on long-term sickness absence. *Journal of Nursing Management, 19,* 752-759.

Ortega, A., Hogh, A., Pejtersen, J., & Olsen, O. (2008). Prevalence and risk groups in the Danish workforce. *International Archives Of Occupational And Environmental Health, 82,* 417-426.

Payne, R. L., Rick, J. T., Smith, G. H., & Cooper, R. G. (1984). Multiple indicators of stress in an active job - Cardiothoracic surgery. *Journal of Occupational Medicine, 26(11),* 805-808.

Pieper, C., LaCroix, A. Z., & Karasek, R. A. (1989). The relation of psychosocial dimensions of work with coronary heart disease risk factors: a meta-analysis of five united states data bases. *American Journal of Epidemiology, 129(3),* 483-494.

Price Spratlen, L. (1995). Interpersonal conflict which includes mistreatment in a university workplace. *Violence and Victims, 10,* 285-297.

Putignano, P., Dubini, A., Toja, P., Invitti, C., Bonfanti, S., Redaelli, G. et al. (2001). Salivary cortisol measurement in normal-weight, obese and anorexic women: comparison with plasma cortisol. *European Journal of Endocrinology, 145,* 165-171.

Putz-Anderson, V., Doyle, G. T., & Hales, T. R. (1992). Ergonomic analysis to characterize task constraint and repetitiveness as risk factors for musculoskeletal disorders in telecommunication office work. *Scandinavian Journal of Work Environment & Health, 18 suppl 2,* 123-126.

Raison, C. L. & Miller, A. H. (2003). When not enough is too much: the role of insufficient glucocorticoid signaling in the pathophysiology of stress-related disorders. *American Journal of Psychiatry, 160,* 1554-1565.

Reme, S. E., Eriksen, H. R., & Ursin, H. (2008). Cognitive activation theory of stress - how are individual experiences mediated into biological systems? *Social Journal of Well-Being and Emotional Health, 6,* 177-183.

Riese, H., van Doornen, L. J., Houtman, I. L., & de Geus, E. J. (2000). Job strain and risk indicators for cardiovascular disease in young female nurses. *Health and Psychology, 19,* 429-440.

Schnorpfeil, P., Noll, A., Schulze, R., Ehlert, U., Frey, K., & Fischer, J. E. (2003). Allostatic load and work conditions. *Soc Sci Med, 57,* 647-656.

Selye, H. (1975). Confusion and controversy in the stress field. *Journal of Human Stress,* 37-44.

Siegrist, J., Starke, D., Chandola, T., Godin, I., Marmot, M., Niedhammer, I. et al. (2004). The measurement of effort-reward imbalance at work: European comparisons. *Soc.Sci.Med., 58,* 1483-1499.

Smith, G. D., Ben Shlomo, Y., Beswick, A., Yarnell, J., Lightman, S., & Elwood, P. (2005). Cortisol, testosterone, and coronary heart disease: prospective evidence from the Caerphilly study. *Circulation, 112,* 332-340.

Steptoe, A., Kunz-Ebrecht, S., Owen, N., Feldman, P. J., Rumley, A., Lowe, G. D. et al. (2003). Influence of socioeconomic status and job control on plasma fibrinogen responses to acute mental stress. *Psychosomatic Medicine, 65,* 137-144.

Strickland, P., Morriss, R., Wearden, A., & Deakin, B. (1998). A comparison of salivary cortisol in chronic fatigue syndrome, community depression and healthy controls. *Journal of Affective Disorders, 47,* 191-194.

Su, C. T. (2001). Association between job strain status and cardiovascular risk in a population of Taiwanese white-collar workers. *Japanese Circulation Journal, 65,* 509-513.

Theorell, T., Ahlberg-Hulten, G., Jodko, M., Sigala, F., & de la Torre, B. (1993). Influence of job strain and emotion on blood pressure in female hospital personnel during workhours. *Scandinavian Journal of Work Environment & Health, 19,* 313-318.

Theorell, T., Ahlberg-Hulten, G., Sigala, F., Perski, A., & Soderholm, M. (1990). A psychosocial and biomedical comparison between men in six contrasting service occupations. *Work and Stress, 4(1),* 51-63.

Thylefors, I. (1987). *Syndabockar. Om utstödning och mobbning i arbetslivet (Scapegoats. About social exclusion and bullying at work).* Stockholm: Natur och Kultur.

Timio, M., Gentili, S., & Pede, S. (1979). Free adrenaline and noradrenaline excretion related to occupational stress. *British Heart Journal, 42,* 471-474.

Touitou, Y., Motohashi, Y., Reinberg, A., Touitou, C., Bourdeleau, P., Bogdan, A. et al. (1990). Effect of shift work on the night-time secretory patterns of melatonin, prolactin, cortisol and testosterone. *European Journal of Applied Physiology, 60,* 288-292.

Tsigos, C. & Chrousos, G. P. (2002). Hypothalamic-pituitary-adrenal axis, neuroendocrine factors and stress. *Journal of Psychosomatic Research, 53,* 865-871.

Tsutsumi, A., Theorell, T., Hallqvist, J., Reuterwall, C., & de Faire, U. (1999). Associations between job characteristics and plasma fibrinogen in a normal working population: A cross sectional analysis in referents of the SHEEP study. *Journal of Epidemiology & Community Health, 53,* 348-354.

Umeda, T., Hiramatsu, R., Iwaoka, T., Shimada, T., Miura, F., & Sato, T. (1981). Use of saliva for monitoring unbound free cortisol levels in serum. *Clinica Chimica Acta, 110,* 245-253.

Ursin, H. & Eriksen, H. R. (2004). The cognitive activation theory of stress. *Psychoneuroendocrinology, 29,* 567-592.

van Eck, M., Berkhof, H., Nicolson, N., & Sulon, J. (1996). The effects of perceived stress, traits, mood states, and stressful daily events on salivary cortisol. *Psychosomatic Medicine, 58,* 447-458.

Vrijkotte, T. G., van Doornen, L. J., & de Geus, E. J. (1999). Work stress and metabolic and hemostatic risk factors. *Psychosomatic Medicine, 61,* 796-805.

Wood, B., Wessely, S., Papadopoulos, A., Poob, L., & Checkly, S. (1998). Salivary cortisol profiles in chronic fatigue syndrome. *Neuropsychobiology, 37,* 1-4.

Wright, C. E. & Steptoe, A. (2005). Subjective socioeconomic position, gender and cortisol responses to waking in an elderly population. *Psychoneuroendocrinology., 30,* 582-590.

Zapf, D. & Einarsen, S. (2005). Mobbing at work: Escalated conflicts in organizations. In S.Fox & P. E. Spector (Eds.), *Counterproductive Work Behavior. Investigations of Actors and Targets* (pp. 237-270). Washington DC: American Psychological Association.

Zapf, D., Knorz, C., & Kulla, M. (1996). On the relationship between mobbing factors, and job content, social work environment, and health outcomes. *European Journal of Work and Organizational Psychology, 5,* 215-237.

Zeier, H. (1994). Workload and psychophysiological stress reactions in air traffic controllers. *Ergonomics, 37,* 525-539.